This book on or before
the last date below.

30 MAY 1997

0 8 OCT 2004

2 6 SEP 1997

3 1 OCT 1997

2 0 FEB 1998

29 MAY 1998

1 6 OCT 1998

2 1 DEC 1999

2 7 OCT 2003

Nursing

RESEARCH

Principles and Methods

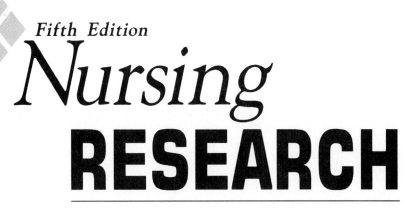

Fifth Edition

Nursing
RESEARCH

Principles and Methods

Denise F. Polit, *Ph.D.*

President
Humanalysis, Inc.
Saratoga Springs, New York

Bernadette P. Hungler, *R.N., Ph.D.*

Boston College School of Nursing
Chestnut Hill, Massachusetts

J.B. LIPPINCOTT COMPANY
Philadelphia

Sponsoring Editor: Margaret Belcher
Coordinating Editorial Assistant: Renee Gagliardi
Project Editor: Amy P. Jirsa
Indexer: Alexandra Nickerson
Design Coordinator: Doug Smock
Cover Designer: Susan Hermansen
Production Manager: Helen Ewan
Production Coordinator: Robert Randall
Compositor: Circle Graphics
Printer/Binder: R. R. Donnelley & Sons Company/Crawfordsville
Cover Printer: R. R. Donnelley & Sons Company/Crawfordsville

5th Edition

6 5 4

Library of Congress Cataloging-in-Publication Data

Polit-O'Hara, Denise.
  Nursing research : principles and methods / Denise F. Polit, Bernadette P. Hungler.—5th ed.
     p.   cm.
  Includes bibliographical references and index.
  ISBN 0-397-55138-X
  1. Nursing—Research—Methodology.   I. Hungler, Bernadette P.   II. Title.
  [DNLM: 1. Nursing Research—methods.   WY 20.5 P769n 1995]
  RT81.5.P64   1995
  610.73'072—dc20
  DNLM/DLC
  for Library of Congress   94-30403
                                                               CIP

Any procedure or practice described in this book should be applied by the healthcare practitioner under appropriate supervision in accordance with professional standards of care used with regard to the unique circumstances that apply in each practice situation. Care has been taken to confirm the accuracy of information presented and to describe generally accepted practices. However, the authors, editors, and publisher cannot accept any responsibility for errors or omissions or for any consequences from application of the information in this book and make no warranty express or implied, with respect to the contents of the book.

Every effort has been made to ensure drug selections and dosages are in accordance with current recommendations and practice. Because of ongoing research, changes in government regulations and the constant flow of information on drug therapy, reactions and interactions, the reader is cautioned to check the package insert for each drug for indications, dosages, warnings and precautions, particularly if the drug is new or infrequently used.

To
JoDoNo

Preface

This fifth edition of *Nursing Research: Principles and Methods* presents the most extensive changes made to this textbook since it was originally written over 15 years ago. This edition retains all of the features that have made this textbook popular in the past, while introducing several innovations that we think will make it even more useful to those learning how to do research.

New material permeates this edition, and much of it is intended to offer practical guidance—guidance on how to translate the abstract notions of research methodology into realistic strategies for conducting research. Nearly every chapter concludes with a series of "tips" for applying the chapter's lessons to real-life situations. The development of these suggestions stems from our belief that there is often a large gap between what gets taught in a research methods textbook and what a researcher needs to know in conducting a study.

Beyond these additions to each chapter, three new chapters have been included in this edition, each of which is designed to promote a smoother transition to actual research situations. All three new chapters are "how to" chapters: how to design a research study; how to develop a data collection plan; and how to develop a data analysis plan. We are enthusiastic about these new chapters and believe that they are important innovations that depart from the standard ways of explaining about research methods.

In addition to these changes, we have continued to update the textbook and to expand the discus-sion of qualitative research. In particular, the issue of assessing data quality in qualitative studies has been given substantially greater coverage, and computer programs for the analysis of qualitative data have been described. Additionally, many of the research examples that enliven the text are now based on qualitative studies.

Despite the numerous improvements, this edition reflects many of the same basic principles that shaped earlier editions. First, we have an unswerving conviction that, more than ever before, the development of research skills is critical to the nursing profession. Second, we firmly believe that research is an intellectually and professionally rewarding enterprise. We try to reflect our enthusiasm for the research process throughout this book. And third, we are persuaded that learning about research methods need be neither intimidating nor dull.

As in the previous four editions, we have tried to present the fundamentals of research methods in a way that both facilitates understanding and stimulates curiosity and interest. We know of no better way to accomplish both aims than to incorporate examples of actual research studies that illustrate concepts under discussion. These illustrations underscore our belief that research methods are not interesting in and of themselves—they are of interest only because they allow us to ask interesting questions and answer them in a meaningful way. We have also maintained other aspects of our basic teaching style: concepts are introduced carefully and systematically; difficult ideas are presented with some redundancy, but from several vantage points; and readers are assumed to have no prior exposure to technical terms.

We have tried to keep in mind the needs of both consumers and producers of nursing research. The uses to which the first four editions have been put suggest that we have reached both audiences. We have paid attention to the problems frequently encountered by students in reading, understanding, and evaluating research reports, and have included in this edition an early discussion on how to "translate" difficult-to-read research reports into a more manageable form. However, as before, the organization of the book is intended as a guide to those nursing students who are learning to conduct their own research.

This edition is organized into six main sections that lead the reader sequentially through the steps in the research process. Part I introduces the reader to the rationale underlying the scientific approach in general, and to the basic aims of nursing research in particular. The early chapters are designed to help students understand and appreciate the manner in which the scientific approach can be applied to solve problems, and to develop an enthusiasm for the kinds of knowledge and discoveries that research can produce. Part II further sets the stage for learning about the research process. The chapters in this part discuss three types of contexts for nursing research: the context of prior knowledge, theoretical and conceptual contexts, and the ethical context. Part III focuses on research design issues, and also introduces students to various types of research, including those that are typically quantitative (e.g., survey research, evaluation research) and qualitative (e.g., ethnographic research, historical research). Part IV covers the major techniques of data collection, as well as principles of measurement. Part V is devoted to the analysis of research data. It includes chapters on qualitative and quantitative analysis, as well as the pathbreaking chapter on the integration of the two that was introduced in the previous edition. The final section of the book focuses on communication in research: writing about research, critiquing written reports, preparing research proposals, and using the results of published studies.

We hope that the content and organization of this book continues to meet the needs of a broad spectrum of nursing students and nurse researchers.

Denise F. Polit, Ph.D.
Bernadette P. Hungler, R.N., Ph.D.

Acknowledgments

This fifth edition, like the previous four editions, depended on the contribution of many individuals. We are deeply appreciative of those who made all five editions possible. In addition to all those who assisted us with the earlier editions, the following individuals deserve special mention.

Many faculty and students who used the text during the past 15 years have made invaluable suggestions for its improvement, and to all of you we are very grateful. In particular, we would like to acknowledge the continuing feedback from the nursing students and faculty at Boston College. Anne Lippman, Marilyn Grant, and the late Mary Pekarski made important contributions to Chapter 4. Several of the examples used in the text and in the accompanying Study Guide were developed from ideas provided by Sarah Cimino, Susan Kelly, and Mary Jane Daly.

We also extend our warmest thanks to those who helped to turn the manuscript into a finished product. Kathy Nolte and Tab Furey served as able assistants in the preparation of this edition. The staff at J. B. Lippincott has been of tremendous assistance in the support they have given us over the years. We are indebted to Margaret Belcher, Kimberly Oaks, Jody DiMatteo, Amy Jirsa, and all the others behind the scenes for their fine contributions.

Finally, we thank our friends and family, who provided ongoing support and encouragement throughout this enterprise.

Contents

Part III
Designs for Nursing Research *137*

Part IV
Measurement and Data Collection 251

Nursing
RESEARCH
Principles and Methods

Part I

THE SCIENTIFIC RESEARCH PROCESS

Chapter 1

Nursing Research and the Scientific Approach

Nursing research involves a systematic search for knowledge about issues of importance to the nursing profession. Nursing research has experienced remarkable growth in the past three decades, providing nurses with an increasingly sound base of knowledge from which to practice. Yet many health care questions remain to be answered by nurse researchers—and many answers remain to be utilized by practicing nurses.

The purpose of this book is to acquaint potential consumers and producers of nursing research with the fundamentals of scientific research methods. In this introductory chapter, we discuss the important role that research plays in establishing a scientific base for the practice of nursing and present an overview of how scientific methods can be used to address problems of concern to nurses.

❖ *NURSING RESEARCH IN PERSPECTIVE*

A consensus has emerged among nursing leaders that nurses at all levels should develop research skills. In this section, we discuss the rationale for this view and present a brief summary of the historical development of nursing research.

The Importance of Research in Nursing

The ultimate goal of any profession is to improve the practice of its members so that the services provided to its clientele will be maximally effective. A profession seeking to enhance its professional stature strives for the continual development of a scientific body of knowledge fundamental to its practice. The emergence of such a body of scientific knowledge can be instrumental in fostering a commitment and accountability to the profession's clientele.

PROFESSIONALISM. Nurses increasingly recognize the need to extend the base of nursing knowledge as part of professional responsibility and endorse scientific investigations as a way to achieve this objective. Moreover, nurses are committed to the evolution of a fairly dis-

Polit DF, Hungler BP: NURSING RESEARCH: PRINCIPLES AND METHODS, 5th ed. © 1995 J. B. Lippincott Company.

tinct body of knowledge that separates nursing from other professions. Nursing is only one of several professions involved in the delivery of health care. Information from nursing investigations helps to define better the unique role that nursing plays.

ACCOUNTABILITY. Gortner (1974) pointed out that the quality of nursing care cannot be improved until scientific accountability becomes as much a part of nursing's tradition as humanitarianism. Nurses who base as many of their clinical decisions as possible on scientifically documented information are being professionally accountable.

SOCIAL RELEVANCE OF NURSING. Nurses today are being asked more than ever before to document their role in the delivery of health services. People are recognizing health care as a right rather than a privilege and, with spiraling costs, are asking various groups of health professionals how their services contribute to the total delivery of health care. This increased interest in examining health care practices makes it essential for nurses to evaluate the efficacy of their practices and to modify or abandon those practices shown to have no effect on client health.

RESEARCH AND DECISION MAKING IN NURSING PRACTICE. Many nurses use the Standards of Nursing Practice established by the American Nurses' Association (ANA) Congress for Practice (1973) both as their method of clinical practice and to evaluate the quality of their nursing care. The process requires nurses to engage in many decision-making activities. What will be assessed? What nursing diagnoses result from the assessment? What plan of care is most likely to produce the desired outcomes? What nursing interventions are necessary? How will the results be evaluated in terms of their effectiveness? Research can play an important role at each phase of the nursing process by helping nurses to make more informed decisions.

The Consumer–Producer Continuum of Nursing Research

Nurses and nursing students have assumed a variety of roles in relation to scientific research, forming a continuum that reflects their degree of active participation in the conduct of research. At one end of the continuum are those nurses whose involvement in research is essentially passive. *Consumers* of nursing research read reports of studies, typically to keep up to date on information that may be relevant to their practice or to develop new skills. Nurses are increasingly expected to maintain, at a minimum, this level of involvement with research.

At the other end of the continuum are the *producers* of nursing research: nurses who actively participate in the design and implementation of scientific studies. At one time, most nurse researchers were academicians who taught in schools of nursing, but research is increasingly being conducted by nurses in practice settings.

Between these two extremes lie a variety of research-related activities in which nurses are engaging, including the following:

- Participation in a *journal club* in a practice setting, which involves regular meetings among nurses to discuss and critique research articles
- Attendance at research presentations at professional conferences
- Formal evaluation of completed research for its possible utilization in the practice setting
- Assistance in the collection of research information (e.g., distributing questionnaires to patients or observing and recording patients' behaviors)
- Review of proposed methods for gathering research information with respect to their feasibility in a clinical setting
- Collaboration in the development of an idea for a research project
- Participation on an institutional committee whose mission is to review the ethical aspects of proposed research before it is undertaken

In all these roles, nurses who have some research skills are in a better position to make a contribution to the nursing profession and to the base of nursing knowledge. Because of this fact, almost all accredited baccalaureate nursing programs include research content as a requirement for nursing students.

Historical Evolution of Nursing Research

Most people would agree that research in nursing began with Florence Nightingale, who recorded detailed observations about the effects of nursing actions during the Crimean War and was able to effect some changes in nursing care based on her observations. During several years after her work, however, little was added to the nursing literature concerning nursing research.

EARLY YEARS. The pattern that nursing research followed subsequent to Florence Nightingale was closely aligned to the problems confronting nursing. For example, most of the studies conducted between 1900 and 1940 concerned nursing education. In 1923, one group, the Committee for the Study of Nursing Education, studied on a national level the educational preparation of nurse teachers, administrators, and public health nurses and the clinical experiences of nursing students. The committee issued what has become known as the Goldmark Report, which identified many inadequacies in the educational backgrounds of the groups studied and concluded that advanced educational preparation was essential. Partly as a result of that study, hospitals began employing registered nurses to give nursing care that freed student nurses from heavy service demands. As more nurses received university-based education, studies concerning students—their differential characteristics, problems, and satisfactions—became more numerous.

THE 1940S. During the 1940s, studies concerning nursing education continued, spurred on by the unprecedented demand for nursing personnel that resulted from World War II. For example, Brown (1948) reassessed nursing education in her study initiated at the request of the National Nursing Council for War Service. The findings from the study, like those of the Goldmark Report, revealed numerous inadequacies in nursing education. Brown recommended that the education of nurses occur in collegiate settings. Many subsequent research investigations concerning the functions performed by nurses, nurses' roles and attitudes, hospital environments, and nurse–patient interactions stemmed from the Brown report.

THE 1950S. A number of forces combined during the 1950s to put nursing research on a rapidly accelerating upswing that is still being experienced today. An increase in the number of nurses with advanced educational degrees, the establishment of a nursing research center at the Walter Reed Army Institute of Research, an increase in the availability of funds from the government and private foundations, and the inception of the American Nurses' Foundation—which is devoted exclusively to the promotion of nursing research—were major forces that provided impetus to the research movement in nursing during this period. The increasing number of research studies being conducted during the 1950s created the need for a journal in which the findings from these studies could be published; thus, *Nursing Research* came into being in 1952. Nursing research took a twist in the 1950s not experienced by research in other professions, at least not to the same extent as in nursing. Nurses studied themselves: Who is the nurse? What does the nurse do? Why do individuals choose to enter nursing? What are the characteristics of the ideal nurse? How do other groups perceive the nurse?

THE 1960S. The 1960s was the period during which terms such as *conceptual framework, conceptual model, nursing process,* and *theoretical base of nursing practice* began to appear in nursing literature and influenced views about the role of theory in nursing research. Funding continued to be available both for the educational preparation of nurses and for nursing research projects. Nursing leaders increasingly expressed concern about the lack of research in nursing practice. Several professional nursing organizations established priorities for research investigations during this period. The Western Interstate Council for Higher Education in Nursing developed content for graduate education in the clinical areas of community health, maternal–child, medical–surgical, and psychiatric nursing and conducted workshops for faculty on the application of scientific knowledge. Finally, the Mugar Library at Boston University established a nursing archive in the late 1960s; one purpose of the archive is to foster nursing research.

THE 1970S. By the 1970s, the growing number of nurses conducting research studies and the discussions of theoretical and contextual issues surrounding nursing research created the need for additional sources of communication. Three additional journals that focus on nursing research—*Advances in Nursing Science, Research in Nursing and Health,* and the *Western Journal of Nursing Research*—were established in that decade. There was also a change in emphasis in nursing research from areas such as teaching, administration, curriculum, recruitment, and nurses themselves to the improvement of client care—signifying a growing awareness by nurses of the need for a scientific base from which to practice. Nursing leaders strongly endorsed this direction for nursing studies. Lindeman (1975), for example, conducted a study to ascertain the views of nursing leaders concerning the focus of scientific nursing studies. Clinical problems were identified as the highest priorities for nursing research. Research skills among nurses continued to improve in the 1970s. The cadre of nurses with earned doctorates steadily increased, especially during the later part of the 1970s. The availability of both predoctoral and postdoctoral research fellowships facilitated advanced preparation in research skills.

THE 1980S. The 1980s brought nursing research to a new level of development. An increase in the number of qualified nurse researchers, widespread availability of computers for the collection and analysis of information, and an ever-growing recognition that research is an integral part of professional nursing led nursing leaders to raise new issues and concerns. Increasing attention was given to the types of questions being asked, the methods of collecting and analyzing that would maximize what could be learned, the linking of research to theory, and the utilization of research findings in practice. Several events provided impetus for nursing research. Of particular importance was the establishment in 1986 of the National Center for Nursing Research (NCNR) at the National Institutes of Health (NIH) by congressional mandate. The purpose of NCNR was to promote—and financially support—research training and research relating to patient care. Additionally, the Center for Research for Nursing was created in 1983 by ANA. The Center's mission is to develop and coordinate a research program to serve as the source of national data for the profession. Several nursing groups developed priorities for nursing research during the 1980s. For example, in 1985, the ANA Cabinet on Nursing Research established priorities that helped focus research more precisely on aspects of nursing practice. Finally, an important new journal was established in the late 1980s: *Applied Nursing Research* includes research reports on studies of special relevance to practicing nurses.

THE 1990S AND THE FUTURE OF NURSING RESEARCH. After a long crusade by nursing organizations, nursing research was strengthened and given more national visibility when NCNR was promoted to full institute status within NIH: in 1993, the National Institute of Nursing Research (NINR) was born. The birth of NINR helps put nursing research more into the mainstream of research activities enjoyed by other health disciplines. Funding for nursing research is also growing. In 1986, the NCNR had a budget of $16.2 million, while in fiscal year 1994, the budget for NINR was about $50 million.

Two more research journals were inaugurated during the 1990s—*Clinical Nursing Research* and *Qualitative Health Research*. These journals emerged in response to the growth in clinically oriented and in-depth research among nurses.

During the 1990s, some of the research undertaken by nurses is being guided by priorities established by prominent nurse scientists, who were brought together by NCNR for two Conferences on Research Priorities (CORP). The priorities established by CORP #1, for research through 1994, were as follows: low birthweight, human immunodeficiency virus (HIV) infection, long-term care, symptom management, nursing informatics, health promotion, and technology dependence. In 1993, CORP #2 established the following as research emphases for a portion of NINR's funding from 1995 through 1999:

- Developing and testing community-based nursing models
- Assessing the effectiveness of nursing interventions in HIV and acquired immunodeficiency syndrome (AIDS)
- Developing and testing approaches to remediating cognitive impairment
- Testing interventions for coping with chronic illness
- Identifying bio-behavioral factors and testing interventions to promote immunocompetence

The future promises to be challenging and exciting for nurse researchers, who are developing an increasingly strong scientific base of knowledge for nursing practice. Studies are more likely to be directed toward the practice of nursing than they were in the past. In addition to pursuing new areas of research, there is a growing interest in building a firmer knowledge base by repeating studies, using the procedures used in previous research but with different clients, in different clinical settings, and at different times. There is also an increasing emphasis on developing mechanisms for utilizing the results of nursing research in actual practice, and this emphasis is likely to become stronger in the years ahead.

❖ THE SCIENTIFIC METHOD

In both our personal and professional lives, we all strive to solve problems, make sense of our experiences, understand regularities, and predict future circumstances. The scientific researcher, similarly, endeavors to understand, explain, predict, or control phenomena. The scientist, however, goes about this task in a more orderly and systematic fashion than is typical of most of our everyday efforts to solve problems. The scientific method involves the formal application of systematic, logical procedures that guide the investigation of phenomena of interest. This section describes some of the fundamental features of the scientific approach.

Sources of Human Knowledge

Human knowledge has many roots. Think for a moment about some facts you have learned relating to the practice of nursing. For example, as nursing students, we learn facts such as "washing hands between patients reduces the spread of bacteria" and "the output of fluids for a patient should be comparable in amount to the intake of fluids per day." What is the source of this and other similar information? Some of the facts we learn are derived from scientific research, but some are not. A brief discussion of some alternative sources of knowledge shows how scientific information is different.

TRADITION

Many questions are answered and problems solved on the basis of inherited customs or tradition. Within our culture, certain "truths" are accepted as given. For example, as citizens of the United States, most of us accept, without demanding proof, that democracy is the highest form of government. This type of knowledge often is so much a part of our heritage that few of us seek verification. The discipline of nursing, like other disciplines, also has its store of information passed on to us by tradition or custom. For example, one of the tasks traditionally performed by nurses is the change of shift report for each and every patient, whether the patient's condition has changed or not. The question of whether it might be more productive or effective under certain circumstances to make a report for only those patients whose conditions have changed has not been seriously addressed.

Tradition offers some advantages as a source of knowledge. It is efficient in the sense that each individual is not required to begin anew in an attempt to understand the world or certain aspects of it. Tradition or custom also facilitates communication by providing a common foundation of accepted truth. Nevertheless, tradition poses some problems for human inquiry. Many traditions have never been evaluated for their validity. Indeed, by their nature, traditions may interfere with the ability to perceive alternatives. Walker's (1967) research on ritualistic practices in nursing suggests that some traditional nursing practices, such as the routine taking of a patient's temperature, pulse, and respirations, may be dysfunctional. The Walker study illustrates the potential value of critical appraisal of custom and tradition before accepting them as truth.

AUTHORITY

In our complex society, there are authorities—people with specialized expertise—in every field. We are constantly faced with making decisions about matters with which we have had no direct experience and, therefore, it seems natural to place our trust in the judgment of people who are authoritative on an issue by virtue of specialized training or experience. As a source of understanding, however, authority has shortcomings. Authorities are not infallible, particularly if their expertise is based primarily on personal experience; yet, like tradition, their knowledge often goes unchallenged. Although

nursing practice would flounder if every piece of advice from nursing educators were challenged by students, nursing education would be incomplete if students never had occasion to pose such questions as: How does the authority (the instructor) *know*? What evidence is there that what I am learning is true?

EXPERIENCE AND TRIAL AND ERROR

Our own experiences represent a familiar and functional source of knowledge. The ability to generalize, to recognize regularities, and to make predictions based on observations is an important characteristic of human behavior. Despite the obvious utility of experience, it has limitations as a basis of understanding. First, each individual's experience may be too restricted to develop generalizations. A nurse may notice, for example, that two or three cardiac patients follow similar postoperative sleep patterns. This observation may lead to some interesting discoveries with implications for nursing interventions, but does the one nurse's observation and experience justify widespread changes in nursing care? A second limitation of experience as a source of knowledge lies in the fact that the same objective event generally is experienced or perceived differently by two individuals. Whose experience constitutes truth?

Closely related to experience is the method of trial and error. In this approach, alternatives are tried successively until we find one that answers our questions or solves our problems. Probably, we have all used the trial and error method at some time in our lives, including in our professional work. For example, many patients dislike the taste of potassium chloride solution. Nurses try to disguise the taste of the medication in various ways until one method meets with the approval of the patient. Trial and error may offer a practical means of securing knowledge, but it is fallible and inefficient. This method is haphazard and unsystematic, and the knowledge obtained is often unrecorded and, hence, inaccessible to subsequent problem solvers.

LOGICAL REASONING

The solutions to many of our perplexing problems are developed by means of logical thought processes. Logical reasoning as a method of knowing combines experience, our intellectual faculties, and formal systems of thought. *Inductive reasoning* is the process of developing generalizations from specific observations. For example, a nurse may observe the anxious behavior of (specific) hospitalized children and conclude that (in general) children's separation from their parents is stressful. *Deductive reasoning* is the process of developing specific predictions from general principles. For example, if we assume that separation anxiety does occur in hospitalized children (in general), then we might predict that the (specific) children in Hospital X whose parents do not room-in would manifest symptoms of stress.

Both systems of reasoning are useful as a means of understanding and organizing phenomena, and both play a role in the scientific approach. Neither system of thought, however, is without limitations when used alone as a basis of knowledge. The quality of knowledge arrived at through inductive reasoning depends highly on *which* specific examples are used as the basis for generalization. The reasoning process itself offers no mechanism for evaluating whether the examples are really typical and has no built-in checks for self-correction. Deductive reasoning is not itself a source of new information; it is, rather, an approach to illuminating relationships as one proceeds from the general (an assumed truth) to the specific. Deductive logic depends, furthermore, on the truth of the generalizations (called *premises*) to arrive at valid conclusions.

SCIENTIFIC RESEARCH

The scientific approach is the most sophisticated method of acquiring knowledge that humans have developed. The scientific method combines important features of induction and deduction, together with several other characteristics, to create a system of obtaining knowledge that, although fallible, is generally more reliable than tradition, authority, experience, or inductive or deductive reasoning alone. One important aspect that distinguishes the scientific approach from other methods of understanding is its capacity for self-evaluation. That is, scientific research uses checks and balances that minimize the possibility that the researcher's emotions or biases will affect the conclusions.

Characteristics of the Scientific Approach

The *scientific approach* to inquiry refers to a general set of orderly, disciplined procedures used to acquire dependable and useful information. *Scientific research*, which represents the application of the scientific approach to the study of a question of interest, may be defined as systematic investigations that are rooted in objective reality and that aim to develop general knowledge about natural phenomena. This definition is complex, so let us briefly examine some characteristics to provide a firmer basis for understanding.

ORDER AND CONTROL

The scientific method is a systematic approach to problem solving and to the expansion of knowledge. In a scientific study, the researcher moves in an orderly and systematic fashion from the definition of a problem, through the design of the study and collection of information, to the solution of the problem. By *systematic*, we mean that the investigator progresses logically through a series of steps, according to a plan of action. An overview of the steps taken in a scientific study is provided in Chapter 2.

Control is another characteristic of the scientific approach. Control involves imposing conditions on the research situation so that biases and confounding factors are minimized. The problems that are of interest to nurse researchers—for example, obesity, compliance with a regimen, or perceptions of pain—are highly complicated phenomena, often representing the effects of various forces. In trying to isolate relationships between phenomena, the scientist attempts to control factors that are not under direct investigation. For example, if a scientist is interested in exploring the relationship between diet and heart disease, steps usually are taken to control other potential contributors to coronary disorders, such as stress and cigarette smoking, as well as additional factors that might be relevant, such as a person's age and gender. The mechanisms of scientific control are the subject of a large part of this book.

EMPIRICISM

Scientific investigations rely on *empirical evidence* that is rooted in objective reality and gathered directly or indirectly through the human senses. This requirement of the scientific approach ensures that the findings of a scientific study are grounded in reality rather than in the personal beliefs of the researcher. Empirical inquiry imposes a certain degree of objectivity on the research situation because ideas or hunches are exposed to testing in the real world.

Empirical evidence, then, consists of observations made known to us by way of our sense organs. The observations are verified through sight, hearing, taste, touch, or smell. Observations of the presence or absence of skin inflammation, the heart rate of a patient, or the weight of a newborn infant are all examples of empirical observations.

GENERALIZATION

An important goal of science is to understand phenomena. This pursuit of knowledge, however, is usually focused not on isolated events or situations but rather on a more generalized understanding of phenomena and how they are interrelated. For example, the scientific researcher is typically not as interested in understanding why Ann Jones has cervical cancer as in understanding what general factors lead to

this form of carcinoma in Ann and in others. Of course, a health practitioner would want to take advantage of the general knowledge obtained in the course of scientific research in an effort to assist a particular individual. The ability to go beyond the specifics of the situation at hand is an important characteristic of the scientific approach. In fact, the degree to which research findings can be generalized to other people or other situations (referred to as the *generalizability* of the research) is a widely used criterion for assessing the quality of an investigation.

Assumptions of the Scientific Approach

Assumptions refer to basic principles that are accepted on faith, or assumed to be true, without proof or verification. This section extends our discussion of the characteristics of the scientific approach by paying specific attention to the assumptions on which science is founded.

THE NATURE OF REALITY

The scientist assumes that there is an objective reality that exists independent of human discovery or observation. That is, the world is assumed to be real and not a creation of the human mind; the processes of the universe would continue to exist even if humans were incapable of observing or recording them.

A related assumption is the belief that nature is basically orderly and regular. Events in nature are assumed to be, at least to a certain extent, consistent. If this principle were not assumed, it would make little sense to conduct scientific research.

DETERMINISM

The assumption of *determinism* refers to the belief that all phenomena have antecedent (preceding) causes. Natural events or conditions are assumed to not be haphazard, random, or accidental. Given the presumed orderliness of nature, events must have causes. If a pregnant woman has a premature delivery, there must be a reason that can potentially be identified and understood. If an individual has a cerebral vascular accident, there must be a cause or perhaps several causes.

Much of the activity in which a scientific researcher engages is directed toward an understanding of cause-and-effect relationships. Scientists believe that antecedent factors relating to all phenomena exist and can be discovered. Science does, however, accept the concept of multiple causation. A particular phenomenon may have several different causes. For example, heart disease may be caused by smoking habits, diet, stress, and additional factors or combinations of factors. The identification of these causes, that is, the search for an explanation of *why* things are the way they are, is one of the chief goals of science.

Purposes of Scientific Research

The scientific approach has been discussed in a general way as a method of problem solving or a system for acquiring knowledge. In this section, we examine some of the more specific reasons for conducting research in the context of the nursing profession.

DESCRIPTION. Many nursing research studies have as their main objective the description of phenomena relevant to the nursing process. The researcher who conducts a descriptive investigation observes, describes, and, perhaps, classifies. Descriptive studies can be of considerable value to the nursing profession. The phenomena that nurse researchers have been interested in describing are varied: stress and coping in patients, pain management, health beliefs, rehabilitation success, and time patterns of temperature readings, to mention only a few.

EXPLORATION. Like descriptive research, exploratory research begins with some phenomenon of interest; but rather than simply observing and recording the incidence of the phenomenon, exploratory research is aimed at exploring the dimensions of the phenomenon, the manner in which it is manifested, and the other factors with which it is related. For example, a descriptive study of patients' preoperative stress might seek to document the degree of stress patients experience before surgery and the incidence of severe stress. An exploratory study might ask the following: What factors are related to a patient's stress level? How does stress manifest itself in patients with different characteristics? Exploratory studies are especially useful when a new area or topic is being investigated.

EXPLANATION. The third basic purpose for conducting research is to provide explanations. Explanatory research is designed to get at the *why* of specific natural phenomena. Explanatory research is often linked to *theories*, which represent a method of organizing and integrating ideas about the manner in which phenomena are interrelated. Whereas descriptive research provides new information, and exploratory research provides promising insights, explanatory research attempts to offer understanding of the underlying causes of phenomena.

PREDICTION AND CONTROL. With our current level of knowledge and theoretical progress, there are numerous problems that defy absolute comprehension and explanation. Yet it is frequently possible to make predictions and to control phenomena based on findings from scientific investigations, even in the absence of complete understanding. For example, research has shown that the incidence of Down syndrome in infants increases with the age of the mother. We can predict that a woman aged 40 years is at higher risk of bearing a child with Down syndrome than a woman aged 25 years. We can partially control the outcome by educating women about the risks and offering amniocentesis to women older than 35 years of age. Note, however, that the ability to predict and control in this example does not depend on the scientist's complete explanation of *why* older women are at a higher risk of having an abnormal child. There are many examples of nursing and health-related studies in which prediction and control are key objectives.

Each of these purposes corresponds to different types of question that the researcher might pose, as shown in Table 1-1. This table also gives an example of an actual research study for each of these four major purposes.

BASIC VERSUS APPLIED RESEARCH. Sometimes the purpose of a scientific inquiry is classified according to the direct practical utility the findings will have. *Basic research* is concerned with making empirical observations that can be used to accumulate information or to formulate or refine a theory. Basic research is not designed to solve immediate problems, but rather to extend the base of knowledge in a discipline for the sake of knowledge and understanding. Of course, many of the findings from basic research endeavors are ultimately applied to practical

problems, but basic research is not directly concerned with the social utility of its findings, and many years may pass before a relevant application is developed. Researchers who engage in *applied research*, by contrast, focus on finding a solution to an immediate problem. Applied research has as its final goal the scientific planning of induced change in a troublesome situation. Just as the possibility of practical application is not ruled out in basic research, applied research may also contribute to general knowledge in a field. It is perhaps more meaningful to think of applied and basic research as two end points on a continuum because, in a given study, there may be multiple goals and multiple lessons. Much of the research conducted in nursing tends to be more applied than basic in nature. Yet nurse researchers are demonstrating increasing interest in the conduct of theory-based research designed to enhance a general understanding of the nursing process and the role of nurses.

Table 1-1.   *Research Purposes and Research Questions*

PURPOSE	TYPES OF QUESTIONS	NURSING RESEARCH EXAMPLE
Description	How prevalent is the phenomenon? What are the characteristics of the phenomenon? What is the process by which the phenomenon is experienced?	What are the categories of activities involved in the at-home care of people with AIDS, and what is the market value of the unpaid caregiving? (Ward & Brown, 1994)
Exploration	What is the full nature of the phenomenon? What is going on? What factors are related to the phenomenon?	What information is used by expert critical care nurses, and how do they structure the information when reasoning and making clinical decisions? (Fonteyn & Grobe, 1994)
Explanation	What is the underlying cause? What does the occurrence of the phenomenon mean? Why does the phenomenon exist?	What are the factors that determine perimenstrual symptom patterns in women? (Mitchell, Woods, & Lentz, 1994).
Prediction and control	If phenomenon *X* occurs, will phenomenon *Y* follow? Can the occurrence of the phenomenon be controlled? Does an intervention result in the intended effect?	What combination of factors best predicts health-promoting behaviors among adults with disabilities? (Stuifbergen & Becker, 1994)

Limitations of the Scientific Method

The scientific approach to inquiry is regarded by many as the highest form of attaining knowledge that humans have devised. This is not to say, however, that scientific research can solve all human problems or that the scientific method is infallible. Several limitations of the scientific approach deserve special mention.

GENERAL LIMITATIONS

Perfectly designed and executed studies are unattainable—virtually every research study contains some flaw. Every research question can be addressed in an almost infinite number of ways. The researcher must make decisions about how best to proceed and, invariably, there are tradeoffs. The best methods are often expensive and time-consuming. Even when tremendous resources are expended, there are bound to be some limitations. This does not mean that small, simple studies are worthless. It means that *no single study can ever definitively prove or disprove our hunches*. Each completed study adds to a body of accumulated knowledge.

Scientists are fundamentally skeptics who challenge unconfirmed observations and tentative conclusions. Scientific researchers (and intelligent consumers of research studies) demand evidence and verification. Verification often comes from repeated studies of the same research problem. If the same question is posed by several researchers, each of whom obtains the same or similar results, increased confidence can be placed in the answer to the question. This is especially true if the researchers' studies have different types of shortcomings. Studies that are repeated for the purpose of verification are known as *replications*.

MORAL OR ETHICAL ISSUES

Moral or ethical issues create limitations for scientific research in two respects. The first concerns constraints on what is considered acceptable in the name of science with regard to the rights of living organisms. Research ethics are discussed in greater detail in Chapter 6.

The second issue concerns the kinds of problems that can be solved using the scientific method. Questions that focus on ethical or value-laden matters cannot be empirically tested. Many of our most persistent and intriguing questions about the human condition fall into the category of moral or ethical problems. Consider, for example, the issue of euthanasia. Descriptive research concerning how nurses feel about euthanasia is certainly possible. Studies concerning the characteristics of nurses with different points of view are also feasible. Similarly, a researcher could explore the extent to which nurses' attitudes concerning euthanasia affect their behavior toward terminally ill patients. All these hypothetical studies lend themselves to a scientific approach, but no study could determine whether euthanasia is right or wrong. Given the many moral issues that are associated with medicine and health care, it is inevitable that the nursing process will never rely exclusively on scientific information.

HUMAN COMPLEXITY

One of the major obstacles confronting nurse researchers using the scientific paradigm is the complexity of the central topic of investigation—humans. This problem is much less troublesome in clinical research dealing with biophysiologic processes than in research concerning human behavior or attitudes. Biologic and physical functioning is considerably more regular and consistent and less susceptible to external influences than is psychological functioning. Each human being is essentially unique with respect to his or her personality, social environment, mental capacities, values, and lifestyle. As a consequence, it is relatively more difficult to detect regularities in, say, human eating behavior than in, say, the functioning of the pancreas. Thus, it has been impossible to achieve the same level of order and discipline over the research situation in studies focusing on human behavior and thought than is the case in studies dealing with biologic or physical phenomena.

The inability of the traditional scientific approach to capture the human experience holistically and meaningfully has led some nurse researchers to reject the traditional model of scientific research, the philosophical underpinnings of which are *logical positivism*. An alternative model of inquiry has emerged that has its intellectual roots in the philosophical tradition known as *phenomenology*. The phenomenological approach rests on different assumptions about the nature of humans and how that nature is to be understood. Phenomenologists emphasize the inherent complexity of humans, the ability of humans to shape and create their own experiences, and the idea that truth is a composite of realities. Investigations in the phenomenological tradition place a heavy emphasis on understanding the human experience as it is actually lived, generally through the careful collection and analysis of narrative, subjective materials. Phenomenologists believe that a major limitation of the classical scientific approach is that it is *reductionist*; that is, it reduces human experience to only the few concepts under investigation, and those concepts are defined in advance by the researcher rather than emerging from the experiences of those under study.

In this book, we take the view that both the phenomenological and the traditional scientific approaches represent valid and important *paradigms* for the study of nursing problems. We have devoted more attention to methods normally associated with the scientific approach because most nursing research studies have adopted this approach, but methods used by phenomenologists are also described.

MEASUREMENT PROBLEMS

Another limitation of the scientific approach that is related to the issue of human complexity concerns problems of measurement. To study a certain phenomenon—for example, patient morale—we must be able to observe or measure it; that is, we must be able to assess whether a patient's morale is high or low, or higher under certain conditions than under others. Although there are reasonably accurate measures of such physiologic phenomena as blood pressure, temperature, and cardiac activity, comparably accurate measures of such psychological phenomena as anxiety, pain, self-confidence, or body image have not been developed. The problems associated with measurement are often the most perplexing in the research process.

CONTROL PROBLEMS

In discussing the characteristics of the scientific approach, we pointed out that the scientist attempts to control the research situation to have confidence in the outcomes. Because scientists accept the principle of multiple causation, and because all potential causes of a phenomenon generally cannot be studied simultaneously, scientists often attempt to control factors that are not under direct investigation. For example, a researcher focusing on the link between prenatal care and low birthweight might want to control—that is, remove the influence of—maternal diet and smoking behavior, both of which have been implicated as contributing to low birthweight.

Adequate control, however, is often difficult to achieve. Confounding factors may be difficult to even identify, let alone control, if the phenomenon of interest is complex. Control over confounding factors is especially problematic in research with humans in naturalistic settings.

PROGRESS IN ADDRESSING OBSTACLES

Despite the various obstacles mentioned earlier, nurse researchers have made outstanding progress in contributing knowledge and understanding about the practice and theory of nursing. Even further progress can be anticipated in the years to come as information accumulates and forms a foundation for more sophisticated theories, as data collection methods and research design become more refined, and as nurses integrate findings from phenomeno-logical and scientific studies.

❖ *METHODS FOR NURSING RESEARCH: QUALITATIVE AND QUANTITATIVE RESEARCH*

The methods that nurse researchers use to study problems of interest in the development of a sci-entific basis for nursing are diverse. This diver-sity, in our view, is critical to the spirit of sci-ence, the basic aim of which is the discovery of knowledge. There is no single right way to un-derstand our complex world. Throughout this book, we discuss alternative ways of asking questions, identifying sources of information, and gathering and analyzing that information. Scientific knowledge would be slim, indeed, if there were not a rich array of alternative ap-proaches available.

A distinction is often made between two broad approaches to gathering and analyzing scientific information: qualitative and quantita-tive. *Quantitative research* involves the system-atic collection of numerical information, often under conditions of considerable control, and the analysis of that information using statistical procedures. *Qualitative research* involves the systematic collection and analysis of more sub-jective narrative materials, using procedures in which there tends to be a minimum of researcher-imposed control. Although most nursing research studies are quantitative, there are a growing number of qualitative investiga-tions. There has also been a recent increase in the number of studies using both qualitative and quantitative methods.

In our view, the selection of an appropri-ate method depends to some degree on the re-searcher's personal taste and philosophy, but it also depends in large part on the nature of the research question. If a researcher asks what the effects of surgery are on circadian rhythms (bio-logic cycles), the researcher really needs to ex-press the effects through the careful quantitative measurement of various bodily processes sub-ject to rhythmic variation. On the other hand, if a researcher inquires about the process by which parents learn to cope with the death of a child, the researcher may be hard pressed to quantify such a process. Personal world views of the researchers generally help to shape the types of questions they ask.

There is a tendency to attach convenient labels to emphasize the distinction between qualitative and quantitative research. For exam-ple, the logical positivist paradigm is most fre-quently associated with quantitative methods. However, many researchers who would con-sider themselves squarely in the logical posi-tivist tradition also collect and analyze qualita-tive data. Ethnographers, who conduct in-depth studies of specific cultures or subcultures, rely heavily on qualitative data but may also use available quantitative data on the members of the culture to provide a context for their inquiry. Similarly, historical researchers often blend qualitative and quantitative information, al-though historical research has traditionally been qualitative.

Although we think that the distinctions be-tween qualitative and quantitative methods have sometimes been exaggerated, it is never-theless true that there tend to be some important differences between these two types of re-search. Quantitative research, which is referred to by some as hard science, tends to emphasize deductive reasoning, the rules of logic, and the measurable attributes of the human experience. Thus, quantitative research does have its roots in logical positivism. Research that uses a quan-titative approach *generally*:

- Focuses on a relatively small number of spe-cific concepts
- Begins with preconceived hunches about how the concepts are interrelated
- Uses structured procedures and formal in-struments to collect information
- Collects the information under conditions of control
- Emphasizes objectivity in the collection and analysis of information

- Analyzes numerical information through statistical procedures

Qualitative research, on the other hand, has sometimes been referred to as soft science. Qualitative researchers tend to emphasize the dynamic, holistic, and individual aspects of the human experience and attempt to capture those aspects in their entirety, within the context of those who are experiencing them. Phenomenological research is almost always exclusively qualitative (although not all qualitative research is phenomenological). Research that uses a qualitative approach *generally*:

- Attempts to understand the entirety of some phenomenon rather than focus on specific concepts
- Has few preconceived hunches; stresses the importance of people's interpretation of events and circumstances, rather than the researcher's interpretation
- Collects information without formal, structured instruments
- Does not attempt to control the context of the research but, rather, attempts to capture it in its entirety
- Attempts to capitalize on the subjective as a means for understanding and interpreting human experiences
- Analyzes narrative information in an organized, but intuitive, fashion

Both qualitative and quantitative approaches have strengths and weaknesses, which are identified throughout this book. It is precisely because the strengths of one approach complement the weaknesses of the other that both are essential to the further development of nursing science.

❖ RESEARCH EXAMPLES

In this section, we present a brief summary of an actual nursing study. Consider this study in terms of the issues that were discussed in this chapter, such as its relevance to nursing, its underlying purpose, its position on the basic–applied continuum, and its status as a qualitative or quantitative study.

Okimi, Sportsman, Rickard, and Fritsche (1991), who were interested in better understanding the roots of glaucoma, designed a study to examine the effects of caffeinated coffee on the intraocular pressure (IOP) of nonglaucomatous individuals. They noted that glaucoma is a condition due to optic nerve damage resulting from increased IOP, but that the factors contributing to elevated IOP levels are not well understood. Twelve individuals who volunteered to participate in the study received three different treatments: caffeinated coffee, hot water, and no fluid. Each person received one treatment per day on three successive mornings, in a totally random order. Each day, their IOP was measured (with an instrument known as a noncontact tonometer) at 1-hour intervals for 3 hours after the treatment. The study revealed that, as a group, the study participants' IOP was higher after ingesting coffee than after receiving the other two treatments. Moreover, the increased IOP was maintained over a 3-hour period. The authors concluded that "there are enough indications of adverse effects of caffeine to advise caution in the use of caffeinated products" (p. 75).

❖ SUMMARY

Research has an important role to play in helping nursing establish a scientific base for its practice. There is a growing consensus that a knowledge of nursing research is needed to enhance the professional practice of all nurses—including both *consumers* of research (who read and evaluate studies) and *producers* of research (who undertake research studies). Nurses may assume a variety of additional research-related roles in the course of their practice.

Nursing research began with Florence Nightingale and gained slow acceptance. The early focus of nursing research closely paralleled the problems faced by the nursing profession: most early research studies were conducted in the areas of nursing education and nursing administration. Nursing research came to be accepted as part of professional nursing behavior during the 1950s, and such acceptance has continued at a rapidly accelerating pace. Since the 1970s, the emphasis in nursing research has been on clinical practice. Nurses are increasingly studying problems such as health promotion, prevention of illness, the efficacy of nursing interventions, and the needs of special health-risk groups. The establishment of the National Institute of Nursing Research at the National Institutes of Health in 1993 attests to the growth and current importance of nursing research.

The scientific approach may be contrasted with other sources of truth and understanding. Certain "truths" are passed on to us by tradition or custom—that is, they are accepted as cultural truths without demands for verification. Authority figures or specialists are another common source of information or knowledge. Our own experiences, together with trial and error procedures, are familiar to all of us as a method of acquiring understanding. Some of our problems can be dealt with by logical reasoning. *Inductive reasoning* is the process of establishing generalizations from specific observations, and *deductive reasoning* is the process of developing specific predictions from general principles. These approaches suffer various limitations as techniques for solving problems. The scientific method offers several advantages as a method of inquiry.

The *scientific approach* may be described in terms of a number of characteristics. It is, first of all, a systematic, disciplined, and controlled process. Scientists base their findings on *empirical* observations, which means that evidence is rooted in objective reality and collected by means of the human senses. Unlike many other problem-solving techniques, the scientific approach strives for *generalizability* and for the development of conceptual explanations or *theories* concerning the relationships among phenomena.

The scientist assumes that there is an objective reality that is not dependent on human observation for its existence. A related belief is that natural phenomena are basically regular and orderly. The assumption of *determinism* refers to the belief that events are not haphazard but, rather, are the consequence of prior causes. The search for an understanding of cause-and-effect relationships is an activity basic to many scientific endeavors.

Scientific research can be categorized in terms of its functions or objectives. Description, exploration, explanation, prediction, and control of natural phenomena represent the most common goals of a research investigation. It is also possible to describe research in terms of the direct practical utility that it aspires to achieve. *Basic research* is designed to extend the base of knowledge in a discipline for the sake of knowledge itself. *Applied research* focuses on discovering solutions to immediate problems.

Although the scientific approach offers a number of distinct advantages as a system of inquiry, it is not without its share of limitations. In general, researchers must make compromises in the face of limited time and resources, so that no single study can ever definitively answer a given question. The design of studies with humans is constrained not only by resources but also by standards of professional ethics. In addition, there are numerous questions of interest to nurse researchers that are difficult to study because they deal with complex social or psychological functioning, such as pain, fear, guilt, anxiety, motivation, and the like. Such phenomena are difficult to accurately measure (in comparison with aspects of biologic functioning such as blood pressure) and difficult to control in a natural setting. In fact, *phenomenologists* have argued that the scientific approach, which has its roots in the tradition of *logical positivism*, is overly reductionist and cannot adequately capture the human experience in all its complexity.

Problems of interest to nurse researchers can be addressed using a wide range of available methods. A distinction is often made between two broad types of methods. *Quantitative research* involves the systematic collection and analysis of numerical information, generally under controlled conditions. *Qualitative research*, which involves the collection and analysis of more subjective, narrative materials, generally attempts to view the experiences of those being studied through their own eyes. Both qualitative and quantitative research have complementary strengths and limitations; both play important roles in the advancement of nursing science.

❖ STUDY SUGGESTIONS

Chapter 1 of the accompanying *Study Guide for Nursing Research: Principles and Methods, 5th ed.*, offers suggested questions for reinforcing concepts presented in this chapter. Additionally, the following study questions can be addressed:

1. What are some of the current changes occurring in the health care delivery system, and how could these changes influence nursing research?

2. Consider one or two nursing "facts" that you possess, and then trace the facts back to some source. Is the basis for your knowledge tradition, authority, experience, or scientific research?

3. Explain the ways in which scientific knowledge differs from knowledge based on tradition, authority, trial and error, and logical reasoning.

4. How does the assumption of scientific determinism conflict with or coincide with superstitious thinking? Take, as an example, the superstition associated with four-leaf clovers or a rabbit's foot.

5. How does the ability to predict phenomena offer the possibility of their control?

6. Below are a few research problems. For each problem, specify whether you think it is essentially a basic or applied research question. Justify your response.
   a. Is the stress level of patients related to the level of information they possess about their medical status?
   b. Do students who get better grades in nursing school become more effective nurses than students with lower grades?
   c. Does the early discharge of maternity patients lead to later problems with breastfeeding?
   d. Can the incidence of decubitus ulcers be affected by a certain massaging technique?
   e. Is individual contraceptive counseling more effective than group-based instruction in minimizing unwanted pregnancies?

❖ SUGGESTED READINGS

METHODOLOGICAL/THEORETICAL REFERENCES

American Nurses' Association Cabinet on Nursing Research. (1985). *Directions for nursing research: Toward the twenty-first century*. Kansas City, MO: Author.

American Nurses' Association Commission on Nursing Research. (1980). Generating a scientific basis for nursing practice: Research priorities for the 1980s. *Nursing Research, 29*, 219.

American Nurses' Association Commission on Nursing Research. (1981). *Guidelines for the investigative function of nurses*. Kansas City, MO: Author.

American Nurses' Association Congress for Practice. (1973). *Standards of nursing practice*. Kansas City, MO: Author.

Braithwaite, R. (1955). *Scientific explanation*. Cambridge, England: Cambridge University Press.

Brown, E. L. (1948). *Nursing for the future*. New York: Russell Sage.

Gortner, S. R. (1974). Scientific accountability in nursing. *Nursing Outlook, 22*, 764–768.

Kuhn, T. S. (1970). *The structure of scientific revolutions* (2nd ed.). Chicago: University of Chicago Press.

Lindeman, C. A. (1975). Delphi survey of priorities in clinical nursing research. *Nursing Research, 24*, 434–441.

Madden, E. H. (Ed.). (1974). *The structure of scientific thought*. Boston: Houghton Mifflin.

Meyers, S. T. (1982). The search for assumptions. *Western Journal of Nursing Research, 4,* 91–98.

Newton, D. E. (1974). *Science and society.* Boston: Holbrook Press.

Oiler, C. (1982). The phenomenological approach in nursing research. *Nursing Research, 31,* 178–181.

Popper, K. R. (1959). *The logic of scientific discovery* (rev. ed.). New York: Harper & Row.

Walker, V. H. (1967). *Nursing and ritualistic practice.* New York: Macmillan.

SUBSTANTIVE REFERENCES

Fonteyn, M. E., & Grobe, S. J. (1994). Expert system development in nursing: Implications for critical care nursing practice. *Heart and Lung, 23,* 80–87.

Mitchell, E. S., Woods, N. F., & Lentz, M. J. (1994). Differentiation of women with three perimenstrual symptom patterns. *Nursing Research, 43,* 25–30.

Okimi, P. H., Sportsman, S., Rickard, M. R., & Fritsche, M. B. (1991). Effects of caffeinated coffee on intraocular pressure. *Applied Nursing Research, 4,* 72–76.

Stuifbergen, A. K., & Becker, H. A. (1994). Predictors of health-promoting lifestyles in persons with disabilities. *Research in Nursing and Health, 17,* 3–13.

Ward, D., & Brown, M. A. (1994). Labor and cost in AIDS family caregiving. *Western Journal of Nursing Research, 16,* 10–22.

Chapter 2

OVERVIEW OF THE RESEARCH PROCESS

❖ BASIC RESEARCH TERMINOLOGY

Scientific research, like nursing or any other discipline, has its own language and terminology. New terms relating to the research process are introduced throughout this textbook. Some terms and concepts are so fundamental, however, that they need to be understood before more complex concepts can be grasped. The purpose of this chapter is to make the rest of this book more manageable by familiarizing readers with the basics of scientific terminology and with the progression of steps that are generally undertaken in a scientific study.

The Scientific Study

When researchers address a problem or answer a question using the scientific approach, it is usually said that they are doing a *study*. Sometimes a study is referred to as an *investigation* or a *research project*.

Research studies with humans involve two sets of people: those who are doing the research and those who are being studied. The people who are being studied are often referred to as the *subjects* (sometimes abbreviated as *ss*) or the *study participants*. When the subjects provide information to the researchers by answering questions directly (e.g., if they participate in an interview), they may be called *respondents* or, sometimes, *informants*.

The person who undertakes the research is called the *researcher, investigator,* or *scientist*. A study is often undertaken by a group of people who work together rather than by a single researcher. For example, a team of nurse researchers and clinical nurses might collaborate on addressing a problem of clinical relevance. When a study is undertaken by a research team, the main person directing the investigation is referred to as the *principal investigator* (PI) or *project director*.

Scientific Concepts, Constructs, and Theories

Conceptualization refers to the process of developing and refining abstract ideas. Scientific

Polit DF, Hungler BP: NURSING RESEARCH: PRINCIPLES AND METHODS, 5th ed. © 1995 J. B. Lippincott Company.

research almost always is concerned with abstract rather than tangible phenomena. For example, the terms good health, pain, emotional disturbance, patient care, and grieving are all abstractions that are formulated by generalizing from particular manifestations of human behaviors or characteristics. These abstractions are referred to as *concepts.*

The term construct is also encountered frequently in the scientific literature. Like the term concept, a *construct* refers to an abstraction or a mental representation inferred from situations, events, or behaviors. Kerlinger (1986) distinguished concepts from constructs by noting that constructs are terms that are deliberately and systematically invented (or constructed) by researchers for a specific scientific purpose. For example, "self-care" in Dorothea Orem's model of health maintenance may be considered a construct. In practice, the terms concept and construct are often used interchangeably.

A *theory* is an abstract generalization that presents a systematic explanation about the interrelationships among phenomena. Concepts are the building blocks of theories. In a theory, concepts (or constructs) are knitted together into an orderly system to explain the way in which our world and the people in it function.

Variables

Within the context of a research investigation, concepts are generally referred to as variables. A *variable* is, as the name implies, something that varies. Weight, height, body temperature, blood pressure readings, and preoperative anxiety levels all are variables. That is, each of these properties varies or differs from one individual to another. When one considers the variety and complexity of humans and their experiences, it becomes clear that nearly all aspects of individuals and the environment can be considered variables. If everyone had black hair and weighed 125 pounds, hair color and weight would not be variables—they would be *constants.* If it rained continuously and the outdoor temperature was always 70°F, weather would

not be a variable. But it is precisely because individuals and conditions *do* vary that most research is conducted. The bulk of all research activity is aimed at trying to understand how or why things vary and to gain insights into how differences in one variable are related to differences in another. For example, lung cancer research is concerned with the variable of lung cancer, which is a variable because not everybody has lung cancer. Researchers in this area are concerned with learning what other variables can be linked to lung cancer. They have discovered that cigarette smoking is related to lung cancer. Again, this is a variable because not everyone smokes. A variable, then, is any quality of an organism, group, or situation that takes on different values.

CONTINUOUS VERSUS CATEGORICAL VARIABLES

Sometimes a variable can take on a range of different values. Age, for instance, can take on values from zero to more than 100 when we are referring to the age in years of humans. Such variables are sometimes referred to as *continuous variables* because their values can be represented on a continuum. Continuous variables can meaningfully take on values that are not whole numbers. For example, a person's weight (another continuous variable) could be designated to the nearest tenth or hundredth of a pound.

Other variables, however, take on a much smaller range of values, representing discrete categories rather than incremental placement along a continuum. The variable gender, for example, has only two values (male or female). Variables of this type, which take on only a handful of discrete values, are referred to as *categorical variables.* Other examples of categorical variables include marital status (married, single, divorced, widowed, other) and blood type (A, B, AB, and O). When categorical variables take on only two values, they are sometimes referred to as *dichotomous variables.* Some additional examples of categorical variables that are dichotomous include pregnant/not pregnant, smoker/nonsmoker, HIV positive/HIV negative, and asleep/awake.

ACTIVE VERSUS ATTRIBUTE VARIABLES

Variables are often inherent characteristics of the research subjects, such as age, health beliefs, weight, or grip strength. Variables such as these are sometimes called *attribute variables*. In many research situations, however, the investigator creates or designs a variable. For example, if a researcher is interested in testing the effectiveness of ice chips as opposed to effervescent ginger ale to refresh the mouth after vomiting, some individuals would be given ice chips and others would receive ginger ale. For the purpose of this study, the type of mouth care is a variable because different individuals receive ice chips or ginger ale. Kerlinger (1986) refers to these variables that the researcher creates or designs as *active variables*.

DEPENDENT VERSUS INDEPENDENT VARIABLES

An important distinction can be made between two types of variables in a research study, and it is a distinction that needs to be mastered before proceeding to later chapters. It is the distinction between the independent variable and the dependent variable. Many research studies are aimed at unraveling and understanding the causes underlying phenomena. Does a drug *cause* improvement of a medical problem? Does a nursing intervention *cause* more rapid recovery? Does smoking *cause* lung cancer? The presumed cause is referred to as the *independent variable* and the presumed effect is referred to as the *dependent variable*.

Variability in the dependent variable is presumed to *depend* on variability in the independent variable. For example, the researcher investigates the extent to which lung cancer (the dependent variable) depends on smoking behavior (the independent variable). Or, an investigator may be concerned with the extent to which patients' perception of pain (the dependent variable) depends on different types of nursing approaches (the independent variable).

The terms independent variable and dependent variable are frequently used to indicate direction of influence rather than a causal connection. For example, let us say that a researcher is studying nurses' attitudes toward abortion and finds that older nurses hold less favorable opinions about abortion than younger nurses. The researcher might be unwilling to infer that the nurses' attitudes were *caused* by their age. Yet the direction of influence clearly runs from age to attitudes. That is, it would make little sense to suggest that the attitudes caused or influenced age. Even though in this example the researcher does not infer a causal relationship between age and attitudes, it is appropriate to conceptualize attitudes toward abortion as the dependent variable and age as the independent variable.

The dependent variable usually is the variable the researcher is interested in understanding, explaining, or predicting. In lung cancer research, it is the carcinoma that is of real interest to the research scientist, not smoking behavior per se. In studies of the effectiveness of therapeutic treatments for alcoholics, it is the drinking behavior of the subjects that is the dependent variable. Although a great deal of time, effort, and resources may be devoted to designing new therapies (the independent variable), they are of interest primarily as they relate to improvements in drinking behavior and overall functioning of alcoholics.

Many of the dependent variables that are studied by researchers have a multiplicity of causes or antecedents. If we are interested in studying the factors that influence people's weight, for example, we might consider their age, height, physical activity, and eating habits as the independent variables. Note that some of these independent variables are attribute variables (age and height), and others (activity and eating patterns) can be influenced by the investigator. Just as a study may examine more than one independent variable, two or more dependent variables may be of interest to the researcher. For example, an investigator may be concerned with comparing the effectiveness of two methods of nursing care delivery (primary versus functional) for children with cystic fibrosis. Several dependent variables could be designated as measures of treatment effectiveness, such as length of stay in the hospital, number of recurrent respiratory infections, presence of cough, dyspnea on exertion, and so forth. In short, it is common to design studies with multiple independent and dependent variables.

The reader should not get the impression that variables are inherently dependent or independent. A variable that is classified as dependent in one study may be considered an independent variable in another study. For example, a researcher may find that the religious background of a nurse (the independent variable) has an effect on the nurse's attitude toward death and dying (the dependent variable). Another study, however, may analyze the extent to which nurses' attitudes toward death and dying (the independent variables) affect their job performance (the dependent variable). To illustrate this point with another example, consider a study that examines the relationship between contraceptive counseling (the independent variable) and unwanted pregnancies (the dependent variable). Yet another research project could study the effect of unwanted pregnancies (the independent variable) on the incidence of child abuse (the dependent variable). In short, the designation of a variable as independent or dependent is a function of the role the variable plays in a particular investigation. Table 2-1 presents some examples of research questions posed by nurse researchers and specifies the dependent and independent variables.

Some researchers use the term *criterion variable* (or criterion measure) rather than dependent variable. In studies that analyze the consequences of a treatment, therapy, or some other type of intervention, it is usually necessary to establish criteria against which the success of the intervention can be assessed—hence, the origin of the expression criterion variable. The term dependent variable, however, is broader and more general in its implications and applicability. Therefore, we use the term dependent variable more frequently than criterion variable, although in many situations the two are equivalent and interchangeable.

HETEROGENEITY

A term that is frequently used in connection with variables is heterogeneity. When an attribute is extremely varied in the group under investigation, the group is said to be *heterogeneous* with respect to that variable. If, on the other hand, the amount of variability is limited, the group is described as relatively *homogeneous*. For example, with respect to the variable height, a group of 2-year-old children is likely to be more homogeneous than a group of 18-year-old adolescents. The degree of *variability* of a group of subjects has implications for the design of a study.

Operational Definitions

Before a study progresses, the researcher usually clarifies and defines the variables under investigation. This is especially likely to be the case in quantitative studies. For the definition to be useful, the researcher should specify how the variable will be observed and measured in the actual research situation. Such a definition has a special name. An *operational definition* is a specification of the operations that the researcher must perform to collect the required information.

Variables differ considerably in the facility with which they can be operationalized. The variable weight, for example, is easy to define and measure. We may use the following as our definition of weight: the heaviness or lightness of an object in terms of pounds. Note that this definition designates that weight will be determined according to one measuring system (pounds) rather than another (grams). The operational definition might specify that the weight of subjects in a research study would be measured to the nearest pound using a spring scale

Table 2-1. *Examples of Independent and Dependent Variables*

RESEARCH QUESTION	INDEPENDENT VARIABLE	DEPENDENT VARIABLE
Do nurses administer greater amounts of narcotic analgesics to men than to women? (McDonald, 1994)	Gender of patients	Amount of narcotic analgesics
What is the effect of hydrogen peroxide rinses on the microbial characteristics of the normal oral mucosa? (Tombes & Gallucci, 1993)	¼-strength vs. ½-strength H_2O_2 rinse vs. normal saline rinse	Bacterial and fungal adherence to buccal epithelial cells
Is tactile stimulation associated with greater physiologic and behavioral arousal in infants with congenital heart disease than verbal stimulation? (Weiss, 1992)	Mode of stimulation	Physiologic and behavioral arousal
What is the effect of activity and bedrest on tissue oxygen tension in healthy adults? (Whitney, Stotts, Goodson, & Janson-Bjerklie, 1993)	Exercise activity vs. bedrest	Subcutaneous oxygen tension ($PscO_2$)
What are the effects of women's adherence to guidelines on exercise during the third trimester of their pregnancy on pregnancy outcomes? (Zeanah & Schlosser, 1993)	Adherence vs. nonadherence to exercise guidelines	Pregnancy outcomes (maternal weight gain, neonatal birthweight)

with the subjects fully undressed after 10 hours of fasting. This operational definition spells out what the investigator must do to measure weight in such a way that a person not associated with the study would know precisely what is meant by the variable weight.

Unfortunately, many of the variables of interest in nursing research are not operationalized as easily and straightforwardly as weight. Often there are multiple methods of measuring a variable, and the researcher must choose the method that best captures the variable as he or she conceptualizes it. For example, patient well-being may be defined in terms of either physiologic or psychological functioning. If the researcher chooses to emphasize the physiologic aspects of patient well-being, the operational definition would involve a measure such as heart rate, white blood cell count, blood pressure, vital capacity, and so forth. If, on the other hand, well-being is conceptualized for the purposes of research as primarily a psychological phenomenon, the operational definition would need to identify the method by which emotional well-being would be assessed, as, for example, the responses of the patient to certain questions or the behavior of the patient as observed by the researcher.

Some readers of a research report may not agree with the way that the investigator has conceptualized and operationalized the variables. Nevertheless, precision in defining the terms conceptually and operationally has the advantage of communicating exactly what the terms mean. If the researcher, is reluctant to be explicit, it will be impossible for others to gauge the full meaning and implications of the research findings. Table 2-2 presents some operational definitions from several nursing research studies.

Table 2-2. *Examples of Operational Definitions*

CONCEPT	OPERATIONAL DEFINITION
Physiological status	The ratio of the Forced Expiratory Volume in 1 second (FEV_1) to Forced Vital Capacity (FVC), i.e., (FEV_1/FVC%), in patients with chronic obstructive pulmonary disease (Narsavage & Weaver, 1994)
Normothermia	Core temperature of 98.4°F, as measured rectally (Howell, MacRae, Sanjines, Burke & DeStefano, 1992)
Total rapid eye movement (REM) density	Total number of eye movments across the period from sleep onset to final morning awakening, divided by total REM time in minutes (Topf & Davis, 1993)
Fatigue	A mood marked by weariness, inertia, listlessness, and/or low energy level, as assessed by Factor F on the Profile of Mood States (Wright, 1991)
Psychological adaptation	A state of well-being related to life satisfaction, as measured by the Affect Balance Scale (Dobratz, 1993)

Qualitative researchers generally do not define in operational terms the concepts in which they are interested before gathering information. This is because of their desire to have the meaning of concepts defined by those being studied themselves. Nevertheless, in summarizing the results of a study, all researchers should be careful in describing the conceptual and methodological basis of key research concepts.

Data

The *data* (singular, datum) of a research study are the pieces of information obtained in the course of the investigation. The researcher identifies the variables of interest, develops operational definitions of those variables, and then collects the necessary data. The variables, because they vary, take on different values. The *actual* values of the study variables constitute the data for a research project. In quantitative research, those values are numbers.

For example, suppose we were interested in studying the relationship between sodium consumption and blood pressure. That is, we want to learn if people who consume more

sodium are particularly susceptible to high blood pressure, or whether these variables are unrelated. The data for the study might consist of three pieces of information for all participants: their average daily intake of sodium (in milligrams), their diastolic blood pressure, and their systolic blood pressure. Some hypothetical data for 10 subjects are shown in Table 2-3. These numerical values associated with the variables of interest represent the data for a research project.

In qualitative studies, the pieces of data are usually narrative descriptions rather than numerical values. Narrative descriptions can be obtained by interviewing subjects, by making detailed notes of how subjects behave in naturalistic settings, or by obtaining narrative records from subjects, such as diaries. These data are referred to as *qualitative data*, while data that are in the form of numerical values are referred to as *quantitative data*.

Relationships

Researchers are rarely interested in single, isolated variables, except in some descriptive studies. As an example of a descriptive study, a

Table 2-3.   *Hypothetical Data for Blood Pressure Study*

SUBJECT NUMBER	DAILY SODIUM INTAKE (MG)	SYSTOLIC BLOOD PRESSURE	DIASTOLIC BLOOD PRESSURE
1	8125	130	90
2	7530	126	80
3	1000	140	90
4	4580	118	78
5	2810	114	76
6	4150	112	78
7	6000	120	80
8	2250	110	70
9	5240	114	76
10	3330	116	74

researcher might focus on the percentage of women who elect to breastfeed their babies. In this example, there is only one variable: breast-feeding versus bottle-feeding. Usually, however, researchers study two or more variables simultaneously. What scientists are most often interested in is the relationship between the independent and dependent variables of a study.

But what exactly is meant by the term relationship in scientific terms? Generally speaking, a *relationship* refers to a bond or connection between two entities. Let us consider as a possible dependent variable a person's body weight. What variables are related to (associated with) a person's weight? Some possibilities include height, metabolism, caloric intake, and exercise. For each of these four independent variables, we can make a tentative relational statement:

Height: Tall people, in general, weigh more than short people.
Metabolism: The lower a person's metabolic rate, the more he or she weighs.
Caloric intake: People with high caloric intake are heavier than those with lower caloric intake.
Exercise: The greater the amount of exercise, the lower is the person's weight.

Each of these statements expresses a presumed relationship between weight and an in-

dependent variable. The terms "more than" and "lower than" imply that as we observe a change in one variable, we are likely to observe a corresponding change in the other. If Nate is taller than Tom, we would expect (in the absence of any other information) that Nate is also heavier than Tom.

Research is often conducted to determine whether relationships exist among variables, as suggested by the following research questions: Is there a relationship between nursing shift assignments and absentee rates? Is there a relationship between the frequency of turning patients and the incidence and severity of decubitus? Is prematurity related to the incidence of nosocomial viral infections? The scientific method can be used to answer questions about whether and to what degree variables are related.

Variables can be related to one another in different ways. Scientists are often interested in what is referred to as *cause-and-effect* (or *causal*) *relationships*. As noted in Chapter 1, the scientist assumes that natural phenomena are not random or haphazard, but rather that all phenomena have antecedent factors or causes, and that these causes are generally discoverable. If variable *X* causes the occurrence or manifestation of variable *Y*, then it can be said that those variables are causally related. For instance, in the previous example, we might say that there is a causal relationship between caloric intake and weight: eating more calories causes increased weight.

Not all relationships between variables can be inferred as cause-and-effect relationships. There is a relationship, for example, between a person's gender and weight; men tend to be heavier than women, on the average. The relationship is not perfect; some women are heavier than some men. Nevertheless, if we had to guess whether Mike Stewart or Gina Stewart were heavier, we would be likely to say Mike because men generally weigh more than women. However, we cannot really say that a person's gender causes his or her weight, despite the relationship that exists between the two variables. This type of relationship is sometimes referred to as a *functional relationship* rather than a causal relationship.

Control

Research control plays a critical role in scientific inquiry, especially in studies that are quantitative. It is a topic to which much of this book is devoted. Chapter 10, in particular, discusses methods of achieving control in scientific research. The concept is so important, however, that some basic ideas about control are presented here.

Essentially, *research control* is concerned with holding constant the possible influences on the dependent variable under investigation so that the true relationship between the independent and dependent variables can be understood. In other words, research control attempts to eliminate any contaminating factors that might otherwise obscure the relationship between the variables that are really of interest. A detailed example should clarify this point.

Let us suppose that a researcher is interested in studying whether teenage women are at higher risk of having low-birthweight infants than are older mothers *because of their age*. In other words, the researcher wants to test whether there is something about the physiologic development of women that causes differences in the birthweights of their babies. Exist-

ing studies have shown that, in fact, teenagers have a higher rate of low-birthweight babies than women in their 20s. The question for this researcher, however, is whether age itself causes this difference or whether there are other mechanisms that can account for or influence the relationship between maternal age and infant birthweight. The researcher in this example would want to design the study in such a way that these other factors are controlled. But what are the other factors? To answer this, one must ask the following critical question:

> *What variables could affect the dependent variable under study while at the same time be related to the independent variable?*

In the current study, the dependent variable is infant birthweight and the independent variable is maternal age. Two variables are prime candidates for concern as contaminating factors (although there are several other possibilities): the nutritional habits of the mother and the amount of prenatal care received. Teenagers tend to be less careful than older women about their eating patterns during pregnancy and are also less likely to obtain adequate prenatal care. Both nutrition and the amount of care could, in turn, affect the baby's birthweight. Thus, if these two factors are not controlled, then any observed relationship between the mother's age and her baby's weight at birth could be caused by the mother's age itself, her diet, or her prenatal care. It would be impossible to know what the underlying cause really is.

These three possible explanations are shown schematically as follows:

1. Mother's age → infant birthweight
2. Mother's age → prenatal care → infant birthweight
3. Mother's age → nutrition → infant birthweight

The arrows here symbolize a causal mechanism or an influence. In examples 2 and 3, the effect of maternal age on infant birthweight is mediated by prenatal care and nutrition, respectively; for this reason, these variables are usually referred to as *mediating variables*. The researcher's task is to design a study in such a way that the true explanation is made clear. Both nutrition and prenatal care must be controlled if the researcher's goal is to learn if explanation 1 is valid.

How can the researcher impose such control? There are a number of ways, as discussed in Chapter 10, but the general principle underlying each alternative is the same: the competing influences—often referred to as the *extraneous variables* of the study—must be held constant. The extraneous variables to be controlled must somehow be handled in such a way that they are not related to the independent or dependent variable. Again, an example should help make this point more clear. Let us say we want to compare the birthweights of infants born to two groups of women: those aged 15 to 19 years and those aged 25 to 29 years. We must then design a study in such a way that the nutritional and prenatal health care practices of the two groups are comparable, even though, in general, the two groups are not comparable in these respects. Table 2-4 illustrates how we might deliberately select subjects for the study in such a way that both older and younger mothers had similar eating habits and amounts of prenatal attention. By building this comparability into the two groups of mothers, we have held nutrition and prenatal care constant. If the babies' birthweights in the two groups differ (as they, in fact, did in Table 2-4), then we might be able to infer that age (and not diet or prenatal care) influenced the birthweight of the infants. If the two

groups do not differ, however, then we might be left to tentatively conclude that it is not the mothers' age per se that causes young women to have a higher percentage of low-birthweight babies, but rather some other variable or set of variables, such as nutrition or prenatal care.

By exercising research control in this example, we have taken a step toward one of the most fundamental aims of science, which is to explain the relationship between variables. Control is essential in firmly establishing cause-and-effect relationships because the world is extremely complex and many variables are interrelated in complicated ways. When studying a particular problem, it is difficult to examine this complexity directly: the researcher must generally be content to analyze a couple of relationships at a time and put the pieces together like a jigsaw puzzle. That is why even modest research studies can make important contributions to science. The extent of the contribution, however, is often directly related to how well a researcher is able to control contaminating influences. A controlled study allows a researcher to understand the nature of the relationship between the dependent and independent variables.

Note that although we have designated prenatal care and nutrition as the extraneous variables in this particular study, they are not at all extraneous to a full understanding of factors influencing infant birthweight. In other studies, nutritional practices and frequency of prenatal care might well be the independent variables.

In the present example, we identified three variables that could affect a baby's birth-

Table 2-4. *Fictitious Example of Controlling Two Variables in a Research Study*

AGE OF MOTHER	RATING OF NUTRITIONAL PRACTICES	NUMBER OF PRENATAL VISITS	INFANT BIRTHWEIGHT
15–19	33% Good	33% 1–3 visits	20% ≤2500 g
	33% Fair	33% 4–6 visits	80% >2500 g
	33% Poor	33% >6 visits	
25–29	33% Good	33% 1–3 visits	9% ≤2500 g
	33% Fair	33% 4–6 visits	91% >2500 g
	33% Poor	33% >6 visits	

weight, but dozens of others could have been suggested, such as maternal stress, mothers' use of drugs or alcohol during pregnancy, sonogram testing, and so on. Researchers need to isolate the independent and dependent variables in which they are interested and then pinpoint from the dozens of possible candidates those extraneous variables that need to be controlled.

It is often impossible to control all the variables that affect the dependent variable and not necessary to do so. It is essential to control a variable only if it is simultaneously related to both the dependent and independent variables. Figure 2-1 illustrates this notion. In this figure, each circle represents the variability associated with a particular variable. The large circle in the center represents the dependent variable, infant birthweight. Overlapping variables indicate the degree to which the variables are related to each other. In this hypothetical example, four variables are shown as being related to infant birthweight: the mother's age, the amount of prenatal care she receives, her nutritional practices, and her smoking practices during pregnancy. The first three variables are also related to each other; this is shown by the fact that these three

circles overlap not only with infant birthweight but also with each other. That is, younger mothers tend to have different patterns of prenatal care and nutrition than older mothers. The mother's prenatal use of cigarettes, however, is unrelated to these three variables. In other words, women who smoke during their pregnancies (according to this hypothetical representation) are as likely to be young as old, to eat properly as not, and to get a lot of prenatal care as not. If this representation is accurate, then it would not be essential to control smoking in a study of the effect of maternal age on infant birthweight. If this scheme is incorrect—if teenage mothers smoke more or less than older mothers—then the mother's smoking practices ideally should be controlled because smoking is related to birthweight.

Figure 2-1 does not represent infant birthweight as being totally determined by the four other variables. The darkened area of the birthweight circle designates unexplained variability in infant birthweight. That is, other circles or determinants of birthweight are needed for us to fully understand what causes babies to be born weighing different amounts. Genetic characteristics, events occurring during the pregnancy,

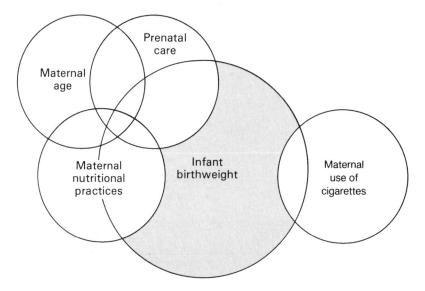

Figure 2-1. *Hypothetical representation of factors affecting infant birthweight.*

and medical treatments administered to the pregnant woman are examples of other factors that contribute to an infant's weight at birth. Dozens, and perhaps hundreds, of circles would need to be sketched onto Figure 2-1 for us to fully understand the complex interrelationships between infant birthweight and other phenomena. In designing a study, we might be interested in the effect of only one variable (such as maternal age) on the dependent variable. This is perfectly respectable—indeed, often necessary. However, researchers should attempt to control those variables that overlap with both the independent and dependent variables to fully understand the relationship between the main variables of interest. In Figure 2-1, if there are other variables that belong in the darkened area that are also related to maternal age, then those extraneous variables ideally should be controlled. Because uncontrolled extraneous variables can lead to erroneous or misleading conclusions, the researcher designing a study must plan how best to control these extraneous variables to maximize the usefulness and validity of the research.

Research rooted in the phenomenological paradigm is less concerned with the issue of control. With its emphasis on a holistic perspective and the individuality of human experience, the phenomenological approach holds that to impose controls on a research setting is to irrevocably remove some of the meaning of reality. However, critics of the phenomenological approach argue that lack of control often makes it impossible to rule out numerous alternative explanations to the findings, in which case, firm conclusions about critical relationships among variables cannot be reached.

❖ MAJOR STEPS IN THE RESEARCH PROCESS

A researcher typically moves from the beginning point of a study (the posing of a question) to the end point (the obtaining of an answer) in a fairly logical progression. In some studies, the steps in this progression overlap; in other cases, some steps are interchangeable; and in yet others, some steps are unnecessary. Still, there is a general flow of activities that is typical of a scientific investigation. This section briefly describes the major phases of a research project and the steps that are typical of each.

Phase 1: The Conceptual Phase

The early steps in a research project typically involve activities with a strong conceptual or intellectual element. These activities involve thinking, reading, rethinking, theorizing, and reviewing ideas with colleagues or advisers. During this phase, the researcher calls on such skills as creativity, deductive reasoning, insightfulness, and a firm grounding in knowledge on a topic of interest.

*STEP 1: FORMULATING
AND DELIMITING THE PROBLEM*

The first step in the scientific process is to develop a research question. Good research depends to a great degree on good questions. Sometimes the importance of securing an interesting and meaningful topic gets lost in the concern for using appropriate and sophisticated research procedures. Yet without a significant, interesting topic, the most carefully and skillfully designed research project will be of no value.

Researchers generally proceed from the selection of broad areas of interest to the development of specific questions that are amenable to empirical inquiry. One of the most common difficulties for beginning researchers is the development of a manageable, researchable problem statement. In developing research problems to be studied, the researcher must consider its substantive dimensions (Is this research question of theoretical or practical significance?); its methodological dimensions (How can this question be studied?); its practical dimensions (Are adequate resources available to conduct the study?); and its ethical dimensions (Can this question be studied in a manner that is consistent with guidelines for the protection of human subjects?).

STEP 2: REVIEWING THE RELATED LITERATURE

Good research does not exist in a vacuum. For research findings to be useful, they should be an extension of previous knowledge and theory as well as a guide for future research activity. For a researcher to build on existing work, it is essential to understand what is already known about a topic. A thorough *literature review* focusing on prior research provides a foundation on which to base new knowledge.

A familiarization with previous studies can also be useful in suggesting research topics or in identifying aspects of a problem about which more research is needed. Thus, in some cases, a literature review precedes the delineation of the problem.

STEP 3: DEVELOPING A THEORETICAL FRAMEWORK

Theory is the ultimate aim of science in that it transcends the specifics of a particular time, place, and set of individuals and aims to identify regularities in the relationships among variables. When research is performed in the context of a theoretical framework, it is more likely that its findings will have long-lasting significance and utility. In many theoretically based studies, the formulation of a problem occurs within the context of a theoretical framework— that is, steps 1 and 3 occur simultaneously.

STEP 4: FORMULATING HYPOTHESES

A *hypothesis* is a statement of the researcher's expectations concerning relationships between the variables under investigation. In other words, a hypothesis is a prediction of expected outcomes; it states the relationships that the researcher expects to find as a result of the study. The problem statement identifies the phenomena under investigation; a hypothesis predicts

how those phenomena will be related. For example, a problem statement might be phrased as follows: Is preeclamptic toxemia in pregnant women associated with stress factors present during pregnancy? This might be translated into the following hypothesis or prediction: Pregnant women with preeclamptic toxemia will report a higher incidence of emotionally disturbing or stressful events during pregnancy than asymptomatic pregnant women. Problem statements represent the initial effort to give a research project direction; hypotheses represent a more formalized focus for the collection and interpretation of data.

Phase 2: The Design and Planning Phase

In the second major phase of a research project, the investigator must make a number of decisions about the methods to be used to address the research question and test the hypotheses and must carefully plan for the actual collection of data. Sometimes the nature of the question dictates the methods to be used, but more often than not, the researcher has considerable flexibility to be creative and must make many decisions. These methodological decisions generally have crucial implications for the validity and credibility of the study findings. If the methods used to collect and analyze the research data are flawed, then little confidence can be put in the conclusions. Much of this book is designed to acquaint readers with a range of methodological options and to give them skills to evaluate their appropriateness for various research problems.

STEP 5: SELECTING A RESEARCH DESIGN

The *research design* is the overall plan for how to obtain answers to the questions being studied and how to handle some of the difficulties encountered during the research process. The design specifies which of the various types of research approach will be adopted and, as appropriate, how the researcher plans to implement a number of scientific controls to enhance the interpretability of the results.

For studies using traditional scientific methods, a wide variety of research designs are available. A basic distinction is the difference between *experimental research* (in which the researcher actively introduces some form of intervention) and *nonexperimental research* (in which the researcher collects data without trying to make any changes or introduce any treatments). For example, if a researcher gave bran flakes to one group of subjects and prune juice to another over a fixed period to evaluate which method facilitated elimination more effectively, then the study would involve an *intervention* (because the researcher intervened in the normal course of things) and would be considered experimental. If the researcher compared elimination patterns of two groups of people whose regular eating patterns differed—for example, some normally took foods that stimulated bowel elimination while others did not—then the study would not involve an intervention and would be considered nonexperimental. Experimental designs generally offer the possibility of greater control over extraneous variables than nonexperimental designs. However, if the researcher's primary interest is understanding some human behavior in naturalistic contexts (as in the case of most qualitative research), the design will inevitably be nonexperimental.

STEP 6: IDENTIFYING THE POPULATION TO BE STUDIED

The term *population* refers to the aggregate or totality of all the objects, subjects, or members that conform to a designated set of specifications. For example, we may specify nurses, that is, registered nurses (RNs), and residence in the United States as the attributes of interest: our study population would then consist of all licensed RNs who reside in the United States. We could in a similar fashion define a population consisting of *all* children under 10 years of age with muscular dystrophy in the state of California, or *all* the patient records in Massachusetts General Hospital, or *all* the individuals who had a fatal coronary in Chicago during a particular year.

The requirement of defining a population for a research project arises from the need to specify the group to which the results of a study can be applied. It is seldom possible to study an entire population unless it is particularly small. Research studies typically involve only a small fraction of the population, referred to as a *sample*. Before one selects actual study participants, it is essential to know what characteristics the subjects should possess.

STEP 7: SPECIFYING METHODS TO COLLECT THE RESEARCH DATA

To address a research problem meaningfully, some method must be developed to observe or measure the research variables as accurately as possible. In most situations, the researcher begins by carefully defining the research variables to clarify exactly what each one means. Then the researcher needs to select or design an appropriate method of measuring the variables—that is, of collecting the data. A variety of measurement and data collection approaches exist. *Biophysiologic measurements* often play an important role in nursing research. Another popular form is *self-reports*, wherein subjects are directly asked about their feelings, behaviors, attitudes, and personal traits. Another method is through *observational techniques*, wherein the researcher collects data by observing people's behavior and recording relevant aspects of it.

Data collection methods vary in the structure imposed on the research subjects. Qualitative methods tend to be loosely structured, permitting subjects full opportunity to express themselves and behave in naturalistic ways. Quantitative approaches are more structured and controlled and generally involve the use of a formal instrument that obtains exactly the same information from every subject. The task of measuring research variables and developing a *data collection plan* is a complex and challenging process that permits a great deal of creativity and choice. Before finalizing the data collection plan, the researcher must carefully evaluate whether the chosen approach is likely to capture the concepts under study accurately.

STEP 8: DESIGNING THE SAMPLING PLAN

Data are generally collected from a sample rather than from an entire population. The advantage of using a sample is that it is more practical and less costly than collecting data from the population. The risk is that the sample selected might not adequately reflect the behaviors, traits, symptoms, or beliefs of the population.

Various methods of obtaining a sample are available to the researcher. These methods vary in cost, effort, and level of skills required, but their adequacy is assessed by the same criterion: the *representativeness* of the selected sample. That is, the quality of the sample is a function of how typical, or representative, the sample is of the population under study with respect to the key research variables. Sophisticated sampling procedures can produce samples that have a high likelihood of being representative. The most sophisticated sampling methods are referred to as *probability sampling*, which uses random procedures for the selection of the sample. In a probability sample, every member of the population has the possibility of being included in the sample. With *nonprobability sampling* techniques, by contrast, there is no way of ensuring that each member of the population could be selected; consequently, the risk of a *biased* (unrepresentative) sample is greater. The design of a *sampling plan* includes the selection of a sampling method, the specification of the sample size, and the selection of procedures for recruiting the subjects.

STEP 9: FINALIZING AND REVIEWING THE RESEARCH PLAN

Normally, researchers have their research plan reviewed by several individuals or groups before proceeding with the actual implementation of the plan. When a researcher is seeking financial support for the conduct of a study, the research plan is generally presented as a formal proposal to a funding source. Even when proposed projects are considered to be of sufficiently high quality for funding, the reviewers generally offer suggestions for improving the study design. Students conducting a study as part of a course or degree requirement must also have their plans reviewed by faculty advisers. Even under other circumstances, however, the researcher is well advised to have individuals external to the project check the preliminary plans. An experienced researcher with a fresh perspective on a research problem can often be invaluable in identifying pitfalls and shortcomings that otherwise might not have been recognized. Finally, before proceeding with a study, researchers often need to have their research plan approved by special committees to ensure that the plan does not violate ethical principles.

STEP 10: CONDUCTING THE PILOT STUDY AND MAKING REVISIONS

Unforeseen problems often arise in the course of a project. The effects of such problems may be negligible but, in other cases, may be so severe that the study has to be stopped so that modifications can be introduced. For this reason, it may be advisable to carry out a *pilot study*, which is a small-scale version, or trial run, of the major study. The function of the pilot study is to obtain information for improving the project or for assessing its feasibility. The pilot study may reveal that revisions are needed in one or more aspects of the project. For example, the pilot study may provide information suggesting that the target population was defined too broadly. Or it may reveal that the initial conceptualization was somehow inadequate or that the hypotheses as stated cannot really be put to a test. From a more practical point of view, a trial run may reveal that it will be impossible to secure the cooperation of people by the intended procedures or that the study is more costly than anticipated. Often the principal focus of a pilot study is the assessment of the adequacy of the data collection plan. The researcher may need to know, for example, if technical equipment is functioning properly. If questionnaires are used, it is important to know whether respondents understand the questions and directions or if they find certain questions objectionable in some way; this is generally referred to as *pretesting* the questionnaire.

A pilot study should be carried out with as much care as the major study so that any weaknesses that are detected will be truly representative of inadequacies inherent in the major study. Subjects for a pilot study should possess the same characteristics as individuals who will compose the main sample. That is, pilot subjects should be chosen from the same population as subjects for the major study. It is often useful to question the individuals who participate in a pilot study concerning their reactions to, and overall impressions of, the project.

When the data from the test run have been collected and scrutinized, the researcher should make the revisions and refinements that in her or his judgment would eliminate or reduce problems encountered during the pilot study. If extensive revisions are required, it may prove advisable to have a second trial run that incorporates those revisions.

Phase 3: The Empirical Phase

The empirical portion of a research study involves the actual collection of research data and the preparation of those data for analysis. In many studies, the empirical phase is the most time-consuming part of the investigation, although the actual amount of time spent varies considerably from project to project. If data are collected by distributing a written questionnaire to intact groups, this task may be accomplished in a day or so. More often, however, the data collection requires several weeks, or even months, of work.

STEP 11: COLLECTING THE DATA

The actual collection of data often proceeds according to a preestablished plan to minimize confusion, delays, and mistakes. The researcher's plan typically specifies procedures for the actual collection of data (e.g., where and when the data will be gathered); for describing the study to participants; for obtaining their consent; and, if necessary, for training the individuals who will be involved in the collection of the research data.

A considerable amount of both clerical and administrative work is required in the data collection task. The investigators must be sure, for example, that enough materials are available to complete the study; that participants are informed of the time and place that their presence may be required; that research personnel (such as interviewers) are conscientious in keeping their appointments; that schedules do not conflict; or that a suitable system of assigning an identification number to maintain subject anonymity has been implemented.

Data collection can occur in a variety of settings that vary in terms of their naturalism. In studies that are done "in the field," the data are collected in the natural settings in which the subjects work and live in their daily lives. At the opposite extreme, some studies are conducted in highly contrived and controlled laboratory settings. Many nursing studies are conducted in settings that fall in between these two extremes (e.g., a hospital setting). Research settings may influence the quality—and quantity—of the data being gathered.

STEP 12: PREPARING THE DATA FOR ANALYSIS

After the data are collected, a few preliminary activities must be performed before the actual analysis of the data can begin. For instance, it is normally necessary to look through questionnaires to determine if they are usable. Sometimes such forms are left almost entirely blank or contain other indications of misinterpretation or noncompliance. Another step that should be taken at this point is to assign identification numbers to the responses or observations of different subjects, if this was not done previously.

Frequently, a step known as coding is required. *Coding* refers to the process of translating verbal data into categories or numerical form. For example, patients' responses to a question about the quality of nursing care they received during hospitalization might be coded into positive reactions, negative reactions, neutral reactions, and mixed reactions. Another preliminary step that is increasingly common is transferring research information from written documents onto computer files so that the data can be analyzed by computer.

Phase 4: The Analytic Phase

The data gathered in the empirical phase are not reported to the consumers of research in raw form. They are subjected to various types of analysis and interpretation, which occurs in the fourth major phase of a project.

STEP 13: ANALYZING THE DATA

The data themselves do not provide us with answers to our research questions. Ordinarily, the amount of data collected in a study is rather extensive and, therefore, needs to be processed and analyzed in some orderly, coherent fashion so that patterns and relationships can be discerned.

Qualitative analysis involves the integration and synthesis of narrative, nonnumerical data. Quantitative information is generally analyzed through statistical procedures. *Statistical analyses* cover a broad range of techniques, from some simple procedures to complex and sophisticated methods. The underlying logic of statistical tests, however, is relatively straightforward and should, therefore, be no cause for concern to the beginning researcher. Computers and pocket calculators have virtually eliminated the need to get bogged down with detailed arithmetic operations.

Although the central focus of the analysis task is the testing of research hypotheses and addressing of the research questions, there are usually a variety of other analytic subtasks. These may include assessments of data quality, assessments of the representativeness of the sample, checks on whether an intervention actually was implemented properly, and supplementary analyses to help in interpreting the findings.

STEP 14: INTERPRETING THE RESULTS

Before the results of a study can be communicated effectively, they must be organized and interpreted in some systematic fashion. By *interpretation*, we refer to the process of making sense of the results and of examining the implications of the findings within a broader context. The process of interpretation begins with an attempt to explain the findings.

If the research hypotheses have been supported, an explanation of the results is usually straightforward because the findings fit into a previously conceived argument. If the hypotheses are not supported, then the investigator must develop some possible explanations. Is the underlying conceptualization wrong or perhaps inappropriate for the research problem? Or do the findings reflect problems with the research methods rather than the theory (e.g., was the measuring tool inappropriate)? To provide sound explanations for obtained findings, then, the researcher must not only be familiar with the literature on a topic and with the conceptual underpinnings of the problem but also must be able to understand the methodological weaknesses of the study. A researcher should be in a position to critically evaluate the decisions that he or she made in designing the study and to recommend alternatives to others interested in the same research problem.

Phase 5: The Dissemination Phase

The previous (analytic) phase brings the researcher full circle: it provides the answers to the questions posed in the first phase of the project. However, the researcher's job is not complete until the results of the study are disseminated.

STEP 15: COMMUNICATING THE FINDINGS

The results of a research investigation are of little utility if they are not communicated to others. Even the most compelling hypothesis, the most careful and thorough study, and the most dramatic results are of no value to the nursing community if they are unknown. Another—and often final—task of a research project, therefore, is the preparation of a *research report* that can be shared with others.

There are various forms of research reports: term papers, dissertations, journal articles, papers for presentation at professional conferences, books, and so on. Journal articles—that is, short reports appearing in such professional journals as *Nursing Research*—are generally the most useful because such reports are available to a broad audience. Nurse researchers have many journals available for publishing their research reports.

STEP 16: UTILIZING THE FINDINGS

Many interesting studies have been conducted by nurses without having any effect on nursing practice or nursing education. Ideally, the concluding step of a high-quality study is to plan for its utilization in the real world. Although nurse researchers are often not themselves in a position to implement a plan for utilizing research findings, they can contribute to the process by including in their research reports recommendations regarding how the results of the study could be incorporated into the practice of nursing and by disseminating their findings to practicing nurses.

❖ ORGANIZATION OF A RESEARCH PROJECT

The steps described in the preceding section represent an idealized conception of what researchers do. The research process rarely follows a neatly prescribed pattern of sequential procedures. Developments in one step, for example, may require alterations in a previously completed activity. This fact does not eliminate the need for careful planning in advance; indeed, it makes careful organization even more important.

Almost all research projects are conducted under some time pressure. Students in research courses may have end-of-term deadlines; government-sponsored research involves funds granted for a specified time. Those who may not have such formal time constraints—such as graduate students working on dissertations—normally have their own goals for project completion. Setting up a timetable in advance may be an important step toward meeting such goals. This means that the investigator should make projections about which tasks should be completed by what point in time. Of course, initial projections often have to be modified, but estimates made at the outset of a project often help in setting intermediary goals. Having deadlines for tasks—even tentative ones—helps to impose some structure and delimits tasks that might otherwise continue indefinitely, such as the selection of a problem and review of the literature.

Unfortunately, it is not possible for us to give even approximate figures for the relative percentage of time that should be spent on each task. Some projects require many months to develop and pilot test the measuring instruments, whereas other studies use previously existing instruments. The write-up of the study may take many months or only a few days. Clearly, however, not all of the steps will be equally time-consuming. If the researcher knew that there was a specified final deadline, it would make little sense to simply divide the time available by the total number of tasks.

Let us suppose that during a 12-month period we were studying the following problem: Does the presence of fathers in the delivery room affect the mothers' perception of pain? Figure 2-2 presents a hypothetical schedule for the research tasks to be completed. The selection of the problem is not included because the research topic has already been identified. Note that many activities overlap and that some tasks are projected to involve little time in terms of time elapsed on the calendar.

In developing a schedule of this sort, a number of considerations should be kept in mind, including the level of knowledge and competence of the researcher. Resources available to the researcher, in the form of research funds and personnel, will greatly influence the time estimates. It is also important to consider the practical aspects of performing the study, which were not all enumerated in the preceding section. Obtaining supplies, securing the necessary permissions, having forms or instruments approved by granting agencies or supervisors, and holding meetings are all time-consuming, but often necessary, activities.

Individuals differ in the kinds of tasks that are appealing to them. Some people greatly enjoy the preliminary phase, which has a strong

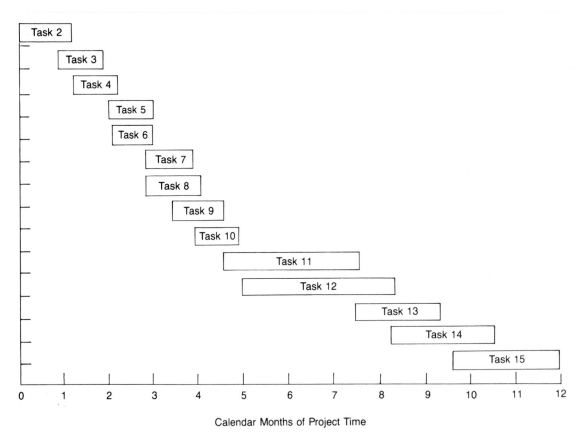

Figure 2-2. *Breakdown of project tasks by time allotted.*

intellectual component, whereas others are more eager to collect the data, a task that is often more interpersonal in nature. The researcher should attempt, however, to allocate a reasonable amount of time to do justice to each activity. Inadequately conceived and hastily designed studies are doomed to failure, or at best mediocrity, no matter how much care and time are given to the collection and analysis of data. On the other hand, the person who lingers too long in the library may never reach the final goal.

❖ RESEARCH EXAMPLES

Below is a brief overview of a clinical study. Think about the key terms that were introduced in this chapter in relation to this study. For example, what are the independent and dependent variables, and how were they operationalized? What is the nature of the relationship under study? Were extraneous variables controlled? Students may wish to consult the full research report in answering these questions.

> Tuten and Gueldner (1991) initiated a study to determine if the patency of the peripheral intermittent intravenous device (PIID) would be maintained as effectively with a sodium chloride solution as with a dilute heparin solution and to determine if a sodium chloride solution could be used with fewer complications. Two groups of subjects (hospitalized patients) were studied: those whose PIIDs were maintained using sodium chloride solution and those whose PIIDs were maintained using dilute heparin solution. Tuten and Gueldner described their variables as follows: "The type of maintenance solution used was the independent variable, and incidence of device complications (coagulation, infiltration, phlebitis) was the dependent variable" (p. 65). Staff nurses completed the PIID Complication Assessment Form, which was used to measure the dependent variable of device complications. The form contained brief descriptions of possible intravenous complications.

❖ SUMMARY

A scientific *study* (or *investigation* or *research project*) is undertaken by one or more *researcher* (or *investigator* or *scientist*). The person in charge of a study is referred to as the *principal investigator* or *project director*. The people who provide information to the researchers are referred to as *subjects*, *study participants*, or—if they answer questions directly—*respondents* or *informants*.

Scientific research focuses on *concepts* or *constructs*, which are abstractions or mental representations inferred from behavior or events. Concepts are the building blocks of *theories*, which present a systematic explanation about the way in which phenomena are interrelated.

In research studies, the concepts under investigation are referred to as *variables*. A variable is a characteristic or quality that takes on different values; that is, a variable is something that varies from one person or object to another. The blood type, blood pressure, grip strength, and hair color of a person are variables. These variables, which are inherent characteristics of a person that the researcher only measures or observes, are referred to as *attribute variables*. When a researcher actively creates or manipulates a variable, as when a special *intervention* or treatment is introduced, the variable may be referred to as an *active variable*. Variables that can take on a range of values along a specified continuum are referred to as *continuous variables* (e.g., height and weight), whereas variables that consist of only several discrete values are *categorical variables* (e.g., gender and blood type).

An important distinction for researchers is differentiation between the dependent and independent variables of a study. The *dependent variable* is the behavior, characteristic, or outcome that the researcher is interested in understanding, explaining, predicting, or affecting. The dependent variable (or *criterion variable*) is the presumed consequence or effect of the independent variable. The *independent variable* is the presumed cause of, antecedent to, or influence on the dependent variable. Groups that are highly varied with respect to some attribute are described as *heterogeneous*; groups with limited *variability* are described as *homogeneous*.

In an actual investigation, the variables are generally clarified and defined in such a way that they are amenable to observation or measurement. The *operational definition* of a concept is the specification of the procedures and tools required to make the needed measurements.

Data are the pieces of information collected during the course of a study. Because variables take on different values, the record of those values for the subjects in the study constitutes the data. Data may take the form of narrative information (*qualitative data*) or numerical values (*quantitative data*).

Except in rare cases, researchers are not interested in studying variables in isolation but rather are interested in learning about the relationship between two or more variables simultaneously. A *relationship* refers to a bond or connection between two variables. Researchers focus on the relationship between the independent and dependent variables. When the independent variable causes the occurrence, manifestation, or alteration of the dependent variable, a *cause-and-effect relationship* is said to exist. Variables that are not causally related can be linked by a *functional relationship*.

In attempting to understand how variables are related, researchers generally attempt to design a study that controls contaminating factors. *Research control* involves holding constant contaminating influences, known as *extraneous variables*, that might otherwise mask the true relationship between the independent and dependent variables.

Although the steps involved in conducting a research project and the sequencing of those steps may vary somewhat from one study to another, many of the activities are fairly standard. The research tasks can be organized into five major phases:

1. *The conceptual phase*—the phase in which the researcher develops the formal question to be studied and places it into some larger context; this phase includes such activities as:
   • Formulating and delimiting the problem to be studied
   • Reviewing the literature relevant to the problem
   • Developing a theoretical framework to place the problem in a broader context
   • Formulating hypotheses to be tested
2. *The design and planning phase*—the phase in which the researcher makes a number of methodological decisions regarding the strategies to be used to collect and analyze the data to address the research question and evaluates those decisions before implementing them; this phase includes such activities as:
   • Selecting a research design appropriate for the study problem
   • Specifying the population on which the study will focus
   • Specifying the methods to measure the research variables and collect the data
   • Designing the plan for selecting and recruiting the sample
   • Finalizing and reviewing all aspects of the research plan
   • Conducting a pilot study and making revisions
3. *The empirical phase*—the phase in which the data are gathered by the researcher according to an established plan, and data are prepared for later analysis; this phase includes:
   • Collecting the research data
   • Preparing the data for analysis through coding and computer preparation
4. *The analytic phase*—the phase in which the researcher organizes, integrates, and makes sense of the data and tests the research hypotheses, encompassing the following tasks:

- Analyzing, through appropriate qualitative or quantitative methods, the research data
- Interpreting the results of the analyses

5. *The dissemination phase*—the phase in which the findings from the study are communicated to others and steps taken to integrate the findings into the practice of nursing; this phase includes:

- Communicating the findings through written or oral presentation
- Undertaking steps to utilize the findings or to promote their utilization

The conduct of research requires careful planning and organization. The preparation of a timetable with expected deadlines for task completion can be extremely useful in establishing subgoals and in helping the researcher to be more realistic in the allocation of time to different tasks.

❖ *STUDY SUGGESTIONS*

Chapter 2 of the accompanying *Study Guide for Nursing Research: Principles and Methods, 5th ed.*, offers various exercises for reinforcing concepts presented in this chapter. Additionally, the following study questions can be addressed:

1. Suggest ways of operationally defining the following concepts: nursing competency, patients' time to first voiding after surgery, aggressive behavior, patients' level of pain, home health hazards, postsurgical recovery, and body image.
2. Name five categorical and five continuous variables; identify which, if any, are dichotomous.
3. Identify which of the following variables could be active variables and which are attribute variables (some may be both): height, degree of fatigue, cooperativeness, noise level on hospital units, length of stay

in hospital, educational attainment, self-esteem, nurses' job satisfaction.

4. In the following research problems, identify the independent and dependent variables:

   a. How do nurses and physicians differ in the way they view the extended role concept for nurses?

   b. Does problem-oriented recording lead to more effective patient care than other recording methods?

   c. Do elderly patients have lower pain thresholds than younger patients?

   d. How are the sleeping patterns of infants affected by different forms of stimulation?

   e. Can home visits by nurses to released psychiatric patients reduce readmission rates?

❖ *SUGGESTED READINGS*

METHODOLOGICAL REFERENCES

Burns, N., & Grove, S. K. (1993). *The practice of nursing research: Conduct, critique, and utilization* (2nd ed.). Philadelphia: W.B. Saunders.

Kerlinger, F. (1986). *Foundations of behavioral research* (3rd ed.). New York: Holt, Rinehart & Winston.

Lindquist, R. (1991). Don't forget the pilot work! *Heart and Lung, 20*, 91–92.

Prescott, P. A., & Soeken, K. L. (1989). The potential uses of pilot work. *Nursing Research, 38*, 60–62.

Wilson, H. S. (1989). *Research in nursing* (2nd ed.). Menlo Park, CA: Addison-Wesley.

SUBSTANTIVE REFERENCES

Dobratz, M. C. (1993). Causal influences of psychological adaptation in dying. *Western Journal of Nursing Research, 15*, 708–723.

Howell, R. D., MacRae, L. D., Sanjines, S., Burke, J., & DeStefano, P. (1992). Effects of two types of head coverings in the rewarming of patients after coronary artery bypass graft surgery. *Heart and Lung, 21,* 1–5.

McDonald, D. D. (1994). Gender and ethnic stereotyping in narcotic analgesic administration. *Research in Nursing and Health, 17,* 45–49.

Narsavage, G. L. & Weaver, T. E. (1994). Physiologic status, coping, and hardiness as predictors of outcomes in chronic obstructive pulmonary disease. *Nursing Research, 43,* 90–94.

Tombes, M. B., & Gallucci, B. (1993). The effects of hydrogen peroxide rinses on the normal oral mucosa. *Nursing Research, 42,* 332–337.

Topf, M., & Davis, J. E. (1993). Critical care unit noise and rapid eye movement (REM) sleep. *Heart and Lung, 22,* 252–258.

Tuten, S. H., & Gueldner, S. H. (1991). Efficacy of sodium chloride versus dilute heparin for maintenance of peripheral intermittent intra-venous devices. *Applied Nursing Research, 4,* 63–71.

Weiss, S. J. (1992). Psychophysiologic and behavioral effects of tactile stimulation on infants with congenital heart disease. *Research in Nursing and Health, 15,* 93–101.

Whitney, J. D., Stotts, N. A., Goodson, W. H., & Janson-Bjerklie, S. (1993). The effects of activity and bed rest on tissue oxygen tension, perfusion, and plasma volume. *Nursing Research, 42,* 349–355.

Wright, S. M. (1991). Validity of the human energy field assessment form. *Western Journal of Nursing Research, 13,* 635–647.

Zeanah, M., & Schlosser, S. P. (1993). Adherence to ACOG guidelines on exercise during pregnancy: Effect on pregnancy outcomes. *Journal of Obstetric, Gynecologic, and Neonatal Nursing, 22,* 329–337.

Chapter 3

RESEARCH PROBLEMS AND HYPOTHESES

A research study begins as a question that a researcher would like to answer or a problem that a researcher would like to solve. For many beginning researchers, the selection of a problem for study is the most difficult task of the research endeavor. The difficulty of selecting a problem for study does not stem from a shortage of study topics. Nothing has been researched in its entirety. Rather, sometimes researchers find it difficult to select a particular topic for study because there are so many things to be known and it is perplexing to choose only one. Other researchers may experience difficulty in selecting a topic because they are unfamiliar with previous research. Beginning researchers may experience an additional dilemma of having to choose a problem for study at a time when they are unsure of what the research process entails and what constitutes a researchable problem.

❖ SOURCES OF RESEARCH PROBLEMS

Beginning researchers often are puzzled and perhaps even threatened by a requirement to develop a research problem. Where do ideas for research problems come from? How can a topic be selected? In this section, we suggest some sources for locating a problem or topic. The four most common sources are experience, the nursing literature, theories, and ideas from others.

Experience

The nurse's everyday experience provides a rich supply of problems for investigation. Whether you are a student nurse, practicing nurse, nurse educator, or nursing administrator, there are sure to be occurrences or situations that you have found puzzling or problematic. If you have ever asked such questions as, "Why are things done this way?" "I wonder what would happen if . . . ?" or "What method would work better?" you may be well along the way to developing a research idea. For the beginning researcher in particular, experience is often the most compelling source for topics. Immediate problems that are in need of solution or that excite the curiosity are relevant and interesting and, thus, may generate more enthusiasm than abstract and distant problems inferred from a theory.

Polit DF, Hungler BP: NURSING RESEARCH: PRINCIPLES AND METHODS, 5th ed. © 1995 J. B. Lippincott Company.

An important ingredient for a successful research project is the investigator's curiosity. If you look around as you are performing your nursing functions, you are bound to find a wealth of research ideas if you are curious about why things are the way they are, or how things could be improved if something were to change.

Nursing Literature

Ideas for research projects often come from reading the nursing literature. The beginning nurse researcher can profit from regularly reading nursing journals, especially ones that report the results of nursing studies, such as *Nursing Research, Clinical Nursing Research, Applied Nursing Research, Research in Nursing and Health,* and the *Western Journal of Nursing Research.* Many nursing specialty journals (e.g., *Heart and Lung* and *Oncology Nursing*) also publish research studies. Reading published reports may help the neophyte researcher to find a problem amenable to scientific investigation and may also help to familiarize the beginning researcher with the wording of research problems and the actual conduct of research studies.

Published research reports may suggest problem areas indirectly by stimulating the reader's imagination or interest in a topic and directly by specifying further areas in need of investigation. For example, Schwartz and Keller (1993) studied unreported chest pain among patients hospitalized with an acute myocardial infarction. They concluded that "studies that further define the role that health care providers play in encouraging or discouraging the reporting of symptoms may prove beneficial" (p. 17).

Inconsistencies in the findings reported in nursing literature often generate ideas for research studies. For example, there are inconsistencies regarding which irrigation fluid (e.g., water, cranberry juice, or cola) is most effective in maintaining the patency of patients' feeding tubes. Such discrepancies could lead to the design of a rigorous study to resolve the matter.

A researcher may also wonder whether a study similar to one reported in a journal article would yield comparable results if applied in a different setting or with different subjects. Replications are needed to establish the validity and generalizability of previous findings.

In summary, a familiarity with existing research, or with problematic and controversial nursing issues that have yet to be understood and investigated scientifically, is an important route to developing a research topic. The student who is actively seeking a problem to study, such as the student required to do an empirical thesis, will find it useful to read widely in areas of interest. In Chapter 4, we deal more extensively with the procedures of doing a research literature review.

Theory

The third major source of research problems lies in the theoretical systems and conceptual schemes that have been developed in nursing and other related disciplines. To be useful in nursing practice, theories must be tested through research for their applicability to the hospital unit, the emergency room, the classroom, and other nursing environments.

If a researcher decides to base a research project on an existing theory, deductions from the theory must be developed. Essentially, the researcher must ask the questions, "If this theory is correct, what kind of behavior would I expect to find in certain situations or under certain conditions?" and "What kind of evidence would support this theory?" This process would eventually result in a specific problem that could be subjected to scientific investigation.

Let us look at an example of how a problem can be derived from a conceptual system. Levine (1973) postulated a conceptual framework for nursing that concerns conservation. She explains nursing as conserving the patient's energy, structural integrity, personal integrity, and social integrity. From this theory, the researcher could formulate specific predictions about expected findings. For example, it might be hypothesized that primary nursing is more effective in conserving the patient's energy and social integrity than team nursing. By developing measures of energy expenditure and social integration, this hypothesis could be tested scientifically.

Ideas From External Sources

External sources can sometimes provide the impetus for a research idea. In some cases, a research topic may be given as a direct suggestion. For example, a faculty member may give students a list of topics from which to choose or may actually assign a specific topic to be studied. Entities that sponsor funded research, such as the federal government, often identify broad or specific topics on which research proposals are encouraged. For example, in recent years, government agencies have requested a variety of AIDS-related research projects. For beginning students, it is often useful to have some guiding suggestions on the development of a research problem. However, even when a research area is suggested, it is better for the researcher to identify the aspect of the problem that is of greatest interest because curiosity is a critical ingredient in successful research.

Research ideas sometimes represent a response to priorities that are established within the nursing profession, examples of which were discussed in Chapter 1. Priorities for nursing research have been established by many nursing specialty practices. Priority lists can often serve as a useful starting point for exploring research topics.

Often, ideas for studies emerge as a result of a brainstorming session. By discussing possible research topics with peers, advisers, or researchers with advanced skills, ideas often become clarified and sharpened, or enriched and more fully developed. Professional conferences often provide an excellent opportunity for such discussions.

❖ DEVELOPING AND REFINING A RESEARCH PROBLEM

Unless a research problem is developed on the basis of theory or an explicit suggestion from an external source, the actual procedures for developing a research topic are difficult to describe. The process is rarely a smooth and orderly one; there are likely to be many false starts, several inspirations, and several setbacks in the initial efforts to devise a problem statement. The few suggestions offered here are not intended to imply that there are techniques for making this first step easy but rather to encourage the beginning researcher to persevere in the absence of instant success.

Selecting a Topic

The development of a research problem is essentially a creative process that depends on imagination, insight, and ingenuity. In the early stages, when research ideas are being generated, it is wise not to be critical of them immediately. It is much better to begin by just relaxing and jotting down general areas of interest as they come to mind. At this point, it matters little if the terms used to remind you of your ideas are abstract or concrete, broad or specific, technical or colloquial—the important point is to put some ideas on paper. Examples of some broad topics that may come to mind include communication with patients, anxiety in hospitalized children, pain among cancer patients, postpartum depression, and postoperative loss of orientation.

After this first step, the ideas can be sorted in terms of interest, knowledge about the topics, and the perceived promise that the topics hold for a research project. When the most fruitful idea has been selected, the rest of the list should not be discarded; it may be necessary to return to it.

Narrowing the Topic

Once you have identified one or more general topics of interest, you will need to begin asking questions that will lead to a researchable problem statement. Some examples of question stems that may help you focus your inquiry include the following:

- What causes . . . ?
- What is the extent of . . . ?
- Why do . . . ?
- When do . . . ?
- What factors lead to . . . ?
- What influences . . . ?
- How intense are . . . ?
- What conditions prevail before . . . ?
- What characteristics are associated with . . . ?
- What are the consequences of . . . ?
- What is the relationship between . . . ?
- How effective is . . . ?
- What differences exist between . . . ?
- What factors contribute to . . . ?

Here again, early criticism of ideas is often counterproductive in this basically creative endeavor. Try not to jump to the conclusion that an idea sounds trivial or uninspired without giving it more careful consideration or without exploring it with fellow students, colleagues, or advisers. It is best not to worry at this point whether another researcher has already done a similar study. Totally original and unique problems are rare, despite the almost infinite range of possible topics. At the same time, no two studies are ever identical, so that every study has the potential of making some contribution to knowledge.

Beginning researchers often develop problems that are too broad in scope or too complex and unwieldy for their level of methodological expertise. The transformation of the general topic into a workable problem is typically accomplished in a number of uneven steps, involving a series of successive approximations. Each step should result in progress toward the goals of narrowing the scope of the problem and sharpening and defining the concepts.

As the researcher moves from a general topic of interest to more specific researchable problems, it is likely that more than one potential problem area will emerge. Let us consider the following example. Suppose you were working on a medical unit and observed that some patients always complained about having to wait for pain medication when certain nurses were assigned to them and, yet, these same patients offered no complaints when other nurses were assigned to them. You wonder why this phenomenon occurs. The general problem area is discrepancy in complaints from patients regarding pain medications administered by different nurses. You might ask, What accounts for this discrepancy? or, How can I improve the situation? Such questions are not actual research questions because they are too broad and vague. They may, however, lead you to ask other questions, such as, How do the two groups of nurses differ? or, What characteristics are unique to each group of nurses? or, What characteristics do the group of complaining patients share? At this point, you may observe that the cultural background of the patients and nurses appears to be a relevant factor. This may direct you to a review of the literature for studies concerning ethnic subcultures in relation to nursing interventions, or it may provoke you to discuss the observations with peers. The result of these efforts may be several researchable problems, such as the following:

Is there a relationship between the ethnic background of nurses and the frequency with which they dispense pain medication?
Is there a relationship between the ethnic background of patients and their complaints of having to wait for pain medication?
Does the number of patient complaints increase when the patient is of dissimilar ethnic background as opposed to of the same ethnic background as the nurse?
Does a nurse's dispensing behaviors change as a function of the similarity between the

nurse's own ethnic background and that of the patient?

All these problems have a similar theme, yet each would be studied in a different manner. How does one choose the final problem to be studied? Tentative problems usually vary in their feasibility and worth. It is at this point that a critical evaluation of ideas is appropriate.

Evaluating Research Problems

No rules have been established for making a final selection of a research problem. Some criteria, however, should be kept in mind in the decision process. The four most important considerations are the significance, researchability, and feasibility of the problem, and its interest to the researcher.

SIGNIFICANCE OF THE PROBLEM

A crucial factor in selecting a problem to be studied is its significance to nursing. The research question should have the potential of contributing to the body of knowledge in nursing in a meaningful way. The researcher should pose the following kinds of questions: Is the problem an important one? Will patients, nurses, or the broader health care community or society benefit by the knowledge that will be produced? Will the results lead to practical applications? Will the results have theoretical relevance? Will the findings challenge (or lend support to) untested assumptions? Will the study help to formulate or alter nursing practices or policies? If the answer to all these questions is no, then the problem should be abandoned.

RESEARCHABILITY OF THE PROBLEM

Not all questions are amenable to study through scientific investigation. Problems or issues of a moral or ethical nature, although provocative, are incapable of being researched. An example of a philosophically oriented question is, Should nurses join unions? The answer to

such a question is ultimately based on a person's values. There are no right or wrong answers, only points of view. The question as stated is more suitable to a debate than to scientific research. To be sure, it is possible to modify the question so that aspects of the issue could be researched. For instance, each of the following questions could be investigated in a research project:

What are nurses' attitudes toward unionization?
Do younger nurses hold more favorable opinions of unions than older nurses?
Does a person's role (nurse versus nursing administrator versus hospital administrator) affect his or her perceptions of the consequences of unions on the delivery of health care?
Is opposition to unionization for nurses based primarily on perceived outcomes to patients and clients or on outcomes to the nursing profession?

The findings from these hypothetical projects would have no bearing, of course, on the answer to the original question of whether or not nurses *should* join unions, but the information could be useful in developing a comprehensive understanding of the issues and in facilitating decision making.

Generally, researchable problems are ones that involve variables capable of being precisely defined and measured. For example, suppose the researcher was trying to determine what effect early discharge had on the general well-being of patients. General well-being is too broad and fuzzy a concept to measure as it is stated. The researcher would have to sharpen the concept so that it could be observed and measured. That is, the researcher would have to establish criteria against which the patients' progress toward well-being could be assessed.

When a new area of inquiry is being pursued, however, it may be impossible to define the concepts of interest in precise terms. In such cases, it may be appropriate to address the problem using in-depth qualitative research. The problem may then be stated in fairly broad terms to permit full exploration of the concept of interest.

FEASIBILITY OF THE PROBLEM

Problems that are both significant and researchable may still be inappropriate if they are not feasible. The issue of feasibility encompasses a variety of considerations. Not all of the following factors are relevant for every problem, but most of them should be kept in mind in making a final decision.

TIME AND TIMING. Most studies have deadlines or at least informal goals for their completion. Therefore, problem must be one that can be adequately studied within the time allotted. This means that the scope of the problem should be sufficiently restricted that enough time will be available for the various steps reviewed in Chapter 2. It is usually wise to be generous in allocating time to the various tasks because research activities often require more time to accomplish than one anticipates. A related consideration is the timing of the project. Some of the research steps—especially data collection—are more readily performed at certain times of the day, week, or year than at other times. For example, if the problem focused on patients with peptic ulcers, the research might be more easily conducted in the fall and spring because of the increase in the number of patients with peptic ulcers during these seasons than in the summer or winter months. When the timing requirements of the tasks do not match the periods available for their performance, the feasibility of the project may be jeopardized.

AVAILABILITY OF SUBJECTS. In any study involving humans, the researcher needs to consider whether individuals with the desired characteristics will be available and willing to cooperate. Securing people's cooperation may in some cases be easy (e.g., getting nursing students to complete a questionnaire in a classroom), but other situations may pose more difficulties for the researcher. Some people may not have the time, others may have no interest in participating in a study that has little personal benefit, and others may not feel well enough to participate. Fortunately, people *are* usually willing to cooperate with a researcher if the demands on their time and comfort are minimal. If the research is time-consuming, additional effort and the payment of a monetary incentive may be necessary to obtain a sufficiently large sample of subjects. An additional problem may be that of identifying and locating subjects with the needed characteristics. For example, if we were interested in studying the health care needs of individuals who had lost a family member through suicide, we would have to develop a plan for identifying prospective subjects.

COOPERATION OF OTHERS. Often it is insufficient to obtain the cooperation of prospective subjects alone. If the sample includes children, mentally incompetent people, or senile individuals, it is almost always necessary to secure the permission of parents or guardians. In institutional settings, such as hospitals, clinics, public schools, or industrial firms, access to clients, members, personnel, or records usually requires administrative approval. Many health care facilities require that any project be presented to a panel of reviewers for approval before permitting the study to be conducted.

FACILITIES AND EQUIPMENT. All research projects have some resource requirements, although in some cases, the needs may be modest. It is prudent to consider what facilities and equipment will be needed and whether or not they will be available before embarking on a project so that disappointments and frustration can be prevented. The following is a partial list of considerations that fall into this category:

- Will space be required and, can it be obtained?
- Will telephones, typewriters, or other office supplies be required?

- If technical equipment and apparatus are needed, can they be secured, and are they functioning properly? Will laboratory facilities be required, and are they available?
- Are duplicating or printing services available, and are they reliable?
- Will transportation needs pose any difficulties?
- Will a computer be required for the collection or analysis of the data, and are computing facilities easily obtainable?

MONEY. Monetary requirements for research projects vary widely, ranging from $10 to $20 for small student projects to hundreds of thousands of dollars for large-scale, federally sponsored research. The investigator on a limited budget should think carefully about projected expenses before making the final selection of a problem. Some major categories of research-related expenditures are the following:

- Literature costs—index cards, books and journals, reproduction of articles, and computerized literature search service charges
- Personnel costs—payments to individuals hired to help with the data collection (e.g., doing interviews), coding, data entry, typing, and so forth
- Subject costs—payment to subjects as an incentive for their cooperation, or to offset their own expenses (e.g., transportation or baby-sitting costs)
- Supplies—paper, envelopes, computer disks, postage, and so forth
- Printing costs—payment to printers for printing forms, questionnaires, subject recruitment notices, and so on
- Equipment—laboratory apparatus, typewriters, calculators, and the like
- Computer service charges
- Laboratory fees for the analysis of biophysiologic data
- Other service charges, such as the costs of duplicating materials
- Transportation costs

EXPERIENCE OF THE RESEARCHER. The problem should be chosen from a field about which the investigator has some prior knowledge or experience. The researcher will have a difficult time in adequately developing a study on a topic that is totally new and unfamiliar. In addition to substantive knowledge, the issue of technical expertise should not be overlooked. A beginning researcher usually has limited methodological skills and, therefore, should avoid research problems that might require the development of sophisticated measuring instruments or that involve complex statistical analyses.

ETHICAL CONSIDERATIONS. A research problem may not be feasible because the investigation of the problem would pose unfair or unethical demands on the participants. The ethical responsibilities of researchers should not be taken lightly. People engaged in research activities should be thoroughly knowledgeable about the rights of human or animal subjects. An overview of major ethical considerations concerning human subjects is presented in Chapter 6 and should be reviewed when considering the feasibility of a prospective project.

INTEREST TO THE RESEARCHER

If the tentative problem passes the tests of researchability, significance, and feasibility, there is still one more criterion for its selection: the researcher's own interest in the problem. Genuine interest in and curiosity about the chosen research problem are important prerequisites to a successful study. A great deal of time and energy are expended in any scientific investigation, and interest and enthusiasm ebb and flow throughout the time required for completion of the project. The problem selected should extend the researcher's personal knowledge as well as the base of knowledge for others.

Personal interest in a research problem is least likely to be high when the topic has been suggested or assigned to the researcher by others. Beginning research students often seek out suggestions and may be grateful for assistance in selecting a topic area; often such assistance can be helpful in getting started. Nevertheless, it is rarely wise to be talked into a research topic toward which you are not personally inclined. If you do not find a problem attractive or stimulating during the beginning phases of a study—when the opportunity for creativity and intellectual reasoning is at its highest—then you are bound to regret your choice later in the project.

❖ STATEMENT OF THE RESEARCH PROBLEM

It is clear that a study cannot progress without the choice of a problem; it is less clear, but nonetheless true, that the problem should be carefully stated in written form before proceeding with the design of the study. Putting one's ideas in writing is often sufficient to illuminate ambiguities and uncertainties.

A good statement of the problem should serve as a guide to the researcher in the course of designing the study. The problem statement should identify the key study variables and their possible interrelationships, and the nature of the population of interest. Researchers have alternative ways of expressing the research problem. The two main forms are statements of purpose and research questions.

Statement of Purpose

Many researchers state their research problem in the declarative form as a broad *statement of purpose*, such as: The purpose of this research is to examine the relationship between the dependency level of renal transplantation patients and their rate of recovery. This statement of purpose indicates the population of interest (renal transplantation patients); the independent variable (dependency level); and the dependent variable (rate of recovery).

Descriptive studies do not always have variables that can be designated as independent or dependent. In such a case, the statement of purpose indicates the nature of the inquiry, the study variables, and the population under study, as in the following example: The purpose of this study is to describe the decision-making process of adult children with regard to the placement of elderly parents in nursing homes.

The researcher who presents a statement of purpose often communicates more than just the nature of the problem. A statement of purpose may suggest the manner in which the researcher is seeking to solve the problem, or the state of knowledge on the topic, through the researcher's selection of verbs. That is, a study whose purpose is to *explore* or *describe* some phenomenon is likely to be an investigation on a little-researched topic; such a study might well use an in-depth qualitative approach. A study whose purpose is to *test* the effectiveness of some intervention or to *compare* two alternative nursing strategies, on the other hand, suggests a study with a more well-established knowledge base, using a quantitative approach and perhaps a design with tight scientific controls. Note that the researcher's choice of verbs in a statement of purpose should connote objectivity. A statement of purpose indicating that the intent of the study is to *prove, demonstrate,* or *show* something suggests a possible bias on the part of the researcher.

Some examples of well-worded statements of purpose from nursing studies are presented in Table 3-1.

Research Questions

Some researchers prefer to present their problem statement in the interrogative form, as a *research question*. The interrogative form of the problems stated in the previous section would be as follows:

- What is the relationship between the dependency level of renal transplantation patients and their rate of recovery?
- What is the process by which adult children make decisions regarding the placement of their elderly parents in a nursing home?

Table 3-1.   *Examples of Statements of Purpose*

STATEMENT OF PURPOSE	SOURCE
The purpose of this study was to examine the influence of attendance and effort in a long-term exercise program on the cognitive and physical functioning of older adults.	Topp & Stevenson, 1994
The purpose of this study was to determine the major physiologic, psychosocial, and lifestyle concerns of women two weeks and eight weeks after an unplanned cesarean delivery.	Miovech, Knapp, Borucki, Roncoli, Arnold, & Brooten, 1994
The purpose of this study was to explore the prevalence and correlates of depressive symptoms among community-dwelling elders 75 years of age and older.	McCurren, Hall, & Rowles, 1993
The purpose of this study was to explore spousal interaction as it pertains to help with diabetes and its management.	Bailey & Kahn, 1993

The question (interrogative) form has the advantage of simplicity and directness. Questions invite an answer and help psychologically to focus the researcher's attention on the kinds of data that would have to be collected to provide that answer. Table 3-2 presents some examples of research questions from the nursing research literature and identifies the independent variable and dependent variable for each.

Many research reports include both a broad statement of purpose and several more specific research questions. The example at the end of this chapter illustrates this approach.

Defining Terms in a Problem Statement

Problem statements such as those presented in Tables 3-1 and 3-2 would be incomplete without an explanation of the variables involved. Sometimes definitions and clarification of concepts can be inserted into the statement of the problem itself, but this usually makes the statement inordinately complex and clumsy.

Dictionary definitions of terms and concepts are almost always inadequate for research purposes. The definition provided by the researcher must imply or specify a method of operationalizing (observing and measuring) the variables. Let us take as an example the following problem statement: Is early discharge for mastectomy patients related to postoperative problems? In this example, early discharge might be defined as "discharged prior to the fourth postoperative day"; and postoperative problems might be defined, in part, as "the patient's inability to comb her hair." If adequate definitions are appended to a well-formulated problem statement, there should be little confusion about what is being studied.

❖ RESEARCH HYPOTHESES

A *hypothesis* is a tentative prediction or explanation of the relationship between two or more variables. Hypotheses translate problem statements into predictions of expected outcomes.

Table 3-2.   *Examples of Nursing Research Questions*

RESEARCH QUESTION	INDEPENDENT VARIABLE	DEPENDENT VARIABLE
Do chronically ill adolescents undergoing hemodialysis and receiving cognitive restructuring and assertive skills training increase their perceptions of self-efficacy? (Beecroft, 1993)	Receipt vs. nonreceipt of training	Perceptions of self-efficacy
Do women who are engaged in anorectic behavior differ in their impressions of their mothers' lives from women who are not? (Korb, 1994)	Women's evaluations of their mothers' lives	Symptoms of anorexia nervosa
Does the administration of analgesics by nurses vs. by patients themselves affect pain intensity during postoperative recovery in older adults? (Duggleby & Lander, 1992)	Source of control over analgesics (nurse vs. patient)	Pain intensity
What is the effect of three different body positions (supine, prone, or prone-free) on oxygenation during fixed-wing transport of neonates with hyaline membrane disease? (Squire & Kirchhoff, 1992)	Body position	Oxygenation (PaO_2 blood gas levels)

Research problems, as we have seen, are often phrased in the form of questions concerning how phenomena are related and interact. Hypotheses, on the other hand, are tentative solutions or answers to such research queries. For instance, the problem statement might ask: Does room temperature affect the optimal placement time of rectal temperature measurements in adults? As a tentative solution to this problem, the researcher might predict the following: Cooler room temperatures require longer placement times for rectal temperature measurements in adults than warmer room temperatures.

Purposes of the Research Hypothesis

Generally speaking, the function of the hypothesis is to guide scientific inquiry. A critical function of hypotheses is to provide direc-

tion to the research design and to the collection, analysis, and interpretation of data. Hypotheses interconnect variables of interest through statements of expected relationships between them; it is these relationships that are subjected to empirical testing.

Hypotheses often follow directly from a theoretical framework. Through deductive reasoning, the scientist develops hypotheses from theories and tests those hypotheses in the real world. Thus, hypotheses are the vehicles through which theories are linked to real-world situations.

Not all hypotheses are derived from theory. Even in the absence of a theoretical framework, the researcher often makes predictions about the outcomes of a study. Well-conceived hypotheses contribute to knowledge because they offer direction and suggest explanations. Even when hypotheses fail to be confirmed, their presence provides a greater possibility for the advancement of understanding than the absence of hypotheses.

Perhaps an example will clarify this point. Suppose we were to hypothesize that nurses who have received a baccalaureate education are more likely to experience stress in their first nursing job than nurses with diploma school education. We could justify our speculation on the basis of theory (e.g., reality shock theory), earlier studies, personal observations, logic, or some combination of these. *The need to develop justifications in and of itself forces the researcher to think logically, to exercise critical judgment, and to tie together earlier research findings.* Now let us suppose the above hypothesis is not confirmed by the evidence collected; that is, we find that baccalaureate and diploma nurses demonstrate an equal amount of stress in their first nursing assignment. *The failure of data to support a prediction forces the investigator to analyze theory or previous research critically, to review the limitations of the study's methods carefully, and to explore alternative explanations for the findings.* The use of hypotheses, in other words, induces critical thinking and, hence, promotes understanding.

To pursue the same example, suppose we conducted the investigation without formulating an explicit prediction and were guided only by a research question: Is there a relationship between a nurse's basic preparation and the degree of stress experienced on the first job? The investigator without a hypothesis is, apparently, prepared to accept any results. The problem is that it is almost always possible to explain something superficially after the fact, no matter what the findings are. Hypotheses guard against superficiality and minimize the possibility that spurious results will be misconstrued.

The reader may be wondering if a hypothesis is always necessary. Most research that can be classified as descriptive proceeds without explicit hypotheses. *Descriptive research,* that is, research that aims predominantly at describing phenomena rather than explaining them, is common in the emerging field of nursing re-search. Examples of descriptive investigations include studies of the health needs of elderly citizens, studies of the coping patterns of mothers of handicapped children, and surveys of the nutritional status of low-income preschool children. This type of study is often extremely important in laying a foundation for later research. When a field is new, it may be difficult to provide adequate justification for the development of explanatory hypotheses because of a dearth of facts or previous findings. Also, most qualitative studies proceed without a hypotheses defined at the outset because their aim is to provide an opportunity for the human experience to be revealed without preconceived restrictions. Thus, there are some studies of a descriptive or exploratory nature for which hypotheses may not be required.

Characteristics of Workable Hypotheses

An essential characteristic of a workable research hypothesis is that it states the predicted relationship between two or more variables. The variables that are related to one another through the hypothesis are the independent variable (the presumed cause, antecedent, or influence) and the dependent variable (the presumed effect or phenomenon of primary interest).

One of the most common flaws of the predictions of beginning researchers is their failure to make a relational statement. The following prediction is not an acceptable research hypothesis: Pregnant women who receive prenatal training will have favorable reactions to the labor and delivery experience. This statement expresses no anticipated relationship; in fact, there is only one variable—the woman's reactions to the labor and delivery experience. A relationship by definition requires at least two variables. This prediction can, however, be altered to make it a suitable hypothesis with an independent and dependent variable: Pregnant women who receive prenatal training will have *more* favorable reactions (the dependent variable) to the labor and delivery experience *than* pregnant women with no prenatal training. Here the second variable (the independent variable) is the woman's status with respect to prenatal training: some will have received it and others will not have received it.

The relational aspect of the prediction is embodied in the phrase *more than.* If a hypothesis lacks a phrase such as more than, less than, greater than, different from, related to, or something similar, it is not amenable to scientific testing. As an example of why this is so, consider the original prediction: Pregnant women who receive prenatal training will have favorable reactions to the labor and delivery experience. How would we know whether the women's reactions are favorable? That is, what absolute standard could be used for deciding whether the women's reactions to their labor and delivery experiences were favorable or not? Perhaps this point will be clearer if we illustrate it more specifically. Suppose we ask a group of women who have taken an 8-week prenatal training course to respond to the question, "On the whole, how would you describe your labor and delivery experience?"

1. Very favorably
2. Favorably
3. Neither favorably nor unfavorably
4. Unfavorably
5. Very unfavorably

Based on this question, how could we compare the actual outcome with the predicted outcome that the women would have favorable responses? Would *all* the women questioned have to respond "very favorably" for the hypothesis to be supported? Would our prediction be supported if 51% of the women said either "very favorably" *or* "favorably"? There is simply no adequate way of testing the accuracy of the prediction. A test is simple, however, if we modify the prediction, as suggested above, to: Pregnant women who receive prenatal training will have more favorable reactions to the labor and delivery experience than pregnant women with

no prenatal training. We could simply ask two groups of women with different prenatal training experiences to respond to the question and then compare the responses of the two groups. The absolute degree of favorability of either group would not be at issue.

Hypotheses, ideally, should be based on a sound, justifiable rationale. The most defensible hypotheses follow from previous research findings or are deduced from a theory. When a new area is being investigated, the researcher may have to turn to logical reasoning or personal experience to justify the predictions. There are, however, few topics for which research evidence is totally lacking.

A good hypothesis should be consistent with an existing body of research findings. This requirement in some cases may be difficult to satisfy because it is not uncommon to find conflicting results on some topics in the research literature. Obviously, when the findings from previous research are inconsistent, it is impossible for the hypothesis to be consistent with all the findings. The researcher must then make a decision, and a good solid basis for such a decision is the critical evaluation of the methods used in earlier studies. The investigator should attempt to understand *why* conflicting results occurred through an examination of the research approach.

The Derivation of Hypotheses

Many students ask the question, How do I go about the task of developing hypotheses? There are no formal rules for deriving hypotheses, but we can offer some suggestions by discussing two broad types of approach. Like the development of research problems, the sources most likely to be fruitful as a basis for the formulation of hypotheses are theoretical systems, personal experience and observations, readings in related literature, and discussions with peers and advisers. However, two basic processes—induction and deduction—constitute the intellectual machinery involved in deriving hypotheses.

An *inductive hypothesis* is a generalization based on observed relationships. The researcher observes certain patterns, trends, or associations among phenomena and then uses these observations as a basis for a tentative explanation or prediction. Related literature should be examined to learn what is already known on a topic, but an important source of ideas for inductive hypotheses is the researcher's own experiences, combined with intuition and critical analysis. For example, a nurse might notice that presurgical patients who ask a lot of questions relating to pain or express many pain-related apprehensions have a more difficult time in learning appropriate postoperative procedures. The nurse could then formulate a hypothesis that could be tested through more rigorous scientific procedures. The following hypothesis might be derived: Patients who are stressed by fears of pain will have more difficulty in deep breathing and coughing after their surgery than patients who are not stressed.

The other mechanism for deriving hypotheses is through deduction. Theories of how phenomena behave and interrelate cannot be tested directly. Through deductive reasoning, a researcher can develop scientific expectations or hypotheses based on general theoretical principles. Inductive hypotheses begin with specific observations and move toward generalizations; *deductive hypotheses* have as a starting point theories that are applied to particular situations.

Although a full explication of deductive logic is beyond the scope of this book, the following syllogism illustrates the reasoning process involved:

All human beings have red and white blood cells.
John Doe is a human being.
Therefore, John Doe has red and white blood cells.

In this simple example, the hypothesis is that John Doe does, in fact, have red and white blood cells, a deduction that could be verified.

If a nurse researcher is familiar with a theory relating to phenomena of interest, the theory can serve as a valuable point of departure for the development of hypotheses. The researcher must ask the question: If this theory is correct or valid, what would the logical consequences be in terms of a situation that interests me? In other words, the researcher deduces that if the general theory is true, specific outcomes or consequences can be expected. The specific predictions derived from general principles must then be subjected to further testing through the collection of empirical data. If these data are in fact congruent with hypothesized outcomes, then the theory is strengthened.

The advancement of scientific research depends on both inductive and deductive hypotheses. Ideally, a cyclical process is set in motion wherein the researcher makes observations; formulates hypotheses inductively; makes systematic, controlled observations; develops theoretical systems; deduces hypotheses; seeks new systematic observations; rethinks the hypotheses or theories; modifies them inductively; and so forth. The scientific researcher needs to be an organizer of concepts (think inductively), a logician (think deductively), and, above all, a critic and a skeptic of resulting formulations.

Testing the Hypothesis

The testing of hypotheses constitutes the heart of most empirical investigations that are quantitative. It must again be emphasized, however, that neither theories nor hypotheses are ever proved in an ultimate sense through hypothesis testing. It is inappropriate to say that the data proved the validity of the hypothesis or that the conclusions proved the worthiness of the theory. Such statements are inappropriate not only because they are incongruent with the limitations of the scientific approach but also because they are inconsistent with the fundamentally skeptical attitudes of scientists. Scientists are basically doubters and skeptics, who are constantly seeking objective, replicable evidence as a basis for understanding natural phenomena. Findings are always considered tentative. Certainly, if the same results are repeatedly produced in a large number of investigations, then greater confidence can be placed in the conclusions. Hypotheses, then, come to be accepted or believed with mounting evidence, but ultimate proof is rarely possible; nor, for that matter, is ultimate falsification of a hypothesis possible.

Let us look more closely at why this is so. Suppose we hypothesize that there is a relationship between height and weight. We predict that, on the average, tall people weigh more than short people. We would then take a sample of people, obtain height and weight measurements, and analyze the data. Now suppose we happened by chance to choose a sample that consisted of short, fat people, and tall, thin people. Our results might then indicate that there is no relationship between an individual's height and weight. Would we then be justified in making the following statement?: This study proved that height and weight in humans are unrelated.

A second example illustrates the converse principle. Suppose we hypothesize that taller people are better nurses than shorter people. This hypothesis is used here only to illustrate a point because, in reality, one might suspect that there is no relationship between height and a nurse's job performance. Now suppose that, by chance again, we hit on a sample of nurses in which the taller nurses happen to receive better job evaluations by their supervisors than short nurses. Could we conclude definitively that height is related to a nurse's performance? These two examples illustrate the difficulty of using observations from a sample to generalize to the broader group (the population) from which the sample has been taken. Other problems, such as the accuracy of our measures, the validity of underlying assumptions, the reasonableness of our logical deductions, and rapid changes in technologies and in society, prohibit us from concluding with finality that our hypotheses are proved.

❖ WORDING THE RESEARCH HYPOTHESIS

A workable hypothesis states a relationship between two (or more) variables and is capable of empirical testing. In this section, we look at how the hypothesis should be stated and provide examples of various kinds of hypotheses.

A good hypothesis is worded in simple, clear, and concise language and provides a definition of the variables in concrete, operational terms. These two requirements may be in conflict if the operational definition needs extensive explanation, in which case the variables should be operationally defined separately. The hypothesis should, however, be specific enough so that the reader understands what the variables are and whom the researcher will be studying.

Simple Versus Complex Hypotheses

For the purpose of this book, we define *simple hypotheses* as hypotheses that express an expected relationship between *one* independent and *one* dependent variable. A *complex hypothesis* refers to a prediction of a relationship between two (or more) independent variables and/or two (or more) dependent variables. Sometimes complex hypotheses are referred to as *multivariate hypotheses* because they involve multiple variables.

We give some concrete examples of both types of hypotheses, but let us first explain the differences in abstract terms. Simple hypotheses state a relationship between a single independent variable, which we will call X, and a single dependent variable, which we will label Y. Our Y variable is the predicted effect, outcome, or consequence of our X variable, which is the presumed cause, antecedent, or precondition. The nature of this relationship is presented in Figure 3-1(A). In Figure 3-1(A), the hatched area of the circles, representing variables X and Y, can be taken to signify the strength of the relationship

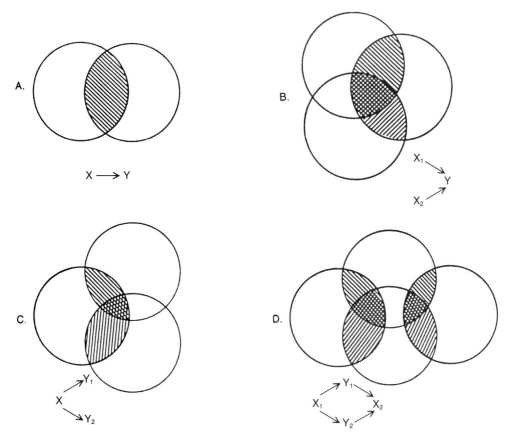

Figure 3-1. *Schematic representation of various hypothetical relationships.*

between these two variables. If there were a one-to-one correspondence between variables X and Y, the two circles would completely overlap, and the entire area would be hatched. If the variables were totally unrelated, the circles would not converge or overlap at all.

In the real world, most phenomena are the result not of one variable but of a complex network of many variables. A person's weight, for example, is affected simultaneously by such factors as the person's height, diet, bone structure, and metabolism. If the dependent variable—Y in Figure 3-1(A)—were weight and the independent variable—X—were a person's caloric intake, we would not be able to explain or understand individual variation in weight completely. Knowing that Matt Jones' daily caloric intake av-

eraged 2500 calories would not allow us a precise prediction of his weight. Knowledge of other factors, such as Matt Jones' height, would improve the accuracy with which his weight could be predicted.

Figure 3-1(B) presents a schematic representation of the simultaneous effect of two independent variables on a single dependent variable. The complex hypothesis would state the nature of the relationship between Y on the one hand and X_1 and X_2 on the other. To pursue the example above, the hypothesis might be: Taller people (X_1) and people with higher caloric intake (X_2) will weigh more (Y) than shorter people and people with lower caloric intake. As the figure shows, a larger proportion of the area of Y is hatched when there are two independent variables than when there is only one. This means that caloric intake *and* height do a better job in helping us understand variations in weight (Y) than caloric intake alone. Complex hypotheses thus have the advantage of allowing researchers to capture some of the complexity of the real world. It is not always possible to design a study with complex hypotheses. A number of practical considerations, including the researcher's technical skills, resources, and time, may render the testing of complex hypotheses impossible or inadvisable. An important goal of research, however, is to explain the dependent variable as thoroughly as possible, and two or more independent variables are typically more successful than one alone.

Just as a phenomenon can be understood as resulting from more than one independent variable, so a single independent variable can have an effect on, or can be antecedent to, more than one phenomenon. Figure 3-1(C) illustrates this type of relationship. A number of studies have found, for example, that cigarette smoking (the independent variable, X) can lead to both lung cancer (Y_1) and coronary disorders (Y_2). This type of complex hypothesis is common in studies that try to assess the impact of a nursing intervention on a variety of criterion measures of patient well-being. Finally, a more complex type of hypothesis,* which links two or more independent variables to two or more dependent variables, is shown in Figure 3-1(D). An example might be a hypothesis that smoking *and* the consumption of alcohol during pregnancy might lead to lower birthweights *and* lower Apgar scores in infants.

Table 3-3 presents five specific examples of simple and complex hypotheses. Most of these hypotheses would need further elaboration in terms of the specification of operational definitions; but each of these hypotheses is potentially testable, and each delineates a predicted relationship.

*A special kind of complex hypothesis, known as the *interaction hypothesis*, is described in Chapter 8.

Although researchers typically adopt a certain style in the phrasing of hypotheses, there is some degree of flexibility allowed. The same hypothesis can generally be stated in a variety of ways as long as the researcher specifies (or implies) the relationship that will be tested. For example, the first hypothesis from Table 3-3 can be acceptably reworded in the following ways:

1. Older nurses are less likely to express approval of the expanding roles of nurses than are younger nurses.
2. There is a relationship between the age of a nurse and approval of the nurse's expanding role.
3. The older the nurse, the less likely it is that he or she approves of the nurse's expanding role.
4. Older nurses differ from younger nurses with respect to approval of the nurse's expanding role.
5. Younger nurses tend to be more approving of the nurse's expanding role than older nurses.
6. Approval of the nurse's expanding role decreases as the age of the nurse increases.

Other variations are also possible. The important point to remember is that the hypothesis should specify the independent and dependent variables and the anticipated relationship between them.

Directional Versus Nondirectional Hypotheses

Sometimes hypotheses are described as being either directional or nondirectional. A *directional hypothesis* is one that specifies the expected direction of the relationship between variables. That is, the researcher predicts not only the existence of a relationship but also the nature of the relationship. In the six versions of the same hypothesis above, versions 1, 3, 5, and 6 are directional because there is an explicit expectation that older nurses will be less approving of the expanding role of nurses than younger nurses.

Table 3-3. *Examples of Hypotheses*

HYPOTHESIS	INDEPENDENT VARIABLE	DEPENDENT VARIABLE	SIMPLE OR COMPLEX
Older nurses are less likely to express approval of the expanding role of nurses than younger nurses.	Age of nurses	Approval of nurses' expanding role	Simple
Infants born to heroin-addicted mothers have lower birthweights than infants with nonaddicted mothers.	Addiction vs. nonaddiction of mother	Birthweight of infant	Simple
Structured preoperative support is more effective in reducing surgical patients' perceptions of pain and requests for analgesics than structured postoperative support.	Timing of nursing intervention	Surgical patients' pain perceptions; requests for analgesics	Complex
Patients who receive a copy of the Patients' Bill of Rights ask more questions about their treatment and diagnosis than do those who do not receive this document	Receipt vs. nonreceipt of Patients' Bill of Rights	Number of questions asked	Simple
Teenagers who have been sexually abused as children are at higher risk of depression and suicide than teenagers with no history of sexual abuse.	History of sexual abuse	Risk of depression; risk of suicide	Complex

A *nondirectional hypothesis,* by contrast, does not stipulate the direction of the relationship. Such a hypothesis predicts that two or more variables are related but makes no projections concerning the exact nature of the association. Versions 2 and 4 in the example illustrate the wording of nondirectional hypotheses. These hypotheses state the prediction that a nurse's age and degree of approval of the nurse's changing role are related; they do not stipulate, however, whether the researcher thinks that older nurses or younger nurses will be more approving.

Deductive hypotheses derived from theory almost always are directional because theories attempt to explain phenomena and, hence, provide a rationale for expecting variables to behave in certain ways. Existing studies also supply, typically, a basis for directional hypotheses. When there is no theory or related research, when the findings of related studies are contradictory, or when the researcher's own experience results in ambivalent expectations, the investigator may use nondirectional hypotheses. Some people argue, in fact, that nondirectional hypotheses are generally preferable because they connote a degree of impartiality or objectivity. Directional hypotheses, it is said, carry the implication that the researcher is intellectually committed to a certain outcome, and such a commitment might lead to bias. This argument fails to recognize that researchers typically do have hunches about the outcomes, whether they state those expectations explicitly or not. Directional hypotheses have three distinct advantages: 1) they demonstrate that the researcher has thought critically and carefully about the phenomena under investigation; 2) they make clear to the readers of a research report the expectations that guided the research; and 3) they may permit a more sensitive statistical test of the hypothesis. This last point, which refers to whether the researcher chooses a one-tailed or two-tailed statistical test, is a fine point that is discussed in Chapter 18.

Research Versus Statistical Hypotheses

Hypotheses are sometimes classified as being either research hypotheses or statistical hypotheses. *Research hypotheses* (also referred to as substantive, declarative, or scientific hypotheses) are statements of expected relationships between variables. All the hypotheses in Table 3-3 are research hypotheses. Such hypotheses indicate what the researcher expects to find as a result of conducting the study.

The logic of statistical inference operates on principles that are somewhat confusing to many beginning students. This logic requires that hypotheses be expressed such that *no* relationship is expected. *Statistical* or *null hypotheses* state that there is no relationship between the independent and dependent variables. The null form of hypothesis 2 in Table 3-3 would be as follows: Infants born to heroin-addicted mothers have birthweights comparable to those of infants born to nonaddicted mothers. As another illustration, the null hypothesis for hypothesis 4 in Table 3-3 would read as follows: Patients who receive a copy of the Patients' Bill of Rights will ask the same number of questions

about their treatment and diagnosis as those who do not receive this document. The null hypothesis might be compared with the assumption of innocence of an accused criminal in our system of justice: the variables are assumed to be "innocent" of any relationship until they can be shown "guilty" through appropriate statistical procedures. The null hypothesis represents the formal statement of this assumption of innocence.

❖ TIPS ON DEVELOPING RESEARCH PROBLEMS AND HYPOTHESES

For those of you who are planning to conduct a study, we offer a few tips on developing research problems and hypotheses:

- As noted earlier in this chapter, your personal experiences as a nurse or nursing student are a provocative source for research topics. Here are some hints on how to proceed:

  Watch for recurring problems and see if you can discern a pattern in situations that lead to the problem.

  Example: Why do many patients complain of being tired after being transferred from a coronary care unit to a progressive care unit?

  Think about aspects of your work that are irksome, frustrating, or do not result in the intended outcome—then try to identify factors contributing to the problem that could be changed.

  Example: Why is supper-time so frustrating in a nursing home?

  Critically examine some of the decisions you make in the performance of your functions. Are these decisions based on tradition, or are they based on scientific evidence that supports their efficacy? Many practices in nursing that have become custom might be challenged.

  Example: What would happen if visiting hours in the intensive care unit were changed from 10 minutes every hour to the regularly scheduled hours existing in the rest of the hospital?

- As an alternative to identifying problematic situations, identify aspects of nursing that you most enjoy or in which you have the greatest interest. For example, think about what course work has been most interesting to you, what rotation you most enjoyed, or what part of your job you like the best. Then do some reading in the research literature on this general area to see if a topic suggests itself.

- In a pinch, do not hesitate to replicate a study that is reported in the research literature. Replications provide a valuable learning experience and have the potential to make valuable contributions because they can corroborate (or challenge) earlier findings.

- If you word your problem statement as a statement of purpose, be careful in your choice of verbs because the verb communicates information about the nature of your research design and possibly about your level of expertise. Among the verb choices are the following: describe, explore, examine, investigate, address, understand, compare, evaluate, test, assess, explain, and predict.

- In wording your research questions or statement of purpose, it may be useful to look at published research reports for models. However, you may find that some reports fail to state unambiguously the problem under investigation. Thus, in some studies, you may have to infer the research problem from several sources, such as the title of the report. In other reports, the problem is clearly stated but may be difficult to locate. Researchers most often state their research problem at the end of the introductory section of the report.

- Although most research studies *do* test hypotheses, only a minority of research reports formally state up front what those hypotheses are. In designing a study of your own, do not be afraid to make a prediction, that is, to state a hypothesis. Being wrong (or having insufficient evidence to demonstrate that you are right) is part of the learning process.

- If you formulate hypotheses, avoid stating them in null form. When statistical tests are performed, the underlying null hypothesis is usually assumed without being explicitly stated.

❖ RESEARCH EXAMPLES

Table 3-4 presents hypotheses that have appeared in several different nursing research reports. These examples illustrate the proper wording of research hypotheses in several areas of interest to nurse researchers. The following investigation, described in detail, is a more fully developed example of how research questions and hypotheses guided an actual study.

Matthews (1991) was interested in studying maternal satisfaction with breastfeeding during the early postpartum period. Matthews noted that other researchers identified the first few days after birth as a critical period in the breastfeeding relationship but that few studies have concentrated on the effect of the neonate's early feeding behavior on the mother's perception of, and satisfaction with, breastfeeding. Matthews' statement of purpose was phrased as follows:

The purpose of this study was to determine how and to what degree the mothers' satisfaction with breastfeeding was influenced by the breastfeeding competence of their neonate (p. 50).

Matthews included four specific research questions: 1) What percentage of feedings are perceived by mothers to be less than satisfactory in the early initiation period of breastfeeding? 2) What is the relationship, if any, between the quality of the breastfeeding performance of the neonate and the mother's pleasure and satisfaction with the feeding? 3) Is there a significant difference between different groups of mothers? and 4) What other effects, if any, did either positive or negative neonatal feeding behaviors have on the mothers?

In the same section of the report, Matthews also posited the following hypothesis:

Table 3-4.   *Examples of Hypotheses From Actual Studies*

HYPOTHESIS	INDEPENDENT VARIABLE	DEPENDENT VARIABLE
There is a positive relationship between mother–daughter attachment and a pregnant woman's maternal–fetal attachment (Zachariah, 1994)	Degree of mother–daughter attachment	Degree of maternal–fetal attachment
Both hypertensive and normotensive men with blood pressure reactivity will engage in less self-disclosure than men with no blood pressure reactivity (Hahn, Brooks, & Hartsough, 1993)	Blood pressure reactivity	Amount of self-disclosure
Solid foam mattress overlays are more effective than convoluted foam overlays in preventing pressure sores in elderly patients (Kemp, Kopanke, Tordecilla, Fogg, Shott, Matthiesen, & Johnson, 1993)	Type of overlay	Incidence of pressure sores
Elderly patients who are taught about their medication regimen visually and verbally will show greater increase in knowledge and compliance than those who are taught verbally only (Hussey, 1994)	Method of instruction (verbal only vs. verbal and visual)	Knowledge about and compliance with a medication regimen
Women with a high-risk obstetrical situation will report lower maternal role competence than low-risk women after the baby's birth (Mercer & Ferketich, 1994)	High-risk vs. low-risk pregnancy	Perceived maternal role competence

Mothers whose neonates are having difficulties with breastfeeding, as evidenced by low scores on the Infant Breastfeeding Assessment Tool, will be less pleased with their neonates' feeding behaviors than mothers whose neonates have high scores and are feeding well.

Matthews collected data from 56 healthy breastfeeding mothers to test this hypothesis and address the research questions.

❖ SUMMARY

The most common sources of ideas for nursing research questions are experience, relevant lit-erature, theory, and external sources such as peers and advisers. Nurses, nursing students, nurse educators, and nursing administrators are likely to have an abundance of experiences in their daily activities that are problematic or pro-voke curiosity and that represent potential re-search topics. Readings in areas of interest con-stitute a second method of generating ideas for a scientific study. Theories and conceptual frameworks often serve as a springboard for empirical studies: the utility of any theory ulti-mately depend on its ability to withstand tests in real-life situations. Finally, research ideas are often generated in interactions with peers or experienced researchers or may be identified by a funding source, by a faculty member, or by the nursing profession through the issuance of research priority statements.

The process of developing a research problem is not a smooth and direct one. The researcher usually starts with the identification of several topics of broad interest. The researcher should be open-minded about the possibilities that are developed at this early phase because a hasty evaluation may result in the rejection of several potentially valuable ideas. After the researcher has tentatively selected a topic, he or she must begin the task of successively narrowing the scope of the problem.

A number of criteria should be considered in making the final selection of the problem. First, the problem should be a significant one that can contribute to nursing practice or nursing theory in a meaningful way. Second, the problem should be researchable. Questions of a moral or ethical nature are inappropriate, and concepts that defy precise definition and measurement should usually be avoided. Third, a problem may have to be abandoned if the investigation is not feasible. Feasibility involves the issues of timing, availability of subjects, cooperation of other individuals, availability of facilities and equipment, monetary requirements, experience and competencies of the researcher, and ethical considerations. Finally, the research question should be one that is of interest to the researcher.

The selected problem should be stated formally (in writing) before proceeding to the design of the study. The problem may be stated in either declarative form as a *statement of purpose* or in interrogative form as a *research question*. The statement of the problem should identify the major variables under consideration and specify the characteristics of the population being studied. The problem statement should be accompanied by a set of clear definitions of the concepts involved.

A *hypothesis* is a statement about predicted relationships among the variables under investigation; that is, hypotheses formally state the expected answers to research questions. Hypotheses are important because they serve as a link between theory and real-world situations, they provide an effective mechanism for extending knowledge, and they offer overall direction for the investigation. Of course, not all investigations are designed to test hypotheses: most qualitative studies, as well as quantitative studies that are descriptive or exploratory, generally proceed without a hypothesis.

A workable hypothesis specifies the anticipated relationship between the independent and dependent variables. A hypothesis that projects a result for only one variable is essentially untestable because there is typically no criterion for assessing absolute, as opposed to relative, outcomes. A good hypothesis should also be justifiable. It should be consistent with existing theory or knowledge (or with the researcher's own experiences) and with logical reasoning. Hypotheses are derived either through *inductive,* observational processes or through *deductive,* theory-based processes.

After hypotheses are developed and refined, they are subjected to an empirical test through the collection, analysis, and interpretation of data. It must be stressed, however, that hypotheses are never proved or disproved in an ultimate sense. Scientists say that hypotheses are accepted or rejected, supported or unsupported. Through replication of studies, hypotheses and theories can gain increasing acceptance, but scientists, who are essentially skeptics, avoid the use of the word proof.

Hypotheses can be classified according to various characteristics. *Simple hypotheses* express a predicted relationship between one independent and one dependent variable; *complex* (or *multivariate*) *hypotheses* state an anticipated relationship between two or more independent and/or two or more dependent variables. Complex hypotheses are powerful because they offer the possibility of mirroring the complexity of the real world. A *directional hypothesis* specifies the expected direction or nature of a hypothesized relationship. *Nondirectional hypotheses* denote a relationship but do not stipulate the precise form that the relationship will take. Directional hypotheses are generally preferable. Sometimes a distinction between research and statistical hypotheses is made. *Research hypotheses* predict the existence of relationships; *statistical (null) hypotheses* express the absence of any relationships. The statistical or null hypothesis is related to the logic of statistical inference and is often assumed without being formally stated.

❖ STUDY SUGGESTIONS

Chapter 3 of the accompanying *Study Guide for Nursing Research: Principles and Methods, 5th ed.*, offers various exercises and study suggestions for reinforcing the concepts presented in this chapter. Additionally, the following study questions can be addressed:

1. Think of a frustrating experience you have had as a nursing student or as a practicing nurse. Identify the problem area. Ask yourself a series of questions until you have one that you feel is researchable. Evaluate the problem in terms of the criteria of a researchable problem discussed in this chapter.

2. Examine the following five problem statements. Are they researchable problems as stated? Why or why not? If a problem statement is not researchable, modify it in such a way that the problem could be studied scientifically.
   a. What are the factors affecting the attrition rate of nursing students?
   b. What is the relationship between atmospheric humidity and heart rate in humans?
   c. Should nurses be responsible for inserting nasogastric tubes?
   d. How effective are walk-in clinics?
   e. What is the best approach for conducting patient interviews?

3. Examine a recent issue of a nursing research journal. Find an article that does not present a formal, well-articulated problem statement. Write a problem statement for that study in both declarative and interrogative form.

4. Below are five hypotheses. For each hypothesis, give a possible problem statement from which the hypothesis might have been developed.
   a. Absenteeism is higher among nurses in intensive care units than among nurses in other wards.
   b. Patients who are not told their diagnosis report more subjective feelings of stress than do patients who are told their diagnosis.
   c. Patients receiving intravenous therapy will report greater nighttime sleep pattern disturbances than patients not receiving intravenous therapy.
   d. Patients with roommates will call for a nurse less often than patients without roommates.
   e. Women who have participated in Lamaze classes will request pain medication less often than will women who have not taken these classes.

5. For each of the five hypotheses in suggestion 4, do the following: (a) indicate whether the hypothesis is simple or complex and directional or nondirectional; (b) state the independent and dependent variables; and (c) state the hypotheses in null form.

❖ SUGGESTED READINGS

METHODOLOGICAL REFERENCES

American Nurses' Association Congress for Practice. (1973). *Standards of nursing practice.* Kansas City, MO: Author.

Armstrong, R. L. (1981). Hypothesis formulation. In S. D. Krampitz, & N. Pavlovich (Eds.), *Readings for nursing research.* St. Louis: C. V. Mosby.

Campbell, J. P., Daft, R. L., & Hulin, C. L. (1982). *What to study: Generating and developing research questions.* Beverly Hills: Sage Publications.

Fuller, E. O. (1982). Selecting a clinical nursing problem for research. *Image: The Journal of Nursing Scholarship, 14*(2), 60–61.

Gordon, M. (1980). Determining study topics. *Nursing Research, 29,* 83–87.

Lewandowski, L. A., & Kositsky, A. M. (1983). Research priorities for critical care nursing. *Heart and Lung, 12,* 35–44.

Lindeman, C. A., & Schantz, D. (1982). The research question. *Journal of Nursing Administration, January,* 6–10.

Moody, L., Vera, H., Blanks, C., & Visscher, M. (1989). Developing questions of substance for nursing science. *Western Journal of Nursing Research, 11,* 393–404.

Valiga, T. M., & Mermel, V. M. (1985). Formulating the researchable question. *Topics in Clinical Nursing, 7*(2), 1–14.

SUBSTANTIVE REFERENCES

Bailey, B. J., & Kahn, A. (1993). Apportioning illness management authority: How diabetic individuals evaluate and respond to spousal help. *Qualitative Health Research, 3,* 55–73.

Beecroft, P. C. (1993). Social skills training and cognitive restructuring for adolescents on hemodialysis. *Clinical Nursing Research, 2,* 188–211.

Bonheur, B., & Young, S. W. (1991). Exercise as a health-promoting lifestyle choice. *Applied Nursing Research, 4,* 2–6.

Duggleby, W., & Lander, J. (1992). Patient-controlled analgesia for older adults. *Clinical Nursing Research, 1,* 107–113.

Hahn, W. K., Brooks, J. A., & Hartsough, D. M. (1993). Self-disclosure and coping styles in men with cardiovascular reactivity. *Research in Nursing and Health, 16,* 275–282.

Hussey L. C. (1994). Minimizing effects of low literacy on medication knowledge and compliance among the elderly. *Clinical Nursing Research, 3,* 132–145.

Kemp, M. G., Kopanke, D., Tordecilla, L., Fogg, L., Shott, S., Matthiesen, V., & Johnson, B. (1993). The role of support surfaces and patient attributes in preventing pressure ulcers in elderly patients. *Research in Nursing and Health, 16,* 89–96.

Korb, M. (1994). Anorexia as symbolic expression of a woman's rejection of her mother's life. *Western Journal of Nursing Research, 16,* 69–80.

Matthews, M. K. (1991). Mothers' satisfaction with their neonates' breastfeeding behaviors. *Journal of Obstetric, Gynecologic, and Neonatal Nursing, 20,* 49–55.

McCurren, C. D., Hall, L. A., & Rowles, G. D. (1993). Community elders: Prevalence and correlates of depressive symptoms. *Clinical Nursing Research, 2,* 128–147.

Mercer, R. T., & Ferketich, S. L. (1994). Predictors of maternal role competence by risk status. *Nursing Research, 43,* 38–43.

Miovech, S. M., Knapp, H., Borucki, L., Roncoli, M., Arnold, L., & Brooten, D. (1994). Major concerns of women after cesarean delivery. *Journal of Obstetric, Gynecologic, & Neonatal Nursing, 23,* 53–59.

Schwartz, J. M., & Keller, C. (1993). Variables affecting the reporting of pain following an acute myocardial infarction. *Applied Nursing Research, 6,* 13–18.

Squire, S. J., & Kirchhoff, K. T. (1992). Positional oxygenation changes in air-transported neonates. *Heart and Lung, 21,* 255–259.

Topp, R., & Stevenson, J. S. (1994). The effects of attendance and effort on outcomes among older adults in a long-term exercise program. *Research in Nursing and Health, 17,* 15–24.

Zachariah, R. (1994). Maternal-fetal attachment: Influence of mother-daughter and husband-wife relationships. *Research in Nursing and Health, 17,* 37–44.

OTHER REFERENCE CITED

Levine, M. E. (1973). *Introduction to clinical nursing* (2nd ed.). Philadelphia: F. A. Davis.

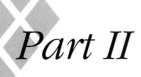

Part II

CONTEXTS FOR NURSING RESEARCH

Chapter 4

THE KNOWLEDGE CONTEXT: LITERATURE REVIEWS

Researchers almost never conduct a study in an intellectual vacuum: their studies are undertaken within the context of an existing knowledge base. Researchers generally undertake a *literature review* to familiarize themselves with that knowledge base.

The term literature review is used in two ways by the research community. The first refers to the activities involved in identifying and searching for information on a topic and developing a comprehensive picture of the state of knowledge on that topic. A researcher may thus say that he or she is "doing a literature review" before conducting a study. The term is also used to designate a written summary of the state-of-the-art on a research problem. Both the search and the write-up are important in the research process.

This chapter discusses several aspects of a literature review: first, the functions that a literature review can play in a research project; second, the kinds of material covered in a literature review; third, suggestions concerning where to find appropriate references and how to record the information once it is located; fourth, tips on

how to read research reports; and finally, the organization and presentation of a written literature review.

❖ PURPOSES OF A LITERATURE REVIEW

Literature reviews serve a number of important functions in the research process. By examining some of their specific functions, we hope to clarify their value.

Source for Research Ideas

Familiarizing oneself with practical or theoretical issues relating to a problem area often helps the researcher to generate ideas or focus on a research topic. A review of the literature may, in some cases, precede the identification of a topic. Readings in areas of general interest can be extremely useful in alerting the researcher to unresolved research problems or to new applications suitable for a project. When a general topic has already been selected, readings on that topic help to bring the problem into sharper focus and aid in the formulation of appropriate research questions.

Orientation to What Is Already Known

One of the major functions of a research literature review is to ascertain what is already known in relation to a problem of interest. For those engaged in doing research, acquaintance with the current state of knowledge should enable them to avoid unintentional duplication of effort and may also lead them to explore aspects of the problem about which there is relatively little knowledge. Of course, there are situations in which a deliberate decision to replicate a study is made, but here too, the researcher needs to be familiar with existing research to make that type of decision.

Nurses who are not researchers also are often interested in learning about the current state of knowledge with regard to a particular issue, as a means of improving their practice or identifying potential solutions to problems. For example, a nurse may be interested in learning about nursing strategies for reducing pain during neonatal circumcision. In such a situation, the nurse would need to turn to the research literature to find out about recent developments. Nurses' ability to utilize research findings in their practice is contingent on their capacity to evaluate the research literature.

Provision of a Conceptual Context

For nurse researchers, a literature review is important for developing a broad conceptual context into which a research problem will fit. It is only within such a context that the findings of a project can make a contribution to a body of knowledge. The more one's study is linked with other research, the more of a contribution it is likely to make. The accumulation of scientific knowledge is analogous to the fitting together of a jigsaw puzzle. Your piece of the puzzle,

small though it may be, may help to join together other parts of the puzzle.

The review also serves the essential function of providing the individual researcher with a perspective on the problem necessary for interpreting the results of his or her study. The comparison of the results of a study with earlier findings is often a good point of departure for suggesting new research either to resolve conflicts or to extend the base of knowledge.

Finally, a written review included in a research report is useful to the nursing community in that it makes explicit to readers the context within which the study was conducted.

Information on the Research Approach

An important role of the literature review, particularly for students engaged in their first research project, is to suggest ways of going about the business of conducting a study on a topic of interest. In other words, the review can be useful in pointing out the research strategies and specific procedures, measuring instruments, and statistical analyses that might be productive in pursuing one's problem. The research literature can also suggest the extraneous variables that should be controlled.

Research reports differ considerably in the amount of detail they include concerning specific methodological procedures, but it is not unusual for a report to provide complete documentation for the investigator's methods, including a description of the measuring instruments used. When the actual instrument is not published with the report, it is almost always possible to obtain a copy by writing to the author.

❖ SCOPE OF A LITERATURE REVIEW

Most readers are undoubtedly familiar with locating library documents and organizing them. However, a review of research literature differs in a number of respects from other kinds of term papers or summaries that students are called on to prepare. In this section, the type of information that should be sought in conducting a research review is examined, and other issues relating to the breadth and depth of the review are considered.

Types of Information to Seek

Written materials vary considerably in their quality, their intended audience, and the kind of information they contain. The researcher performing a review of the literature ordinarily comes in contact with a wide range of documents and, thus, has to be selective in deciding what to examine or include. How are such decisions to be made? There is, unfortunately, no easy answer to this question, but we can offer a number of suggestions that may prove useful.

The first step in selecting appropriate materials is to make sure that you have been thorough in tracking down most of the relevant references. It is annoying to learn of good references *after* the completion of a study. The next main section of this chapter addresses the issue of locating good source materials.

The type of information included in academic or other nonfictional documents can be classified roughly into five categories: 1) facts, statistics, or findings; 2) theory or interpretation; 3) methods and procedures; 4) opinions, beliefs, or points of view; and 5) anecdotes, clinical impressions, or narrations of incidents and situations. Table 4-1 summarizes the functions that each type of information normally serves in a literature review. A brief description of the utility of the various kinds of information follows.

1. *Research findings.* This category of information represents the results of research investigations; it clearly constitutes one of the most important types of information for a research review. Research findings provide information on what is already known on a topic, based on empirical investigations using the scientific approach. As Table 4-1 indicates, published studies can also inspire new research ideas and can help in the development of the conceptualization and design of new research. Normally, research findings are available in a variety of sources, including books, encyclopedias, conference proceedings, and, especially, scholarly journals such as *Nursing Research.* Depending on the topic, it is usually useful to review research findings in the nursing literature as well as in the literature of related disciplines, such as sociology, psychology, medicine, or physiology. Because research reports are often difficult for beginning students to understand, a section of this chapter is devoted to suggestions on reading published research studies.

2. *Theory.* The second type of information deals with broader, more conceptual issues of relevance to the topic of interest.

Table 4-1. *Summary of the Uses of Various Types of Information*

TYPE OF INFORMATION	REVIEW FUNCTION			
	Source of Research Ideas	*Information on What Is Known*	*Conceptual Context*	*Research Approach*
Research findings	√	√	√	√
Theoretical explications	√		√	
Methodology				√
Opinions	√			
Clinical anecdotes	√			

Descriptions of theory are useful in providing a conceptual context for a research problem but may also be useful for suggesting a research topic. Sometimes discussions of a body of theory are briefly presented in research reports and journal articles, but they are more likely to be found in developed form in books.

3. *Methodology.* The third type of information that should be sought in a literature review concerns the methods of conducting a study on the topic of interest. That is, in reviewing the literature, the researcher should pay attention not only to what has been found but also to *how* it was found. What approaches have other researchers used? How have they measured their variables and gathered their data? How have they controlled the research situation to enhance interpretation? What procedures have they used to analyze their data? Although modification of existing approaches and instruments may be necessary, it usually is possible to find techniques that can serve as a foundation for research activities. Research reports concerning similar problems are especially useful. Journal articles and textbooks on methods and statistics may be helpful. References that deal exclusively with various tests, measures, and instruments also may be useful. Several of these sources are cited in the suggested readings of the chapters in Part IV.

4. *Opinions and viewpoints.* The general and specialty nursing literature contains numerous papers and articles that focus on an author's opinions or attitudes concerning a topic of interest. Such articles are inherently subjective, presenting the suggestions and points of view of the authors. Opinion articles are often an important source of ideas for studies that focus on controversial or emerging issues in nursing.

5. *Anecdotes and clinical descriptions.* Numerous reports of an anecdotal nature appear frequently in nursing, medical, and health-related literature. These articles relate the experiences and clinical impressions of the authors. For instance, Rittman and her coauthors (1993), in an article that appeared in the *American Journal of Nursing,* described their "never again" experiences—stories about difficult situations in which the patient's treatment did not proceed as it best might have. Anecdotes or other types of nonresearch literature (such as opinion articles) may serve to broaden the researcher's understanding of the problem, particularly if the researcher is relatively unfamiliar with the underlying issues. Such sources may also illustrate a point or demonstrate a need for rigorous research. However, these two categories have limited utility in literature reviews for research studies because of their highly subjective nature. Beginning researchers should avoid the temptation of relying heavily on such sources in their review of the literature, particularly if they are preparing a written review. This is not to say that such materials are uninteresting or unimportant, but generally they are inappropriate in summarizing scientific knowledge and theories concerning a research question.

Depth and Breadth of Literature Coverage

Beginning students often are troubled by the question of how limited or broad their literature review should be. Once again, there is no convenient formula giving a precise number of references to be tracked down. The extensiveness of the literature review depends on a number of factors. For written reviews, one determinant is the nature of the document being prepared. Doctoral dissertations often include a thorough and extensive review that covers materials directly and indirectly related to the problem area. Reports in research journals, on the other hand, tend to have a much more selective bibliography covering only highly pertinent findings from other studies. Another factor to consider is the researcher's own level of knowledge and expertise. Inexperienced researchers who are relatively unfamiliar with a topic may have to cover more materials than more experienced researchers to feel secure about their level of understanding.

The breadth of a literature review depends to a great extent on how well researched the topic is. If there have been 20 published studies on a specific problem, it would be difficult for the researcher to come to conclusions about the current state of knowledge on a topic without reading all 20 reports. However, it is not necessarily true that the literature task is more easily accomplished if the topic has not been heavily researched. Literature reviews on new topics or little-researched problems may need to involve reviews of a broad spectrum of peripherally related studies to develop a meaningful context.

Students embarking on their first research review should strive for relevancy and quality rather than quantity in selecting references for a written review of the literature. A common misconception is that the quality of the review depends on the number of references included. A small review covering pertinent studies and organized in a coherent fashion is of more value than a rambling presentation of questionably relevant information.

With respect to the depth of coverage in a written review, the most important criterion is, once again, relevancy. Research that is highly related to the problem or theory usually merits detailed coverage, including a description of the purpose, research approach, instruments, sample, target population, findings, and conclusions. Studies that are only indirectly related can often be summarized in a sentence or two.

Primary and Secondary Sources

References can be categorized as being either primary or secondary sources. Although this distinction probably is familiar to most readers, it is sufficiently important to merit a comment here. A *primary source,* from the point of view of the research literature, is the description of an investigation written by the person who conducted it. For example, most of the articles appearing in journals such as *Nursing Research, Research in Nursing and Health, Applied Nursing Research,* and the *Western Journal of Nursing Research* are original research reports and, therefore, are primary sources. A *secondary source* is a description of a study or studies prepared by someone other than the original researcher. Review articles that summarize the literature on a topic are secondary sources. When you have completed and written up a review of the literature on a topic, your document will be considered a secondary reference. If you go on to collect new data on the same topic, however, your description of the research problem, methods, and results of the study will be a primary source reference for others doing a literature review.

Primary and secondary sources play important, but different, roles in the literature review task. Secondary sources are useful in providing bibliographical information on relevant primary sources. However, secondary descriptions of studies should not be considered substitutes for the primary sources. Secondary sources typically fail to provide sufficient detail about research studies. An even more serious limitation of secondary sources is that it is rarely possible to achieve complete objectivity in summarizing and reviewing written materials. We must accept our own values and biases as one filter through which information passes— although we should certainly make every effort to control such biases. However, we should not have to accept as a second filter the biases of the person who prepared a summary of research studies. The literature review task should use primary sources whenever possible.

❖ LOCATING RESEARCH REPORTS

The ability to identify and locate documents on a topic of interest is an important skill that is not as easily acquired as one might suspect. It is, nevertheless, a skill worth cultivating because it is clearly indispensable for nurse researchers, as well as practicing nurses, to know how to access previous findings on a topic. In this section, some general issues concerning the mechanics of locating references are discussed, and some specific major sources commonly used by nurse researchers are presented.

Bibliographical Aids for Nursing Research Problems

The number of individual books, journals, and reports that could be consulted in compiling information on a nursing research topic is overwhelming. Fortunately, various indexes, abstracting services, and other retrieval mechanisms can facilitate the process of locating pertinent references. Several major sources that can be consulted in performing the review of the literature are identified here. However, these materials by no means exhaust the possibilities; for example, we do not discuss manual and computerized card files that allow readers to access library holdings. Librarians are a particularly valuable resource inasmuch as they are knowledgeable about the literature, literature retrieval tools, and services in their own libraries. Librarians also are familiar with additional resources available through the community, state, and regional libraries and the National Library of Medicine, which make up the Health Science Library Network in the United States.

Table 4-2 is designed to assist students in the selection of an appropriate literature retrieval source for locating references from books, periodicals, government documents, and abstracts. The table indicates whether the source can be searched by computer. The table is not meant to be exhaustive but is intended to aid the beginning researcher who is initiating a literature search.

INDEXES

Health sciences *indexes* are the key to the vast health sciences literature. Several indexes

particularly useful to nurse researchers are the *International Nursing Index, Cumulative Index to Nursing and Allied Health, Nursing Studies Index, Index Medicus, Hospital Literature Index,* and *Current Index to Journals in Education.*

1. The *International Nursing Index* is one of the major sources for locating references from both nursing and nonnursing journals. Articles from more than 275 nursing journals, as well as nursing articles appearing in more than 2700 nonnursing journals, are listed alphabetically by subject heading and author. Foreign journal articles appear at the end of each subject heading and are enclosed in brackets.

    Although the *International Nursing Index* is primarily a periodical index, it also lists in special appendixes publications of professional organizations and agencies, nursing books published during the year, and doctoral dissertations by nurses. It is published quarterly with an annual cumulative index and covers articles from 1966 to the present.

    The procedure for locating references through an index is described in the preliminary pages of each volume. Because the procedures tend to be similar for various indexes, only those for accessing information in the *International Nursing Index* are described here. The *International Nursing Index* begins with a *thesaurus,* which lists commonly used terms or *key words.* The thesaurus directs the reader to actual subject headings by means of a "see" reference if the term is not one used. For example, suppose you are looking for references on nursing care plans. This phrase, although common in nursing, is not one of the subject headings. Nursing Care Plans is listed in the thesaurus and followed by a "see" reference, directing you to look under the subject headings of Nursing Process or Patient Care Planning.

    In addition to "see" references, the thesaurus also suggests, at times, other subject *(text continues on page 78)*

Table 4-2. *A Quick Guide to Selected Abstracts and Indexes for Nursing and Related Subjects*

TITLE	Index	Abstract	FRE-QUENCY	DATE COVERAGE	Medicine	Nursing	Hospital	Other	Books	Studies	Technical report	Periodical	ANA/NLN Publ	Gov't Publ	Pamphlet	Dissertation	Book review	Data Base NAME	Data Base DATE
Books																			
Card catalog of the library	●								●				X	X	X	X			
National Library of Medicine current catalog @	●		Qa	1880	●	●	●		●				X	X	X	X		CATLINE	1801–
Catalog to the Sophia F. Palmer Memorial Library, AJN Co.	●		2 vol.	1922–1973	●	●	●		●	●	●		●						
Medical Books in Print	●		A	1986		●		H	●									Books in Print	Current
Periodicals*																			
Annual or cumulative indexes to individual periodical titles (e.g., AJN, Public Health Nursing)	●				●	●						●	X	X	X		X		
International Nursing Index	●		Qa	1966		●			○			●	○	○	○	○		MEDLINE	1966–
CINAHL (Cumulative Index to Nursing and Allied Health Literature) @	●		B-Ma	1956		●			○			●	+	○	○			CINAHL	1983–
Nursing Studies Index (V. Henderson)	●		4 vol.	1900–1959		●			●	●		●	+	+	+	+			

(continued)

Table 4-2. *A Quick Guide to Selected Abstracts and Indexes for Nursing and Related Subjects (continued)*

TITLE	TYPE OF INDEX — Index	TYPE OF INDEX — Abstract	FRE-QUENCY	DATE COVERAGE	SUBJECT COVERAGE — Medicine	SUBJECT COVERAGE — Nursing	SUBJECT COVERAGE — Hospital	Other	MATERIAL — Books	MATERIAL — Studies	MATERIAL — Technical report	MATERIAL — Periodical	MATERIAL — ANA/NLN Publ	MATERIAL — Gov't Publ	MATERIAL — Pamphlet	MATERIAL — Dissertation	MATERIAL — Book review	Data Base — NAME	Data Base — DATE
Periodicals																			
Index Medicus/ Cumulated Index Medicus @	●		Ma	1927–	●	+	+				○	●						MEDLINE	1966–
Hospital Literature Index/Cumulative Index of Hospital Literature	●		Qa	1945		+	●	H	○			●						HEALTH	1975–
History of Nursing Index to Adelaide Nutting, Teachers' College, Columbia U. collection	●		1 vol.			●			●										
Bibliography of Bioethics			A	1973, 75–				M	●	+	+	+	+	+	+			BIOETHICS	1973–
Bibliography of the History of Medicine			Aa	1965–	●	●		e	●	+		●	X	+	+			HISTLINE	1970–
Government																			
NTIS—SRIM Index to Health Planning	●		Qa	1978–	+	+		H		●	●			+	+			NTIS	1964–
MEDOC	●		Qa	1968–	+	+	+	H						●				MEDOC	1976–1979
Monthly Catalog, U.S. Government Publications	●		Msa	1895–	+	+	+	M						●				Monthly catalog	1976–

Abstracts

Title	Frequency	Dates	Subject Coverage	Computerized database	Database dates
Annual Review of Nursing Research	A	1983–			
Nursing Research Abstracts	B-Ma	1979–			
Abstracts of Reports of Studies in Nursing (in each issue of *Nursing Research*)	B-M	1960–1978			
Abstracts of Studies in Public Health Nursing (in *Nursing Research, 8, 1957*)		1924–1957			
Nursing Research Abstracts (UK)	Qa	1979–			
Abstracts of Health Care Management Studies @	Qa	1965–		PARADEX (offline)	
ERIC (Education Resources Information Center)	Qa	1966–	E	ERIC	1966–
Psychological Abstracts	Msa-a	1927–	P	PSYCH ABS	1967–
Dissertation Abstracts International @	Ma	1938–		DISS ABS	1861–
Excerpta Medica	Msa	1947–	M	EXCERPTA MEDICA	1974–

Frequency

A—annual

M—monthly

B-M—bimonthly

Q—quarterly

a—with annual or multiyear cumulation

sa—with semiannual cumulation

Subject Coverage

e—ethics

E—education

H—health

M—multidiscipline

P—psychology/psychological aspects

*Some titles listed in this chart under periodical indexes also include books and other materials. This table is printed with the permission of its author, M. L. Pekarski, previously Coordinator, Special Projects, O'Neill Library (which contains a nursing collection), Boston College, Chestnut Hill, MA 02167.

headings that are pertinent to your particular topic. It does this by means of a "see also" reference. Sometimes both "see" and "see also" references appear for a particular term.

The researcher then proceeds to the subject section of the index.* The subject heading lists the actual references. Each reference contains the following information: title of the article, author, journal, volume number, issue number, page numbers, and date of issue. A recent reference found under Patient Care Planning is:

Title   *Author*

Determinants of health-promoting lifestyles in older persons. Duffy ME. Image J Nurs Sch 1993 Spring; 25(1): 23-8.

Journal   *Date of Issue*

Volume   *Issue*   *Page Numbers*

A list of journal abbreviations cited in the references appears in the section "Journals Indexed" at the beginning of each issue of the *International Nursing Index.* In the above example, "Image J Nurs Sch" represents the journal *Image: Journal of Nursing Scholarship.*

Each researcher must decide, based on the title of the articles, whether the references cited may be pertinent to the topic under study. Once relevant references are identified, the particular articles can be obtained and reviewed.

2. The *Cumulative Index to Nursing and Allied Health Literature* (CINAHL) is published bimonthly with an annual cumulation. It indexes more than 500 nursing, allied health, and health-related journals published in English and also the publications of the American Nurses' Association and the National League for Nursing. It includes pertinent articles from the biomedical journals indexed in *Index Medicus* and

relevant material from popular journals. CINAHL started publication in 1956, before the *International Nursing Index,* and is the only index to nursing journals from 1960 to 1965. Articles unavailable through local sources or the Regional Medical Library and its area libraries may be obtained for a fee from the CINAHL or American Journal of Nursing Libraries.

3. The *Nursing Studies Index* is a four-volume index prepared by Virginia Henderson and others. It is an annotated guide to reported studies, research methods, and historical and biographical materials in periodicals, books, and pamphlets published in English before 1960. The *Nursing Studies Index* constitutes the only means of access to nursing literature for the 1900 to 1959 period. Originally published by J. B. Lippincott, this index is now available in reprint format from Garland Publishing.

4. The *Index Medicus* is one of the most well-known biomedical indexes. More than 3000 worldwide biomedical journals are indexed. A small number of nursing journals are also indexed. It is published monthly and cumulated annually. Foreign language articles appear at the end of a subject and are enclosed in brackets. An additional feature included as a separate entity in both the monthly and annual cumulated volumes is the *Bibliography of Medical Reviews,* an index to the latest review articles that have appeared in biomedical journals.

5. The *Hospital Literature Index* is published four times annually, with the final issue containing an annual cumulation of listings. This index, which covers primarily administrative aspects of health care delivery, has been published since 1945. It includes citations from more than 1000 English-language journals.

6. Educational Resources Information Center (ERIC) was established in 1964 by the U.S. Office of Education and is useful to the nurse researcher concerned with educa-

---

* When the researcher is seeking articles published by a particular author, the procedure is to go directly to the author section of the index.

tional issues. Access to ERIC is by *The The-saurus of ERIC Descriptors* found in most libraries. The *Current Index to Journals in Education* is a monthly publication produced by ERIC. The index references articles, by subject and author, from more than 700 educational journals.

ABSTRACTS

Abstract journals summarize articles that have appeared in other journals. Abstracting services are generally more useful than indexes in that they provide a summary (abstract) of a study rather than just a title. The title of an article often does not fully indicate its contents. Having an abstract helps in deciding whether a particular reference is worth retrieving.

1. *Nursing Abstracts* is a bimonthly publication that was first published in 1979. The periodical presents abstracts of articles from more than 80 nursing journals. Entries in *Nursing Abstracts* are indexed by subject, author, and journal. An example of an entry from this periodical is presented in Box 4-1.

2. Abstracts of books and journal articles in the field of psychology and other behavioral and social sciences appear in *Psychological Abstracts*. Articles from selected nursing journals (e.g., *Nursing Research*) that are psychologically oriented are abstracted. To use this tool, the researcher first looks up the appropriate subject heading in the cumulative index. Under each subject heading are listed, in alphabetical order, the titles of research reports pertaining to the subject area of interest and an abstract number. The abstract can then be located by this number in the abstract section of this periodical.

3. *Sociological Abstracts* covers more than 1000 publications in the field of sociology and related behavioral and social sciences. This abstract periodical is published five times a year, with an annual cumulative index. Because the fields of medical sociology and the sociology of illness are growing, there may be many relevant references in this abstract journal.

4. *Research in Education,* another monthly publication of ERIC, abstracts reports of research projects funded by the U.S. Office of Education. These abstracts are indexed by subject and author.

BOOKS AND BIBLIOGRAPHIES

Books should not be overlooked when conducting a literature search. Although period-

---

BOX 4-1.   EXAMPLE OF AN ENTRY FROM *NURSING ABSTRACTS**

#933005
A Follow-up Study of Patients with Implantable Cardioverter Defibrillators
Bremmer, Siobhan M., et al
J Cardiovas Nurs, 7:3, Apr 93, pp 40–51

This study describes clinical characteristics and experiences of 381 patients over a 9-year follow-up period in terms of the occurrence of implantable cardioverter defibrillator discharge and the relationship of discharge to potential risk factors for sudden cardiac death. Shocks were categorized as appropriate, indeterminate, or inappropriate. Definitions of these categories and their occurrence are discussed and the characteristics and experiences of these patients are described.

*This entry was from Volume 15, Issue 3 (1993) of *Nursing Abstracts.*

icals contain more up-to-date information than books, books do provide more extensive coverage of a particular topic by treating more than one facet or aspect of the issue in depth. Books are a particularly valuable resource for locating discussions of theoretical issues. Books are also useful in that they usually contain numerous references to other sources of information. Books can be identified through library card catalogs and the computerized data bases corresponding to those catalogs.

Bibliographies are compilations of references found in books, periodicals, and reports on some particular topic. Annotated bibliographies provide comments concerning the purposes or findings of the references and sometimes concerning their quality. If a bibliography on a topic of interest is available, it is an invaluable resource.

Computer Searches

As an alternative to searching indexes or abstracts manually, computerized literature searches have become increasingly popular. A *computer search* provides the researcher with a list of references with complete bibliographical information and, in many cases, abstracts as well. Computer searches are particularly useful when multiple concepts need to be linked. For example, there may be many references in *Index Medicus* for the key word anorexia, but if the research problem of interest concerned eating disorders in adolescents, you could direct the computer to identify only those references that had both anorexia and adolescents as key words. Another advantage of computer searches is that references to new literature may be available by way of the computer up to 1 month before their appearance in the printed index or abstract. Computer searches save some of the researcher's time and energy, thereby providing more time for reading the original publications.

No knowledge of computers is necessary for requesting a computer literature search. The researcher typically fills out a request form indicating the topic of interest and any limitations

on the search, such as dates of publication. If the researcher has done some manual searching of the literature, subject headings found to be useful can be indicated. The librarian confers with the researcher, devises the best search strategy, and then performs the actual search.

Most computer searches are able to produce an immediate search, generating references at the same time the request is received. This is called an *on-line search*. If more than a small number of citations is obtained, the bulk of them may be printed *off-line* because this process is less expensive. The off-line printout is sent by mail and usually arrives several days after the computer search is conducted. The cost of a computer search varies depending on the type of search (the extensiveness of the bibliography requested) and the data base used in the search.

Table 4-2 includes a selected listing of data bases available for computer literature searches relevant for nursing. MEDLINE, the data base most commonly used by nurse researchers, is one of the largest data bases in the world. MEDLINE centers are located at the libraries of major research centers, medical schools, nursing schools, and hospitals. MEDLINE covers all areas of biomedical literature and corresponds to *Index Medicus* with added coverage of nursing, hospital, and dental literature. All journals currently indexed in the *International Nursing Index* are included in MEDLINE. Several subfiles relating to specific subject areas or types of materials are also included. For example, CANCERLINE contains literature on all aspects of cancer, and AIDSLINE cites references relating to acquired immunodeficiency syndrome.

CINAHL, the resource mentioned earlier in the section on indexes, is also a bibliographical retrieval system available for on-line searching. The Combined Health Information Database is a combination of files of books, periodicals, and other materials from various clearinghouses on arthritis, diabetes, health, digestive diseases, and high blood pressure. Other data bases that may be useful include PSYCHOLOGICAL ABSTRACTS (psychological literature); SOCABS (sociologic literature); ERIC (educational materials); and NTIS, the data base that covers technical reports released by more than 250 government and other agencies.

Although the traditional data base search systems generally require the services of a librarian, a new and intensifying trend is end-user searching. *End-user systems* are designed to allow researchers without computer expertise to conduct their own computer search in the library or in other locations with a personal computer or terminal, without the assistance of a search specialist. Selected examples of end-user systems include BRS AFTER DARK, BRS COLLEAGUE, BRS BRKTHRU, DIALOG KNOWLEDGE, DIALOG MEDICAL CONNECTION, GRATEFUL MED, PAPER CHASE, and SILVERPLATTER. These commercial systems can be used to access many data bases, including MEDLINE and CINAHL. Many data bases are now available in CD-ROM (compact disc-read only memory) format.

A recent innovation is NurseSearch, a unique bibliographical retrieval system. NurseSearch can be used to search a list of citations from 60 nursing journals from the CINAHL data base. This system provides subscribers with both the computer program that provides the searching (which can be used on personal computers) and the actual data base on floppy diskettes. This means that the users of NurseSearch do not incur any on-line costs to access the data base.

Tips on Locating Research Reports

Locating all relevant information on a research problem is a bit like being a detective. The various manual and computerized literature retrieval tools are a tremendous aid, but there inevitably needs to be some digging for, and a lot of sifting and sorting of, the clues to knowledge on a topic. Here are a few suggestions:

- If you plan to do a computerized search, it is a good idea to do a little manual exploring first to become acquainted with relevant key words and major subject headings. Authors

of research reports, or the people coding reports for entry into the computer data base, may conceptualize the research problem somewhat differently from you and may therefore use different key words by which to access the study.

- If you are interested in identifying all major research reports on a topic, you will need to be flexible and to think broadly about the key words and subject headings that could possibly be related to the topic in which you are interested. For example, if you are interested in anorexia in adolescents, you should look under *anorexia, eating disorders*, and *adolescence*, and perhaps under *nutrition, diet, bulimia, weight*, and *body image.*

- If you are doing a completely manual search, it is a wise practice to begin the search for relevant references with the most recent issue of the index or abstract journal, and to proceed backward.

- It is rarely possible to identify all relevant studies if you rely on literature retrieval mechanisms exclusively. An excellent method of identifying additional research reports is to find several recently published studies and examine the references at the end. Researchers who are conducting studies on a topic are usually knowledgeable about other research on that topic and refer to major relevant studies as a means of providing context for their own investigations.

❖ READING RESEARCH REPORTS

Once the researcher has identified potential references, he or she must proceed to locate the actual references. Academic libraries (i.e., libraries in colleges and universities) are likely to contain many of the references identified in the initial literature search. If a reference cannot be located, it is wise to check with a librarian because most academic libraries have interlibrary loan capabilities that make it possible to obtain a reference from another cooperating library.

For research literature reviews, relevant information will be found mainly in research reports in professional research journals, such as *Nursing Research* or *Research in Nursing and Health*. Before discussing how to prepare a written review, we briefly present some suggestions on how to read a research report.

What Are Research Journal Articles?

Research *journal articles* are reports that summarize the highlights of a scientific investigation. Because journal space is limited, the typical research article is relatively brief—generally only 10 to 25 typewritten double-spaced pages. This means that the researcher must condense a lot of information into a very short space.

Research reports are accepted by journals on a competitive basis and are critically reviewed before acceptance for publication. Readers of research journal articles thus have some assurance that the studies have already been scrutinized for their scientific merit. Nevertheless, the publication of an article does not mean that the research findings can be uncritically accepted as true, because the validity of the findings depends to a large degree on how the study was conducted; this is why both producers and consumers of research can profit from gaining some knowledge about research methods.

Research reports in journals tend to follow a certain format for the presentation of material and tend to be written in a particular style. The next two sections discuss the content and style of research reports.

Content of Research Reports

Research reports in professional journals typically consist of six major sections: an abstract, an introduction, a methods section, a results section, a discussion, and references. These sections are briefly described next to provide some guidelines for what to expect in a scientific report.

THE ABSTRACT

The *abstract* is a brief description of the study placed at the beginning of the journal article. (When the description is placed at the end, it is called a summary rather than an abstract). The abstract answers, in about 100 to 200 words, the following questions: What were the research questions? What methods did the researcher use in answering those questions? and What did the researcher discover? Readers can readily review an abstract to assess whether the entire report should be read. (The author's abstract is generally the source for the entries appearing in abstract journals, discussed in the previous section.)

THE INTRODUCTION

The purpose of the introductory section of a research report is to acquaint readers with the research problem and its context. Generally, the introduction consists of four elements:

1. The statement of purpose, research questions, or hypotheses to be tested
2. A review of the related literature
3. The theoretical framework
4. The significance of and need for the study

The purpose of the introduction is to set the stage for a description of what the researcher did and what the researcher discovered. In essence, the introduction communicates the decisions the researcher made and the activities undertaken in steps 1 through 4 of the research process, as described in Chapter 2.

THE METHODS SECTION

The purpose of the methods section is to communicate to readers exactly what the researcher did to solve the research problem or answer the research questions. This section tells readers about the researcher's methodologic decisions (steps 5 through 10 of the research process). Generally, the methods section describes the following:

1. The research subjects, that is, the study population, sampling plan, and the number and characteristics of the subjects
2. The research design, including any methods used to control extraneous variables
3. The methods of data collection and measurement of variables
4. Study procedures, including a description of any interventions

The methods section often provides a discussion of not only *what* was done but also *why* it was done. In other words, the researcher may defend his or her methodological decisions by articulating a rationale.

THE RESULTS SECTION

The results section presents the key *research findings*, that is, the results obtained in the analysis of the data. This section is typically the core focus of the article for the person doing a literature review.

In qualitative studies, the results section generally presents a description of the themes that emerge in the analysis of the narrative materials, together with a summary of the researcher's theoretical integration of those materials. The researcher often includes direct excerpts from the data to illustrate important points.

In quantitative studies, the researcher often begins by providing basic descriptive information for the key variables, using simple statistics. For example, in a study of the effect of prenatal drug exposure on the birth outcomes of infants, the results section might begin by describing the characteristics of the mothers in the sample, such as the average age of the mothers or the percentage who failed to obtain any prenatal care. In quantitative studies, the results section typically reports the following additional types of information (often summarized in tables):

1. *The name of the statistical test used.* A *statistical test* is, simply, a procedure for evaluating the believability of the findings. For example, if the average birthweight of the

infants in the sample of drug-exposed infants is computed, how likely is it that the average accurately reflects the birthweight of all drug-exposed infants? Statistical tests provide an answer to questions such as this. Dozens of statistical tests exist, but they are all based on common principles; readers do not have to know the names of all statistical tests to comprehend the findings.

2. *The value of the calculated statistic.* Computers are used almost universally to process the research data and compute a value for the particular test used. The value allows the researcher to draw conclusions about the meaning of the results. The actual numerical value of the statistic, however, is not inherently meaningful and need not concern readers of research reports.

3. *The significance of the statistical test.* Perhaps the most important piece of information in the results section is whether the results are significant (not to be confused with important). If a researcher reports that the results are *statistically significant*, it means that, according to the statistical test, the findings are likely to be valid and replicable with a completely new sample of subjects. Research reports also indicate the *level of significance*, which is an index of how probable it is that the findings are reliable. For example, if a report indicates that a finding was significant at the .05 level, this means that only 5 times out of 100 would the obtained result be spurious or haphazard. In other words, 95 times out of 100, similar results would be obtained, and the researcher can therefore have a high degree of confidence that the findings are reliable.

DISCUSSION

In the discussion section of a journal article, the researcher draws conclusions about the meaning and implications of the study. This section tries to unravel what the results mean and why things turned out the way they did. The discussion typically incorporates the following elements:

1. An interpretation of the results
2. A discussion of study limitations
3. The implications of the study for research and practice

REFERENCES

Research journal articles conclude with a list of the books, reports, and other journals articles that were cited in the text of the report. For those interested in pursuing additional reading on a substantive topic, the reference list of a current research study is an excellent place to begin.

Style of a Research Report

Research reports tell a story. The style in which most research journal articles is written, however, often makes it difficult for beginning researchers or research consumers to become interested in the story that is being reported. To unaccustomed audiences, research reports often sound stuffy and pedantic. Three factors contribute to this impression:

1. *Compactness.* Because journal space is limited, authors must try to compress many ideas and concepts into the short space available. Some of the interesting, personalized aspects of the investigation cannot be reported. Furthermore, the need for efficiency means that tables must be used rather than text to present an array of information.
2. *Jargon.* The authors often use complex scientific terms that are assumed to be part of the reader's vocabulary. Often the jargon can be translated into everyday terms but at the expense of efficiency and, in some cases, precision.
3. *Objectivity.* The writer of a research report generally strives to present findings in a manner that suggests neutrality and the ab-

sence of personal biases. The scientist is primarily an observer and recorder of natural phenomena, and, therefore, researchers often take pains to avoid any impression of subjectivity. Because of this, research stories are often told in a way that makes them sound impersonal. Typically, for example, a research article is written in the passive voice—that is, personal pronouns such as *I* and *we* are avoided. Use of the passive voice tends to make a report less inviting and lively than the use of the active voice and tends to give the impression that the researcher did not actually *do* anything in conducting the study.

4. *Statistical information.* Numbers and statistical symbols may intimidate readers who do not have strong mathematic interest or training. Most nursing studies are quantitative, and thus most research journal articles summarize the results of statistical analyses. Indeed, nurse researchers have become increasingly sophisticated over the past decade and have begun to use more powerful and complex statistical tools.

Tips on Reading Research Reports

As students progress through this textbook, they will acquire skills with which to evaluate critically various aspects of research reports. Some preliminary hints on digesting research reports and dealing with the issues described previously follow.

•   Grow accustomed to the style of research reports by reading them frequently, even though you may not at this point understand many technical points. Try to keep the underlying rationale for the style of research reports (as just described) in mind as you are reading.
•   We recommend that, at least initially, you read research journal articles slowly; it may be useful to first skim the article to get the

major points, and then reread the article more carefully a second time.

- Try not to get bogged down in—or scared away by—the statistical information. Try to grasp the gist of the story without letting formulas and numbers frustrate you.

- Until you become more accustomed to the style and jargon of scientific writing, you may want to translate research articles mentally. You can do this by translating compact paragraphs into looser constructions, by translating jargon into more familiar phrases and terms, by recasting the report into an active voice to get a better sense of the researcher's dynamic role in the research process, and by summarizing the findings with words rather than with numbers. As an example of such a translation, Box 4-2 presents a brief summary of a fictitious study. The top panel is written in the style typically found in research journal articles. The bottom panel presents a translation of the summary that recasts the information into language that is more digestible to students and novice consumers.

- Although we have described the major sections of the report as the introduction, methods section, results section, and discussion, not all research reports present their content under exactly these headings. In particular, many reports do not specifically label their introductory materials with the heading "Introduction." There is considerable variation in how authors present the background of their studies, but in general the information appearing before the methods section is part of the introduction to the study.

- Although it is certainly important to read research reports with understanding, it is also important to read them critically, especially when you are preparing a written literature review. A critical reading involves an evaluation of the researcher's major conceptual and methodological decisions. Unfortunately, it is difficult for students to criticize these decisions before they have gained some conceptual and methodological skills themselves. These skills will be strengthened as you

progress through this book, but sometimes common sense and thoughtful analysis suggest to beginning students flaws in a study. Some of the key questions to ask include the following: Does the way the researcher conceptualized the problem make sense—for example, do the hypotheses seem sensible? Did the researcher design the study in such a way that the relationship between the independent and dependent variables could be understood? Were the major research variables measured in a reasonable way or would an alternative method have been better? Did the researcher choose subjects in such a way that they are representative of the group being studied, and was the sample large enough that the results are likely to be replicable? Additional guidelines for critiquing various aspects of a research report are presented in Chapter 25.

❖ *PREPARING A WRITTEN LITERATURE REVIEW*

A number of steps are involved in preparing a written review, as summarized in Figure 4-1. As the figure shows, after identifying potential sources, the reader must locate the references and screen them for their relevancy to the topic being reviewed. References that appear appropriate are read and notes are taken, and inappropriate references can be discarded. Frequently, one reference will provide citations to many other relevant references, which sends the reader back to locate additional sources. After all relevant references have been reviewed, the researcher can proceed to organize, analyze, and integrate the body of literature. The written review can then be prepared. This section provides some advice on the last few steps in preparing a written review.

Abstracting and Recording Notes

Once a document has been determined to be relevant, the entire report should be read

---

BOX 4-2.   SUMMARY OF A FICTITIOUS STUDY AND A "TRANSLATION"*

Original Version

The potentially negative sequelae of having an abortion on the psychological adjustment of adolescents has not been adequately studied. The present study sought to determine whether alternative pregnancy resolution decisions have different long-term effects on the psychological functioning of young women.

Three groups of low-income pregnant teenagers attending an inner-city clinic were the subjects in this study: those who delivered and kept the baby; those who delivered and relinquished the baby for adoption; and those who had an abortion. There were 25 subjects in each group. The study instruments included a self-administered questionnaire and a battery of psychological tests measuring depression, anxiety, and psychosomatic symptoms. The instruments were administered upon entry into the study (when the subjects first came to the clinic) and then one year after termination of the pregnancy.

The data were analyzed using analysis of variance. The ANOVA tests indicated that the three groups did not differ significantly in terms of depression, anxiety, or psychosomatic symptoms at the initial testing. At the posttest, however, the abortion group had significantly higher scores on the depression scale and were significantly more likely than the two delivery groups to report severe tension headaches. There were no significant differences on any of the dependent variables for the two delivery groups.

The results of this study suggest that young women who elect to have an abortion may experience a number of long-term negative consequences. It would appear that appropriate efforts should be made to follow-up abortion patients to determine their need for suitable treatment.

Translated Version

As researchers, we wondered whether young women who had an abortion had any emotional problems in the long run. It seemed to us that not enough research had been done to know whether any actual psychological harm resulted from an abortion.

We decided to study this question ourselves by comparing the experiences of three types of teenagers who became pregnant—first, girls who delivered and kept their babies; second, those who delivered the babies but gave them up for adoption; and third, those who elected to have an abortion. All the teenagers in the sample were poor, and all were patients at an inner-city clinic. Altogether, we studied 75 girls—25 in each of the three groups. We evaluated the teenagers' emotional state by asking them to fill out a questionnaire and to take several psychological tests. These tests allowed us to assess things like the girls' degree of depression and anxiety and whether or not they had any complaints of a psychosomatic nature. We asked them to fill out the forms twice: once when they came into the clinic, and then again a year after the abortion or the delivery.

We learned that the three groups of teenagers looked pretty much alike in terms of their emotional states when they first filled out the forms. But when we compared how the three groups looked a year later, we found that the teenagers who had abortions were more depressed and were more likely to say they had severe tension headaches than teenagers in the other two groups. The teenagers who kept their babies and those who gave their babies up for adoption looked pretty similar one year after their babies were born, at least in terms of depression, anxiety, and psychosomatic complaints.

Thus, it seems that we may be right in having some concerns about the emotional effects of having an abortion. Nurses should be aware of these long-term emotional effects, and it even may be advisable to institute some type of follow-up procedure to find out if these young women need additional help.

*The "findings" summarized here are not necessarily accurate.

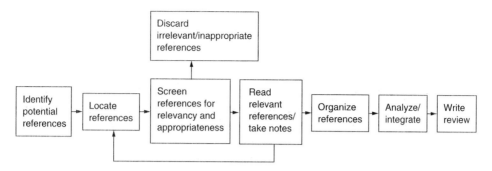

Figure 4-1. *Flow of tasks in a literature review.*

carefully and critically, identifying material that is sufficiently important to warrant note taking as well as observing flaws or gaps in the report. Notes should be taken (ideally on index cards) to remind the reviewer of the content of the report and its strengths and limitations. The following kinds of information should usually be recorded: the *full* citation for inclusion in your bibliography, the problem statement or hypotheses, the theoretical framework, key features of the research methods, and the major findings and conclusions.

Organizing the Review

If the end product of your literature search is to be a written review, a critical task is the organization of the gathered information. Several devices may help in the successful accomplishment of this task. When the literature on a topic is extensive, it is sometimes useful to organize the findings from studies in a summary table. The table could include columns with headings such as "Author," "Number of Subjects," "Type of Design," "Method of Measuring Variables," and "Key Findings." Such a table provides a quick overview that allows the reviewer to make sense of a large mass of information. As an example, Tuten and Gueldner (1991), in the introduction to their study of the effectiveness of sodium chloride versus dilute heparin for maintenance of peripheral intermittent intravenous devices, present an excellent table summarizing earlier research.

Most writers find it helpful to work from an outline. If the review is lengthy and complex, it is useful to write out the outline. For shorter reviews, a mental outline may be sufficient. The important point is to sit back for a minute before starting to write and work out a structure so that the presentation has a meaningful and understandable flow. Lack of organization is a common weakness in students' first attempts at writing a literature review.

Once the main topics and their order of presentation have been determined, a review of the notes is in order. This will not only help recall materials read earlier but also lay the groundwork for decisions about where (if at all) a particular reference fits in terms of the outline. If certain references do not seem to fit anywhere, the outline may need to be revised or the reference discarded. Students should avoid the temptation to force a reference into the review if it does not make a contribution. The number of references used in the review is much less important than the relevance of the references, the quality of the summary, and the overall organization.

Content of the Written Literature Review

A written review of the literature should be neither a series of quotes nor a series of abstracts. The central task is to organize and summarize the references so they reveal the current state of knowledge on the selected topics and, in the context of a new study, to lay a systematic foundation for the research. The review should point out both consistencies and contradictions in the literature as well as offer possible explanations for the inconsistencies, for example, different conceptualizations or methods.

Studies that are particularly relevant should be described in some detail. However, reports that result in comparable findings can often be grouped together and briefly summarized, as in the following fictitious example:

> A number of studies have found that the incidence of phlebitis is directly related to the method of administering intravenous infusions and to certain parameters of materials used in the infusions (Altes, 1993; Baum & Schwerin, 1994; Trattles, 1993).

It is important to paraphrase, or summarize, a report in one's own words. The review should demonstrate that thoughtful consideration has been given to the materials. Stringing together quotes from various documents fails to show that previous research and thought on the topic have been assimilated and understood.

Another point to bear in mind is that the review should be as objective as possible. Studies that conflict with personal values should not be omitted. It is not unusual to find studies with contradictory results. The review should not deliberately ignore a study simply because its findings contradict other studies. Analyze inconsistent results and evaluate the supporting evidence as objectively as possible.

The literature review should conclude with a summary or overview of the state-of-the-art knowledge regarding the problem under consideration. The summary should not only point out what has been studied and how adequate the investigations have been but also should make note of any gaps or areas of research inactivity. The summary requires some critical judgment concerning the extensiveness and dependability of information on a topic. If the literature review is conducted as part of a research project, this critical summary should demonstrate the need for the new study and

should clarify the context within which the hypotheses will be developed.

Style of a Research Review

One of the most frequent problems for the student researcher preparing a written research review for the first time is adjusting to the style of writing that is used in research reviews. There is a tendency, for example, for students to accept the results of previous research as a fact or as proof that a finding is conclusive or a theory is correct. This tendency is understandable; it is the style of presentation commonly used in many textbooks, opinion articles, and other nonresearch papers. This style stems partly from a desire for clarity and lack of ambiguity for pedantic purposes, but it is also, in part, the result of a common misunderstanding about the degree of conclusiveness that can be achieved through empirical research. *No hypothesis or theory can be definitively proved or disproved by empirical testing.* Every study has some limitations, the severity of which depends to a great extent on the researcher's methodologic decisions. The fact that theories and hypotheses cannot be ultimately proved or disproved does not, of course, mean that we must disregard evidence or challenge every idea we encounter. The problem is partly a semantic one: hypotheses are not *proved*, but they are *supported* by research findings; theories are not *verified* or *confirmed*, but they may be tentatively *accepted* if there is a substantial body of evidence demonstrating their legitimacy. The reviewer must learn to adopt this language of tentativeness in presenting the review of the literature.

A related stylistic problem is the inclination of novice reviewers to liberally intersperse opinions (their own or someone else's) with the findings of research investigations. The review should use statements of opinions sparingly, if at all, and should be explicit about the source of the opinion. A description of the point of view of a knowledgeable or influential individual may be useful in establishing the need to investigate the problem or in providing a perspective on the topic, but it should occupy a relatively small section of the review. The researcher's own opinions do not belong in a review section, with the exception of an assessment of the quality of existing studies.

The left-hand column of Table 4-3 presents several examples of the kinds of stylistic difficulties we have been discussing in this section. The right-hand column offers some recommendations for rewording the sentences to conform to a more generally acceptable form for a research literature review. Many alternative ways of phrasing these sentences are possible.

❖ RESEARCH EXAMPLES

Because of space limitations in journals, most literature reviews that appear in research reports are fairly brief (although occasionally an entire journal article is devoted to a research literature review). Table 4-4 contains brief excerpts from the literature review sections of three research reports. These examples should help to acquaint beginning researchers with the style and

content considered appropriate for written literature reviews as well as illustrate the range of research problems in which nurse researchers have been interested. In addition, we present an expanded excerpt below.

Shapiro (1993) conducted a study to examine the judgments of neonatal intensive care unit nurses regarding pain intensity in full-term and preterm newborns, using both qualitative and quantitative methods. The following excerpt represents essentially the entire literature review section of Shapiro's research report, which appeared in the *Journal of Obstetric, Gynecologic, and Neonatal Nursing.**

> Knowledge about pain in the neonatal population to date has been relatively limited. Because it is unethical to inflict pain inten-

* Reprinted from Shapiro, C. R. (1993). Nurses' judgments of pain in term and preterm newborns. *Journal of Obstetric, Gynecologic, and Neonatal Nursing, 22,* 41–47, copyright 1989 by the Association of Women's Health, Obstetric, and Neonatal Nurses, with permission. The reader is referred to this source for the full article and references in the literature review.

Table 4-3. *Examples of Stylistic Difficulties for Research Reviews**

INAPPROPRIATE STYLE OR WORDING	RECOMMENDED CHANGE
1. It is known that unmet expectations engender anxiety.	1. A number of commentators have asserted that unmet expectations engender anxiety. (Abraham, 1993; White, 1992)
2. The woman who does not undertake preparations for childbirth classes tends to manifest a high degree of stress during labor.	2. Previous studies have demonstrated that women who participate in preparation for childbirth classes manifest less stress during labor than those who do not. (Andrew, 1993; Chase, 1992)
3. Studies have proved that doctors and nurses do not fully understand the psychobiologic dynamics of breastfeeding.	3. The studies by O'Hara (1993) and Carson (1992) suggest that doctors and nurses do not fully comprehend the psychobiologic dynamics of breastfeeding.
4. Attitudes cannot be changed overnight.	4. Attitudes, presumably, are enduring attributes that cannot be changed overnight.
5. Responsibility is an intrinsic stressor.	5. Responsibility is an intrinisic stressor, according to Doctor A. Cassard, an authority on stress. (Cassard, 1994).

*All references are fictitious.

Table 4-4.   *Excerpts From Published Literature Reviews in Research Reports*

PROBLEM STATEMENT	LITERATURE REVIEW EXCERPT*
What are the effects of ovarian hormone cessation, hormone supplementation, and dietary fiber on body weight, appetite and intestinal transit in rats? (Bond, Heitkemper, & Jarrett, 1994)	Dietary fiber, often recommended for symptomatic women, is associated with altered GI function, including motility. Among changes attributed to fiber are delayed gastric emptying (1), altered intestinal transit (2, 3), increased colon and intestinal lengths and weights (4), altered histology, such as epithelial proliferation (5), and altered nutrient absorption (6). The mechanism by which fiber modulates GI function may be mechanical, hormonal, or a combination of these.
What is the prevalence of alcohol use, and what are the factors that predict alcohol use among rural sixth- and seventh-grade children? (Long & Boik, 1993)	The importance of self-concept in relation to the likelihood of adolescent alcohol abuse has been examined in several studies. The data suggest that positive self-concept is associated with less alcohol abuse (1–3). Beliefs about the effects and consequences of alcohol use have been found to correlate with the alcohol use and abuse behaviors of adolescents (4–5). Mann, Chassin, and Shur (1987) found that adolescents who expected alcohol to relieve tension and enhance functioning were particularly likely to engage in alcohol-abusing behavior.
What are the experiences of older adults and their female caregivers related to adult day care? (Scott, 1993)	Research related to the caregiving of the elderly has expanded over the past few decades. Generally, this research found that (a) "families" constitute the majority of informal caregivers to the elderly (1–7); (b) caregiving to elderly is often a burdensome affair (8–11); and (c) the burden of the relationship is primarily borne by the caregiver (12–16). The intensity of the caregiving burden is often correlated with the mental health status or dependency needs of the older adult (17–21).

*The number in parentheses designate the bibliographic references, which are not cited in full here because of space constraints.

tionally on a newborn child for the sake of study, researchers have used an alternative methodology to study acute pain in this population: naturalistic observation of neonates undergoing painful procedures in the course of routine medical care. Among the neonatal behavioral signs that observers have suggested are measures of pain such as crying, facial expression, and body movement (Frank, 1986; Grunau & Craig, 1987; Johnson & Strada, 1986). Physiologic variables such as heart rate, oxygenation status, palmar sweat response, and serum hormone levels also have been examined (Anand, Sippell, & Aynsley-Green, 1987; Beaver, 1987; Harpin & Rutter, 1982).

Although the researchers' studies have contributed important baseline information on healthy fullterm newborns and infants beyond the neonatal period who have been exposed to brief procedural pain, the studies did not extend beyond this population and were carried out by social scientists, physicians, and nurses, but not staff nurses. In contrast to earlier work, one recently published study has explored the behavioral symptoms and physiologic signs of pain in newborns from a staff nurse perspective (Jones, 1989).

Jones (1989) distributed a pain sensitivity questionnaire to a group of neonatal nurses in a tertiary-care hospital in the American midwest. The nurses were provided with a list of 34 physiologic signs and behavioral symptoms suggestive of the possibility of pain in a newborn. A large number of these were identified by the nurses as useful; however, only 3 of the 34 symptoms were selected with high frequency: fussiness, crying, and grimacing.

In another study, Pigeon, McGrath, Lawrence, and MacMurray (1989) used a questionnaire to examine neonatal nurses' perceptions of the indicators and causes of different intensities of pain in neonates under their care in the NICU. They reported that nurses use similar classes of behavior (e.g., general state, crying, and limb movement) to identify pain in neonates, but the frequency of each varies for different levels of pain.

The work of Penticuff (1989) was based on content analysis of interviews of 20 nurses in three NICUs over a 6-year period. The nurses all reported experiencing emotional distress when the therapies that newborns under their care received resulted in suffering without proportional benefit.

No research has been reported that has considered whether differences exist between how nurses judge and interpret pain in preterm versus full-term neonates. It is this important and neglected area that the current study addresses.

❖ SUMMARY

The task of reviewing research literature involves the identification, selection, critical analysis, and written description of existing information on the topic of interest. It is usually advisable to undertake a *literature review* on a subject before actually conducting a research project. Such a review can play a number of important roles. First, in the start-up phase of a project, a review of work conducted in an area of general interest can help in the formulation or clarification of a research problem. Second, a scrutiny of previous work acquaints the researcher with what has been done in a field, thereby minimizing the possibility of unintentional duplication. Third, the review provides a conceptual context or framework for the researcher and for the research community, thereby facilitating the cumulation of scientific knowledge. Fourth, the researcher may be in a better position to assess the feasibility of a proposed study by becoming familiar with related work. Finally, the review can be highly useful in providing methodological suggestions for the actual conduct of the investigation.

The kinds of information available in written documents can be categorized into five broad classes: facts, findings, or results; theory; research procedures or methods; opinions, points of view, or personal commentaries; and anecdotes or impressions of a particular event or situation. Another way of categorizing literature is in terms of its being either a primary or secondary source. A *primary source* with respect to the research literature is the original description of a study prepared by the researcher who conducted it; a *secondary source* is a description of the study by a person unconnected with the investigation. Primary sources should be consulted whenever possible in performing the literature review task.

The search for existing writings on a topic is greatly facilitated by the use of various *indexes* and *abstract journals*, such as *CINAHL* or *Index Medicus*. An important bibliographical development to emerge in recent years is the increasing availability of various computerized information retrieval systems, such as MEDLINE. *End-user systems*, which allow individuals to do their own search rather than rely on a librarian, have become more popular with the widespread availability of personal computers.

After the researcher has identified and located references, he or she must screen them for relevance and then read them critically. For research reviews, most references are likely to be found in professional journals. Research *journal articles*, which present concise descriptions of scientific investigations, typically contain six major sections: the *abstract* (a brief summary of the study); the introduction (which explains the study problem and its context; the methods (the strategy the researcher used to address the research problem); the results (the actual research *findings*); the discussion (the interpretation and implications of the findings); and the bibliographical references.

The compactness of research journal articles, the use of technical scientific terms, their impersonal style, and the description of *statistical tests* often make research articles difficult for students to read. Students may need to translate the ideas contained in a research article before trying to digest them.

Skillful note taking and organization can greatly simplify the task of analyzing, summarizing, and evaluating literature on a given topic. In preparing a written review, it is important to organize materials in a logical, coherent fashion. The preparation of an outline is recommended, and the development of summary charts often helps in integrating diverse studies. The written review should not be a succession of quotes or abstracts. The role of the reviewer is to point out what has been studied to date, how adequate and dependable those studies are, what gaps there seem to be in the existing body of research, and what contribution a new study would make. The reviewer should present facts and findings in the tentative language that befits scientific inquiry and should remember to identify the source of opinions, points of view, and generalizations.

❧ STUDY SUGGESTIONS

Chapter 4 of the accompanying *Study Guide for Nursing Research: Principles and Methods, 5th ed.*, offers various exercises and study sugges-

tions for reinforcing the concepts presented in this chapter. Additionally, the following study suggestions can be addressed:

1. Read the study by Keeling and her colleagues (1994) entitled, "Postcardiac catheterization time-in-bed study: Enhancing patient comfort through nursing research," *Applied Nursing Research, 7,* 14–17. Write a summary of the problem, methods, findings, and conclusions of the study. Your summary should be capable of serving as notes for a review of the literature.

2. Suppose that you were planning to study counseling practices and programs for rape trauma victims. Make a list of several key words relating to this topic that could be used with indexes or information retrieval systems for identifying previous work.

3. Below are five sentences from literature reviews that require stylistic improvements. Rewrite these sentences to conform to considerations mentioned in the text. (Feel free to give fictitious references if desired.)

   a. Children are less distressed during immunization when their parents are present.

   b. Young adolescents are unprepared to cope with complex issues of sexual morality.

   c. More structured programs to use part-time nurses are needed.

   d. Intensive care nurses need so much emotional support themselves that they can provide insufficient support to patients.

   e. Most nurses have not been adequately educated to understand and cope with the reality of the dying patient.

4. Suppose you are studying factors relating to the discharge of chronic psychiatric patients. Obtain five bibliographical references for this topic. Compare your references and sources with those of other students.

❖ *SUGGESTED READINGS*

METHODOLOGICAL REFERENCES

American Psychological Association. (1983). *Publication manual* (3rd ed.). Washington, DC: Author.

Cooper, H. M. (1984). *The integrative research review.* Beverly Hills, CA: Sage.

Fox, R. N., & Ventura, M. R. (1984). Efficiency of automated literature search mechanisms. *Nursing Research, 33,* 174–177.

Ganong, L. H. (1987). Integrative reviews of nursing research. *Research in Nursing and Health, 10,* 1–11.

Light, R. J., & Pillemer, D. B. (1984). *Summing up: The science of reviewing research.* Cambridge, MA: Harvard University Press.

Saba, V. K., Oatway, D. M., & Rieder, K. A. (1989). How to use nursing information sources. *Nursing Outlook, 37,* 189–195.

Smith, L. W. (1988). Microcomputer-based bibliographic searching. *Nursing Research, 37,* 125–127.

Turabian, K. L. (1980). *A manual for writers of term papers, theses, and dissertations* (6th ed.). Chicago: University of Chicago Press.

SUBSTANTIVE REFERENCES

Bond, E. F., Heitkemper, M. M., & Jarrett, M. (1994). Intestinal transit and body weight responses to ovarian hormones and dietary fiber in rats. *Nursing Research, 43,* 18–24.

Long, K. A., & Boik, R. J. (1993). Predicting alcohol use in rural children. *Nursing Research, 42,* 79–86.

Scott, C. B. (1993). Circular victimization in the caregiving relationship. *Western Journal of Nursing Research, 15,* 230–245.

Shapiro, C. R. (1993). Nurses' judgments of pain in term and preterm newborns. *Journal of Obstetric, Gynecologic, and Neonatal Nursing, 22,* 41–48.

Tuten, S. H., & Gueldner, S. H. (1991). Efficacy of sodium chloride versus dilute heparin for maintenance of peripheral intermittent devices. *Applied Nursing Research, 4,* 63–71.

OTHER REFERENCE CITED

Rittman, M. R., Nedoma, N., Quesenberry, L., Gallimore, I., Cox-Henley, M., & Smith, L. (1993). Learning from "never again" stories. *American Journal of Nursing, 93,* 40–43.

Chapter 5

CONCEPTUAL AND THEORETICAL CONTEXTS

Good research generally builds on existing knowledge. Links between new research and existing knowledge are developed through a thorough review of the prior research on a topic (see Chapter 4) and through efforts to identify an appropriate theoretical framework. These activities are important because they provide a conceptual context for a scientific investigation—and because they help the reader to define and delimit the problem to be studied. This chapter discusses theoretical and conceptual contexts for nursing research problems.

❖ THEORIES, CONCEPTUAL FRAMEWORKS, AND MODELS

The term *theory* is used in many ways. For example, nursing instructors and students frequently use the term to refer to the content covered in classrooms, as opposed to the actual practice of performing nursing activities. Sometimes the term is used to refer to someone's hunches or ideas, as in: My theory is that if you smile at patients and establish rapport with them, they will be more compliant. In both lay and scientific usage, the term theory almost always connotes an abstraction or a generalization.

Even within research circles, however, the term theory is used differently by different authors. Classically, scientists have used theory to refer to an abstract generalization that presents a systematic explanation about how phenomena are interrelated. Thus, the traditional definition requires that a theory embody at least two concepts that are related to one another in a manner that the theory purports to explain.

Others, however, use the term theory less restrictively to refer to a broad characterization of some phenomenon. According to this less restrictive definition, a theory can account for (i.e., thoroughly describe) a single phenomenon. Some authors specifically refer to this type of theory as *descriptive theory*. For example, Fawcett and Downs (1992) define descriptive theories as empirically driven theories that "describe or classify specific dimensions or characteristics of individuals, groups, situations, or events by summarizing commonalities found in discrete

Polit DF, Hungler BP: NURSING RESEARCH: PRINCIPLES AND METHODS, 5th ed. © 1995 J. B. Lippincott Company.

observations" (p. 7). Descriptive theory plays an especially important role in qualitative studies. Qualitative researchers often strive to develop a conceptualization of the phenomena under study that is grounded in the actual observations made by the researcher. As discussed in Chapter 22, these researchers seek to develop what is referred to as a *grounded theory*—an empirically based conceptualization for integrating and making sense of a process or phenomenon.

In this textbook, we use theory primarily in the traditional sense. We distinguish between theories and other less formal systems of conceptualization, which are also discussed in this chapter. However, the distinction is seldom of great importance. Both theoretical and other frameworks represent important avenues for making research findings more intelligible and for observing patterns and regularities in the world.

Theories

As traditionally defined, scientific theories involve a series of propositions regarding the interrelationships among concepts, from which a large number of empirical observations can be deduced. In the writings on scientific theory, one encounters a variety of terms such as proposition, postulate, premise, axiom, law, principle, and so forth, some of which are used interchangeably, and others of which introduce subtleties that are too complex for the beginning researcher. Here we present a simplified analysis of the components of a theory for the sake of clarity.

COMPONENTS OF A TRADITIONAL THEORY

Theories comprise, first of all, a set of concepts. As we noted in Chapter 2, *concepts* are abstract characteristics of the objects that are being studied. Examples of nursing concepts are adaptation, health, anxiety, nurse–client interaction, and social support. Concepts are the basic ingredients in the formulation of a theory.

Second, theories comprise a set of statements or propositions, each of which indicates a relationship among the concepts. Relationships are denoted by such terms as "is associated with," "varies directly with," or "is contingent on." Third, the propositions must form a logically interrelated deductive system. This means that the theory must provide a mechanism for logically arriving at new statements from the original propositions.

Let us consider the following example, which illustrates these three points. Selye (1978) developed a theory of adaptation to stress. This theory postulates that a person's body responds to the nonspecific demands of stress by means of the General Adaptation Syndrome (GAS), which continues until adaptation occurs or death ensues. Stress may be internal or external to the individual and is manifested by the syndrome, which consists of nonspecifically induced changes occurring within the person's body. The GAS consists of three phases—the alarm phase, the phase of adaptation or resistance, and the phase of exhaustion—all of which are reversible if adjustment to stress occurs. A greatly simplified construction of Selye's theory might consist of the following propositions:

1. Humans seek to attain a desired state (e.g., the reduction of stress) by mobilizing the body's general defense mechanisms to overact to maintain life.
2. When the specific defense mechanism is identified by the body for dealing with the sources of stress (such as increased muscular activity), the overactivity of the general mechanisms subsides, and the specific mechanisms overact (such as increasing the oxygen supply in muscular activity).
3. If the specific defense mechanisms are unable to cope with the stress, then the general defense mechanisms reactivate to help the body adjust, or death ensues.
4. During the alarm and exhaustion phases, there is an increase in the production of adrenocortical hormones, which subsides during the resistance phase when specific defense mechanisms come into play.

The concepts that form the basis of Selye's theory include stress, the GAS, the body's general defense mechanisms, and the body's specific defense mechanisms. His theory postulates that relationships occur between stress and the body's defense mechanisms, which are activated to cope with the stress. For example, the theory claims that the level of adrenocortical hormones varies with the stage of the GAS. Selye's propositions readily lend themselves to empirical verification by providing a mechanism for deductive hypothesis generation. We might hypothesize on the basis of Selye's theory that the level of adrenocorticotropic hormone (ACTH) will be greater before a meal than it is after a meal or that ACTH production is less during an intravenous infusion than immediately before its inception. On the basis of his theory, we should be able to identify how well the person is coping with the stress by measuring changes in ACTH production. Several nursing studies have been based on Selye's theory of stress and adaptation. For example, Erickson and Swain (1982) studied hospitalized medical–surgical patients to determine the relationship between their adaptive potential and length of hospital stay. Henneman (1989) used Selye's concepts of stress response to evaluate the effect of direct nursing contact on patients.

TYPES OF TRADITIONAL THEORIES

Theories differ extensively in their level of generality. So-called *grand theories* or *macrotheories* purport to describe and explain large segments of the environment or of human experience. Some learning theorists, such as Clark Hull, or sociologists, such as Talcott Parsons, have developed highly general theoretical systems that claim to account for broad classes of behavior and social functioning. On the whole, macrotheories have not been shown to be particularly useful in the behavioral and applied sciences.

Within nursing and fields such as psychology, sociology, and education, theories are usually somewhat restricted in scope, focusing only on a narrow range of phenomena. Theories that focus on only a piece of reality or human experience and that incorporate a selected number of concepts are sometimes referred to as *middle-range theories*. For example, there are middle-range theories that attempt to explain such phenomena as decision-making behavior, leadership behavior, compliance, and attitude change. This limited scope is consistent with the state of scientific developments in many fields dealing with human behavior and is, therefore, appropriate and realistic. In the physical sciences, macrotheories such as the theory of mechanics are feasible and provide a goal toward which the younger social and applied sciences may aspire.

Theories also vary in their complexity. Here we refer to the number and intricacy of the concepts involved and the complexity of relationships presumed. Theories in the sciences dealing with humans often tend to be complex not only because the subject matter is inherently complex but also because conditional relationships and multiple variables are required at the current level of understanding and conceptualization.

Conceptual Frameworks

Conceptual frameworks, conceptual models, or *conceptual schemes* (we use the terms interchangeably here) represent a less formal attempt at organizing phenomena than theories. As the name implies, conceptual frameworks deal with abstractions (concepts) that are assembled by virtue of their relevance to a common theme. Both conceptual schemes and theories use concepts as building blocks. What is absent from conceptual schemes is the deductive system of propositions that assert a relationship between the concepts. Like theories, however, conceptual frameworks can serve as a springboard for the generation of research hypotheses and can provide an important context for scientific research. Many existing conceptual frameworks are likely to serve as the preliminary steps in the construction of more formal theories.

Much of the conceptual work that has been done in connection with nursing practice falls into the category we have designated as conceptual frameworks. These frameworks often represent world views about the nature of nursing and the nurse–patient relationship. A subsequent section of this chapter describes a few of the major conceptual models in nursing and illustrates how they have been used in nursing research.

Schematic and Statistical Models

The term *model* is sometimes used to denote a symbolic representation of conceptualizations of phenomena. Within a research context, the models that one is most likely to encounter are mathematic (or statistical) models and schematic models. These *models,* like conceptual frameworks, are constructed representations of some aspect of our environment. They use abstractions (i.e., concepts) as the building blocks, but they attempt to represent reality with a minimal use of words. A visual or symbolic representation of a theory or conceptual framework often helps to express abstract ideas in a more readily understandable or graphic form than the original conceptualization.

Schematic models are common and undoubtedly are familiar to all readers. A schematic model (also referred to as a *conceptual map*) represents the phenomena of interest figuratively. Concepts and the linkages between them are represented diagrammatically through the use of boxes, arrows, or other symbols. An example of a schematic model is presented in Figure 5-1. This model, known as the Health Promotion Model, is described by its developer as "a multivariate paradigm for explaining and predicting the health-promotion component of lifestyle" (Pender, Walker, Sechrist, & Frank-Stromborg, 1990, p. 326). Schematic models of this type can be useful in the research process in clarifying concepts and their associations, in enabling researchers to place a specific problem into an appropriate context, and in revealing areas where further inquiry is needed.

Statistical models are playing a growing role in research endeavors in nursing and related sciences. These models use symbols to express quantitatively the nature of relationships among variables. There are few relationships in the behavioral sciences that can be summarized as elegantly as in the mathematic model $F = ma$ (force = mass $\times$ acceleration). Because human behavior is so complex and subject to so many influences as yet poorly understood, it is typically possible to model it only in a probabilistic manner. This means that we are not able to develop equations, such as the example of force from mechanics, in which a human behavior can be simply described as the product of two other phenomena. What we can do, however, is describe the probability that a certain behavior or characteristic will exist, given the occurrence of other specified phenomena. This is the function of statistical models. An example of a statistical model is shown below:

$$Y = \beta_1 X_1 + \beta_2 X_2 + \beta_3 X_3 + \beta_4 X_4 + e$$

where Y = nursing effectiveness, as measured by a supervisor's evaluation

X_1 = nursing knowledge, as measured by a standardized test

X_2 = past achievement, as measured by grades in nursing school

X_3 = decision-making skills, as measured by number of nursing diagnoses made

X_4 = empathy, as measured by timing between the patient's request for pain medication and actual administration of pain medication

e = a residual, unexplained factor

$\beta_1, \beta_2, \beta_3,$ and β_4 = weights indicating the importance of $X_1, X_2, X_3,$ and X_4, respectively, in determining nursing effectiveness

Each term in this model is quantified or quantifiable; that is, every symbol can be re-

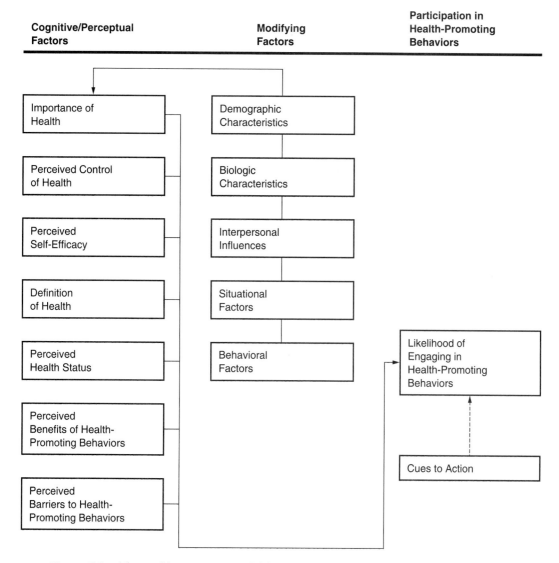

Figure 5-1. *The Health Promotion Model (Pender, N. J., Walker, S. N., Sechrist, K. R. & Frank-Stromborg, M. [1990]. Predicting health-promoting lifestyles in the workplace.* Nursing Research, 39, [331]).

placed by a numerical value, such as an individual's score on a standardized test of knowledge (X_1).

What does this equation mean and how does it work? This model constitutes a proposed mechanism for understanding and predicting nursing effectiveness. The model proposes that on-the-job effectiveness is affected primarily by four factors: the nursing knowledge, past achievement, decision-making skill, and empathy of the nurse. These influences are not presumed to be equally important. The weights (βs) associated with each factor represent a recipe for designating the relative importance of each. If empathy were much more important than past achievement, for example, then the weights might be 2 to 1, respectively (i.e., two parts empathy to one part past achievement). The *e* (or *error term*) at the end of the model represents all those unknown or unmeasurable other attributes that affect one's performance as a nurse. In the quantitative equation, *e* would be set equal to some constant value; it would not vary from one nurse to another because it really constitutes an unknown element in the equation. Once the values of the weights and *e* have been established (through statistical procedures), the model can be used to predict the nursing effectiveness of any nurse for whom we have gathered information on the four *X*s (standardized test scores and so forth). Our prediction of who will make an especially effective nurse will not always be perfectly accurate, in part because of the influence of those unknown factors summarized by *e*. Perfect forecasting is seldom attainable with probabilistic statistical models. However, such a model makes prediction of nursing effectiveness less haphazard than mere guesswork or intuition.

❖ THE NATURE OF THEORIES AND CONCEPTUAL FRAMEWORKS

Theories and conceptual frameworks have much in common, including their origin, general nature, purposes, and role in the research process. In this section, we examine some of the general characteristics of frameworks that provide contexts for nursing research. In this section, we use the term theory in its least restrictive sense.

Origin of Frameworks

Theories and conceptual frameworks are not discovered by researchers and scientists; they are created and invented by them. The building of a framework depends not only on the observable facts in our environment but also on the scientist's ingenuity in pulling those facts together and making sense of them. Thus, theory construction is a creative and intellectual en-

terprise that can be engaged in by anyone who has imagination, a solid base of knowledge, and the ability to knit together observations and existing knowledge into an intelligible pattern.

Tentative Nature of Frameworks

Theories and conceptual frameworks can never be proved or confirmed. A theory represents a scientist's best efforts to describe and explain phenomena; today's successful theory may be relegated to tomorrow's intellectual junk yard. This may happen if new evidence or observations discredit or undermine a previously well-accepted framework. It is also possible that a new theoretical system can integrate new observations with the observations on which the old theory was based and result in a more parsimonious explanation of the phenomena in question.

Theories and frameworks that are not congruent with a culture's values and philosophical orientation also may be discredited over time. It is not unusual for a theory to lose supporters because its implications are not in vogue. For example, psychoanalytic and structural social theories, which had widespread support for decades, have come to be challenged and revised as a result of the emergence of feminism and changes in society's views about the roles of women. This link between theory and values may surprise those who think of science as being completely objective. It should be remembered, however, that frameworks are deliberately invented by humans; thus, they can never be freed totally from the human perspective, which is amenable to change over time.

Thus, no framework or theory, no matter what its subject matter, can ever be considered final and verified. There always remains the possibility that a theory will be modified or discarded. Many theories in the physical sciences have received considerable empirical support, and their well-accepted propositions are often referred to as *laws,* such as Boyle's law of gases. Nevertheless, we have no way of knowing the ultimate accuracy and utility of any theory and should, therefore, treat all theories as tentative. This caveat is nowhere more relevant than in the emerging sciences such as nursing.

Purposes of Theories and Frameworks

Theoretical and conceptual frameworks play several interrelated roles in the progress of a science. Their overall purpose is to make scientific findings meaningful and generalizable. Theories allow scientists to knit together observations and facts into an orderly scheme. Frameworks are efficient mechanisms for drawing together and summarizing accumulated facts, sometimes from separate and isolated investigations. The linkage of findings into a coherent structure makes the body of accumulated knowledge more accessible and, thus, more useful both to practitioners who seek to implement findings and to researchers who seek to extend the knowledge base.

In addition to summarizing, theories and frameworks can guide the scientist's understanding of not only the *what* of natural phenomena but also the *why* of their occurrence. Theories often provide a basis for predicting the occurrence of phenomena. Prediction, in turn, has implications for the control of those phenomena. A utilitarian framework is one that has potential to bring about desirable changes in people's behavior or the environment.

Theories and conceptual frameworks help to stimulate research and the extension of knowledge by providing both direction and impetus. Many nursing studies have been generated explicitly to examine aspects of a conceptual model of nursing. Thus, frameworks may serve as a springboard for scientific advances.

Relationship Between Theory and Research

The relationship between theory and research is a reciprocal and mutually beneficial one. Frameworks are built inductively from observations, and an excellent source for those observations is prior scientific research. Concepts and relations that are validated in the empirical arena become the foundation for theory development. The theory, in turn, must be tested by subjecting deductions from it (hypotheses) to further scientific inquiry. Thus, research plays a dual and continuing role in theory building and testing. Theory guides and generates ideas for research; research assesses the worth of the theory and provides a foundation for new ones.

It would be unreasonable to assert that research without a specific theoretical framework cannot make a contribution to knowledge. In nursing research, many facts still need to be accumulated, and purely descriptive inquiries may well form the basis for subsequent theoretical developments. Research that does not test a theory can potentially be linked to a framework at a later time. However, although it is not always easy to place one's research problems into a theoretical context, it is advantageous for the advancement of nursing science to do so. Some suggestions for linking a study to a conceptual framework are presented later in this chapter.

❖ CONCEPTUAL FRAMEWORKS USED IN NURSING RESEARCH

Nurse researchers have used both nursing and nonnursing frameworks to provide a conceptual context for their studies. This section briefly summarizes several frameworks that have been found useful by nurse researchers.

Conceptual Models of Nursing

In the past few decades, nurses have formulated a number of conceptual frameworks and models of nursing practice. These models constitute formal explanations of what the nursing discipline is according to the model developer's point of view. As Fawcett (1989) has noted, four central concepts are central to models of nursing:

- Person
- Environment

- Health
- Nursing

The various conceptual models, however, define these concepts differently, link them in diverse ways, and give different emphasis to the relationships among them.

The conceptual models were not developed primarily as a base for nursing research. Indeed, these models have thus far had more impact on nursing education, administration, and clinical practice than on nursing research. Nevertheless, nurse researchers are turning increasingly toward these conceptual frameworks for their inspiration and theoretical foundations in formulating research questions and hypotheses. In this section, we briefly examine some of the major conceptual frameworks of nursing and give examples of research that claimed their intellectual roots in these models.

JOHNSON'S BEHAVIORAL SYSTEMS MODEL

Johnson's (1980) model focuses on a behavioral system (the patient), its subsystems, and its environment. According to this model, each individual behavioral system is a collection of seven interrelated subsystems (attachment, dependency, ingestion, elimination, sexuality, aggression, and achievement), the response patterns of which form an organized and integrated whole. Each subsystem carries out specialized tasks for the integrated system, and each is structured by four motivational elements: goal, set, choice, and action/behavior. The model is concerned primarily with behavioral functioning that results in the equilibrium of the integrated system. In Johnson's model, the function of nursing is to help restore the balance of each subsystem in the event of disequilibrium and to help prevent future system disturbances. Several researchers have designated Johnson's Behavioral Systems Model as their conceptual basis. For example, Holaday (1987) focused on Johnson's concept of behavioral set in her study of the vocal and visual interactions occurring between mothers and their chronically ill infants.

KING'S OPEN SYSTEM MODEL

King's conceptual model (1981) includes three types of dynamic, interacting systems: personal systems (represented by individuals); interpersonal systems (represented by such dyadic interactions as nurse–patient dialogue); and social systems (represented by larger institutions such as hospitals and families). The social system provides a context in which nurses work. Within King's model, the domain of nursing includes promoting, maintaining, and restoring health. Nursing is viewed as "a process of action, reaction, and interaction whereby nurse and client share information about their perceptions of the nursing situation" (King, 1981, p. 2). King herself (1981) conducted a descriptive observational study of nurse–client encounters that yielded a classification of elements in nurse–client interactions. The study provided preliminary support for the proposition that goal attainment was facilitated by accurate nurse–client perceptions, satisfactory communication, and mutual goal setting. Hanucharurnkui and Vinyanguag (1991) employed King's concept of goal attainment in their study of the effects of participation in self-care on postoperative recovery and satisfaction with care. Kemppainen (1990) used King's framework in her case study of a psychotic patient with HIV infection.

LEVINE'S CONSERVATION MODEL

Levine's (1973) model focuses on individuals as holistic beings, and the major area of concern for nurses is maintenance of the person's wholeness. The model identifies adaptation as the process by which the integrity or wholeness of individuals is maintained. Levine's model identifies several principles of conservation that aim to facilitate patients' adaptation processes. Through these principles, the model emphasizes the nurse's responsibility to maintain the client's integrity in the threat of assault through illness or environmental influences. Foreman (1989) categorized variables associated with confusion in the elderly according to

Levine's conservation principles. Schaefer and Potylycki (1993) based their study of fatigue associated with congestive heart failure on Levine's conservation model.

NEUMAN'S HEALTH CARE SYSTEMS MODEL

Neuman's (1989) model focuses on the person as a complete system, the subparts of which are interrelated physiologic, psychological, sociocultural, spiritual, and developmental factors. In this model, the person maintains balance and harmony between internal and external environments by adjusting to stress and by defending against tension-producing stimuli. Wellness is equated with equilibrium. The primary goal of nursing is to assist in the attainment and maintenance of client system stability. Nursing interventions include activities to strengthen flexible lines of defense, to strengthen resistance to stressors, and to maintain adaptation. Ross and Bourbonnais (1985) described the interpersonal, intrapersonal, and extrapersonal stressors identified in the home care of a man after a myocardial infarction. They developed nursing interventions directed toward strengthening the flexible lines of defense and resistance.

OREM'S MODEL OF SELF-CARE

Orem's (1985) model focuses on each individual's ability to perform self-care, defined as "the practice of activities that individuals initiate and perform on their own behalf in maintaining life, health, and well-being" (p. 35). One's ability to care for oneself is referred to as *self-care* agency, and the ability to care for others is referred to as *dependent-care* agency. In Orem's model, the goal of nursing is to help people meet their own therapeutic self-care demands. Orem identified three types of nursing systems: 1) wholly compensatory, wherein the nurse compensates for the patient's total inability to perform self-care activities; 2) partially compensatory, wherein the nurse compensates for the patient's partial inability to perform these activi-

ties; and 3) supportive–educative, wherein the nurse assists the patient in making decisions and acquiring skills and knowledge. Orem's Self-Care Model has generated considerable interest among nurse researchers. For example, Jirovec and Kasno (1993) studied the predictors of self-care abilities among the institutionalized elderly. Monsen (1992) compared the autonomy, coping styles, and self-care agency of healthy adolescents and adolescents with spina bifida. Hartweg (1993) studied the self-care actions that healthy middle-aged women perform to promote well-being.

PARSE'S MODEL OF MAN–LIVING–HEALTH

Parse's (1987) model views a human being as an open system freely able to choose from among a series of options in giving meaning to a situation. Humans and the environment remain independent entities during interchanges, and together they co-create meaning and patterns. The goal of the Man–Living–Health model in nursing practice is to encourage a client to share his or her thoughts and feelings about the meaning of a situation. The explication of the meaning changes the situation, and new meaning occurs. As new meanings arise, the patterns co-created by client and environment change. Clients may then be guided to plan for change from the known health patterns to new health patterns. The Parse framework is a relatively young one but has already generated several applications in the research literature, particularly among qualitative researchers. For example, Banonis (1989) relied on the Parse model in her study of the experience of recovering from an addiction. Smith (1990) used the Parse framework for exploring the experience of struggling through a difficult time among people who are unemployed.

ROGERS' MODEL OF THE UNITARY PERSON

Rogers' model (1970, 1986) focuses on the individual as a unified whole in constant interaction with the environment. The unitary person is viewed as an energy field that is more than, as well as different from, the sum of the biologic, physical, social, and psychological parts. In Rogers' model, nursing is concerned with the unitary person as a synergistic phenomenon. Nursing science is devoted to the study of the nature and direction of unitary human development. Nursing practice helps individuals achieve maximum well-being within their potential. Schodt (1989) applied Rogers' principle of integrality in her study of the nature of interactions between fathers and their unborn children. Alligood (1991) tested Rogers' principle of accelerating change in her study of the relationships among creativity, actualization, and empathy over the life course.

ROY'S ADAPTATION MODEL

In Roy's Adaptation Model (1984, 1991), humans are biopsychosocial adaptive systems who cope with environmental change through the process of adaptation. Within the human system, there are four subsystems: physiologic needs; self-concept; role function; and interdependence. These subsystems constitute adaptive modes that provide mechanisms for coping with environmental stimuli and change. The goal of nursing, according to this model, is to promote patient adaptation during health and illness. Nursing also regulates stimuli affecting adaptation. Nursing interventions generally take the form of increasing, decreasing, modifying, removing, or maintaining internal and external stimuli that affect adaptation. Roy's model has provided a conceptual framework for many nursing studies. Based on Roy's concepts, Christian (1993) studied the relationship between women's symptoms of endometriosis and self-esteem. Fawcett and Weiss (1993) used Roy's adaptation principles in their study of cross-cultural adaptation to cesarean birth. Samarel and Fawcett (1992) developed an innovative approach to cancer support groups based on the Roy Adaptation Model.

Other Models Used by Nurse Researchers

Many of the phenomena in which nurse researchers are interested involve concepts that are not unique to nurses, and therefore their studies are sometimes linked to conceptual frameworks that are not models of nursing. Three conceptual models that have frequently been used in nursing research investigations are the Health Belief Model (HBM), the Health Promotion Model (HPM), and Lazarus' Model of Stress and Coping. These models—and examples of nursing studies that were based on them—are briefly described next.

THE HEALTH BELIEF MODEL

The HBM has become a popular conceptual framework in nursing, especially in studies focusing on patient compliance and preventive health care practices. The model postulates that health-seeking behavior is influenced by a person's perception of a threat posed by a health problem and the value associated with actions aimed at reducing the threat (Becker, 1978). The major components of the HBM include perceived susceptibility, perceived severity, perceived benefits and costs, motivation, and enabling or modifying factors. Perceived susceptibility refers to a person's perception that a health problem is personally relevant or that a diagnosis of illness is accurate. Even when one recognizes personal susceptibility, action will not occur unless the individual perceives the severity to be high enough to have serious organic or social implications. Perceived benefits refer to the patients' beliefs that a given treatment will cure the illness or help prevent it, and perceived costs refer to the complexity, duration, and accessibility of the treatment. Motivation includes the desire to comply with a treatment and the belief that people should do what is prescribed by health care personnel. Among the modifying factors that have been identified are personality variables, patient satisfaction, and sociodemographic factors. Nurse researchers have used the HBM in connection with studies of women's practice of breast self-examination (Wyper, 1990; Champion & Scott, 1993), women's decisions regarding estrogen replacement therapy (Logothetis, 1991), and gender differences in leisure-time physical exercise (Hawkes & Holm, 1993).

THE HEALTH PROMOTION MODEL

The theoretical work of Becker has been extended by Pender (1987), whose model focuses on explaining health-promoting behaviors. A major difference between the two models is that the HPM uses a wellness orientation; the threat of disease is not identified as a determinant of a person's health-promoting behavior. According to the model, a schematic model of which is shown in Figure 5-1, *health promotion* is defined as activities directed toward the development of resources that maintain or enhance an individual's well-being. The HPM encompasses two phases: a decision-making phase and an action phase. In the decision-making phase, the model emphasizes seven cognitive–perceptual factors that compose primary motivational mechanisms for acquisition and maintenance of health-promoting behaviors (e.g., perceived barriers to health-promoting behaviors) and five modifying factors that indirectly influence patterns of health behavior (e.g., situational influences). In the action phase, both barriers and cues to action trigger activity in health-promoting behavior. According to the model, people move back and forth in a reciprocal fashion between the two phases. Nurse researchers have applied the HPM to study the determinants of exercise and aerobic fitness among outpatients with arthritis (Neuberger, Kasal, Smith, Hassanein, & DeViney, 1994), the effect of health-promoting behaviors on life satisfaction among elderly African Americans (Foster, 1992), and factors predictive of health-promoting lifestyles among people with disabilities (Stuifbergen & Becker, 1994). A more

detailed example of a study using this model is presented at the end of this chapter.

LAZARUS' STRESS AND COPING MODEL

Lazarus' model (Lazarus, 1966; Folkman & Lazarus, 1988) represents an effort to explain people's methods of dealing with stress, that is, environmental and internal demands that tax or exceed a person's resources and endanger his or her well-being. The model posits that coping strategies are learned, deliberate responses to stressors that are used to adapt to or change the stressors. According to this model, a person's perception of mental and physical health is related to the ways he or she evaluates and copes with the stresses of living. Many nurses have conducted research within the context of this model, including studies of coping effectiveness in postmyocardial infarction patients (Bennett, 1993), stress and coping among family members responsible for a nursing home placement (Kammer, 1994), coping and emotional stress associated with artificial insemination (Prattke & Gass-Sternas, 1993), and coping and adaptation to chronic illness (White, Richter, & Fry, 1992).

❖ TESTING, USING, AND DEVELOPING A THEORY OR FRAMEWORK

In a previous section, we described the strong interrelationship between theory and research. The manner in which theory and conceptual frameworks are used by researchers is elaborated on in the following section. In the discussion, the term theory is used in its broadest sense. In other words, the procedures discussed are almost always equally applicable to conceptual frameworks and models as well as to formal theories.

Testing a Theory

As noted earlier, theories often stimulate new research investigations. For example, a nurse might read several papers relating to Orem's Self-Care Model. As the nurse's reading progresses, the following types of conjectures might arise: "If Orem's self-care model is valid, then one might expect that nursing effectiveness can be enhanced in environments more conducive to self-care (e.g., a birthing room versus a delivery room)" or "Given this conceptual framework, it might be expected that the dependency level of patients (in terms of either their physical or psychologic characteristics) would influence the nature and intensity of effective interventions." These conjectures, derived from a theory or conceptual framework, can serve as a point of departure for testing the adequacy of the theory.

In testing a theory, the researcher deduces implications (as in the preceding example) and develops research hypotheses. These hypotheses are predictions about the manner in which variables would be related, if the theory were correct and useful. The hypotheses are then subjected to empirical testing through systematic research. A theory is never tested directly. It is the hypotheses deduced from a theory that are subjected to scientific investigations.

Comparisons between the observed outcomes of research and the relationships predicted by the hypotheses are the major focus of the testing process. Through this process, the theory is continually subjected to potential disconfirmation. Repeated failures of research endeavors to disconfirm a theory result in increasing support for and acceptance of a theoretical position. The testing process continues until pieces of evidence cannot be interpreted within the context of the theory but *can* be explained by a new theory that also accounts for all previous findings. From the point of view of theory testing, the goals of a serviceable research project are to devise logically adequate deductions from theory, to develop a research design that reduces the credibility of alternative explanations for observed relationships, and to select methods that assess the theory's validity under maximally heterogeneous situations so that potentially competing theories can be ruled out.

Testing Two Competing Theories

Researchers who directly test two competing theories to explain some phenomenon are in a particularly good position to advance scientific knowledge. Almost all phenomena can be explained in alternative ways, as suggested by the alternative conceptual models of nursing. There are also competing theories for such phenomena as stress, compliance, child development, learning, and grieving. All these phenomena are of great importance to nursing. Each competing theory for these phenomena suggests alternative approaches to facilitating a positive outcome or minimizing a negative one. It is therefore important to know which explanation has more validity, if we are to design maximally effective nursing interventions.

Typically, researchers have opted to test a single theory in a research investigation. Then, to evaluate the worth of competing theories, they must compare the results of different studies. However, such comparisons are often difficult to make because study designs rarely lend themselves to direct comparisons. For example, one study of stress might use a sample of college students, another might use military personnel in a combat situation, and yet another might use terminally ill cancer patients. Each of these studies might use an alternative approach to measuring stress. If the results of these studies support alternative theories of stress to different degrees, it would be difficult to know the extent to which the results reflected differences in the study design rather than differences in the validity of the theories.

The researcher who directly tests two (or more) competing theories, using a single sample of subjects and comparable measures of the key research variables, is in a position to make powerful and meaningful comparisons. Such a study typically requires considerable advance planning and the inclusion of a wider array of measures than would otherwise be the case, but such efforts are to be commended. In recent years, a growing number of nursing investigators have used this approach to generate and refine our knowledge base and to provide promising new leads for further research. For example, Campbell (1989) tested a "grief model" and a "learned helplessness" model to explain women's responses to battering. She found that both theories had some support, but that the "learned helplessness" concepts had not been sufficiently operationalized in her study and required further investigation. Mahon and Yarcheski (1992) tested two alternative explanations for loneliness in adolescents: an explanation dependent on situational factors, and one linking loneliness to characterological or personality traits. The findings suggested that the situational explanation had substantially more support for older adolescents than for younger ones.

Fitting a Problem to a Theory

The preceding sections addressed the situation in which a researcher begins with one or more specific theories or conceptual frameworks and uses the theories as the basis for developing a research problem and design. Circumstances sometimes arise in which the problem is formulated before consideration is given to a theoretical framework. Even in such situations, researchers may wish to (or may be required to) devise a theoretical context in an effort to enrich the value and interpretability of their inquiry. Although we recognize that this situation sometimes occurs, we must nevertheless caution that an after-the-fact linkage of theory to a research question is usually considerably less meaningful than the testing of a particular theory of interest. This is especially true for neophyte researchers who may lack a thorough grounding in the theoretical positions of their own or related disciplines.

The search for relevant existing theories can be greatly facilitated by first conceptualizing on a sufficiently abstract level what the nature of the problem is. For example, take the research question, "Do daily telephone conversations between a psychiatric nurse and a patient for 2 weeks following discharge from the hospital result in lower rates of readmission by short-term

psychiatric patients?" This is a relatively concrete research problem but might profitably be viewed as a subproblem for Orem's Self-Care Model, for a theory of reinforcement, a theory of social influence, or a theory of crisis resolution. Part of the difficulty in finding a theory is that a single phenomenon of interest can be conceptualized in a number of ways and, depending on the manner chosen, may refer the researcher to conceptual schemes from a wide range of disciplines.

Once the researcher has conceptualized the research problem on an abstract level, the search for a suitable framework can proceed. Textbooks, handbooks, and encyclopedias in the chosen discipline usually are a good starting point for the identification of a framework. These sources usually summarize the status of a theoretical position and document the efforts to confirm and disconfirm it. Journal articles contain more current information but are usually restricted to descriptions of specific studies rather than to broad expositions or evaluations of theories. When a theoretical position has been developed at length or has been supported by extensive empirical observations, entire books may be devoted to its description.

Once a potential conceptual framework has been identified, its utility should be carefully evaluated in terms of its congruity with the problem to be studied and its congruity with the researcher's own philosophy and world view. If the framework is judged to be adequate on these grounds, it then becomes the researcher's job to design the study in such a way that it fits the framework.

The task of fitting a problem to a theory should be done with caution. It is true that having a theoretical context enhances the meaningfulness of a research study, but artificially cramming a problem into a theory is not the route to scientific utility. There are many published studies that purport to have a conceptual framework when in fact the post hoc nature of the conceptualization is all too evident. If a conceptual framework is really linked to a research problem, then the design of the study, the selection of appropriate data collection strategies, the data analysis, and (especially) the interpretation of the findings *flow* from that conceptualization. We advocate a balanced and reasoned perspective on this issue: *Researchers should not shirk their intellectual duties by failing to make an attempt to link their problem to broader theoretical concerns, but there is no point in fabricating such a link when it does not exist.*

Developing a Framework

Many beginning researchers may think of themselves as unqualified to develop a theory or conceptual scheme of their own. But theory development depends much less on one's knowledge of research methods and experience in the conduct of investigations than on one's powers of observation, understanding of a problem, and readings about a substantive issue. There is, therefore, nothing to prevent an imaginative and sensitive person from formulating an original conceptual framework for a study. The conceptual scheme may or may not be a full-fledged formal theory with well-articulated postulates; the scheme should, however, place the issues of the study into some broader perspective. In the field of nursing research, in which there has not yet been extensive theoretical work, the beginning researcher may have an easier task in devising an original framework than in finding one that is appropriate for the problem of interest.

The basic intellectual process underlying theory development is *induction,* which refers to the process of reasoning from particular observations and facts to generalizations. The inductive process involves integrating what one has experienced or learned into some concise and general conclusion. If one has observed that Morgan P., Brooke L., Shanley I., and Daniel S. (all of whom are tonsillectomy patients) have refused to eat their first postoperative meal, one might conclude that loss of appetite characterizes those who have just had a tonsillectomy operation. The observations used in the inductive

process need not be personal observations; they may be (and often are in formal theories) the findings and conclusions from research investigations. When relationships among variables are arrived at this way, one has the makings of a theory that can be put to a more rigorous scientific test. The first step in theory development, then, is to formulate a generalized scheme of relevant concepts, that is, to perform a conceptual analysis. The product of this step should be a conceptual framework, whose worth can be assessed through the collection of empirical information.

Let us consider the following simple example. Suppose that we were interested in understanding the factors influencing enrollment in a prenatal education program. We might begin by considering two basic sets of forces: those that promote enrollment and those that hinder it. After reviewing the literature, discussing the problem with colleagues, and developing ideas from our own experiences, we might arrive at a conceptual scheme such as the one presented in Figure 5-2. This framework is undoubtedly incomplete and imperfect, but it does allow us to study a number of research questions *and* to place those problems in perspective. For example, the conceptual scheme suggests that as the availability of social supports declines, the obstacles to participation in a prenatal education program increase. We might then make the following hypothesis: "Single pregnant women are less likely to participate in a prenatal education program than married pregnant women," on the assumption that husbands are an important source of social support to women in their pregnancy.

Many nursing studies involve a conceptual framework developed by the researchers. For example, Ferrell, Rhiner, Cohen, and Grant (1991) evolved a conceptual model, guided by findings from their own previous research, to explain the impact of pain on a person's overall quality of life. Janson-Bjerklie, Ferketich, and Benner (1993) tested their own conceptual model to predict psychosocial and morbidity outcomes in adults with chronic asthma.

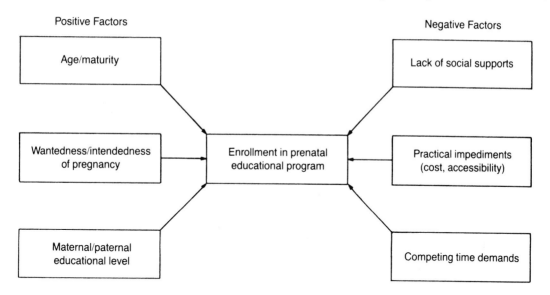

Figure 5-2. *Conceptual model—factors that influence enrollment in a prenatal education program*

Theoretical Contexts and Nursing Research

Theory and research have reciprocal, beneficial ties. Fawcett (1978) described the relationship between theory and research as a double helix, with theory as the impetus of scientific investigations and findings from research shaping the development of theory. However, this relationship has not always characterized the progress of nursing science. Many have criticized nurse researchers for producing numerous pieces of isolated research that are not placed in a theoretical context.

This criticism was more justified a decade ago than it is today. Many researchers are developing studies on the basis of conceptual models of nursing. Nursing science is still struggling, however, to integrate accumulated knowledge within theoretical systems. This struggle is reflected, in part, in the number of controversies surrounding the issue of theoretical frameworks in nursing.

One of these controversies concerns whether there should be one single, unified model of nursing or multiple, competing models. Fawcett (1989) has argued against combining different models, noting that "before all nurses follow the same path, the competition of multiple models is needed to determine the superiority of one or more of them" (p. 9). Research can play a critical role in testing the utility and validity of alternative nursing models.

Another controversy involves the desirability and utility of developing theories unique to nursing. Some commentators argue that theories relating to humans developed in other disciplines, such as physiology, psychology, and sociology (so-called *borrowed theories*), can and should be applied to nursing problems. Others advocate the development of unique nursing theories, claiming that only through such development can knowledge to guide nursing practice be produced.

Until these controversies are resolved, nursing research is likely to continue on its current path of conducting studies within a multidisciplinary and multitheoretical perspective. We are inclined to see the use of multiple frameworks as a healthy and unavoidable part of the development of nursing science.

❖ TIPS ON USING FRAMEWORKS IN NURSING STUDIES

Most published nursing studies are not explicitly linked to a conceptual framework or theory—despite the widespread acknowledgment that research without theory often undermines the utility of the knowledge gained. In this section, we offer some suggestions on how to strengthen the conceptual basis of nursing studies.

- Although most nursing studies are not theory-driven, virtually all studies have an unacknowledged conceptual basis. Concepts (which become research variables) are by definition abstractions of observable phenomena, and our world view and views on nursing shape how those concepts are defined and operationalized. What often happens, however, is that researchers fail to clarify the conceptual underpinnings of their research variables, thereby making it more difficult to integrate research findings. Consider, for example, the concept of *caring*. Caring can be conceptualized as a human trait, a moral ideal, an affect, an interaction, or an intervention (Morse, Solberg, Neander, Bottorff, & Johnson, 1990). A researcher undertaking a study concerned with caring should make clear which perspective on caring he or she has adopted. Thus, even if you are not testing a specific theory, it is wise to clarify the conceptual perspective you have on key constructs.
- If you begin with a research problem and are trying to identify a suitable conceptual framework, it is probably wise to confer with others—especially with people who may be familiar with a broad range of theoretical perspectives. By having an open discussion, you are more likely to become aware of your own conceptual perspectives and are thus in a better position to identify an appropriate framework.
- It is often suggested that a theory first be evaluated before it is used as a basis for a research project—a suggestion that may be dif-

ficult for many beginning researchers. However, some basic evaluative criteria are fairly easy to apply, including the following:

Is the theory one that has significance—that is, does it address a problem of particular interest to nurses or society?

Does the theory offer the possibility of explaining or systematically describing some phenomenon?

Is the theory testable—that is, can the concepts be observed and measured, and can hypotheses be deduced?

For the advanced student, Stevens (1984), Chinn and Jacobs (1991), and Fawcett and Downs (1992) present more extensive and more rigorous criteria for assessing conceptual frameworks in nursing.

- If you begin with a research question and then subsequently identify an appropriate framework, be willing to adapt or augment your original research problem as you gain greater understanding of the framework. The linking of theory and research question often requires an iterative approach.
- If you are basing your study on a specific theory or conceptual framework, be sure to read about the theory from a primary source. It is important to understand fully the conceptual perspective of the theorist. If this perspective is not congruent with your own, it may be that an alternative theory or framework would be more appropriate.
- It may also be very useful to read research reports of other studies that were based on the selected framework—even if the research problem is not similar to your own. By reading other studies, you will be better able to judge how much empirical support the theory has received and perhaps how the theory should be adapted.
- Once you have identified an appropriate framework, it is important to strive for maximal congruity between the theory and its components, the research problem and hypotheses, the definition and operationalization of the concepts, and the selection of re-

search design. If you are really testing the utility of the framework, the framework should drive many of your research decisions as well as your interpretation of the findings.

additional examples of nursing studies that used other less widely used frameworks as their conceptual bases. A study based on the Health Promotion Model is described in greater detail next.

❖ *RESEARCH EXAMPLES*

Throughout this chapter, we have described studies that used various widely used conceptual and theoretical models. Table 5-1 provides

Pender and her colleagues (1990) used the HPM to predict health-promoting lifestyles among employees enrolled in six employer-sponsored health-promotion programs. The researchers noted that when workplace health promotion programs are initially introduced, employee enrollment tends to be

Table 5-1.   *Examples of Other Theories and Models Used by Nurse Researchers*

RESEARCH QUESTION	THEORY OR MODEL
To what extent is regimen compliance behavior among hypertensive patients influenced by intention to comply, attitude, perceived beliefs of others, and motivation to comply? (Miller, Wikoff, & Hiatt, 1992)	Theory of Reasoned Action (Fishbein)
What are the relative contributions of positive outcome expectancies, smoking to cope, general coping skills, and nicotine intake in predicting nicotine dependence among African American women cigarette smokers? (Ahijevych & Wewers, 1993)	Social Learning Theory (Bandura)
To what extent do health experiences, family functioning, self-esteem, intrinsic motivation, and health perception explain the positive health behaviors of preadolescent children? (Farrand & Cox, 1993)	Interaction Model of Client Health Behavior (Cox)
What are the behaviors of first-born children before and after the birth of a sibling? (Gullicks & Crase, 1993)	Attachment Theory (Bowlby)
What is the value of nurse caring behaviors as perceived by patients in different triage categories in an emergency department? (Huggins, Gandy, & Kohut, 1993)	Care Theory (Watson)
What is the relationship between physical health and psychological well-being in elderly women? (Heidrich, 1993)	Life-span Development and Aging (Ryff)
What is the relationship between uncertainty and coping after coronary bypass surgery? (Redeker, 1992)	Uncertainty in Illness Theory (Mishel)
To what extent do social context, disease-related stressors, coping, and social support explain levels of strain in the caregivers of patients receiving chemotherapy? (Schumacher, Dodd, & Paul, 1993)	Stress Process Model (Pearlin)

high. However, over time, erratic participation and a high dropout rate tend to characterize many such programs, a situation that concerns both the employers and the health professionals responsible for operating the programs.

Pender and her co-researchers noted that most studies of the determinants of healthy lifestyles have used a prevention-oriented model in which fear of the consequences of illness are viewed as the primary motivation for health-related behavior. In contrast, these researchers used a wellness-oriented framework, the HPM, in their investigation. The model tested by this team of researchers is shown in Figure 5-1. The arrows in this figure denote the hypothesized direction of causal influences. The model includes seven cognitive/perceptual factors that are hypothesized to be influenced by five modifying factors. The cognitive/perceptual factors, which are viewed as directly affecting participation in health-promoting behaviors, are considered to be amenable to change—an important feature of factors proposed as a basis for the design of interventions to promote healthy lifestyles. These seven factors are as follows:

- *Importance of health*—the value placed on health in relation to other personal values
- *Perceived control of health*—the perception of whether health is self-determined, influenced by powerful others, or the result of chance factors
- *Perceived self-efficacy*—the belief that one has the competence and skills to carry out specific actions
- *Definition of health*—the personal meaning of health to each individual
- *Perceived health status*—the self-evaluation of current health as a subjective state
- *Perceived benefits of health-promoting behavior*—the perceived desirability of behavioral outcomes
- *Perceived barriers to health-promoting behaviors*—the perceived hindrances to taking action

Pender and her colleagues tested the utility of the HPM in explaining health-promot-

ing lifestyles among employees who had enrolled in a workplace health promotion program (thereby suggesting an intent to change their health habits) but who varied greatly in their level of participation in the program. With a sample of nearly 600 subjects, the researchers assessed each of the cognitive/perceptual factors as well as several of the modifying factors. The dependent variable, participation in health-promoting behaviors, was measured by the Health-Promoting Lifestyle Profile, a 48-question scale focusing on such behaviors as health responsibility, exercise, nutrition, and stress management.

The findings provided some support for the HPM model. In particular, perceptions of control of health, personal efficacy, definition of health, and health status emerged as a constellation of HPM constructs most closely associated with health-promoting lifestyle behaviors among employees enrolled in a worksite health-promotion program. However, other hypothesized factors (e.g., valuing health) were not significant determinants of a health-promoting lifestyle.

❖ SUMMARY

Theoretical and conceptual frameworks provide an important context for a scientific investigation. In its least restrictive sense, a theory is a broad and abstract characterization of some phenomenon. According to this broad definition, a theory can be descriptive—that is, it can describe or classify dimensions of phenomena by summarizing abstract commonalities. As classically defined, however, a *theory* is an abstract generalization that systematically explains the relationships among phenomena.

The basic components of a theory are concepts. In its classical sense, theories consist of a set of statements, each of which expresses a relationship among the concepts. The statements are arranged in a logically interrelated system that permits new statements to be derived from them. Theories vary in their level of generality and level of complexity. Some theories attempt to describe large segments of the environment and are called *grand theories* or *macrotheories,* whereas other theories are more restricted in scope. Theories that are more specific to certain phenomena are sometimes referred to as *middle-range theories.*

Conceptual frameworks or *schemes* are less fully developed attempts at organizing phenomena than are theories. Concepts are the basic elements of a conceptual scheme, as in theories. However, in a conceptual framework, the concepts are not linked to one another in a logically ordered deductive system. Much of the conceptual work in nursing is more rightfully described as conceptual schemes than as theories. Conceptual frameworks are highly valuable in that they often serve as the springboard for theory development.

Models are symbolic representations of phenomena. Models depict a theory or conceptual scheme through the use of symbols or diagrams. Two types of models frequently used in research are mathematic or *statistical models* and *schematic models* (or *conceptual maps*). Models are useful to scientists because they use a minimal amount of words, which tend to be ambiguous, in representing reality.

The overall objective of theories and frameworks is to make scientific findings meaningful and generalizable. In addition, they help to summarize existing knowledge into coherent systems and stimulate new research by providing both direction and impetus. Theories and conceptual frameworks are created or developed by scientists. Their creation requires imagination on the part of the scientist and congruence with reality and existing knowledge. All theories and frameworks are considered tentative and are never proved.

Nursing research is increasingly drawing on conceptual frameworks and models in its efforts to integrate accumulated knowledge and advance nursing science. Many investigations are based on *borrowed theories* from other disciplines (such as the Health Belief Model), but an increasing number of studies have conceptual models of nursing as their frameworks.

Among the major conceptual models of nursing are Johnson's Behavioral System Model, King's Interacting Systems Model, Levine's Conservation Model, Neuman's Health Care Systems Model, Orem's Self-Care Model, Parse's Model of Man–Living–Health, Rogers' Model of the Unitary Human Being, and Roy's Adaptation Model.

Conceptual schemes and theories can be integrated with empirical research in a number of ways. The investigator may design a scientific study specifically to test a theory of interest or to test two or more competing theories. In other situations, a problem may be developed first and a theory selected to fit the problem. An after-the-fact selection of a theory usually is more problematic and less meaningful than the systematic testing of a particular theory.

❖ *STUDY SUGGESTIONS*

Chapter 5 of the accompanying *Study Guide for Nursing Research: Principles and Methods, 5th ed.,* offers various exercises and study suggestions for reinforcing the concepts presented in this chapter. Additionally, the following study questions can be addressed:

1. Read the following article:
    Salazar, M. K., & Carter, W. B. (1993). Evaluation of breast self-examination beliefs using a decision model. *Western Journal of Nursing Research, 15,* 403–418.

    What theoretical basis does the author develop for health conception and health behavior choice? Would you classify the theoretical basis as a theory or as a conceptual framework? Draw a schematic model of the major concepts used in the study.

2. Select one of the nursing conceptual frameworks or models described in this chapter. Formulate a research question and two hypotheses that could be used to empirically test the utility of the conceptual framework or model in nursing practice.

3. Four researchable problems are as follows:
   a. What is the relationship between angina pain and alcohol intake?
   b. What effect does rapid weight gain during the second trimester have on the outcome of pregnancy?
   c. Do multiple hospital readmissions affect the achievement level of children?
   d. To what extent do coping mechanisms of individuals differ in health and illness?

   Abstract a generalized issue or issues for each of these problems. Search for an existing theory that might be applicable and appropriate.

❖ SUGGESTED READINGS

THEORETICAL REFERENCES

Andrews, H. A., & Roy, C. (1986). *Essentials of the Roy Adaptation Model.* Norwalk, CT: Appleton-Century-Crofts.

Batey, M. V. (1977). Conceptualization: Knowledge and logic guiding empirical research. *Nursing Research, 26,* 324–329.

Becker, M. (1978). The Health Belief Model and sick role behavior. *Nursing Digest, 6,* 35–40.

Chinn, P. L., & Jacobs, M. (1991). *Theory and nursing: A systematic approach* (3rd ed.). St. Louis: C. V. Mosby.

Craig, S. L. (1980). Theory development and its relevance for nursing. *Journal of Advanced Nursing, 5,* 349–355.

Fawcett, J. (1978). The relationship between theory and research: A double helix. *Advances in Nursing Science, 1,* 49–62.

Fawcett, J. (1989). *Analysis and evaluation of conceptual models of nursing* (2nd ed.). Philadelphia: F. A. Davis.

Fawcett, J., & Downs, F. (1992). *The relationship between theory and research.* (2nd ed.). Philadelphia: F. A. Davis.

Flaskerud, J. H. (1984). Nursing models as conceptual frameworks for research. *Western Journal of Nursing Research, 6,* 153–155.

Flaskerud, J. H., & Halloran, E. J. (1980). Areas of agreement in nursing theory development. *Advances in Nursing Science, 3,* 1–7.

Folkman, S., & Lazarus, R. S. (1988). Coping as a mediator of emotion. *Journal of Personality and Social Psychology, 54,* 466–475.

Hardy, M. E. (1974). Theories: Components, development, evaluation. *Nursing Research, 23,* 100–107.

Homans, G. C. (1964). Contemporary theory in sociology. In R. E. L. Farris (Ed.), *Handbook of modern sociology* (pp. 951–977). Chicago: Rand McNally.

Hurley, B. A. (1979). Why a theoretical framework in nursing research? *Western Journal of Nursing Research, 1,* 28–41.

Johnson, D. E. (1980). The Behavioral System Model for nursing. In J. P. Riehl, & C. Roy (Eds.), *Conceptual models for nursing practice* (2nd ed.). Norwalk, CT: Appleton-Century-Crofts.

King, I. M. (1981). *A theory for nursing: Systems, concepts, and process.* New York: John Wiley and Sons.

Lazarus, R. (1966). *Psychological stress and the coping response.* New York: McGraw-Hill.

Levine, M. E. (1973). *Introduction to clinical nursing* (2nd ed.). Philadelphia: F. A. Davis.

Marriner-Tomey, A. (1993). *Nursing theorists and their work* (3rd ed.). St. Louis: C. V. Mosby.

McFarlane, E. A. (1980). Nursing theory: The comparison of four theoretical proposals (King, Rogers, Roy, Orem). *Journal of Advanced Nursing, 5,* 3–19.

Morse, J. M., Solberg, S. M., Neander, W. L., Bottorff, J. L., & Johnson, J. L. (1990). Concepts of caring and caring as a concept. *Advances in Nursing Science, 13,* 1–14.

Neuman, B. (1989). *The Neuman systems model* (2nd ed.). Norwalk, CT: Appleton & Lange.

Orem, D. E. (1985). *Concepts of practice* (3rd ed.). New York: McGraw-Hill.

Parse, R. R. (1987). *Nursing science: Major paradigms, theories, and critiques.* Philadelphia: W. B. Saunders.

Pender, N. (1987). *Health promotion in nursing practice* (2nd ed.). Norwalk, CT: Appleton & Lange.

Rogers, M. E. (1970). *An introduction to the theoretical basis of nursing.* Philadelphia: F. A. Davis.

Rogers, M. E. (1986). Science of unitary human beings. In V. Malinski (Ed.), *Explorations on Martha Rogers' science of unitary human-beings.* Norwalk, CT: Appleton-Century-Crofts.

Roy, C. (1984). *Introduction to nursing: An adaptation model* (2nd ed.). Englewood Cliffs, NJ: Prentice-Hall.

Roy, C. Sr., & Andrews, H. (1991). *The Roy adaptation model: The definitive statement.* Norwalk, CT: Appleton & Lange.

Sandelowski, M. (1993). Theory unmasked: The uses and guises of theory in qualitative research. *Research in Nursing and Health, 16,* 213–218.

Selye, H. (1978). *The stress of life* (2nd ed.). New York: McGraw-Hill.

Stevens, B. J. (1984). *Nursing theory: Analysis, application, evaluation* (2nd ed.). Boston: Little, Brown.

SUBSTANTIVE REFERENCES

Ahijevych, K., & Wewers, M. E. (1993). Factors associated with nicotine dependence among African American women cigarette smokers. *Research in Nursing and Health, 16,* 283–292.

Alligood, M. R. (1991). Testing Rogers's theory of accelerating change: The relationships among creativity, actualization, and empathy in persons 18 to 92 years of age. *Western Journal of Nursing Research, 13,* 84–96.

Banonis, B. C. (1989). The lived experience of recovering from addiction. *Nursing Science Quarterly, 2,* 37–47.

Bennett, S. J. (1993). Relationships among selected antecedent variables and coping effectiveness in postmyocardial infarction patients. *Research in Nursing and Health, 16,* 131–139.

Campbell, J. C. (1989). A test of two explanatory models of women's responses to battering. *Nursing Research, 38,* 18–24.

Champion, V., & Scott, C. (1993). Effects of a procedural/belief intervention on breast self-examination practices. *Research in Nursing and Health, 16,* 163–170.

Christian, A. (1993). The relationship between women's symptoms of endometriosis and self-esteem. *Journal of Obstetric, Gynecologic and Neonatal Nursing, 22,* 370–376.

Erickson, H., & Swain, M. A. (1982). A model for assessing potential adaptation to stress. *Research in Nursing and Health, 5,* 93–101.

Farrand, L. L., & Cox, C. L. (1993). Determinants of positive health behavior in middle childhood. *Nursing Research, 42,* 208–213.

Fawcett, J., & Weiss, M. E. (1993). Cross-cultural adaptation to cesarean birth. *Western Journal of Nursing Research, 15,* 282–294.

Ferrell, B. R., Rhiner, M., Cohen, M. Z., & Grant, M. (1991). Pain as a metaphor for illness. Part I: Impact of cancer pain on family caregivers. *Oncology Nursing Forum, 18,* 1303–1309.

Foreman, M. D. (1989). Confusion in the hospitalized elderly: Incidence, onset, and associated factors. *Research in Nursing and Health, 12,* 21–29.

Foster, M. F. (1992). Health promotion and life satisfaction in elderly black adults. *Western Journal of Nursing Research, 14,* 444–463.

Gullicks, J. N., & Crase, S. J. (1993). Sibling behavior with a newborn: Parents' expectations and observations. *Journal of Obstetric, Gynecologic and Neonatal Nursing, 22,* 438–444.

Hanucharurnkui, S., & Vinya-nguag, P. (1991). Effects of promoting patients' participation in self-care on postoperative recovery and satisfaction with care. *Nursing Science Quarterly, 4,* 14–20.

Hartweg, D. L. (1993). Self-care actions of healthy middle-aged women to promote well-being. *Nursing Research, 42,* 221–227.

Hawkes, J. M., & Holm, K. (1993). Gender differences in exercise determinants. *Nursing Research, 42,* 166–172.

Heidrich, S. M. (1993). The relationship between physical health and psychological well-being in elderly women: A developmental perspective. *Research in Nursing and Health, 16,* 123–130.

Henneman, E. A. (1989). Effect of nursing contact on the stress response of patients being weaned from mechanical ventilation. *Heart and Lung, 18,* 483–489.

Holaday, B. (1987). Patterns of interaction between mothers and their chronically ill infants. *Maternal-Child Nursing Journal, 16,* 29–45.

Huggins, K. N., Gandy, W. M., & Kohut, C. D. (1993). Emergency department patients' perception of nurse caring behaviors. *Heart and Lung, 22,* 356–364.

Janson-Bjerklie, S., Ferketich, S., & Benner, P. (1993). Predicting the outcomes of living with asthma. *Research in Nursing and Health, 16,* 241–250.

Jirovec, M. M., & Kasno, J. (1993). Predictors of self-care abilities among the institutionalized elderly. *Western Journal of Nursing Research, 15,* 314–323.

Kammer, C. H. (1994). Stress and coping of family members resposnsible for nursing home placement. *Research in Nursing and Health, 17,* 89–98.

Kemppainen, J. K. (1990). Imogene King's theory: A nursing case study of a psychotic patient with human immunodeficiency virus infection. *Archives of Psychiatric Nursing, 4,* 384–388.

Logothetis, M. L. (1991). Women's decisions about estrogen replacement therapy. *Western Journal of Nursing Research, 13,* 458–474.

Mahon, N., & Yarcheski, A. (1992). Alternate explanations of loneliness in adolescents: A replication and extension study. *Nursing Research, 41,* 151–156.

Miller, P., Wikoff, R., & Hiatt, A. (1992). Fishbein's Model of Reasoned Action and compliance behavior of hypertensive patients. *Nursing Research, 41,* 104–109.

Monsen, R. B. (1992). Autonomy, coping, and self-care agency in healthy adolescents and in adolescents with spina bifida. *Journal of Pediatric Nursing, 7,* 9–13.

Neuberger, G. B., Kasal, S., Smith, K. V., Hassanein, R., & DeViney, S. (1994). Determinants of exercise and aerobic fitness in outpatients with arthritis. *Nursing Research, 43,* 11–17.

Pender, N. J., Walker, S. N., Sechrist, K. R., & Frank-Stromborg, M. (1990). Predicting health-promoting lifestyles in the workplace. *Nursing Research, 39,* 326–332.

Prattke, T. W., & Gass-Sternas, K. A. (1993). Appraisal, coping, and emotional health of infertile couples undergoing artificial insemination. *Journal of Obstetric, Gynecologic and Neonatal Nursing, 22,* 516–527.

Redeker, N. S. (1992). The relationship between uncertainty and coping after coronary bypass surgery. *Western Journal of Nursing Research, 14,* 48–60.

Ross, M. M., & Bourbonnais, F. F. (1985). The Betty Neuman Systems Model in nursing practice: A case study approach. *Journal of Advanced Nursing, 10,* 199–207.

Samarel, N., & Fawcett, J. (1992). Enhancing adaptation to breast cancer: The addition of coaching to support groups. *Oncology Nursing Forum, 19,* 591–596.

Schaefer, K. M., & Potylycki, M. J. S. (1993). Fatigue associated with congestive heart failure: Use of Levine's Conservational Model. *Journal of Advanced Nursing, 18,* 260–268.

Schodt, C. M. (1989). Parental-fetal attachment and couvade: A study of patterns of human–environment integrity. *Nursing Science Quarterly, 2,* 88–97.

Schumacher, K. L., Dodd, M. J., & Paul, S. M. (1993). The stress process in family caregivers of persons receiving chemotherapy. *Research in Nursing and Health, 16,* 395–404.

Smith, M. C. (1990). Struggling through a difficult time for unemployed persons. *Nursing Science Quarterly, 3,* 18–28.

Stuifbergen, A. K., & Becker, H. A. (1994). Predictors of health-promoting lifestyles in persons with disabilities. *Research in Nursing and Health, 17,* 3–14.

White, N. E., Richter, J. M., & Fry, C. (1992). Coping, social support, and adaptation to chronic illness. *Western Journal of Nursing Research, 14,* 211–224.

Wyper, M. A. (1990). Breast self-examination in the Health Belief Model: Variation on a theme. *Research in Nursing and Health, 13,* 421–428.

Chapter 6

*T*HE ETHICAL CONTEXT
OF NURSING RESEARCH

Nurses continually face ethical dilemmas in their practice: the prolongation of life by artificial means, the institution of tube feedings when patients are unable to sustain oral nourishment, and the testing of new products to monitor care are but a few examples. Dilemmas such as these have led to an increasing number of discussions and debates concerning ethical issues in the delivery of nursing care.

The proliferation of research involving human subjects has led to similar ethical concerns and debates regarding the protection of the rights of people who participate in nursing research. Ethical concerns are especially prominent in the field of nursing because the line of demarcation between what constitutes the expected practice of nursing and the collection of research information has become less distinct as research by nurses increases. Furthermore, ethics poses particular problems to nurse researchers in some situations because ethical requirements sometimes conflict with the rigors of the scientific approach. This chapter discusses the ethical context of scientific research.

❖ THE NEED FOR ETHICAL GUIDELINES

When humans are used as subjects in scientific investigations—as they usually are in nursing research—great care must be exercised in ensuring that the rights of those humans are protected. The requirement for ethical conduct may strike you as so self-evident as to require no further comment, but the fact is that ethical considerations have not always been given adequate attention. In this section, we consider some of the reasons that the development of ethical guidelines became imperative.

Historical Background

As modern, civilized humans, we might like to think that systematic violations of moral principles among scientists occurred centuries ago rather than in recent times, but this is not the case. The Nazi medical experiments of the 1930s and 1940s are the most famous example of recent disregard for ethical conduct. The Nazi

Polit DF, Hungler BP: NURSING RESEARCH: PRINCIPLES
AND METHODS, 5th ed. © 1995 J. B. Lippincott Company.

program of research involved the use of prisoners of war and racial "enemies" in numerous experiments designed to test the limits of human endurance and human reaction to diseases and untested drugs. The studies were unethical not only because they exposed the human subjects to permanent physical harm and even death but also because the subjects were not given an opportunity to refuse participation.

Unfortunately, some recent examples are closer to home. For instance, between 1932 and 1972, a study known as the Tuskegee Syphilis Study, sponsored by the U.S. Public Health Service, investigated the effects of syphilis among 400 men from a poor black community. Medical treatment was deliberately withheld to study the course of the untreated disease. Another well-known case of unethical research involved the injection of live cancer cells into elderly patients at the Jewish Chronic Disease Hospital in Brooklyn, without the consent of those patients. Even more recently, it was revealed in 1993 that U.S. federal agencies, such as the Atomic Energy Commission, have sponsored radiation experiments since the 1940s on hundreds of human beings, many of them prisoners or elderly hospital patients. Many other examples of studies with ethical transgressions—often much more subtle than these examples—have emerged to give ethical concerns the high visibility they have today.

Ethical Dilemmas in Conducting Research

Research that violates ethical principles is rarely done specifically to be cruel or immoral, but more typically occurs out of a conviction that knowledge is important and potentially life-saving or beneficial (usually to others) in the long run. There are, unfortunately, research problems in which the rights of subjects and the demands of science are put in direct conflict, resulting in *ethical dilemmas* for the researcher. Here are some examples of situations in which the scientist's need for rigor can be compromised by ethical considerations:

Research question: How empathic are nurses in their treatment of patients in intensive care units?

Ethical dilemma: Ethical research generally involves explaining the study to subjects and obtaining their consent to participate in the study. Yet if the researcher in this example informs the nurses serving as subjects that their treatment of patients will be observed, will their behavior be "normal"? If the nurses' behavior is altered because of their awareness of being observed, the entire value of the study could be undermined.

Research question: What are the feelings and coping mechanisms of parents whose children have a terminal illness?

Ethical dilemma: To fully answer this question, the researcher may need to intrusively probe into the psychological state of the parents at a highly vulnerable time in their lives; such probing could be painful and even traumatic. Yet knowledge of the parents' coping mechanisms could help to design more effective ways of dealing with parents' grief and anger.

Research question: Does a new medication prolong life in cancer patients?

Ethical dilemma: The best way to test the effectiveness of interventions is to administer the intervention to some subjects but withhold it from others to see if differences between the groups emerge. However, if the intervention is untested (e.g., a new drug), the group receiving the intervention may be exposed to potentially hazardous side effects. On the other hand, the group not receiving the drug may be denied a beneficial treatment.

Research question: What are the familial characteristics that are predictive of child sexual abuse?

Ethical dilemma: In identifying factors that place children at high risk of sexual exploitation, the researcher would ideally like to study a typical sample of families with child victims. However, ethical considerations might restrict the sample to families who volunteer to participate in the study, and these volunteering families are likely to be atypical, in which case the results might be inaccurate and misleading.

As these examples suggest, researchers involved with human subjects are sometimes in a bind: they are obligated to advance knowledge, using the most scientifically rigorous procedures available, but they must also adhere to the dictates of ethical rules that have been developed to protect the rights of subjects. Another type of dilemma arises from the fact that nurse researchers may be confronted with conflict-of-interest situations, in which their expected behavior as nurses comes into conflict with the expected behavior of scientists (e.g., deviating from a standard research protocol to give needed assistance to a patient). It is precisely because of such conflicts and dilemmas that codes of ethics are so important in guiding the efforts of researchers.

Codes of Ethics

Over the past four decades, largely in response to the human rights violations described earlier, various *codes of ethics* have been developed. One of the first internationally recognized efforts to establish ethical standards is referred to as the Nuremberg Code, developed after the Nazi atrocities were made public in the Nuremberg trials. Several other international standards have subsequently been developed, the most notable of which is the Declaration of Helsinki, which was adopted in 1964 by the World Medical Assembly and then later revised in 1975.

Most disciplines have established their own code of ethics. The American Nurses' Association (1975) put forth a document entitled *Human Rights Guidelines for Nurses in Clinical and Other Research*. The American Sociological

Association published its *Code of Ethics* in 1984. Guidelines for psychologists were published by the American Psychological Association (1982) in *Ethical Principles in the Conduct of Research With Human Participants*. Although there is considerable overlap in the basic principles articulated in these documents, each deals with problems of particular concern to their respective disciplines.

An especially important code of ethics was adopted by the National Commission for the Protection of Human Subjects of Biomedical and Behavioral Research (1978). The commission, established by the National Research Act (Public Law 93-348), issued a report in 1978 that served as the basis for regulations affecting research sponsored by the federal government. The report, sometimes referred to as the *Belmont Report*, also served as a model for many of the guidelines adopted by specific disciplines. The *Belmont Report* articulated three primary ethical principles on which standards of ethical conduct in research are based: beneficence, respect for human dignity, and justice.

❖ THE PRINCIPLE OF BENEFICENCE

One of the most fundamental ethical principles in research is that of *beneficence*, which encompasses the maxim: Above all, do no harm. Most researchers consider that this principle contains multiple dimensions.

Freedom From Harm

Exposing research participants to experiences that result in serious or permanent harm is unacceptable. Research should only be conducted by scientifically qualified people, especially if potentially dangerous technical equipment or specialized procedures are used. The researcher must be prepared at any time during the study to terminate the research if there is reason to suspect that continuation would result in injury, disability, undue distress, or death to study participants. When a new medical procedure or drug is being tested, it is almost always advisable to first experiment with animals or tissue cultures before proceeding to tests with humans. (Ethical guidelines relating to the treatment of animal subjects should be consulted for research on animals).

Although protecting human subjects from physical harm is in many cases clearcut, some psychological consequences of participating in a study may be subtle and thus require closer attention and sensitivity. Sometimes, for example, people are asked questions about their personal views, weaknesses, or fears. Such queries might require individuals to admit to aspects of themselves that they dislike and would perhaps rather forget. The point is not that the researcher should refrain from asking any questions but, rather, that it is necessary to think carefully about the nature of the intrusion on people's psyches. Researchers strive to avoid inflicting psychological harm by carefully considering the phrasing of questions, by having *debriefing* sessions that permit subjects to ask questions after their participation, and by providing subjects with written information on how they may later contact the researchers.

The need for sensitivity on the part of the researcher may be heightened in qualitative studies, which often involve in-depth exploration into highly personal areas. In-depth probing may actually expose deep-seated fears and anxieties that the study participants had previously repressed. Qualitative researchers must thus be especially vigilant in anticipating such problems.

Freedom From Exploitation

Involvement in a research study should not place subjects at a disadvantage or expose them to situations for which they have not been explicitly prepared. Subjects need to be assured that their participation, or the information they might provide to the researcher, will not be used against them in any way. For example, a subject describing his or her economic circumstances to a researcher should not be exposed to the risk of losing Medicaid benefits; the person reporting drug abuse should not fear exposure to criminal authorities.

The subject enters into a special relationship with the researcher, and it is critical that that relationship not be exploited in any way. Exploitation may be overt and malicious (e.g., sexual exploitation, use of subjects' identifying information to create a mailing list, and use of donated blood for the development of a commercial product), but it is more likely to be subtle. For example, subjects may agree to participate in a study requiring 30 minutes of their time. The researcher may then decide 1 year later to go back and talk to the subjects to follow their progress or circumstances. Unless the researcher had previously warned the subjects that there might be a follow-up study, the researcher might be accused of not adhering to the agreement previously reached with subjects and of exploiting the researcher–subject relationship.

In qualitative research, the risk of exploitation may become especially acute because the psychological distance between the investigator and the study participant typically diminishes dramatically as the study progresses. The emergence of a pseudotherapeutic relationship between the investigator and study participants is not uncommon, and this imposes additional responsibilities on the researcher—and additional risks that exploitation could inadvertently occur.

Nurse researchers must be especially thoughtful in balancing potentially competing obligations. Because nurse researchers may have a nurse–patient (in addition to a researcher–subject) relationship, special care may need to be exercised to avoid exploitation of people's vulnerabilities.

Benefits From Research

Subjects agree to participate in scientific investigations for a number of reasons. They may perceive that there are some direct personal benefits. More often, however, any benefits from the research accrue to society in general or to other individuals. Thus, many subjects may participate in a study out of a desire to be helpful. The researcher should strive insofar as possible to maximize benefits and to candidly communicate the potential benefits to subjects.

The Risk/Benefit Ratio

In deciding to conduct a study, the researcher must carefully assess the risks and benefits that would be incurred. The assessment should weigh the risks and benefits that individual subjects might experience, and the assessment should be shared with the subjects so that they can evaluate whether it is in their best interest to participate. Box 6-1 summarizes some of the more salient benefits and costs to which research subjects might be exposed. In evaluating the anticipated *risk/benefit ratio*, the researcher might want to consider how comfort-

able he or she would feel if it were family members participating in the study.

The risk/benefit ratio should also be considered in terms of whether the risks to research subjects are commensurate with the benefit to society and the nursing profession in terms of the knowledge produced. The general guideline is that the degree of risk to be taken by those participating in the research should never exceed the potential humanitarian benefits of the knowledge to be gained. Thus, the selection of a significant topic for study is the first step in ensuring that research is ethical.

All research involves some risks, but in many cases, the risk is minimal. *Minimal risk*, according to federal guidelines, is defined as anticipated risks that are no greater than those ordinarily encountered in daily life or during the performance of routine physical or psychological tests or procedures. When the risks are not minimal, the researcher must proceed with great

---

BOX 6-1. POTENTIAL BENEFITS AND COSTS OF RESEARCH TO PARTICIPANTS

Major Potential Benefits

- Access to an intervention to which they otherwise may not have access
- Comfort in being able to discuss their situation or problem with an objective and nonjudgmental researcher
- Increased knowledge about themselves or their conditions, either through opportunity for introspection or though direct interaction with the researcher
- Enhanced self-esteem resulting from special attention or treatment
- Escape from normal routine, excitement of being part of a scientific study, and satisfaction of curiosity about what it is like to participate in a study
- Knowledge that the information subjects provide may help others with similar problems or conditions
- Direct monetary or material gains

Major Potential Costs

- Physical harm, including unanticipated side effects
- Physical discomfort, fatigue, or boredom
- Psychological or emotional distress resulting from self-disclosure, introspection, fear of the unknown or interacting with strangers, fear of eventual repercussions, anger at the type of questions being asked, and so on
- Loss of privacy
- Loss of time
- Monetary costs (e.g., for transportation, baby-sitting, time lost from work, or charges for additional procedures and tests associated with the research)

caution, taking every step possible to reduce risks and maximize benefits. If the perceived risks and costs to subjects outweigh the anticipated benefits of the research, the research should be either abandoned or redesigned.

In quantitative studies, most of the details of the study are usually spelled out in advance, and therefore a reasonably accurate risk/benefit assessment can be developed. However, qualitative studies are often less structured and are likely to evolve as data are gathered. It may thus be more difficult to assess all risks at the outset of a study. Qualitative researchers thus must remain sensitive to potential risks throughout the research process.

❖ THE PRINCIPLE OF RESPECT FOR HUMAN DIGNITY

Respect for the human dignity of subjects is the second ethical principle articulated in the *Belmont Report*. This principle includes the right to self-determination and the right to full disclosure.

The Right to Self-Determination

Humans should be treated as autonomous agents, capable of controlling their own activities and destinies. The principle of *self-determination* means that prospective subjects have the right to voluntarily decide whether or not to participate in a study, without the risk of incurring any penalties or prejudicial treatment. It also means that subjects have the right to decide at any point to terminate their participation, to refuse to give information, or to ask for clarification about the purpose of the study or specific study procedures.

A person's right to self-determination includes freedom from coercion of any type. *Coercion* involves explicit or implicit threats of penalty from failing to participate in a study or excessive rewards from agreeing to participate. The obligation to honor and protect individuals

from coercion may require careful thought when the researcher is in a position of authority, control, or influence over potential subjects, as might often be the case in a nurse–patient relationship. The ideal of noncoercion may also require thoughtful consideration even when there is not a preestablished relationship. For example, a monetary incentive offered to an economically disadvantaged group—such as the homeless—might be considered mildly coercive; its acceptability might have to be evaluated in terms of the risk/benefit ratio. That is, if risks are high relative to any benefits and the subjects are poor, monetary incentives (sometimes referred to as *subject stipends*) may place undue pressure on prospective subjects.

The Right to Full Disclosure

The principle of respect for human dignity encompasses people's right to make informed voluntary decisions about their participation in a study. Such decisions cannot be made without full disclosure. *Full disclosure* means that the researcher has fully described the nature of the study, the subject's right to refuse participation, the researcher's responsibilities, and the likely risks and benefits that would be incurred. The right to self-determination and the right to full disclosure are the two major elements on which informed consent is based. Procedures for obtaining informed consent from research subjects are discussed in a later section of this chapter.

Although full disclosure is normally provided to subjects before their participation in a study, there is often a need for further disclosure after the subjects have participated, either in debriefing sessions or in written communications. For example, issues that arise during the course of collecting information from subjects may need to be clarified, or the participant may want aspects of the study explained once again. Many investigators also offer to send participants summaries of the research findings after the information has been analyzed. In qualitative studies, researchers sometimes share preliminary findings with subjects and invite their comments about the researcher's interpretations, as a means of validation.

Issues Relating to the Principle of Respect

Although almost all researchers would, in the abstract, endorse subjects' right to self-determination and full disclosure, there are circumstances that make these standards difficult to adhere to in practice. One issue concerns the inability of certain individuals to make well-informed judgments about the costs and benefits associated with participation. Children, for example, may be unable to give truly informed consent. The issue of groups that are vulnerable within a research context is discussed in a subsequent section of this chapter.

Other circumstances occur in which the researcher may feel that the right to full disclosure and self-determination must be violated for the research to yield meaningful information. Researchers concerned with the validity of the study findings are sometimes worried that full disclosure might result in two types of biases: 1) the bias resulting from distorted information; and 2) the bias resulting from failure to recruit a representative sample.

Let us suppose that a researcher were studying the relationship between men's drinking patterns and spouse abuse. That is, the researcher wants to know if men who abuse their wives are heavier users and more regular users of alcohol than men who do not abuse their wives. If the researcher approached potential subjects and fully explained the purpose of the study, many people might refuse to participate. The problem is that nonparticipation would be highly selective; one would expect, in fact, that the people least likely to volunteer for such a study would be men who had abused their wives or men who were heavy drinkers—the very groups of primary interest in the research. Moreover, by knowing the focus of the study, those who did volunteer to participate might be less inclined to give candid responses. The researcher in such a situation might argue that full disclosure would totally undermine his or her ability to conduct the study productively.

Researchers who feel that full disclosure is incompatible with the conduct of rigorous scientific research sometimes use two techniques. The first is *covert data collection* or *concealment*, which means the collection of information without the subjects' knowledge and, thus, without their consent. This might happen, for example, if a researcher wanted to observe naturalistic behavior in a real-world setting and was concerned that doing so openly would result in changes in the behavior of interest. In such a situation, the researcher might obtain the information through concealed methods, such as by audiotaping or videotaping subjects through hidden equipment, observing through a one-way mirror, or observing while pretending to be engaged in other activities. As another example of covert data collection, hospital patients might unwittingly become subjects in a study through the researcher's use of existing hospital records. In general, covert data collection may be acceptable as long as the risks to the subjects are negligible and the subjects' right to privacy has not been violated. Covert data collection is least likely to be ethically acceptable if the research is focused on sensitive aspects of the subjects' behavior, such as drug use, sexual conduct, or illegal acts.

The second, and more controversial, technique is the researcher's use of *deception*. Deception can involve either withholding information about the study or providing subjects with false information. For example, the researcher studying spouse abuse might describe the research as a study of marital relationships, which is a mild form of misinformation.

The practice of deception is problematic from an ethical standpoint because it interferes with the subjects' right to make a truly informed decision regarding the personal costs and benefits of participation. Some people argue that the use of deception is never justified. Others, however, believe that if the study involves minimal risk to subjects and if there are anticipated benefits to science and society, then deception may be justified to enhance the validity of the findings. The American Psychological Association's (1982) code of ethics offers the following guideline regarding the use of deception and concealment:

> Methodological requirements of a study may make the use of concealment or deception necessary. Before conducting such a study, the investigator has a special responsibility to 1) determine whether the use of such techniques is justified by the study's prospective scientific, education, or applied value; 2) determine whether alternative procedures are available that do not use concealment or deception; and 3) ensure that the participants are provided with sufficient explanation as soon as possible. (pp. 35–36)

❖ THE PRINCIPLE OF JUSTICE

The third broad principle articulated in the *Belmont Report* concerns justice. This principle includes the subjects' right to fair treatment and their right to privacy.

The Right to Fair Treatment

Subjects have the right to fair and equitable treatment both before, during, and after their participation in the study. Fair treatment includes the following features:

- The fair and nondiscriminatory selection of subjects such that any risks and benefits will be equitably shared; subject selection should be based on research requirements and not based on the convenience, gullibility, or compromised position of certain types of people
- The nonprejudicial treatment of individuals who decline to participate or who withdraw from the study after agreeing to participate
- The honoring of all agreements made between the researcher and the subject, including adherence to the procedures outlined in advance and the payment of any promised stipends

- Subjects' access to research personnel at any point in the study to clarify information
- Subjects' access to appropriate professional assistance if there is any physical or psychological damage
- Debriefing, if necessary, to divulge information that was withheld before the study or to clarify issues that arose during the study
- Respectful and courteous treatment at all times

The Right to Privacy

Virtually all research with humans constitutes some type of intrusion into the subjects' personal lives. Researchers need to ensure that their research is not more intrusive than it needs to be and that the subjects' privacy is maintained throughout the study.

Subjects have the right to expect that any information collected during the course of a study will be kept in strictest confidence. This can occur either through anonymity or through other confidentiality procedures. *Anonymity* occurs when even the researcher cannot link a subject with the information for that subject. For example, if questionnaires were distributed to a group of nursing home residents and the questionnaires were returned without any identifying information on them, the responses would be considered anonymous. As another example, if a researcher reviewed hospital records from which all identifying information (e.g., name, address, social security number, and so forth) had been expunged, anonymity would again protect the subjects' right to privacy. Whenever it is possible to achieve anonymity, the researcher should strive to do so.

In situations in which anonymity is impossible, appropriate confidentiality procedures need to be implemented. A *promise of confidentiality* to subjects is a guarantee that any information that the subject provides will not be publicly reported in a manner that identifies the subject or made accessible to parties other than those involved in the research. This means that research information should not be shared with strangers nor with people known to the subjects, such as family members, counselors, physicians, and other nurses, unless the researcher has been given explicit permission to share the information.

Researchers can take a number of steps to safeguard the confidentiality of subjects, including the following:

- Obtain identifying information (e.g., name, address, etc.) from subjects only when it is essential to do so.
- Assign an identification (ID) number to each subject and attach the ID number rather than other identifiers to the actual research information.
- Maintain any identifying information and lists of ID numbers with corresponding identifying information in a locked file.
- Restrict access to identifying information to a small number of individuals on a need-to-know basis.
- Enter no identifying information onto computer files.
- Destroy identifying information as quickly as is feasible.
- Have all research personnel who have contact with the research information or identifiers sign pledges of confidentiality.
- Report research information in the aggregate; if information for a specific subject is reported, take steps to disguise the person's identity, such as through the use of a fictitious name together with sparing use of descriptors of the individual.

Qualitative researchers sometimes find that extra precautions are needed to safeguard the privacy of their research participants. Anonymity is almost never possible in qualitative research because the researcher typically is interjected deeply into the lives of those being studied. Moreover, because of the in-depth nature of many qualitative studies, there may be a greater invasion of privacy than is true in quantitative research. Researchers who spend time in the home of a study participant, for example, may have difficulty segregating the public be-

haviors that the study participant is willing to share from the private behaviors that unfold unwittingly during the course of data collection. A final thorny issue that many qualitative researchers face is adequately disguising study participants in their research reports. Because the number of respondents is typically small and because rich descriptive information is typically obtained, it may be difficult to protect the identities of the participants adequately.

❖ INFORMED CONSENT

Prospective subjects who are fully informed about the nature of the research and potential costs and benefits to be incurred are in a position to make thoughtful decisions regarding participation in the study. *Informed consent* means that subjects have adequate information regarding the research; are capable of comprehending the information; and have the power of free choice, enabling them to voluntarily consent to or decline participation in the research. This section discusses procedures for obtaining informed consent.

The Content of Informed Consent

Fully informed consent involves the disclosure of the following pieces of information to subjects:

1. *Subject status.* Prospective subjects should be informed that any data they provide will be used in a scientific study. Patients should be told which health care activities are routine and which are implemented specifically for the purposes of the research.
2. *Study purpose.* The overall purpose of conducting the research should be stated, preferably in lay rather than technical terms. The use to which the research information will be put should also be described.
3. *Type of data.* Prospective subjects should be told the type of data that will be col-

lected from them during the course of the study.

4. *Nature of the commitment.* Information regarding the duration of the study should be provided together with an estimated time commitment at each point of contact.

5. *Sponsorship.* Information on who is sponsoring or funding the study should be mentioned; if the research is a course or degree requirement, this information should be shared.

6. *Subject selection.* The researcher should explain how the prospective subjects came to be selected for recruitment into the study; the explanation may also indicate how many subjects will be involved in the study.

7. *Procedures.* Prospective subjects should be given a description of the procedures that will be used to collect the data and of the procedures involved in any special or experimental treatment.

8. *Potential risks or costs.* Prospective subjects should be informed of any potential foreseeable risks (physical, psychological, or economic) or costs that might be incurred as a result of participation. The possibility of unforeseeable risks should also be discussed, if appropriate. If injury or damage is possible, treatments that will be made available to subjects should be described. (In qualitative research, it may not always be possible to assess fully all risks at the outset because the study design often evolves as the data are collected. It may thus be necessary for the researcher to provide study participants continually with updated information about potential costs as emergent risks are identified.)

9. *Potential benefits.* Specific benefits to subjects, if any, should be described together with information on possible benefits to others. If subject stipends are to be paid, they should be discussed.

10. *Confidentiality pledge.* Prospective subjects should be assured that their privacy will at all times be protected.

11. *Voluntary consent.* The researcher should clearly indicate that participation is strictly voluntary and that failure to comply will not result in any penalties or loss of benefits.

12. *Right to withdraw.* Prospective subjects should be informed that even after consenting to cooperate they will have the right to withdraw from the study and to refuse to provide any specific piece of information. Additionally, researchers may, in some cases, need to provide subjects with a description of circumstances under which the researcher will terminate their participation or the overall study.

13. *Alternatives.* If appropriate, the researcher should provide information regarding alternative procedures or treatments, if any, that might be advantageous to subjects.

14. *Contact information.* The researcher should provide information on whom the subjects could contact in the event of further questions, comments, or complaints relating to the research.

Comprehension of Informed Consent

The information just described is normally presented to prospective subjects orally while they are being recruited to participate in a study. As discussed in the next section, researchers often present this information to prospective subjects in writing as well. However, a written form should not take the place of an oral explanation of critical information about the study (unless the study does not involve face-to-face contact with subjects). Oral presentations provide opportunities for greater elaboration and for subject questioning. Because informed consent is based on a person's evaluation of the potential costs and benefits of participation, it is important that the critical information be not only communicated but also understood.

Researchers preparing statements for prospective subjects should be careful to use simple language, avoiding jargon and technical terms whenever possible. Written statements should be consistent with the subjects' reading levels and educational attainment. For subjects from a general population (e.g., patients in a hospital), the statement should be written at about the seventh- or eighth-grade reading level.

For studies involving more than minimal risk, researchers need to make special efforts to ensure that prospective subjects understand what participation in the research will involve. In some cases, this might involve testing the subjects for their comprehension of the informed consent material before ruling them eligible for participation.

Documentation of Informed Consent

In most cases, researchers should document the informed consent process by having subjects sign a *consent form*. Federal regulations covering studies conducted under the sponsorship of government agencies require written consent, except under two circumstances: 1) when the consent document would be the only record linking the subject and the research information, and subjects agree that documentation can be foregone in the interest of protecting their privacy; or 2) when the study involves minimal risk and involves no procedures for which written consent would normally be needed. For example, for studies involving the completion of a questionnaire, informed consent documentation is normally optional.

The consent form should contain all the information essential to informed consent, as described earlier. An example of a written consent form is presented in Figure 6-1. The prospective subject should have ample time to review the written document before signing it. The document should also be signed by the researcher, and a copy should be retained by both parties.

If the informed consent information is lengthy, government regulations give researchers whose study is funded by federal agencies the option of presenting the full information orally and then summarizing essential

information in a *short form*. However, if a short form is used, the oral presentation must be witnessed by a third party, and the signature of the witness must appear on the short consent form. The signature of a third-party witness is also advisable in studies involving more than minimal risk, even when a long and comprehensive consent form is used.

❖ VULNERABLE SUBJECTS

Adherence to ethical standards such as those discussed thus far is, in most cases, straightforward. However, the rights of special vulnerable groups may need to be protected through additional procedures and heightened sensitivity on the part of the researcher. *Vulnerable subjects* may be incapable of giving fully informed consent (e.g., mentally retarded people) or may be at high risk of unintended side effects because of their circumstances (e.g., pregnant women). Researchers interested in studying high-risk groups should become acquainted with laws and guidelines governing informed consent, risk/benefit assessments, and acceptable procedures for research involving the group of interest. In general, research with vulnerable groups should be undertaken only when the researcher has determined that the risk/benefit ratio is low or when there is no alternative (e.g., studies of childhood development require child subjects).

Among the groups that nurse researchers should consider as being especially vulnerable are the following:

- *Children.* Legally and ethically, children do not have the competence to give their informed consent. Generally, the informed consent of children's parents or legal guardians should be obtained. If the child is developmentally mature enough to understand the basic information involved in informed consent (e.g., a 13-year-old), it is advisable to obtain written consent from the child as well, as evidence of respect for the child's right to self-determination.

In signing this document, I am giving my consent to be interviewed by an employee of Humanalysis, Inc., a nonprofit research organization based in Saratoga Springs, New York. I understand that I will be part of a research study that will focus on the experiences and needs of mothers of young children in the United States. This study, supported by a grant from the U.S. Department of Health and Human Services, will provide some guidance to people who are trying to help mothers and their children.

I understand that I will be interviewed in my home at a time convenient to me. I will be asked some questions about my experiences as a parent, my feelings about how to raise children, the health and characteristics of my oldest child, and my use of community services. I also understand that the interviewer will ask to have my oldest child present during at least some portion of the interview. The interview will take about $1\frac{1}{2}$ to 2 hours to complete. I also understand that the researcher may contact me for more information in the future.

I understand that I was selected to participate in this study because I was involved in a study of young mothers at the time of my oldest child's birth. At that time, I was recruited into the study, along with about 500 other young mothers, through a hospital or service agency.

This interview was granted freely. I have been informed that the interview is entirely voluntary, and that even after the interview begins I can refuse to answer any specific questions or decide to terminate the interview at any point. I have been told that my answers to questions will not be given to anyone else and no reports of this study will ever identify me in any way. I have also been informed that my participation or nonparticipation or my refusal to answer questions will have no effect on services that I or any member of my family may recieve from health or social services providers.

This study will help develop a better understanding of the experiences of young mothers and the services that can be most helpful to them and their children. However, I will receive no direct benefit as a result of participation. As a means of compensating for any fatigue, inconvenience, or monetary costs associated with participating in this study, I have received $25 for granting this interview.

I understand that the results of this research will be given to me if I ask for them and that Dr. Denise Polit is the person to contact if I have any questions about the study or about my rights as a study participant. Dr. Polit can be reached through a collect call at (518) 587-3994.

_____   _____
Date   Respondent's Signature

                                                  _____
                                                  Interviewer's Signature

Figure 6-1. *Sample consent form.*

- *Mentally or emotionally disabled people.* Individuals whose disability makes it impossible for them to weigh the risks and benefits of participation and make an informed decision (e.g., people affected by mental retardation, senility, mental illness, unconsciousness, and so on) also cannot legally or ethically be expected to provide informed consent. In such cases, the researcher should obtain the written consent of each person's legal guardian. However, the researcher should be sensitive to the fact that the legal guardian may not necessarily have the person's best interests in mind. In such cases, informed consent should also be obtained from a person whose primary interest is the person's welfare. As in the case of children, informed consent from prospective subjects themselves should be sought to the extent possible in addition to consent from the guardian.

- *Physically disabled people.* For certain physical disabilities, special procedures for obtaining consent may be required. For example, with deaf subjects, the entire consent process may need to be in writing. For people who have a physical impairment preventing them from writing or for subjects who cannot read and write, alternative procedures for documenting informed consent (such as audio-taping or videotaping the consent proceedings) should be used.

- *Institutionalized people.* Nurses often conduct studies using hospitalized or institutionalized people as subjects. Special care may be required in recruiting such subjects because they often depend on health care personnel and may feel pressured into participating or may feel that their treatment would be jeopardized by their failure to cooperate. Inmates of prisons and other correctional facilities, who have lost their autonomy in many spheres of activity, may similarly feel constrained in their ability to give free consent. The government has issued special regulations for the additional protection of prisoners as subjects (see Code of Federal Regulations, 1983). Researchers studying institutionalized groups need to emphasize the voluntary nature of participation.

- *Pregnant women.* The government has issued stringent additional requirements governing research with pregnant women (Code of Federal Regulations, 1983). These requirements reflect a desire to safeguard both the pregnant woman, who may be at heightened physical and psychological risk, and the fetus, who cannot give informed consent. The regulations stipulate that a pregnant woman cannot be involved in a study unless the purpose of the research is to meet the health needs of the pregnant woman and risks to her and the fetus are minimized or there is only a minimal risk to the fetus.

❖ EXTERNAL REVIEWS AND THE PROTECTION OF HUMAN RIGHTS

Researchers may not be objective in their assessment of the risk/benefit ratio or in their development of procedures to protect the rights of subjects. Biases may arise as a result of the researchers' commitment to an area of knowledge and their desire to conduct a study with as much scientific rigor as possible. Because of the risk of a biased evaluation, the ethical dimensions of a study should normally be subjected to external review.

Most hospitals, universities, and other institutions where research is conducted have established formal committees and protocols for reviewing proposed research plans and procedures before they are implemented. These committees are sometimes called *human subjects committees* or *research advisory panels.* If the institution receives federal funds that help to pay for the costs of research, it is likely that the committee will be called an *Institutional Review Board* (IRB).

Research involving human subjects that is sponsored through federal funds (including federally sponsored fellowships) is subject to strict guidelines for evaluating the treatment of human subjects. Before undertaking such a study, the researcher must submit research plans to the IRB (see Appendix A for an example). The duty of the IRB is to ensure that the proposed plans meet the federal requirements for ethical research. An IRB can approve the proposed plans, require modifications, or disapprove the plans. IRB decisions are usually documented on an approval form, such as the one shown in Figure 6-2. The main requirements governing IRB decisions may be summarized as follows (Code of Federal Regulations, 1983):

- Risks to subjects are minimized.
- Risks to subjects are reasonable in relation to anticipated benefits, if any, to subjects, and the importance of the knowledge that may reasonably be expected to result.
- Selection of subjects is equitable.
- Informed consent will be sought, as required.
- Informed consent will be appropriately documented.
- Adequate provision is made for monitoring the research to ensure the safety of subjects.
- Appropriate provisions are made to protect the privacy of subjects and the confidentiality of data.

REVIEW OF SAFEGUARDS FOR HUMAN SUBJECTS

Proposal/Project Number: Internal ——————————— Sponsor: ———————————

Proposal/Project Title: ————————————————————————————

————————————————————————————

Type of review:

—— Determination of Exemption   —— Full Board Proposal Review
—— Expedited Review   —— Ongoing research in certifi-
                                    cation of change

—— Other (Specify): ————————————————————————————

————————————————————————————

After reviewing the above proposal/project:

Exemption   ——   The institutional official has determined that the research is
                     exempt under 45 CFR 46.101 (b) or

Safeguards   ——   This Institutional Review Board (or member signing below
                     in the case of expedited review) has determined by unani-
                     mous vote of the members present that:

               ——   Risks to subjects are minimized and are reasonable in rela-
                     tion to anticipated benefits. Selection of subjects is equita-
                     ble, and the privacy of the subjects and confidentiality of the
                     data are adequately protected. Approval is given.

               ——   Approval is given under the following conditions:

               ——   Approval is not given, for the following reasons:

Where applicable, attach summary of controverted issues and their resolution.

————————————————————————————

Date: ———————————————

Names of Members Present: *Signatures of Members Present:*

————————————————   ————————————————

————————————————   ————————————————

————————————————   ————————————————

————————————————   ————————————————

————————————————   ————————————————

Figure 6-2. *Sample Institutional Review Board review/approval form.*

- When vulnerable subjects are involved, appropriate additional safeguards are included to protect the rights and welfare of these subjects.

Many research projects require a full review by the IRB. For a full review, the IRB convenes meetings at which most IRB members must be present. An IRB must consist of five or more members, at least one of whom is not a researcher (e.g., a member of the clergy or a lawyer may be appropriate). One member of the IRB must also be a person who has no affiliation with the institution and is not a family member of a person affiliated with the institution. The IRB cannot comprise entirely men, women, or members from a single profession. These requirements are designed to safeguard against the possibility of various biases.

For certain kinds of research involving no more than minimal risk to human subjects, the IRB can use expedited review procedures, which do not require that a meeting be convened. In an *expedited review*, a single IRB member (usually the IRB chairperson or another member designated by the chairperson) carries out the review. Examples of the kinds of research activities that qualify for an expedited IRB review include the following:

- Recording of information from subjects 18 years old or older using noninvasive procedures routinely employed in clinical practice (e.g., weighing, testing sensory acuity, electrocardiography, and thermography)
- Collection of blood samples by venipuncture, in amounts not exceeding 450 milliliters, in an eight-week period from subjects at least 18 years old, in good health, and not pregnant
- Collection of excreta and external secretions, including sweat, uncannulated saliva, placenta removed at delivery, and amniotic fluid at the time of rupture of the membrane before or during delivery
- The study of existing documents, records, pathologic specimens, or diagnostic specimens

- Research on individual behavior or characteristics when the researcher does not manipulate the subjects' behavior and when the study will not involve stress to the subjects

The federal regulations also allow certain types of research to be totally exempt from IRB review. These are studies in which there are no apparent risks to human subjects. Box 6-2 summarizes the types of research for which investigators can request an exemption from the IRB review process.

❖ TIPS ON ADDRESSING ETHICAL ISSUES IN A RESEARCH STUDY

Not all nurse researchers face ethical dilemmas in their research, but they all must give adequate attention to the protection of the rights of their subjects. Below are some suggestions for addressing the ethical aspects of a study.

- Researchers need to give careful thought to ethical requirements during the planning of a research project and to ask themselves continuously whether planned safeguards for protecting human subjects are sufficient. Once the study procedures have been developed, researchers should undertake a self-evaluation of those procedures to determine if they meet ethical requirements. Box 25-15 in Chapter 25 provides some guidelines for such a self-evaluation.
- Not all research is subject to federal guidelines, and so not all studies are reviewed by IRBs or other formal committees. Nevertheless, researchers have a responsibility to ensure that their research plans are ethically acceptable and are thus encouraged to seek an outside opinion regarding the ethical dimensions of a study before it is underway. Advisers may include faculty members, the clergy, representatives from the group that would be asked to participate in the research, or advocates for that group.

BOX 6-2.   TYPES OF RESEARCH EXEMPT FROM INSTITUTIONAL REVIEW BOARD REVIEW

Research activities in which the only involvement of human subjects will be in one or more of the following categories are ordinarily exempt from IRB review:

1. Research conducted in established or commonly accepted educational settings, involving normal educational practices
2. Research involving the use of educational tests (cognitive, diagnostic, achievement), if information taken from these sources is recorded such that the identity of subjects is not divulged.
3.* Research involving survey or interview procedures, *except* where all the following conditions are met:
   a. Responses are recorded in such a way that the human subjects can be identified.
   b. The subject's responses, if they became known, could place the subject at risk of criminal or civil liability or financial loss.
   c. The research deals with sensitive aspects of the subject's own behavior, such as illegal conduct, sexual behavior, or use of alcohol.
4. Research involving the observation of public behavior, except when all of the three conditions described above in (3) exist
5. Research involving the collection or study of existing data, documents, records, pathological specimens, if the sources are publicly available or if the information is recorded such that the subject cannot be identified
6. Unless specifically required by statute, research and demonstration projects that are conducted or approved by the U.S. Department of Health and Human Services that are designed to study or evaluate the following:
   a. Programs under the Social Security Act or other public benefit or service programs
   b. Procedures for obtaining benefits or services under those programs
   c. Possible changes in or alterations to those programs or procedures
   d. Possible changes in methods or levels of payment for benefits or services under those programs

*The exemption does not apply when the subjects are minors. Also, all survey research is exempt, without exception, when the subjects are elected or appointed public officials or are candidates for public office.

These exemptions are based on guidelines appearing in the Code of Federal Regulations, revised as of March 8, 1983.

- If the research is being conducted within an institution (or if clients are being referred by an institution), it is important to find out early what the institution's requirements are regarding ethical issues. Many clinical agencies have specific protocols and forms for submitting human subjects' protection information. Because nursing students are often under fairly stringent time constraints to complete research projects, they should consult with the nurse researcher or nursing administration personnel at the agency as quickly as possible to determine the appropriate procedures to follow, the schedule of human subjects committee meetings, and the anticipated date for receiving information regarding the committee's decision.
- There are no firm rules regarding the payment of subject stipends. In general, stipends are used as incentives to increase the rate of subject participation in a study; they appear to be especially effective when the group under study is known to be difficult to recruit or when the study is extremely time-consuming or tedious. Stipends range from one dollar to hundreds of dollars, but most stipends are in the range of 10 to 25 dollars. Some federal agencies that sponsor research do not

allow the payment of an outright stipend but will allow for the reimbursement of certain expenses (e.g., for the subjects' travel, child care, or lunch money).

❖ RESEARCH EXAMPLES

Because researchers generally attempt to report the results of their research as succinctly as possible, they rarely describe in much detail the efforts they have made to safeguard the rights of their subjects. (The absence of any mention of such safeguards does not, of course, imply that no precautions were taken.) Researchers are es-

pecially likely to discuss their adherence to human subjects guidelines when the study involves more than minimal risk or when the group of people being studied is a vulnerable one. Table 6-1 outlines the procedures used in several studies in which the authors described some of the steps taken to protect human rights. The following is a summary of a study in which safeguards were described in considerable detail. You may need to review the actual research report to assess fully the adequacy of the researcher's efforts to safeguard the subjects.

Holdcraft and Williamson (1991) studied levels of hope among psychiatric and chemi-

Table 6-1.   *Examples of Procedures To Protect Human Subjects*

PRINCIPLE	STUDY QUESTION	PROCEDURES
Informed consent IRB review Privacy Risk reduction Exclusion of at-risk subjects	What are the experiences of hospitalized patients who have resuscitation option discussions with a health care professional?	Approval for the study was obtained from both the Human Subjects Committee and IRB. Subjects were informed about the study purpose before consenting to participate. Interviews were conducted without family members or health care professionals present. Participants were told to conclude the interview if they experienced angina symptoms. Only alert and oriented patients with stable vital signs were included. (Larson, 1994)
Informed consent of minors	What are the behavior patterns of children with Turner syndrome in comparison to those of children with learning disabilities?	Informed consent was obtained from the parents of 8- to 15-year-old children. The children also consented. (Williams, 1994)
Informed consent IRB review Risk reduction Exclusion of vulnerable subjects	What are the effects of different temperature cooling blankets in humans with fever in terms of time to cool, shivering, and perceived discomfort?	Subjects were informed of the study purpose and signed a consent form. Vulnerable subjects (e.g., pregnant women) were excluded. All equipment was carefully tested before the study. IRB approval was secured (Caruso, Hadley, Shukla, Frame, & Khoury, 1992)
Informed consent Anonymity IRB review	What is the difference between users and nonusers of estrogen replacement therapy with regard to perceived susceptibility to menopausal problems?	Women were asked to volunteer to participate in the study after being told the study's purpose. A woman's consent was indicated by her return of a completed, anonymous questionnaire. IRB approval was obtained. (Logothetis, 1991)

cally dependent in-patients, noting that hospitalization for these patients may be a time of crisis or despair. Patients in a large general hospital were asked to participate in the study and complete the Miller Hope Scale. Patients in the mental unit were approached within the first 3 days after admission or transfer to the unit. Patients on the chemical dependency unit were told about the study during their transition from the detoxification phase of their treatment. For both groups, the study was explained and informed consent was obtained. Subjects who agreed to participate completed the questionnaire and returned it in a sealed envelope. The subjects were asked to complete the questionnaire a second time, to determine if levels of hope changed over the course of their treatment. The subjects received the materials and instructions to complete the second questionnaires at discharge. The subjects' names were not used on any study materials, except on the consent forms and on a master list of names and code numbers. Consent forms and the list of names were filed in a separate office and destroyed at the completion of the study.

❖ SUMMARY

Research that involves human subjects requires a careful consideration of the procedures to be used to protect their rights. Because scientific research has not always been conducted ethically and because of the genuine *ethical dilemmas* that researchers often face in designing studies that are both ethical and scientifically rigorous, *codes of ethics* have been developed to guide researchers. The three major ethical principles that are incorporated into most guidelines are beneficence, respect for human dignity, and justice.

Beneficence encompasses the maxim: Above all, do no harm. This principle involves the protection of subjects from physical and psychological harm, protection of subjects from exploitation, and the performance of some good. In deciding to conduct a study, the re-

searcher must carefully weigh the costs and benefits of participation to individual subjects and must also weigh the risks to the subjects against the potential benefits to society.

The principle of respect for human dignity includes the subjects' right to *self-determination*, which means that subjects have the freedom to control their own activities, including their voluntary participation in the study. The respect principle also includes the subjects' right to full disclosure. *Full disclosure* means that the researcher has fully described to prospective subjects the nature of the study and subjects' rights. Because full disclosure can lead to potentially misleading and distorted study findings, researchers sometimes feel that this principle can be violated in the name of good science. When full disclosure poses the risk of biased results, researchers sometimes use *covert data collection* or *concealment*, which means the collection of information without the subjects' knowledge or consent. In other research situations, researchers have used *deception* (either withholding information from subjects or providing false information) to avoid biases. When deception or concealment is necessary, extra precautions are usually needed to minimize risks and protect the other rights of subjects.

The third principle, justice, includes the *right to fair treatment* (both in the selection of subjects and during the course of the study) and the *right to privacy*. Privacy of subjects can be maintained through *anonymity* (wherein not even the researcher knows the identity of the subjects) or through formal *confidentiality procedures*.

Most studies should involve *informed consent* procedures designed to provide prospective subjects with sufficient information to make a reasoned decision about the potential costs and benefits of participation. Informed consent normally involves having the subject sign a *consent form*, which documents the subject's voluntary decision to participate after receiving a full explanation of the research.

Certain people, sometimes referred to as *vulnerable subjects*, require additional safeguards to protect their rights. These subjects may be vulnerable because they are not competent with regard to making an informed decision about participating in a study (e.g., children or mentally retarded people); because their circumstances make them feel that free choice is constrained (e.g., an institutionalized group of subjects); or because their circumstances heighten their risk for physical or psychological harm (e.g., pregnant women).

External review of the ethical aspects of a study is highly recommended and, in many cases, is required by either the agency funding the research or the organization in which the research is being conducted. Most institutions have special review committees for such purposes. Research funded through the federal government is normally reviewed by the *Institutional Review Board* (IRB) of the institution with which the researcher is affiliated. In studies in which risks to subjects are minimal, an *expedited review* (review by a single member of the IRB) may be substituted for a full board review; in cases in which there are no anticipated risks, the research may be exempted from review. However, researchers are always advised to consult with at least one external adviser whose perspective allows him or her to evaluate objectively the ethics of a proposed study.

❖ *STUDY SUGGESTIONS*

Chapter 6 of the accompanying *Study Guide for Nursing Research: Principles and Practice, 5th ed.*, offers suggested questions and exercises for reinforcing concepts relating to research ethics. Additionally, the following questions can be addressed:

1. Point out the ethical dilemmas that might emerge in the following studies:
   a. A study of the relationship between sleeping patterns and acting-out behaviors in hospitalized psychiatric patients
   b. A study of the effects of a new drug on human subjects
   c. An investigation of an individual's psychological state after an abortion
   d. An investigation of the contraceptive decisions of high school students at a school-based clinic
2. For each of the studies described in question 1, indicate whether you think the study would require a full IRB review or an expedited review, or whether it would be totally exempt from review.
3. For the study described in the research example section (the study by Holdcraft and Williamson, 1991), prepare an informed consent form that includes required information, as described in the section on informed consent.

❖ *SUGGESTED READINGS*

REFERENCES ON RESEARCH ETHICS

American Nurses' Association. (1975). *Human rights guidelines for nurses in clinical and other research.* Kansas City, MO: Author.

American Nurses' Association. (1985). *Code for nurses with interpretive statements.* Kansas City, MO: Author.

American Psychological Association. (1982). *Ethical principles in the conduct of research with human participants.* Washington, DC: Author.

American Sociological Association. (1984). *Code of ethics.* Washington, DC: Author.

Code of Federal Regulations. (1983). *Protection of human subjects: 45CFR46* (revised as of March 8, 1983). Washington, DC: Department of Health and Human Services.

Cowles, K. V. (1988). Issues in qualitative research on sensitive topics. *Western Journal of Nursing Research, 10,* 163–179.

Damrosch, S. P. (1986). Ensuring anonymity by use of subject-generated identification codes. *Research in Nursing and Health, 9,* 61–63.

Davis, A. J. (1989a). Clinical nurses' ethical decision-making in situations of informed consent. *Advances in Nursing Science, 11,* 63–69.

Davis, A. J. (1989b). Informed consent process in research protocols: Dilemmas for clinical nurses. *Western Journal of Nursing Research, 11,* 448–457.

Munhall, P. L. (1988). Ethical considerations in qualitative research. *Western Journal of Nursing Research, 10,* 150–162.

National Commission for the Protection of Human Subjects of Biomedical and Behavioral Research. (1978). *Belmont report: Ethical principles and guidelines for research involving human subjects.* Washington, DC: U.S. Government Printing Office.

Ramos, M. C. (1989). Some ethical implications of qualitative research. *Research in Nursing and Health, 12,* 57–64.

Rempusheski, V. F. (1991a). Elements, perceptions, and issues of informed consent. *Applied Nursing Research, 4,* 201–204.

Rempusheski, V. F. (1991b). Research data management: Piles into files—locked and secured. *Applied Nursing Research, 4,* 147–149.

Silva, M. C., & Sorrell, J. M. (1984). Factors influencing comprehension of information for informed consent. *International Journal of Nursing Studies, 21,* 233–240.

Thurber, F. W., Deatrick, J. A., & Grey, M. (1992). Children's participation in research: Their right to consent. *Journal of Pediatric Nursing, 7,* 165–170.

Watson, A. B. (1982). Informed consent of special subjects. *Nursing Research, 31,* 43–47.

SUBSTANTIVE REFERENCES

Caruso, C. C., Hadley, B. J., Shukla, R., Frame, P., & Khoury, J. (1992). Cooling effects and comfort of four cooling blanket temperatures in humans with fever. *Nursing Research, 41,* 68–72.

Fahs, P. S. S., & Kinney, M. R. (1991). The abdomen, thigh, and arm as sites for subcutaneous sodium heparin injections. *Nursing Research, 40,* 204–207.

Holdcraft, C., & Williamson, C. (1991). Assessment of hope in psychiatric and chemically dependent patients. *Applied Nursing Research, 4,* 129–133.

Larson, D. E. (1994). Resuscitation discussion experiences of patients hospitalized in a coronary care unit. *Heart and Lung, 23,* 53–58.

Lemmer, C. M. (1991). Parental perceptions of caring following perinatal bereavement. *Western Journal of Nursing Research, 13,* 475–493.

Logothetis, M. L. (1991). Women's decisions about estrogen replacement therapy. *Western Journal of Nursing Research, 13,* 458–474.

Williams, J. K. (1994). Behavioral characteristics of children with Turner syndrome and children with learning disabilities. *Western Journal of Nursing Research, 16,* 26–35.

Part III

DESIGNS FOR NURSING RESEARCH

Chapter 7

SELECTING A RESEARCH DESIGN

A researcher's overall plan for obtaining answers to the research questions or for testing the research hypotheses is referred to as the *research design*. The research design spells out the basic strategies that the researcher adopts to develop information that is accurate and interpretable.

The research design incorporates some of the most important methodological decisions that the researcher makes in conducting a research study. Other aspects of the study—the data collection plan, the sampling plan, and the analysis plan—also involve important decisions, but the research design stipulates the fundamental form that the research will take. For this reason, it is important to have a good understanding of design options when embarking on a research project. The purpose of this chapter is to provide an overview of various considerations in selecting a research design. Subsequent chapters cover research design issues in greater depth.

❖ ASPECTS OF RESEARCH DESIGN

The researcher's overall plan for addressing the research problem covers multiple aspects of the study's organizational structure. The key factors that are incorporated into a research design are discussed in this section.

Intervention

In some studies, nurse researchers want to test the effects of a specific intervention (e.g., an innovative program to promote breast self-examination or new procedures for monitoring infants in the neonatal intensive care unit). In such studies, which are called *experimental studies*, the researcher plays an active role by introducing the intervention. In other studies, referred to as *nonexperimental studies*, the researcher observes phenomena as they naturally occur without intervening in any way. The distinction between experimental and nonexperimental designs is discussed at length in Chapter 8.

When the study is experimental, the research design specifies the full nature of the intervention. Among the questions that would be addressed are the following:

- What exactly *is* the intervention? How does it differ from the more usual methods of care?
- What are the procedures to be used with those receiving—and with those *not* receiving—the intervention?

Polit DF, Hungler BP: NURSING RESEARCH: PRINCIPLES
AND METHODS, 5th ed. © 1995 J. B. Lippincott Company.

- Who will receive the intervention, and who will not? How will each group be selected or designated?
- What is the dosage or intensity of the intervention?
- Over how long a period will the intervention be administered? When will the treatment begin (e.g., 2 hours after operation)?
- Who will administer the intervention? What are their credentials, and what type of special training or preparation will they receive?
- Will those administering the intervention be fully informed about the nature of the study? Will subjects be fully informed?
- Under what conditions will the intervention be withdrawn or altered?

Comparisons

Generally, researchers try to develop some type of comparison within their studies so that their results will be interpretable. In designing the research, the researcher needs to specify the nature of the comparisons. Comparisons in research studies can be of various types, the most common of which are as follows:

- *Comparison between two or more groups.* For example, suppose a researcher wanted to study the emotional consequences of having an abortion. To do this, the researcher might compare the emotional status of women who had an abortion with women from the same health clinic who had an unintended pregnancy but who nevertheless delivered the baby.
- *Comparison of a single group at two or more points in time.* For example, the researcher might want to assess patients' levels of stress before and after introducing a new procedure intended to reduce preoperative stress.
- *Comparison of a single group under different circumstances or experiences.* For example, a researcher might compare the heart rates of subjects undergoing one type of exercise and then a second type.

- *Comparison based on relative rankings.* Researchers addressing questions about relationships among variables are really making comparisons, although this may not be obvious. For example, if the research question asks whether there is a relationship between the amount of pain experienced by cancer patients and their level of hopefulness (the dependent variable), the researcher is essentially asking whether patients with high levels of pain feel less hopeful than patients with low levels of pain. Thus, the research question involves a comparison of those with different rankings (high versus low) on the independent variable: the amount of pain.
- *Comparison with samples from other studies.* Sometimes researchers directly compare their results with results from other studies, sometimes using statistical procedures. This type of comparison typically supplements rather than replaces other types of comparisons. It is useful primarily when the measure of the dependent variable is a widely used and accepted measure (e.g., blood pressure measures or scores on a standard measure of depression).

Comparisons are sometimes the central focus of the research, but even when they are not, they provide a context for understanding the findings. In the example in which the researcher was interested in the emotional status of women who had an abortion, the inclusion of a comparison group allows the researcher to better interpret the findings for the women who had an abortion. If the researcher did not use a comparison group, it would be difficult to know whether the emotional status of the abortion group members was unusual in any way.

In some studies, a natural comparison group suggests itself. For example, if a researcher were testing the effectiveness of a new nursing procedure for a group of nursing home residents, a natural comparison group would be nursing home residents who were exposed to the standard procedure rather than to the innovation. In other cases, however, the comparison group to be used is less clearcut, and the researcher's decision about a comparison group can have serious consequences for the interpretability of the findings. In the example about the emotional consequences of an abortion, the researcher decided to use women who delivered a baby as the comparison group. This reflects a comparison focusing on the *outcome* of the pregnancy (i.e., pregnancy termination versus live birth). An alternative comparison group might be women who had a miscarriage. In this case, the comparison focuses not on the outcome (in both groups the outcome is pregnancy loss) but rather on the *determinant* of the outcome. Thus, in designing a study, the researcher often must be careful to select a comparison group that will best illuminate the central issue under investigation. Of course, in some cases, it may be desirable to include two or more comparison groups, but this usually increases the cost of undertaking the study.

Some examples of comparisons incorporated into the design of actual nursing studies are presented in Table 7-1.

Controls for Extraneous Variables

As noted in Chapter 2, the complexity of relationships among human characteristics often makes it difficult to answer research questions unambiguously unless efforts are made to isolate the independent and dependent variables and to control other factors extraneous to the research question. Thus, in structured quantitative studies, an important feature of the research design is the specification of steps that will be taken to control extraneous variables. The methods used to enhance research control are discussed in Chapter 10.

In designing a study, the researcher must carefully consider which extraneous variables need to be controlled. If the researcher is using

Table 7-1.   *Examples of Studies With Various Types of Comparisons*

RESEARCH QUESTION	NATURE OF THE COMPARISON
What are the effects of music and muscle relaxation on patient anxiety in the coronary care unit? (Elliott, 1994)	Three groups of patients compared: those receiving music relaxation treatment, those receiving muscle relaxation treatment, and those receiving neither
What is the effect of a coronary artery risk evaluation (CARE) program on serum lipid values and cardiovascular risk levels? (Bruce & Grove, 1994)	One group, compared before and after participation in the CARE program
Are there differences in cardiac output with iced injectate (0°C–6°C) versus refrigerated injectate (10°C–16°C) after cardiac surgery? (Price & Fowlow, 1993)	One group, compared after injection with two temperatures of injectate (half the subjects got the refrigerated injectate first, half got the iced injectate first)
What are the characteristics of women with high versus low levels of anxiety after an abnormal Pap smear result? (Nugent, Tamlyn-Leaman, Isa, Reardon, & Crumley, 1993)	Relative rankings, comparing higher versus lower scorers on a measure of anxiety; also, comparison with samples in other studies

a sophisticated research design or analytic strategy, it may be possible to control for a whole host of extraneous variables, but beginning researchers are more likely to be able to control for only one or two. Familiarity with the research literature often helps to identify especially important candidates.

Timing of Data Collection

In most studies, data are collected from subjects at a single point in time. For example, patients might be asked on a single occasion to complete a questionnaire about their nutritional practices. However, some designs call for multiple contacts with subjects, either to determine how things have changed over time, to determine the stability of some phenomenon, or to establish a baseline against which the effect of some treatment can later be compared. Thus, in designing a study, the researcher must decide on the number of times data will be collected.

The research design also designates *when,* relative to other events, the data will be collected. For example, the design might call for a sample of pregnant women to be interviewed in the 16th and 30th weeks of gestation; or for blood samples to be drawn after 10 hours of fasting; or for patients to be observed 1 day after surgery. The timing should make sense in terms of the overall research objectives.

Research Setting

The research design must specify the setting for the research study. That is, the researcher needs to decide where the interventions (if any) will be implemented and where the data will be collected. Because the setting can influence the way people behave or feel and how they respond to questions, the selection of an appropriate setting is important.

Sometimes studies take place in *naturalistic settings*, such as in people's homes or places of employment. In-depth qualitative studies are especially likely to occur in natural settings because qualitative researchers usually are inter-ested in studying the full context within which their research subjects live or work.

At the other extreme, some studies are conducted in highly controlled *laboratory settings.* By laboratory, we do not necessarily mean a setting in which scientific equipment is installed. Here, the term is used in a general sense to refer to a physical location apart from the routine of daily living, which is used by the researcher as the site for the collection of data and where subjects report to participate in the research project.

For nurse researchers, studies are often conducted in quasi-natural settings such as hospitals, clinics, or other institutional facilities. These are settings that are not necessarily natural to the subjects (unless the primary subjects are nurses), but neither are they highly contrived and controlled research laboratories. Nevertheless, it may be important to consider whether the research subjects are being influenced by being in a setting that may be anxiety-provoking or foreign to their usual experiences.

Research sometimes occurs in more than one location. One prominent reason is that the use of multiple settings can often ensure a larger and more representative sample. For example, in a study of a new nursing intervention, the researchers may wish to implement the intervention in both a public and a private hospital or in both an urban and a rural location. Multiple settings are especially common in longitudinal studies. For example, the eating and sleeping patterns of burn patients may first be studied while they are hospitalized, with follow-up information gathered once the patients have returned home.

Table 7-2 describes the settings of several actual nursing studies.

Communication With the Subjects

In designing the study, the researcher must decide how much information will be provided to the subjects. As discussed in Chapter 6, full disclosure to research subjects before obtaining their consent to participate is highly de-

Table 7-2. *Examples of Studies Conducted in Various Settings*

RESEARCH QUESTION	SETTING
What are the factors that are perceived to contribute to the ability to initiate and maintain behavior changes among patients with a recent myocardial infarction? (McSweeney, 1993)	Homes of the informants
What are the self-perceived health concerns among the homeless, and what are the conditions under which they would use health services? (Kinzel, 1991)	Homeless shelters, the streets
What are the risk factors and pregnancy outcomes among pregnant incarcerated women? (Fogel, 1993)	A women's maximum security prison
What topics do patients with bipolar disorder (manic depression) raise in group therapy sessions for in-patients? (Pollack, 1993)	A 250-bed state and county hospital
What are the health consequences of loneliness in adolescents? (Mahon, Yarcheski, & Yarcheski, 1993)	Elementary, high school, and college classrooms
Is nap therapy effective in improving alertness and reducing the frequency of sleep attacks among narcoleptic patients? (Rogers & Aldrich, 1993)	A hospital sleep disorder laboratory

sirable from an ethical standpoint but may in some cases undermine the value of the research. The researcher should consider the costs and benefits of various alternative means of communicating information to subjects. Among the issues that should be addressed are the following:

- How much information about the specific study aims will be provided to prospective subjects while they are being recruited to participate?
- How much information about the study aims will be provided to subjects during the informed consent process?
- How will information be provided—orally or in writing?
- Who will provide the information, and what instructions will be given to the provider regarding answers to additional questions the subjects may ask?

- Will there be any debriefing sessions after the data are collected to explain more fully the study purpose or answer subjects' questions?
- Will subjects be provided with a written summary of the study results?

Because the nature of the communication with subjects can affect the study results, these issues should be given careful consideration in designing the research.

❖ OVERVIEW OF RESEARCH DESIGN TYPES

There is no single, easy-to-describe typology of research designs. Research designs vary along a number of dimensions, some of which are related to the factors discussed in the preceding section. This section describes the major dimensions along which research designs can vary—the major exception being the experimental/nonexperimental dimension, which is covered at length in the next chapter.

Structured Versus Unstructured Designs

Research designs vary with regard to how much structure the researcher imposes on the research situation and how much flexibility is allowed in making structural changes once the study is underway. The research designs of most quantitative studies are highly structured and are spelled out in advance of any data collection. In a typical quantitative study, the researcher specifies the nature of any intervention, the nature of the comparisons, the methods to be used to control extraneous variables, the timing of data collection, the study setting, and the information to be given to subjects—all before a single piece of data is gathered. Once data collection is underway, modifications to the research design are rarely instituted. Indeed, when changes are found to be needed, it is usually the result of a discovery that some aspect of the design did not work. The researcher may then decide to discard all the data gathered before implementing the change—essentially treating the first part of the study as pilot work.

Research design in a qualitative study tends to be more fluid. The qualitative researcher often wants to make deliberate modifications that are sensitive to what is being learned as the data are gathered. For example, interesting types of comparisons may potentially be identified during the collection of data and may drive subsequent data collection decisions. Or the researcher may discover that certain types of settings work better than others for encouraging candor or for observing certain types of natural behavior and may at that point alter the setting for future data collection. The fluidity of the research design in qualitative studies is consistent with their basically exploratory and investigative nature.

The Time Dimension

As mentioned in the previous section, the research design generally specifies when and how often data will be collected in a study. There are four situations in which it might be appropriate to design a study with multiple points of data collection:

1. *Time-related processes.* Certain research problems specifically focus on phenomena that evolve over time. Examples include such phenomena as healing, learning, growth, recidivism, and physical development.
2. *Time-sequenced phenomena.* It is sometimes important to correctly ascertain the temporal sequencing of phenomena. For example, if it is hypothesized that infertility results in depression, then it would be important to determine that the depression did not precede the fertility problem.
3. *Comparative purposes.* Sometimes a time dimension is useful for placing findings in a broader context, to determine if changes have occurred over time. For example, a study might be concerned with documenting trends in the incidence of child abuse over a 10-year period. Another example of collecting data over time for comparative purposes is a study in which the intent is to see if changes over time can reasonably be attributed to some intervention.
4. *Enhancement of research control.* Some research designs involve the collection of data at multiple points to enhance the interpretability of the results. For example, when two groups are being compared with regard to the effects of alternative interventions, the collection of data before any intervention occurs allows the researcher to detect—and control—any initial differences between groups.

Because of the importance of the time dimension in designing research, studies are often categorized in terms of how they deal with time. The major distinction is between cross-sectional and longitudinal designs.

CROSS-SECTIONAL DESIGNS

Cross-sectional designs involve the collection of data at one point in time. The phenomena under investigation are captured, as they manifest themselves, during one period of data collection. Cross-sectional studies are especially appropriate for describing the status of phenomena or for describing relationships among phenomena at a fixed point in time. For example, a researcher might be interested in determining whether psychological symptoms in menopausal women are correlated contemporaneously with physiologic symptoms.

Cross-sectional designs are sometimes used for time-related purposes, but the resulting design is often much weaker than longitudinal designs. As an example, cross-sectional data are sometimes used to infer a causal, temporal chain. For instance, a researcher might test the hypothesis, using cross-sectional data, that a determinant of excessive alcohol consumption is low impulse control, as measured by a psychological test. However, when both alcohol consumption and impulse control are measured concurrently, it is difficult to know which variable influenced the other, if either. Cross-sectional data can most appropriately be used to infer temporal sequencing under two circumstances: 1) when there is evidence or logical reasoning to ensure that one variable preceded the other (e.g., in a study of the effects of low birthweight on morbidity in school-aged children, there would be no confusion over whether birthweight, the independent variable, came first); and 2) when there is a strong theoretical framework guiding the analysis.

Cross-sectional studies can also be designed in such a way that processes evolving over time can be inferred, such as when the measurements capture the process at different points in its evolution with different individuals. As an example, suppose we were interested in studying the changes in nursing students' professionalism as they progress through a 4-year baccalaureate program. One way to investigate this issue would be to survey students when they are freshmen and survey them again every year until they graduate; this would be a longitudinal design. On the other hand, we could use a cross-sectional design by surveying members of the four classes at one point and then comparing the responses of the four groups. If seniors manifested stronger professionalism than freshmen, it might be inferred that nursing students become increasingly socialized professionally by their educational experiences. To make this kind of inference, the researcher must assume that the senior students would have responded as the freshmen responded had they been questioned 3 years earlier, or, conversely, that freshmen students would demonstrate increased professionalism if they were surveyed 3 years later.

The main advantage of cross-sectional designs in such situations is that they are practical: they are relatively economical and easy to manage. There are, however, a number of problems in inferring changes and trends over time using a cross-sectional design. The overwhelming number of social and technological changes that characterizes our society frequently makes it questionable to assume that differences in the behaviors, attitudes, or characteristics of different age groups are the result of the passage through time rather than the result of cohort or generational differences. In the nursing students example, seniors and freshmen may have different attitudes toward the nursing profession, independent of any experiences during their 4 years of education. In such cross-sectional studies, there are frequently several alternative explanations for the research findings.

LONGITUDINAL DESIGNS

Research projects that are designed to collect data at more than one point in time use a *longitudinal design*. In this section, we discuss several types of longitudinal studies to present new terminology and to acquaint students with alternative designs.

Trend studies are investigations in which samples from a general population are studied over time with respect to some phenomenon. Different samples are selected at repeated intervals, but the samples are always drawn from the same population. Trend studies permit researchers to examine patterns and rates of change over time and to predict future directions. For example, trend studies have been initiated to analyze the number of students entering nursing programs and to forecast future supplies of nursing personnel.

Cohort studies are a particular kind of trend study in which specific subpopulations are examined over time. The samples are drawn from specific subgroups that are often age-related. For example, the cohort of women born from 1946 to 1950 may be studied at regular intervals with respect to health care utilization. As another example, the cohort of nursing students receiving their bachelor's degree in the 1960s may be periodically surveyed to determine their employment/unemployment patterns.

A sophisticated design known as the *cross-sequential design* combines the features of cohort studies with a cross-sectional approach. In cross-sequential studies, two or more different age cohorts are studied longitudinally so that both changes over time and generational or cohort differences can be detected. For example, a researcher might compare the development of AIDS awareness over time for both a younger and older cohort of teenagers.

In *panel studies,* the *same* subjects are used to supply data at two or more points in time. The term *panel* refers to the sample of subjects involved in the study. Panel studies typically yield more information than trend studies because the investigator can usually reveal patterns of change and reasons for the changes. Because the same individuals are contacted at two or more points in time, the researcher can identify the subjects who did and did not change and then isolate the characteristics of the subgroups in which changes occurred. As an example, a panel study could be designed to explore over time the antecedent characteristics of people who were later able to quit smoking. Panel studies also allow the researcher to examine how conditions and characteristics at time 1 influence characteristics and conditions at

time 2. For example, health outcomes at time 2 could be studied among individuals with different health-related practices at time 1. A panel study is intuitively appealing as an approach to studying change and temporal sequencing but is extremely difficult and expensive to manage. The most serious problem is the loss of participants at different points in the study—a problem that is known as *attrition.* Attrition is problematic for the researcher because those who drop out of the study may differ in important respects from the individuals who continue to participate, resulting in potential biases to the results.

Follow-up studies are similar in design to panel studies. Follow-up investigations are generally undertaken to determine the subsequent development of individuals who have a specified condition or who have received a specified intervention—unlike panel studies, which have samples drawn from a general population. For example, patients who have received a particular nursing intervention or clinical treatment may be followed up to ascertain the long-term effects of the treatment. As another example, samples of premature babies may be followed up to assess their later perceptual and motor development.

In sum, longitudinal designs are appropriate for studying the dynamics of a variable or phenomenon over time. The number of data collection periods and the time intervals in between the data collection points depend on the nature of study. When change or development is rapid, numerous time points at short intervals may be required to document the pattern and make accurate forecasts.

Many nursing studies involve a time dimension. Table 7-3 presents a brief description of several nursing studies that have used different research designs to address time-related research questions.

Retrospective Versus Prospective Designs

Many scientific studies are undertaken in an effort to better understand the underlying causes of phenomena. In studies that are non-

Table 7-3. *Examples of Studies With a Time Dimension*

RESEARCH QUESTION	DESIGN	SAMPLE
What is the pattern of development of nutritive sucking in very low birthweight (VLBW) infants of different gestational ages? (Medoff-Cooper, Verklan, & Carlson, 1993)	Cross-sectional	50 VLBW infants born at 27 to 32 weeks of gestational age
What are the trends in the academic achievement, values, and personal attributes of college freshmen aspiring to nursing careers from the 1960s to the 1980s? (Williams, 1988)	Trend study	Samples of 500 college freshmen surveyed in 1966, 1972, 1982, 1983, 1984, and 1985
What are the factors that contribute to turnover, absenteeism, and reduced work schedules in hospital nurses? (Wise, 1993)	Cohort study	A cohort of 404 nurses hired in a 2-year period in five hospitals
What is the level of experienced burnout, depression, and substance abuse among nursing students in different years of school? (Haack, 1988)	Cross-sequential	238 sophomore and junior nursing students, surveyed twice at a 1-year interval
What are the correlates of alcohol use among rural sixth- and seventh-grade children? (Long & Boik, 1993)	Panel study	625 children in rural Montana surveyed in third and fourth grade, then 3 years later
What are the levels of anxiety, anger, denial, depression, and heart rate variability during recovery from a myocardial infarction? (Buchanan, Cowan, Burr, Waldron, & Kogan, 1993)	Follow-up study	21 men assessed in first 4 days and 6 months after acute myocardial infarction

experimental—that is, in which the researcher does not introduce an intervention—there are two basic types of design that can be used to explore causality.

RETROSPECTIVE DESIGNS

Studies with a *retrospective design* are investigations in which some phenomenon existing in the present is linked to other phenomena that occurred in the past, before the study was initiated. That is, the investigator is interested in some presently occurring outcome and attempts to shed light on antecedent factors that have caused it. Many epidemiological studies are retrospective in nature, and this approach has been used by medical researchers for more than

a century. Most of the early cigarette smoking–lung cancer studies were retrospective. In such studies, the researcher would begin with a group of lung cancer victims and another group of people without the disease. The researcher would then look for differences between the two groups in antecedent behaviors or conditions, such as smoking habits. In nursing research, as in medical research, retrospective studies are fairly common.

PROSPECTIVE DESIGNS

A study with a nonexperimental *prospective design* starts with presumed causes and then goes forward in time, longitudinally, to the presumed effect. For example, a researcher might want to test the hypothesis that the incidence of rubella during pregnancy is related to malformations in the offspring. To test this hypothesis prospectively, the investigator would begin with a sample of pregnant women, including some who contracted rubella during their pregnancy and others who did not. The subsequent occurrence of congenital anomalies would be observed and the researcher would then be in a position to test whether women who contracted the disease during pregnancy were more likely to bear malformed babies than women who did not have rubella when pregnant.

Prospective studies are usually more costly than retrospective studies and perhaps are less common for this reason. Prospective research often requires large samples, particularly if the dependent variable of interest is rare, as in the example of malformed babies and maternal rubella. Another difficulty with prospective studies is that a substantial follow-up period may be necessary before the phenomenon or effect under investigation manifests itself, as is the case in prospective studies of cigarette smoking and lung cancer.

Despite these problems, prospective studies are considerably stronger than retrospective studies. For one thing, any ambiguity concerning the temporal sequence of phenomena usually is resolved in prospective research. In addition, samples are more likely to be representative, and investigators may be in a position to impose numerous controls to rule out competing explanations for observed effects.

Some actual research examples of retrospective and prospective designs are presented in Table 7-4.

❖ CHARACTERISTICS OF GOOD DESIGN

In selecting a research design, the researcher should be guided by one overarching consider-

Table 7-4. *Examples of Retrospective and Prospective Designs*

RESEARCH QUESTION	INDEPENDENT VARIABLE/TIMING	DEPENDENT VARIABLE/TIMING
PROSPECTIVE		
What are the predictors of the concerns and coping strategies of cancer chemotherapy outpatients? (Dodd, Dibble, & Thomas, 1993)	Predictive factors: time 1	Concerns and coping strategies: 6 months after time 1
What are the interdependent contributions of hemodynamics, gas exchange, and pulmonary mechanics to the prediction of weaning outcome in cardiac surgery patients? (Hanneman, 1994)	Cardiopulmonary predictive factors: time 1, two hours after surgery	Ability to be weaned from mechanical ventilation, several hours later
RETROSPECTIVE		
What are the antecedent factors associated with nicotine dependence among African American women cigarette smokers? (Ahijevych & Wewers, 1993)	Antecedent factors: time 1	Nicotine dependence: time 1
What antecedent factors are associated with battering by a partner during pregnancy? (Campbell, Poland, Waller, & Ager, 1992)	Antecedent factors: time 1	Battering status: time 1

ation: whether the design does the best possible job of providing reliable answers to the research questions. In this section, we briefly examine more specific characteristics of good research design.

Appropriateness to the Research Question

The requirement that the research design should be appropriate to the question being asked seems so obvious that it may be overlooked. Generally, a given research problem can be handled adequately with a number of different designs so that the researcher typically has some flexibility in selecting a design. Yet many designs are completely unsuitable for dealing with the research problem. For example, a loosely structured research design such as those often used in qualitative studies might be inappropriate to address the question of whether nonnutritive sucking opportunities among premature infants facilitate early oral feedings. On the other hand, a tightly controlled study may unnecessarily restrict the researcher interested in understanding the processes by which nurses make diagnoses. There are many research questions of interest to nurses for which highly structured designs are unsuitable.

Lack of Bias

A second characteristic of good research design in traditional scientific studies is that it results in data that are not biased. *Bias*, which refers to an influence that can distort the results of a study, can operate in a variety of ways, some of which are particularly subtle.

A common source of bias stems from differences among subjects in groups that are being compared. When groups are formed on a nonrandom basis, the risk of bias is always present. For example, in studies of the effects of smoking on lung cancer, an important concern is that smokers and nonsmokers may differ in ways that have little to do with smoking habits per se. The problem is that these other differ-

ences, rather than smoking, are potentially the real cause of the cancer. Unless these other differences (extraneous variables) are controlled, the resulting biases may make it difficult for the researcher to conclude with confidence that there is a causative link between smoking and lung cancer.

In studies in which the data are collected by means of observation, the researcher's preconceptions might unconsciously bias the objective collection of data. In such a case, the researcher should take a number of steps to minimize this risk. For example, *double-blind* procedures are often useful in this regard. The double-blind technique removes observer biases by virtue of the fact that neither the subject nor the person collecting the data knows the specific research objectives (nor, if groups are being compared, the group the subject is in) and thus cannot systematically distort the data. When this approach is not feasible, it is a good practice to have two or more observers so that at least an estimation of the biases can be made.

Bias can enter the data whenever there is an opportunity for something other than the independent variable of interest to affect the outcomes in a systematic way. Chapter 10 presents a number of techniques that can be used to eliminate or reduce problems of bias.

Although techniques of research control are often mechanisms for controlling bias, there are situations in which too much control can introduce bias. For example, if the researcher tightly controls the ways in which the key study variables can be manifested, it is possible that the true nature of those variables will be obscured. When the key variables are phenomena that are poorly understood or whose dimensions have not been clarified, then a design that allows some flexibility is better suited to the study aims.

Precision

The researcher should generally try to design a study to achieve the highest possible *precision*, which is achieved through control over extraneous variables. Research control actually concerns control over variability in the dependent measures. This concept can best be understood through a specific example.

Suppose we were interested in studying the effect of admission into a nursing home on the level of depression among the elderly. Depression may be the result of various influences; that is, depression varies from one elderly person to another for a variety of reasons. In the present study, we are interested in isolating—as precisely as possible—the portion of the variation in depression that is attributable to nursing home admission. Mechanisms of research control that reduce the variability attributable to extraneous factors can be built into the research design, thereby enhancing precision.

What the researcher is attempting to assess may be expressed in the following ratio:

$$\frac{\text{Variation in depression due to nursing home admission}}{\substack{\text{Variation in depression due to other factors} \\ \text{(e.g., age, pain, medical prognosis, social support, etc.)}}}$$

This ratio, although greatly simplified here, captures the essence of many statistical procedures. The researcher wants to make the variability in the numerator (the upper half) as large as possible relative to the variability in the denominator (the lower half) to evaluate most clearly the relationship between nursing home admission and levels of depression. The smaller the variability in depression that is due to extraneous variables such as the elderly person's age and prognosis, the easier it will be for the researcher to detect differences in depression between those who were and those who were not admitted to a nursing home. Designs that enable the researcher to reduce the variability caused by the extraneous variables are said to increase the precision of the research. As a purely hypothetical illustration of why this is so, we will attach some numerical values* to the ratio:

---

* The reader should not be concerned at this point with how these numbers can be obtained in a real analysis. The procedure will be explained in Chapter 18.

$$\frac{\text{Variability due to nursing home admission}}{\text{Variability due to extraneous variables}} = \frac{10}{4}$$

Now, if we can make the bottom number smaller, say changing it from 4 to 2, then we will have a purer and more precise estimate of the effect of nursing home admission on depression, relative to other influences.

How can a research design help to reduce the variability caused by extraneous variables? Several approaches are discussed in Chapter 10, but we illustrate here with a simple example. The total variability in levels of depression can be conceptualized as having three components:

Total variability in depression =
Variability due to nursing home admission +
Variability due to age + Variability due to other extraneous variables

This equation can be taken to mean that part of the reason why some elderly individuals are depressed and others are not is that some were admitted to a nursing home and others were not; some were older and some were younger; and other factors such as level of pain, medical prognosis, availability of social supports, and so forth also had an effect on depression.

One way to increase the precision in this study would be to control age, thereby removing the variability in depression that is the result of differences in the subjects' ages. We could do this, for example, by including in our sample only elderly people within a fairly narrow age range (e.g., only those older than 80 years of age). By limiting the age of the sample, the variability in levels of depression due to age would be reduced or eliminated. As a result, the effect of nursing home admission on depression becomes greater, relative to the remaining extraneous variability. Thus, we can say that this design has enabled us to get a more precise estimate of the effect of nursing home admission on level of depression. Research designs differ considerably in the sensitivity with which effects under study can be detected with statistical tools. Lipsey (1990) has prepared an excellent guide to assist researchers in enhancing the sensitivity of their research designs.

Power

We use *power* here to describe the ability of a research design to detect relationships among variables. Precision contributes to the power of a design. Power is also increased when a large sample is used. This aspect of power is discussed in Chapters 11 and 19.

One other aspect of a powerful design concerns the construction or definition of the independent variable. For both statistical and theoretical reasons, results are clearer and more conclusive when the differences between groups that are being compared are large. The researcher should generally aim to maximize group differences on the dependent variables by maximizing differences on the independent variable. In other words, the results are likely to be more clearcut if the groups are as different as possible. This advice is more easily followed in experimental than in nonexperimental research. In experiments, the investigator can devise interventions that are distinct and as strong as time, money, ethics, and practicality permit. However, even in nonexperimental research, there are frequently opportunities to operationalize the independent variables in such a way that power to detect differences is enhanced.

❖ TIPS ON DESIGNING RESEARCH

If you are planning to undertake a study, you will need to make a number of important decisions regarding the study's overall design. These decisions will affect your ability to interpret the data and the overall believability of your findings. In some cases, the decisions will affect whether you receive funding (if you are seeking financial support for your study) or whether you are able to publish your research report (if you plan to submit it to a professional journal). Therefore, a great deal of care and thought

should go into these decisions. The following tips may be useful in designing a study:

- When deciding between various alternative design strategies, make a written list of the pros and cons. For example, in the hypothetical study about the emotional consequences of an abortion, what are the advantages and disadvantages of using as a comparison group women who delivered the baby versus women who had a miscarriage?

- In making design decisions, you will often need to balance a number of considerations, such as time, cost, ethical issues, and the integrity of the study. Try to get a firm understanding of what your upper limits are before making final design decisions. That is, what is the most money that can be spent on the project? What is the maximal amount of time available for conducting the study? What is the limit of acceptability with regard to ethical issues, given the risk/benefit ratio of the study? These limits often eliminate a number of design options. With these constraints in mind, the central focus should be on designing a study that maximizes the accuracy and interpretability of the data.

- In designing a study, try to anticipate alternative findings and consider whether design adjustments might affect the results. For example, suppose we hypothesized that environmental factors such as light and noise affected the incidence of acute confusion among the hospitalized elderly. With a preliminary design for such a study in mind, try to imagine findings that *fail* to support the hypothesis. Then ask yourself what could be done to decrease the possibility of these negative results. Can power be increased by making differences in environmental conditions sharper? Can precision be increased by controlling additional extraneous variables? Can bias be eliminated by better training of research personnel?

- Do not try to make all design decisions single-handedly. Seek the advice of professors, colleagues, research consultants, and so on.

- Once you have made your design decisions, it may be useful to write out a rationale for your choices. Share the rationale with those you have consulted to see if they can find any flaws in your reasoning or if they can make suggestions for further improvements.

❖ RESEARCH EXAMPLES

We conclude this chapter with examples of two research studies that highlight some of the points made. The first example illustrates a structured design that involved the collection of data at two points in time. The second example describes a qualitative study with a substantially more flexible design. In reading these brief summaries, consider the strengths and weaknesses of the designs in terms of the study's objectives, referring as needed to the original journal articles.

Example of a Structured, Prospective Design

Winkelstein and Feldman (1993) used a theoretical model that combined elements from the Health Belief Model with psychosocial elements from other models to predict the consumption of sweet-tasting high-calorie foods after smoking cessation. A total of 203 men and women who were participating in Freedom From Smoking programs agreed to participate in the study.

During the first round of data collection, which occurred at the first program session, subjects completed a questionnaire and were observed in a "snack choice" exercise. The questionnaire included measures of the factors hypothesized to be predictive of the consumption of sweets after smoking cessation (e.g., the previous consumption of sweets, intention to avoid sweets, attitudes toward eating sweets, self-efficacy). Follow-up data were obtained at the sixth program session, which was 5 weeks after the first session (2 weeks after smoking cessation). The 114 subjects who were present at the

follow-up completed another questionnaire and again made snack choices. The dependent variable was based on three follow-up questions regarding the recent consumption of sweets as well as on the number of sweet snacks consumed in the second snack choice exercise.

The results indicated that subjects who stopped smoking reported eating more sweets than those who did not stop, regardless of prior habit of eating sweets. However, prior habit and self-efficacy as reported in the initial questionnaire were strong predictors of eating sweet-tasting, high-calorie foods after smoking cessation.

Example of a Flexible Research Design

Kidd (1993) conducted a study to better understand factors contributing to motor vehicle crashes (MVCs). A flexible design was used to qualitatively explore the variables surrounding an MVC and their interrelationships.

Kidd's design decisions evolved as new data were gathered and interpreted. The basic sample consisted of 18 MVC trauma patients, who were all interviewed during their hospitalization. Kidd decided to reinterview a subset of three informants while they were still in the hospital, to confirm certain of her findings. She also added three former trauma patients to her sample, who were interviewed in the community at varying lengths of time after their MVC injury. Kidd's development of data for comparative purposes also evolved during the course of the study. For example, after reflecting on some of her early data, Kidd decided to make an active effort to include informants with negative as well as positive blood alcohol levels, to determine whether pretrauma perceptions differed between these two groups. She also decided to augment her interview data by analyzing automobile advertisements in several periodicals and by analyzing favorite songs, commercials, and actors cited by her informants.

Based on her various sources of data, Kidd began to develop a theory of self-protection. She found that self-protecting strategies were contingent on the driver evaluating loss of control during the MVC. Kidd's self-protection theory postulates that if motor vehicle control was perceived to have been lost and such control is desired, then self-protecting strategies to enhance future control will be adopted.

❖ SUMMARY

The *research design* is the researcher's overall plan for answering the research question. The design indicates whether there is an intervention, and what the intervention is; the nature of any comparisons to be made; the methods to be used to control extraneous variables and enhance the study's interpretability; the timing and frequency of data collection; the setting in which the data collection is to take place; and the nature of communications with subjects.

Although there is no clearcut typology of research designs, designs can be described along various dimensions, such as whether there is an intervention (experimental versus nonexperimental designs). Another dimension concerns the degree of structure imposed on the design in advance. Most quantitative studies tend to be highly structured, with major features of the design specified before a single piece of data is collected. The designs in most qualitative studies, by contrast, are more fluid, with design changes permitted—and even encouraged—to take advantage of information gathered early in the study.

Another important dimension concerns the study's handling of the time dimension. *Cross-sectional designs* involve the collection of data at one point in time, whereas *longitudinal designs* collect data at two or more points in time. Research problems that involve trends, changes, or development over time or that intend to demonstrate temporal sequencing of phenomena are best addressed through longitudinal designs. *Trend studies* investigate a particular phenomenon over time by repeatedly drawing different samples from the same general population. *Cohort studies* are ones in which a particular subpopulation (typically a specific age cohort) is studied over time with respect to some phenomenon. Longitudinal studies in which the *same* sample of subjects is questioned twice (or more often) are known as *panel studies. Follow-up studies* similarly deal with the same subjects studied at two or more points in time and generally refer to those investigations in which subjects who have received a treatment or who have a particular characteristic of interest are followed to study their subsequent development. Longitudinal studies are typically expensive, time-consuming, and beset with such difficulties as *attrition* (loss of subjects over time) but are often extremely valuable with respect to the information they produce.

Many studies attempt to elucidate cause-and-effect relationships. Nonexperimental studies with such an aim use either a retrospective or prospective design. *Retrospective designs* are ones in which the researcher observes the manifestation of some phenomenon (the dependent variable) and tries to retrospectively identify its antecedents or causes (the independent variable). *Prospective studies* start with an observation of presumed causes and then go forward in time longitudinally to observe the consequences. Prospective research is typically initiated after evidence of important relationships is produced by retrospective investigations.

A good research design must be appropriate to the question being asked. It must also minimize or avoid *biases* that can distort the results of the study. Another feature of a good design is that it attempts to enhance *precision*, which refers to the sensitivity with which the effects of the independent variable, relative to the effects of extraneous variables, can be detected. Finally, the design should deal adequately with the issue of *power*, which concerns the ability of the design to create maximal contrasts among groups being compared.

❖ *STUDY SUGGESTIONS*

Chapter 7 of the accompanying *Study Guide for Nursing Research: Principles and Methods, 5th ed.*, offers various exercises and study suggestions for reinforcing the concepts presented in this chapter. Additionally, the following study questions can be addressed:

1. Suppose you were planning to conduct a nonexperimental study concerning the effects of three types of ambulation devices (a cane, a walker, and a crutch) on feelings of control or security for people requiring such assistive devices. What types of extraneous variables relating to characteristics of the subjects would be important to consider and, if possible, control?
2. Suppose you wanted to study how nurses' attitudes toward death change as a function of years of nursing experience. Design a cross-sectional study to research this question, specifying the samples that you would want to include. Now design a longitudinal study to research the same problem. Identify the problems and strengths of each approach.
3. Read one of the studies cited in Table 7-4. If you have chosen a prospective study, indicate how the study might have been conducted retrospectively, and vice versa. Compare the strengths and weaknesses of the new design with the design used in the actual study.

❖ *SUGGESTED READINGS*

METHODOLOGICAL REFERENCES

Given, B. A., Keilman, L. J., Collins, C., & Given, C. W. (1990). Strategies to minimize attrition in longitudinal studies. *Nursing Research, 39,* 184–186.
Kelly, J. R., & McGrath, J. E. (1988). *On time and method.* Newbury Park, CA: Sage.
Kerlinger, F. N. (1986). *Foundations of behavioral research* (3rd ed.). New York: Holt, Rinehart & Winston.

Lipsey, M. W. (1990). *Design sensitivity: Statistical power for experimental research.* Newbury Park, CA: Sage.
Spector, P. E. (1981). *Research designs.* Beverly Hills, CA: Sage.
Weekes, D. P., & Rankin, S. H. (1988). Life-span developmental methods: Application to nursing research. *Nursing Research, 37,* 380–383.

SUBSTANTIVE REFERENCES

Ahijevych, K., & Wewers, M. E. (1993). Factors associated with nicotine dependence among African American women cigarette smokers. *Research in Nursing and Health, 16,* 283–292.
Bruce, S. L., & Grove, S. K. (1994). The effect of a coronary artery risk evaluation program on serum lipid values and cardiovascualr risk levels. *Applied Nursing Research 7,* 67–74.
Buchanan, L. M., Cowan, M., Burr, R., Waldron, C., & Kogan, H. (1993). Measurement of recovery from myocardial infarction using heart rate variability and psychological outcomes. *Nursing Research, 42,* 74–78.
Campbell, J. C., Poland, M. L., Waller, J. B., & Ager, J. (1992). Correlates of battering during pregnancy. *Research in Nursing and Health, 15,* 219–226.
Dodd, M. J., Dibble, S. L., & Thomas, M. L. (1993). Predictors of concerns and coping strategies of cancer chemotherapy outpatients. *Applied Nursing Research, 6,* 2–7.
Elliott, D. (1994). The effects of music and muscle relaxation on patient anxiety in a coronary care unit. *Heart and Lung, 23,* 27–35.
Fogel, C. I. (1993). Pregnant inmates: Risk factors and pregnancy outcomes. *Journal of Obstetric, Gynecologic, and Neonatal Nursing, 22,* 33–39.
Haack, M. R. (1988). Stress and impairment among nursing students. *Research in Nursing and Health, 11,* 125–134.
Hanneman, S. K. (1994). Multidimensional predictors of success or failure with early weaning from mechanical ventilation after cardiac surgery. *Nursing Research, 43,* 4–10.
Kidd, P. S. (1993). Self-protection: Trauma patients' perspectives of their motor vehicle crashes. *Qualitative Health Research, 3,* 320–340.
Kinzel, D. (1991). Self-identified health concerns of two homeless groups. *Western Journal of Nursing Research, 13,* 181–190.

Long, K. A., & Boik, R. J. (1993). Predicting alcohol use in rural children: A longitudinal study. *Nursing Research, 42,* 79–86.

Mahon, N. E., Yarcheski, A., & Yarcheski, T. J. (1993). Health consequences of loneliness in adolescents. *Research in Nursing and Health, 16,* 23–32.

McSweeney, J. C. (1993). Making behavior changes after a myocardial infarction. *Western Journal of Nursing Research, 15,* 441–455.

Medoff-Cooper, B., Verklan, T., & Carlson, S. (1993). The development of sucking patterns and physiologic correlates in very-low-birthweight infants. *Nursing Research, 42,* 100–105.

Nugent, L. S., Tamlyn-Leaman, K., Isa, N., Reardon, E., & Crumley, J. (1993). Anxiety and the colposcopy experience. *Clinical Nursing Research, 2,* 267–277.

Pollack, L. E. (1993). Content analysis of groups for inpatients with bipolar disorder. *Applied Nursing Research, 6,* 19–27.

Price, P., & Fowlow, B. (1993). Thermodilution cardiac output determinations: A comparison of iced and refrigerated injectate temperatures in patients after cardiac surgery. *Heart and Lung, 22,* 266–274.

Rogers, A. E., & Aldrich, M. S. (1993). The effect of regularly scheduled naps on sleep attacks and excessive daytime sleepiness associated with narcolepsy. *Nursing Research, 42,* 111–117.

Williams, R. P. (1988). College freshmen aspiring to nursing careers: Trends from the 1960s to the 1980s. *Western Journal of Nursing Research, 10,* 94–97.

Winkelstein, M. L., & Feldman, R. H. L. (1993). Psychosocial predictors of consumption of sweets following smoking cessation. *Research in Nursing and Health, 16,* 97–105.

Wise, L. C. (1993). The erosion of nursing resources: Employee withdrawal behaviors. *Research in Nursing and Health, 16,* 67–75.

Chapter 8

EXPERIMENTAL, QUASI-EXPERIMENTAL, AND NONEXPERIMENTAL DESIGNS

In the previous chapter, we discussed various aspects of research design. This chapter focuses on research designs that vary along an important dimension: whether the researcher actively controls the independent variable. We begin with a discussion of research designs that offer the greatest amount of control: experimental studies.

❖ EXPERIMENTAL RESEARCH

Experiments differ from nonexperiments in one important respect: the researcher is an active agent in experimental work rather than a passive observer. Early physical scientists learned that although observation of natural phenomena is valuable and instructive, the complexity of the events occurring in the natural state often obscures understanding of important relationships. This problem was handled by isolating the phenomenon of interest in a laboratory setting and controlling the conditions under which

it occurred. The procedures developed by physical scientists were profitably adopted by biologists during the 19th century, resulting in many achievements in physiology and medicine. The 20th century has witnessed the use of experimental methods by scholars and researchers interested in human behavior and psychological phenomena.

Characteristics of True Experiments

The controlled experiment is considered by many to be the ideal of science. Except for purely descriptive research, the aim of scientific research is to understand the nature of relationships among phenomena. For example, does a certain drug cause the cure of a certain disease? Do certain nursing techniques produce a decrease in patient anxiety? The strength of the true experiment over other methods lies in the fact that the experimenter can achieve greater confidence in the genuineness and interpreta-

Polit DF, Hungler BP: NURSING RESEARCH: PRINCIPLES AND METHODS, 5th ed. © 1995 J. B. Lippincott Company.

bility of relationships because they are observed under carefully controlled conditions. As we pointed out in Chapter 3, hypotheses are never ultimately proved or disproved by scientific methods, but true experiments offer the most convincing evidence concerning the effects one variable can have on another.

A true experiment is a scientific investigation characterized by the following properties:

- *Manipulation*—the experimenter *does* something to at least some of the subjects in the study
- *Control*—the experimenter introduces one or more controls over the experimental situation, including the use of a control group
- *Randomization*—the experimenter assigns subjects to a control or experimental group on a random basis

Each of these properties is discussed more fully below.

MANIPULATION

Manipulation involves *doing* something to at least one group of subjects. The introduction of that "something" (often referred to as the experimental *treatment* or experimental *intervention*) constitutes the independent variable. The experimenter manipulates the independent variable by administering a treatment to some subjects and withholding it from others (or by administering some other treatment, such as a placebo). The experimenter, in other words, consciously *varies* the independent variable and observes the effect that the manipulation has on the dependent variable of interest.

For example, let us say we have hypothesized that the color of a pediatric nurse's uniform affects the degree to which children display positive affective behaviors such as smiling and laughing during hospitalization. The independent or presumed causative variable in this example is uniform color, which could be manipulated by assigning some nurses white uniforms (for instance) and other nurses brightly colored uniforms. Thus, in this study we might compare, 24 hours after hospitalization, the affective behavior (the dependent variable) of two groups of children: 1) those cared for by white-uniformed nurses; and 2) those cared for by nurses in colored uniforms.

CONTROL

The notion of control in an experimental context actually summarizes all the major experimental activities: control is acquired by manipulating, by randomizing, by carefully preparing the experimental protocols, and by using a control group. This section focuses on the function of the control group in experiments.

Obtaining scientific evidence about relationships requires making at least one comparison. If we were to supplement the diet of a group of premature infants with a particular combination of vitamins and other nutrients every day for 2 weeks, the weight of those infants at the end of the 2-week period would give us absolutely no information about the effectiveness of the treatment. At a bare minimum, we would need to compare their posttreatment weight with their pretreatment weight to determine if, at least, their weight had increased. But let us assume for the moment that we find an average weight gain of 1 pound. Does this finding support the conclusion that there is a causative relationship between the nutritional supplements (the independent variable) and weight gain (the dependent variable)? No, it does not. Babies normally gain weight as they mature. Without a control group—a group that does *not* receive the nutritional supplements—it is impossible to separate the effects of maturation from those of the treatment. The term *control group,* in other words, refers to a group of subjects whose performance on a dependent variable is used as a basis for evaluating the performance of the *experimental group* (the group that receives the treatment of interest to the researcher) on the same dependent variable.

In some biologic, medical, and psychological research, the experimenter administers the treatment of interest to the experimental group, while the control group receives no treatment at all and is merely observed with respect to behavior on the dependent variable. This kind of situation probably is not feasible for many nursing research projects because it may be impossible to isolate a control group and do nothing to those subjects. For example, if we wanted to evaluate the effectiveness of some nursing intervention on hospital patients, it would be unlikely that we would devise an experiment in which the control group of patients received no nursing care at all. We would have to evaluate our new intervention not against the total absence of care but rather against a control group receiving conventional methods of care.

RANDOMIZATION

Randomization (also referred to as *random assignment*) involves the placement of subjects in groups on a random basis. Random essentially means that every subject has an equal chance of being assigned to any group. If subjects are placed in groups randomly, there is no *systematic bias* in the groups with respect to attributes that may affect the dependent variable under investigation.

Before discussing the mechanics of random assignment, we should pause to consider its function. Suppose a researcher wishes to study the effectiveness of a hospital-based contraceptive counseling program for a group of multiparous women who have just given birth. Two groups of subjects are established, one of which will be counseled and the other of which will receive no counseling. The women in the sample may be expected to differ from one another on a number of characteristics, such as age, marital status, financial situation, attitudes toward child-rearing, and the like. Any of these characteristics could have an effect on the diligence with which a woman practices contraception, independent of whether or not she receives counseling. The researcher needs to have the "counsel" and "no counsel" groups equal with respect to these extraneous characteristics to properly assess the impact of the experimen-

tal counseling program on the women's subsequent pregnancies. The random assignment of subjects to one group or the other is designed to perform this equalization function. One method might be to flip a coin for each woman (more elaborate procedures are discussed later). If the coin is "heads," the woman would be assigned to one group; if the coin is "tails," she would be assigned to the other group.

Although randomization is the preferred scientific method for equalizing groups, there is no guarantee that they will, in fact, be equal. Let us take as an extreme example the case in which only 10 women, all of whom have given birth to at least four children, constitute the entire sample for the study. Five of the 10 women are aged 35 years or older, and the remaining five are younger than 35 years of age. One would anticipate that a random assignment of women to an experimental or control group would result in about two or three women from the two age ranges in each group. But let us suppose that, by chance, the older five women all ended up in the experimental group. Because these women are nearing the end of their child-bearing years, the likelihood of their conceiving is diminished. Thus, follow-up of their subsequent reproductive behavior (the dependent variable) might suggest that the counseling program was successful for the experimental group; however, a higher pregnancy rate for the control group may only reflect the age and fecundity differences and not the lack of exposure to counseling.

Despite this possibility, randomization remains the most trustworthy and acceptable method of equalizing groups. Unusual or deviant assignments such as this one are rare, and the likelihood of obtaining markedly unequal groups is reduced as the number of subjects increases.

Students often wonder why the researcher does not consciously control those characteristics of subjects that are likely to affect the experimental outcome. The procedure that is sometimes used to accomplish this is known as *matching*. For example, if matching were used in the contraceptive counseling study, the researcher might want to ensure that if there were a married, 38-year-old woman with six children in the experimental group, there would be a married, 38-year-old woman with six children in the control group as well. There are two serious problems with matching, however. First of all, to match effectively, we must know what are the characteristics that are likely to affect the dependent variable. This information is not always known. Second, even if we knew the relevant traits, the complications of matching on more than three or four characteristics simultaneously are prohibitive. With random assignment, on the other hand, *all* possible distinguishing characteristics—age, gender, intelligence, blood type, religious affiliation, and so on—are likely to be equally distributed in all groups. Over the long run, the groups tend to be counterbalanced with respect to an infinite number of biologic, psychological, economic, or social traits.

To demonstrate how random assignment is actually performed, we turn to another example. Suppose we have 15 children who are about to have a tonsillectomy and we are interested in testing the effectiveness of two alternative nursing interventions with regard to the child's level of preoperative anxiety. One intervention focuses on structured information regarding the activities of the surgical team (procedural information); the other focuses on structured information regarding what the child will feel (sensation information). A third group will receive no special intervention. Five children will be in each of the three groups. Because there are three groups, we can no longer use the flip of a coin to decide the group to which an individual will be assigned. One possibility would be to write the names of the individuals on slips of paper, put the slips into a hat, and then draw names. The first five individuals whose names were drawn would be assigned to group I, the second five would be assigned to group II, and the remaining five would be assigned to group III.

Pulling names from a hat involves considerable work, especially if there are many sub-jects. Researchers typically use a *table of random numbers* to facilitate the randomization process. A portion of such a table is reproduced in Table 8-1. A random number table is set up by using the digits from 0 to 9 in such a way that each number is equally likely to follow any other. These tables are often generated by computers. Going in any direction from any point in the table produces a random sequence.

In our example, we would number the 15 subjects from 1 to 15, as shown in the second column of Table 8-2, and then draw numbers between 1 and 15 from the random number table. A simple procedure for finding a starting point is to close your eyes and let your finger fall at some point on the table. For the sake of following the example, let us assume that we have followed this procedure and that the starting point is at number 52 as circled on Table 8-1. We can now move from that point in any direction in the table. Our task is to select the first five numbers that fall between 01 and 15. Let us move from the starting point to the right, looking at two-digit combinations to be sure to get numbers from 10 to 15. The next number to the right of 52 is 06. The person whose number is 06, that is, Nathan O., is assigned to group I. Moving along in the table, we find that the next number within the range of 01 to 15 is 11. Katy M., whose number is 11, is also assigned to group I. When we get to the end of the row, we move down to the next row, and so forth. To find numbers in the required range, we may have to bypass many numbers. The next three numbers we find are 01, 15, and 14. Thus Megan B., Thomas N., and Kevin K. are all put into group I. The next five numbers between 01 and 15 that emerge in the random number table are used to assign five individuals to group II in the same fashion, as shown in the third column of Table 8-2. The remaining five people are put into group III. Note that numbers that have already been used often reappear in the table before our randomization task is completed. For example, the number 15 appeared four times during the randomization procedure. This is perfectly normal because the numbers are

Table 8-1. *Small Table of Random Digits*

46 85 05 23 26	34 67 75 83 00	74 91 06 43 45
69 24 89 34 60	45 30 50 75 21	61 31 83 18 55
14 01 33 17 92	59 74 76 72 77	76 50 33 45 13
56 30 38 73 15	16 (52) 06 96 76	11 65 49 98 93
81 30 44 85 85	68 65 22 73 76	92 85 25 58 66
70 28 42 43 26	79 37 59 52 20	01 15 96 32 67
90 41 59 36 14	33 52 12 66 65	55 82 34 76 41
39 90 40 21 15	59 58 94 90 67	66 82 14 15 75
88 15 20 00 80	20 55 49 14 09	96 27 74 [82] 57
45 13 46 35 45	59 40 47 20 59	43 94 75 16 80
70 01 41 50 21	41 29 06 73 12	71 85 71 59 57
37 23 93 32 95	05 87 00 11 19	92 78 42 63 40
18 63 73 75 09	82 44 49 90 05	04 92 17 37 01
05 32 78 21 62	20 24 78 17 59	45 19 72 53 32
95 09 66 79 46	48 46 08 55 58	15 19 11 87 82
43 25 38 41 45	60 83 32 59 83	01 29 14 13 49
80 85 40 92 79	43 52 90 63 18	38 38 47 47 61
80 08 87 70 74	88 72 25 67 36	66 16 44 94 31
80 89 07 80 02	94 81 33 19 00	54 15 58 34 36
93 12 81 84 64	74 45 79 05 61	72 84 81 18 34
82 47 42 55 93	48 54 53 52 47	18 61 91 36 74
53 34 24 42 76	75 12 21 17 24	74 62 77 37 07
82 64 12 28 20	92 90 41 31 41	32 39 21 97 63
13 57 41 72 00	69 90 26 37 42	78 46 42 25 01
29 59 38 86 27	94 97 21 15 98	62 09 53 67 87
86 88 75 50 87	19 15 20 00 23	12 30 28 07 83
44 98 91 68 22	36 02 40 08 67	76 37 84 16 05
93 39 94 55 47	94 45 87 42 84	05 04 14 98 07
52 16 29 02 86	54 15 83 42 43	46 97 83 54 82
04 73 72 10 31	75 05 19 30 29	47 66 56 43 82

Reprinted from *A Million Random Digits with 100,000 Normal Deviates.* New York: The Free Press, 1955. Used with permission of the Rand Corporation, Santa Monica, CA.

random. After the first time a number appears and is used, subsequent appearances can be ignored.

It might be useful to look at the three groups to see if they are about equal with respect to one readily discernible characteristic, that is, the gender of the subject. We started out with eight girls and seven boys in the total group. The gender breakdown of the three groups is presented in Table 8-3. As this table shows, the randomization procedure did a good job of allocating boys and girls about equally across the three groups. We must accept on faith the probability that other characteristics are fairly well distributed in the randomized groups as well.

One more step in the randomization process must be completed before the experiment begins. Note that in the previous discussion we did not state that the five subjects in group I would be assigned to the procedural information group. This is because it is a good strategy to randomly assign groups to treatments as well as individuals to groups. To continue

Table 8-2. *Example of Random Assignment Procedure*

NAME OF SUBJECT	NUMBER	GROUP ASSIGNMENT
Megan B.	1	I
Billy M.	2	III
Claire L.	3	III
Lauren C.	4	II
Rebecca C.	5	II
Nathan O.	6	I
Lindsey S.	7	III
Jevan F.	8	III
Chad C.	9	II
Rosanna D.	10	III
Katy M.	11	I
Emily B.	12	II
Alex H.	13	II
Kevin K.	14	I
Thomas N.	15	I

with our example, we give the procedural information, sensation information, and control conditions the numbers 1, 2, and 3, respectively. Finding a new starting point in the random number table, we look for the numbers 1, 2, or 3. This time we can look at one digit at a time, because the range of values we are seeking does not include a two-digit number. Let us say that we start at number 8 in the ninth row of the table, which is indicated by a rectangle. Reading *down* this time, we find the number 1. We therefore assign group I to the procedural information condition. Further along in the same column we come to the number 3. Group III, therefore, is assigned to the second condition, sensation information, and the remaining group, group II, is assigned to the control condition.

In most cases, randomization involves the assignment of individual subjects to different groups on a random basis. However, an important alternative is *cluster randomization,* which involves randomly assigning groups or clusters of individuals to different treatment groups (Hauck, Gilliss, Donner, & Gortner, 1991). There are several advantages to such an approach, the most important of which is enhancing the feasi-

bility of conducting a true experiment. Groups of patients who enter a hospital unit at the same time, or groups of patients from different medical practices, can be randomly assigned to a treatment condition as a unit—thus ruling out, in some situations, some practical impediments to randomization. This approach also reduces the possibility of *contamination* between two different treatments, that is, the co-mingling of subjects in the groups, which could reduce the effectiveness of the manipulation. The main disadvantages of cluster randomization are that the statistical analysis of data obtained through this approach is somewhat more complex, and usually sample size requirements are greater for a given level of accuracy.

Experimental Designs

There are numerous types of experimental design. The most commonly used designs are discussed in this section.

BASIC EXPERIMENTAL DESIGNS

At the beginning of this chapter, we described an example of testing hospitalized children's affective behavior after being cared for by nurses wearing different color uniforms. This example illustrates a simple design that is sometimes referred to as an *after-only* or *posttest-only* experimental design because data on the dependent variable are only collected once—after the experimental treatment has been introduced.

A second basic design is slightly more complex. Let us suppose that we are interested

Table 8-3. *Breakdown of the Gender Composition of the Three Groups*

SEX	GROUP I	GROUP II	GROUP III
Boys	3	2	2
Girls	2	3	3

	Before the Treatment	After the Treatment
Experimental Group	Pretest	Posttest
Control Group	Pretest	Posttest

Figure 8-1.   *Before–after (pretest-posttest) experimental design.*

in investigating the effect on heart rate of being physically restrained by Posey belt. We might choose to begin our experimentation with some subhuman species such as the rat. We decide to use an experimental scheme such as the one shown in Figure 8-1. This design involves imposing restraint by Posey belt on one group of rats (the experimental group) while imposing no restraint on another (the control group). In this design, the dependent variable is measured at two points in time: before and after the experimental intervention. This scheme permits us to examine what changes in heart rate were produced as a result of being physically restrained, which is our independent variable. This design, because of its two measurement points, is referred to as a *before–after* or *pretest–posttest* experimental design. In such designs, the initial measure of the dependent variable is often referred to as the *baseline measure.* (Some researchers involved in experimental research refer to the posttest measure of the dependent variable as the *outcome measure*—that is, the measure that captures the outcome of the experimental intervention).

SOLOMON FOUR-GROUP DESIGN

When data are collected both before and after an intervention, the pretest (initial) measure sometimes has the potential to distort the results. That is, the posttest measures may be affected not only by the treatment but also by exposure to the pretest. For example, if our intervention was a workshop to improve nurses'

attitudes toward AIDS patients, a pretest attitudinal measure may in itself constitute a sensitizing treatment and could obscure an analysis of the workshop's effect. Such a situation might call for the *Solomon four-group design,* which consists of two experimental groups and two control groups. One experimental group and one control group would be administered the pretest and the other groups would not, thereby allowing the effects of the pretest measure and intervention to be segregated. Figure 8-2 illustrates the Solomon four-group design.

FACTORIAL DESIGN

The discussion to this point has considered designs in which the experimenter systematically varies or manipulates only one independent variable at a time. It is, however, possible to manipulate two or more variables simultaneously. Suppose that we are interested in com-

	Data Collection	
Group	**Before**	**After**
Experimental—with pretest	X	X
Experimental—without pretest		X
Control—with pretest	X	X
Control—without pretest		X

Figure 8-2.   *Solomon four-group experimental design.*

paring two therapeutic strategies for premature infants: one method involves tactile stimulation, and the second approach involves auditory stimulation. At the same time, however, we are interested in learning if the daily amount of stimulation is related to the progress of the infant. The dependent variables for the study will be various measures of infant development, such as weight gain, cardiac responsiveness, and so forth. Figure 8-3 illustrates the structure of this experiment.

This type of study is known as a *factorial experiment*. Factorial designs permit the testing of multiple hypotheses in a single experiment. In this example, the three research questions being addressed are as follows:

1. Does auditory stimulation have a more beneficial effect on the development of premature infants than tactile stimulation?
2. Is the duration of stimulation (independent of type) related to infant development?
3. Is auditory stimulation most effective when linked to a certain dose and tactile stimulation most effective when coupled with a different dose?

The third question demonstrates a major strength of factorial designs: they permit us to evaluate not only *main effects* (effects resulting from experimentally manipulated variables, as exemplified in questions 1 and 2) but also *interaction effects* (effects resulting from combining the treatment methods). We may feel that it is insufficient to say that auditory stimulation is preferable to tactile stimulation (or vice versa) and that 45 minutes of stimulation per day is more effective than 15 minutes per day. Rather, it is how these two variables interact (how they behave in combination) that is of interest. Our results may indicate that 15 minutes of tactile stimulation and 45 minutes of auditory stimulation are the most beneficial treatments. We could *not* have obtained these results by conducting two separate experiments that manipulated only one independent variable and held the second one constant.

In factorial experiments, subjects are assigned at random to a specific combination of conditions. In the example that Figure 8-3 illustrates, the premature infants would be assigned randomly to one of the six cells. A *cell* in exper-

TYPE OF STIMULATION

		Auditory A1	Tactile A2
DAILY EXPOSURE	15 min. B1	A1 B1	A2 B1
	30 min. B2	A1 B2	A2 B2
	45 min. B3	A1 B3	A2 B3

Figure 8-3. *Schematic diagram of a factorial experiment.*

imental research refers to a treatment condition; it is represented in a schematic diagram as a box (cell) in the design.

Figure 8-3 can also be used to define some design terminology sometimes encountered in the research literature. The two independent variables in a factorial design are referred to as the *factors*. The type-of-stimulation variable is factor A and the amount-of-daily-exposure variable is factor B. Each factor must have two or more *levels* (if there were only one level, the factor would not be a variable). Level one of factor A is auditory and level two of factor A is tactile. When describing the dimensions of the design, researchers refer to the number of levels. The design in Figure 8-3 would be described as a 2 × 3 design: two levels in factor A times three levels in factor B. If a third source of stimulation, such as visual stimulation, were added, and if a daily dosage of 60 minutes were also added, the design would be referred to as a 3 × 4 design.

Factorial experiments can be performed with three or more independent variables (factors). However, designs with more than three factors are rare because the analysis becomes complex and because the number of subjects required becomes prohibitive.

REPEATED MEASURES DESIGN

Thus far we described experimental studies in which the subjects who are randomly assigned to different treatments are different people. For instance, in the previous example, infants exposed to 15 minutes of auditory stimulation were not the same infants as those exposed to the other five possible treatment conditions. In some studies, however, the same subjects are exposed to more than one treatment, in what is known as a *repeated measures design* (sometimes referred to as a *crossover design*). This type of design has the advantage of ensuring the highest possible equivalence among subjects exposed to different conditions—the groups being compared are obviously equal with respect to age, weight, psychological state, and so on because they are composed of the same people.

In repeated measures experimental designs, the subjects are randomly assigned to different ordering of treatments. For example, if a repeated measures design were used to compare the effects of auditory and tactile stimulation on the development of premature infants, some infants would be randomly assigned to receive auditory stimulation first, while others would be randomly assigned to receive tactile stimulation first. In such a study, the three conditions for an experiment have been met: there is manipulation, randomization, and control—with subjects serving as their own control group.

Although repeated measures designs are extremely powerful, they are sometimes inappropriate for certain research questions because of the problems of carry-over effects. When subjects are exposed to two different treatments or conditions, they may be influenced in the second condition by their experience in the first condition. As one example, drug studies rarely use a repeated measures design because drug B administered after drug A is not necessarily the same treatment as drug B administered after drug A.

RANDOMIZED CLINICAL TRIALS

Medical researchers and epidemiologists often evaluate an innovative treatment through the use of a randomized clinical trial (sometimes referred to simply as a clinical trial). *Clinical trials* typically use either a before–after or an after-only design. The term clinical trial, then, does not refer so much to a distinctive design as to an application of a design. Clinical trials always involve the testing of a clinical treatment; the random assignment of subjects of experimental and one or more control conditions; the collection of information on outcomes of the treatment from subjects in all groups, sometimes after a long period has elapsed; and generally, the use of a large and heterogeneous sample of subjects, frequently selected from multiple, geographically dispersed sites to ensure that the findings are not unique to a single setting.

When clinical trials involve the withholding of a potentially beneficial treatment from the control group or the administration of a potentially risky new treatment to the experimental group, researchers are sometimes reluctant to allocate subjects to groups on an equal basis. For example, for evaluating a promising new drug for the treatment of AIDS, researchers may randomly allocate 75% of the subjects to the experimental group and 25% to the control group. This unequal allocation has obvious advantages from an ethical point of view, but it is generally more costly because when subjects are not equally divided among treatment groups, the total number of subjects needed is greater to achieve the same level of power in performing statistical tests.

Advantages and Disadvantages of Experiments

Controlled experiments are often considered the ideal of science. In this section, we explore the reasons why experimental methods are held in high esteem and examine some of their limitations.

EXPERIMENTAL ADVANTAGES

True experiments are the most powerful method available to scientists for testing hypotheses of cause-and-effect relationships between variables. Because of its special controlling properties, the scientific experiment offers greater corroboration than any other research approach that, *if* the independent variable (e.g., diet, drug dosage, or teaching approach) is manipulated in a certain way, *then* certain consequences in the dependent variable (e.g., weight loss, recovery of health, or learning) may be expected to ensue. This "if . . . then" type of relationship is important to nursing and medical researchers because of its implications for prediction and control. The great strength of exper-

iments, then, lies in the confidence with which causal relationships can be inferred.

Paul Lazarsfeld (1955), a sociologist, identified three criteria for causality. The first criterion is temporal: a cause must precede an effect in time. If we were testing the hypothesis that saccharin causes bladder cancer, it would obviously be necessary to demonstrate that the subjects had not developed cancer before exposure to saccharin. The second requirement is that there be an empirical relationship between the presumed cause and the presumed effect. In the saccharin and cancer example, the researcher would have to demonstrate an association between the ingestion of saccharin and the presence of a carcinoma, that is, that a higher percentage of saccharin users than nonusers developed cancer. The final criterion for establishing a causal relationship is that the relationship cannot be explained as being the result of the influence of a third variable. Suppose, for instance, that people who use saccharin tend also to drink more coffee than nonusers of saccharin. There would then be a possibility that any empirical relationship between saccharin use and bladder cancer in humans reflects an underlying causal relationship between a substance in coffee and bladder cancer. It is particularly because of this third criterion that the experimental approach is so strong. Through the controls imposed by manipulation, comparison, and randomization, alternative explanations to a causal interpretation can often be ruled out or discredited.

EXPERIMENTAL DISADVANTAGES

Despite the overwhelming advantages of experimental research, this approach has several limitations. First of all, there are a number of constraints that make an experimental approach impractical or impossible in some situations. These constraints are discussed later in this chapter.

Sometimes experiments are criticized for their artificiality. Part of the difficulty lies in the requirement for randomization and then equal treatment within groups. In ordinary life, the way in which we interact with people is not random. For example, within the nursing field, certain aspects of the patient (e.g., age, physical attractiveness, personality, or severity of illness) will cause us to modify our behavior and, hence, our care. The differences may be extremely subtle, but they undoubtedly are not random. Another aspect of experiments that is considered artificial by phenomenologists is the focus on only a handful of variables, while attempting to hold all else constant. This requirement is criticized as being reductionist and as artificially constraining human experience.

Another problem with experiments is the *Hawthorne effect,* which is a kind of placebo effect. The term is derived from a series of experiments conducted at the Hawthorne plant of the Western Electric Corporation in which various environmental conditions such as light and working hours were varied to determine their effect on worker productivity. Regardless of what change was introduced, that is, whether the light was made better or worse, productivity increased. Thus, it appears that the knowledge of being included in a study may be sufficient to cause people to change their behavior, thereby obscuring the effect of the variable of interest. In a hospital situation, the researcher might have to contend with a double Hawthorne effect. For example, if an experiment to investigate the effect of a new postoperative patient routine were conducted, nurses and hospital staff, as well as patients, might be aware of their participation in a study, and both groups might alter their actions accordingly. It is precisely for this reason that double-blind experiments, in which neither the subjects nor those who administer the treatment know who is in the experimental or control group, are so powerful. Unfortunately, the double-blind approach is not feasible for some types of nursing research because nursing interventions are more difficult to disguise than medications.

In sum, despite the clearcut superiority of experiments in terms of their ability to test research hypotheses, they are subject to a number of limitations that make them difficult to apply to many real-world problems. Nevertheless, the fact that experimental conditions may be difficult to establish does not mean that all attempts to achieve them should be abandoned.

Research Example of an Experimental Design

Nurse researchers are increasingly using experimental designs to test their hypotheses. Table 8-4 summarizes some recent examples. An experimental study described in more detail follows.

Hastings-Tolsma and her colleagues (1993) used an interesting design to study differences in tissue response to warm versus cold applications to infiltrated intravenous sites. The researchers also wanted to investigate the effect of warm versus cold applications in the resolution of infiltrated solutions of three different levels of osmolarity (½ saline, normal saline, and 3% saline). The dependent variables included measures of pain intensity, erythema and induration, and interstitial fluid volume.

The sample consisted of 18 healthy adults. Six subjects were sequentially assigned to each of the three different solutions, in order of recruitment into the study. The experimental procedure (i.e., infiltration, application of a thermostat pad, and measurements of the dependent variable) was performed twice on each subject—once with a cold application (0°C) and once with a warm application (43°C), on alternate arms. Randomization was used to determine which application would be done first (cold or warm) and which arm would be used first (left or right). Measurements of pain intensity, surface induration, and fluid volume were obtained three times: at 12, 42, and 72 minutes after infiltration.

Given the complexity of design and measures used, the study yielded many findings. For example, the researchers found that the cold versus warm applications did not yield any significant differences in terms of pain intensity or surface induration, but there

Table 8-4.   *Examples of Studies Using Experimental Designs*

RESEARCH QUESTION	MANIPULATED VARIABLE	SUBJECTS
DESIGN: AFTER-ONLY How effective is a medication discharge planning program for patients with congestive heart failure in terms of reducing hospital readmissions? (Schneider, Hornberger, Booker, Davis, & Kralicek, 1993)	Participation versus nonparticipation in medication discharge planning program	26 patients in experimental program; 28 patients in control group
DESIGN: BEFORE–AFTER What is the relative efficacy of specialized and traditional AIDS education programs grams on behavioral and psychological outcomes among poor women of color? (Nyamathi, Leake, Flaskerud, Lewis, & Bennett, 1993)	Specialized versus traditional AIDS education program	448 women in specialized program; 410 in traditional program
DESIGN: FACTORIAL What is the effect of informational interventions on mothers' and childrens' ability to cope with an unplanned childhood hospitalization? (Melnyk, 1994)	Receipt of child behavioral information versus nonreceipt; receipt of parental role information versus nonreceipt	26 in child behavioral information group; 22 in parental role information group; 23 in group with neither; 27 in group with both
DESIGN: REPEATED MEASURES What is the effect of boomerang pillows on the respiratory capacity of hospitalized patients? (Roberts, Brittin, Cook, & deClifford, 1994)	Placement of patients on boomerang pillows versus straight pillows	42 patients exposed to both types of pillows in random order

were differences in interstitial fluid volume. For all three solutions, the volume was less with warm than with cold application. A difference in pain intensity by solution was found, with the highest pain ratings resulting in the 3% saline condition. There were no interaction effects between type of solution, warm versus cold application, and time of measurement on pain intensity.

❖ QUASI-EXPERIMENTAL RESEARCH

Research that uses a quasi-experimental design often looks much like an experiment. *Quasi-*

experiments, like true experiments, involve the manipulation of an independent variable, that is, the institution of an experimental treatment. However, quasi-experimental designs lack at least one of the other two properties that characterize true experiments: randomization or a control group.

Quasi-Experimental Designs

The basic difficulty with the quasi-experimental approach is its weakness, relative to experiments, in allowing us to make causal inferences. The problems inherent in quasi-exper-

R = Randomization
O = Observation or measurement
X = Treatment or intervention

$$R \quad O_1 \quad X \quad O_2$$
$$R \quad O_1 \quad \quad O_2$$

Figure 8-4. *Symbolic representation of a pretest–posttest (before-after) experimental design.*

iments are most easily discussed using examples of specific designs. Before presenting these examples, however, it is useful to introduce some notation to facilitate our discussion.* Figure 8-4 presents a symbolic representation of a pretest–posttest experimental design, identical to the design shown in Figure 8-1. According to the notation used in Figure 8-4, R means that there has been a random assignment to separate treatment groups. O represents an observation, that is, the collection of data on the dependent variable. X stands for the exposure of a group to an experimental treatment. Thus, the top line in Figure 8-4 represents the experimental group that has had subjects randomly assigned to it (R), has had both a pretest (O_1) and a posttest (O_2), and has been exposed to the experimental treatment of interest (X). The second row in the figure represents the control group, which differs from the experimental group only by the absence of exposure to the experimental treatment. We are now equipped to examine a few quasi-experimental designs.

NONEQUIVALENT CONTROL GROUP DESIGNS

Suppose that we wished to study the effect of introducing primary nursing as the method of delivering nursing care on nursing staff morale. The system is being implemented in a 600-bed hospital in a large metropolitan area. Because the new system of nursing care delivery is being implemented throughout the hospital, randomization is not possible. Therefore, we decide to find another hospital with similar characteristics (size, geographic location,

and the like) that is not instituting primary nursing. We decide to collect baseline data by administering a staff morale questionnaire in both hospitals before the change is made (the pretest). We would again collect data on nurses' morale after the system is installed in the experimental hospital (the posttest).

Figure 8-5 depicts this study symbolically. The top row is our experimental (primary nursing) hospital; the second row is the hospital using traditional nursing care. A comparison of this diagram with the one in Figure 8-4 shows that they are identical, except that subjects have not been randomly assigned to treatment groups in the second diagram. The design in Figure 8-5 is the weaker of the two because *it can no longer be assumed that the experimental and comparison groups† are equal.* Because of the inability to randomize subjects, our study is quasi-experimental rather than truly experimental. The design is, nevertheless, a strong one because the collection of pretest data allows us to determine whether the groups were initially similar in terms of their morale. If the morale of the two groups is very different at the start, our interpretation of the posttest data will be difficult, although there are statistical procedures that can help. If the comparison and experimental groups respond similarly, on the average, on their pretest questionnaire, then we can

---

† In quasi-experiments, the term *comparison group* is generally used in lieu of *control group* to refer to the group against which outcomes in the treatment group will be evaluated.

---

* The notation, as well as most of the concepts in this section, are derived from Campbell and Stanley's (1963) classic monograph.

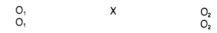

Figure 8-5. *Nonequivalent control group pretest–posttest design (quasi-experimental).*

be relatively confident that any posttest group differences in self-reported morale are the result of the new method of nursing care.

Suppose that we had not thought to or had been unable to collect pretest data before the new method of nursing care delivery was introduced. The resulting study could be diagrammed to show the scheme in Figure 8-6. This design has a flaw that is difficult to remedy. We have no basis on which to judge the initial equivalence of the two nursing staffs. If we find that, at the posttest, the morale of the experimental hospital staff is lower than that of the control hospital staff, can we conclude that the new method of delivering care *caused* a decline in staff morale? There could be several alternative explanations for the posttest differences. In particular, it might be that the morale of the employees in the two hospitals differed even at the outset. Campbell and Stanley (1963), in fact, would call the design shown in Figure 8-6 *pre-experimental* rather than quasi-experimental because of its essentially irreconcilable weaknesses. Thus, although quasi-experiments lack some of the controlling properties inherent in true experiments, the hallmark of the quasi-experimental approach is the effort to introduce other controls to compensate for the absence of either the randomization or control group component.

TIME SERIES DESIGNS

The designs reviewed in the previous section illustrate studies in which a control group was used but randomization was not, but some designs have neither. In some studies in which both characteristics are absent, there are inherent weaknesses that seriously jeopardize the validity of the findings. However, there are several designs that offer the researcher some measure of protection against these problems.

Let us suppose that a hospital decides to adopt a requirement that all its nurses accrue a certain number of continuing education units before being considered for a promotion or raise. The nursing administrators want to assess some of the positive and negative consequences of this mandate. Some of the indicators they might examine include turnover rate, absentee rate, qualifications of new employee applicants, number of raises and promotions awarded, and so on. For the purposes of this example, let us assume that there is no other comparable hospital that could reasonably serve as a comparison for this study. In such a case, the only kind of comparison that could be made is a before–after contrast. If the requirement were inaugurated in January, one could compare the turnover rate, for example, for the 3-month period before the new rule with the turnover rate for the subsequent 3-month period. The schematic representation for such a study is shown in Figure 8-7.

Although this design appears logical and straightforward, there actually are numerous problems with it. What if either of the 3-month periods is atypical, apart from the new regulation? What about the effects of any other hospital rules inaugurated during the same period? What about the effects of external factors that influence employment patterns, such as employment opportunities at other nearby hospitals? The design in Figure 8-7 offers no way of controlling for any of these problems. This design is also pre-experimental because it fails to control for many possible extraneous factors.

A design that can assist us in this case is known as the *time series design* (sometimes referred to as the interrupted time series design) and is diagrammed in Figure 8-8. The basic notion underlying the time series design is the col-

<table>
<tr><td style="text-align:center">X</td><td style="text-align:center">O
O</td></tr>
</table>

Figure 8-6. *Nonequivalent control group posttest only design (pre-experimental).*

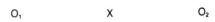

O_1 X O_2

Figure 8-7. *One-group pretest–posttest design (pre-experimental).*

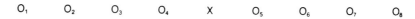

O_1 O_2 O_3 O_4 X O_5 O_6 O_7 O_8

Figure 8-8.   *Time series design (quasi-experimental).*

lection of information over an extended period and the introduction of an experimental treatment during the course of the data collection period. In the figure, O_1 through O_4 represent four separate instances of observation or data collection on a dependent variable before treatment; X represents the treatment (the introduction of the independent variable); and O_5 through O_8 represent four posttreatment observations. In our present example, O_1 might be the number of nurses who left the hospital in January through March in the year before the new continuing education rule, O_2 the number of resignations in April through June, and so

forth. After the rule is implemented, data on turnover are similarly collected for four consecutive 3-month periods, giving us observations O_5 through O_8.

Even though the time series design does not eliminate all the problems of interpreting changes in turnover rate, the extended time perspective immensely strengthens our ability to attribute any change to our experimental manipulation, which in this case is the continuing education requirement. Figure 8-9 attempts to demonstrate why this is so. The two diagrams (A) and (B) in the figure show two possible outcome patterns for the eight measures of nurse

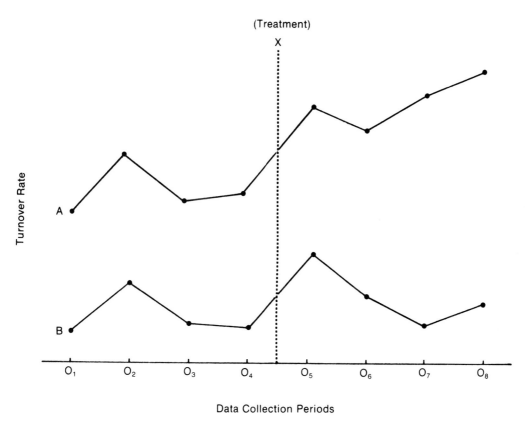

Figure 8-9.   *Two possible time series outcome patterns.*

turnover. The vertical dotted line in the center represents the time at which the continuing education rule was implemented. Both (*A*) and (*B*) reflect a feature that is common to most time series studies, and this is the fluctuation from one observation or measurement to another. These fluctuations are, of course, perfectly normal. One would not expect that, if 48 nurses resigned from a hospital in 1 year, the resignations would be spaced evenly during the course of the year with exactly four resignations per month. It is precisely because of these fluctuations that the design shown in Figure 8-7, with only one observation before and after the experimental treatment, is so weak.

Let us compare the kind of interpretations that can be made for the outcomes reflected in Figure 8-9(*A*) and (*B*). In both cases, the number of resignations increases between O_4 and O_5, that is, immediately after the introduction of the continuing education requirement. In (*B*), however, the number of resignations falls at O_6 and continues to decrease at O_7. The increase at O_5, therefore, looks similar to other apparently haphazard fluctuations in the turnover rate at other periods. Therefore, it probably would be erroneous to conclude that the treatment had an effect on resignations. In (*A*), on the other hand, the number of resignations increases at O_5 and remains relatively high for all subsequent periods of data collection. It is true, of course, that there may be other explanations for a change in turnover rate from one year to the next. The time series design, however, does permit us to rule out the possibility that the data reflect an unstable measurement of resignations made at only two points in time. If we had used the design in Figure 8-7 to study this problem, it would have been analogous to obtaining the measurements at O_4 and O_5 of Figure 8-9 only. The outcomes in both Figure 8-9(*A*) and (*B*) look similar at these two points in time. Yet the use

of a broader time perspective leads us to draw different conclusions about the nature of the changes from one pattern of outcomes to the next.

A particularly powerful design results when the time series and nonequivalent control group designs are combined, as diagrammed in Figure 8-10. In the example just described, a *time series nonequivalent control group design* would involve the collection of data over an extended period from both the hospital introducing the continuing education mandate and another hospital not imposing the mandate. This use of information from another hospital with similar characteristics would make any inferences regarding the effects of the mandate more convincing because trends influenced by external factors would presumably be observed in both groups.

Numerous variations on the simple time series design are possible and are being used by nurse researchers. For example, additional evidence regarding the effects of a treatment can be achieved by instituting the treatment at several different points in time, strengthening the treatment over time, or instituting the treatment at one point in time and then *withdrawing* the treatment at a later point, sometimes with *reinstitution of treatment*. These three designs are diagrammed in Figures 8-11 through 8-13. Nurse researchers are often in a good position to use such time series designs because measures of patient functioning are generally routinely made at multiple points over an extended period.

Advantages and Disadvantages of the Quasi-Experimental Approach

The great strength of quasi-experiments lies in their practicality, feasibility, and, to a certain extent, their generalizability. In the real

O_1	O_2	O_3	O_4	X	O_5	O_6	O_7	O_8
O_1	O_2	O_3	O_4		O_5	O_6	O_7	O_8

Figure 8-10. Time series nonequivalent control group design (quasi-experimental).

$$O_1 \quad O_2 \quad X \quad O_3 \quad O_4 \quad X \quad O_5 \quad O_6 \quad X \quad O_7 \quad O_8$$

Figure 8-11. *Time series with multiple institutions of treatment (quasi-experimental).*

$$O_1 \quad O_2 \quad X \quad O_3 \quad O_4 \quad X+1 \quad O_5 \quad O_6 \quad X+2 \quad O_7 \quad O_8$$

Figure 8-12. *Time series with intensified treatment (quasi-experimental).*

$$O_1 \quad O_2 \quad X \quad O_3 \quad O_4 \quad (-X) \quad O_5 \quad O_6 \quad X \quad O_7 \quad O_8$$

Figure 8-13. *Time series with withdrawn and ·einstituted treatment (quasi-experimental).*

world, it is often impractical, if not impossible, to conduct true experiments. A good deal of the research that is of interest to nurses occurs in natural settings. Frequently, it is difficult to deliver an innovative treatment to only half of a group, and randomization may be even less feasible. The inability to randomize, or even to secure a control group, need not force a researcher to abandon all hopes of conducting a respectable investigation. Quasi-experimental designs are research plans that introduce some controls over extraneous variables when full experimental control is lacking.

It is precisely because the control inherent in true experiments *is* absent in quasi-experiments that the researcher needs to be acquainted with the weaknesses of this approach. When a researcher uses a quasi-experimental design, there may be several *rival hypotheses* competing with the experimental manipulation as explanations for observed results. Take as an example the case in which we administer certain medications to a group of babies whose mothers are heroin addicts to assess whether this treatment results in a weight gain in these typically low-birthweight babies. If we use no comparison group or if we use a nonequivalent control group and then observe a weight gain, we must ask the questions: Is it *plausible* that some other factor caused or influenced the gain? Is it *plausible* that pretreatment differences between the experimental and comparison groups of babies resulted in differential gain? Is it *plau-*

sible that the babies could have gained the weight simply as a result of maturation? If the answer is "yes" to any of these questions, then the inferences we can make about the effect of the experimental treatment are weakened considerably. The plausibility of any one threat cannot, of course, be answered unequivocally. It is generally a situation in which judgment must be exercised. It is because quasi-experiments ultimately depend in part on human judgment, rather than on more objective criteria, that the validity of cause-and-effect inferences can be challenged. We must hasten to add that the quality of a study is not necessarily a function of its design. There are many excellent quasi-experimental investigations as well as weak experiments.

Research Example of a Quasi-Experimental Study

Table 8-5 briefly summarizes the characteristics of several studies conducted by nurse researchers in which a quasi-experimental or pre-experimental design was used. A more detailed description of a quasi-experimental study follows. It may be helpful to consult the full journal article for more information about the research design.

Pickler and her colleagues (1993) used a strong quasi-experimental design to examine the effects of nonnutritive sucking on the

Table 8-5. *Examples of Studies Using Quasi-Experimental and Pre-Experimental Designs*

RESEARCH QUESTION	MANIPULATED VARIABLE	SUBJECTS
DESIGN: ONE GROUP, BEFORE–AFTER		
Is a special community-based mental health training program effective in increasing primary nurses' knowledge and skills relating to depression? (Badger, Mishel, Biocca, & Cardea, 1991)	Nurses' participation in the special program	237 primary care nurses
DESIGN: NONEQUIVALENT CONTROL GROUP, AFTER-ONLY		
How do four different methods of securing endotracheal tubes in orally intubated patients compare in terms of tube stability, facial skin integrity, and patient satisfaction? (Kaplow & Bookbinder, 1994)	Method of securing endotracheal tubes (Lillihie harness, Comfit, Dale, and SecureEasy)	120 intensive care unit patients (30 per method)
DESIGN: NONEQUIVALENT CONTROL GROUP, BEFORE–AFTER		
What is the relative effectiveness of two different educational methods (a comprehensive class and an information session with a brochure) in encouraging breast self-examination among rural women? (Kuhns-Hastings, Brakey, & Marshall, 1993)	Participation in a comprehensive (experimental) class versus information session	50 women in experimental group; 53 women in comparison group
DESIGN: TIME SERIES		
What is the effect of a dietary fiber and fluid intervention on the number of bowel movements and frequency of elimination among residents of a long-term health care facility? (Rodrigues-Fisher, Bourguignon, & Good, 1993)	Participation in a dietary fiber and fluid program	15 laxative-dependent nursing home residents
DESIGN: TIME SERIES, WITHDRAWN AND REINSTITUTED TREATMENT		
Is an individualized speech therapy program effective in increasing communication skills in aphasic and dysarthric patients? (Buckwalter, Cusack, Sidles, Wadle, & Beaver, 1989)	Speech therapy versus withdrawal of speech therapy versus systematic attention without therapy	36 brain-damaged patients with diagnoses of aphasia, dysarthria, or both
DESIGN: TIME SERIES WITH NONEQUIVALENT CONTROL GROUP		
Does an intervention based on the nursing mutual participation model reduce the stress of parents with children in the pediatric intensive care unit? (Curley, 1988)	Parents enrolled in a special nursing program versus parents receiving usual nursing care in the pediatric intensive care unit	16 parents in the experimental group; 17 parents in the comparison group

physiologic and behavioral stress reactions of preterm infants at early bottle feedings. The sample consisted of 20 preterm infants, 10 of whom were provided nonnutritive sucking for 5 minutes before and 5 minutes after an early bottle feeding. The 10 infants who served as a comparison group (and who received no nonnutritive sucking) were matched to the experimental group on the basis of gender, race, birthweight, and gestational age.

Physiologic stress was measured in terms of heart rate and oxygen saturation rate. For each, mean rates were computed for three periods: the 5 minutes before feeding, the first 5 minutes of bottle feeding, and the 5 minutes after total feeding. Behavioral stress was measured by observation of the infant's behavioral state at four points: immediately before the 5-minute prefeeding period, immediately after the initiation of bottle feeding, immediately after the conclusion of bottle feeding, and immediately after the conclusion of the 5-minute postfeeding period.

The results indicated that infants who received nonnutritive sucking before and after bottle feedings were more likely to be in a quiescent behavior state 5 minutes after feeding. However, there were no treatment, time, or time × treatment interaction effects for heart rate. Oxygen saturation was unaffected by the treatment but did change between different measurements in time.

❖ NONEXPERIMENTAL RESEARCH

Many research problems do not lend themselves to an experimental or quasi-experimental design, that is, to experimental manipulation of the independent variable. Let us suppose, for example, that we were interested in studying the effect of widowhood on physical and psychological functioning. We could use as our dependent variables various physiologic and medical measures, such as blood pressure, heart rate, and so on, as well as standard psychological diagnostic tests, such as the Center for Epidemiological Studies Depression Scale. Our independent

variable is widowhood versus nonwidowhood. Clearly, we would be unable to manipulate widowhood. Spouses become widows or widowers by a process that is neither random nor subject, ethically, to research control. Thus, we must proceed by taking two groups as they naturally occur (those who are widowed and those who are not) and comparing them in terms of psychological and physical well-being.

Reasons for Undertaking Nonexperimental Research

Many research studies involving human subjects, including most nursing research investigations, are nonexperimental in nature. There are many different reasons for choosing a nonexperimental approach. First, a vast number of human characteristics are inherently not subject to experimental manipulation (e.g., blood type, personality, health beliefs, medical diagnosis) and thus the effects of these characteristics on some phenomenon of interest cannot be studied experimentally.

A second issue is that in nursing research, as in other fields in which human behavior is of primary interest, numerous variables could technically be manipulated but should not be manipulated for ethical reasons. If the nature of the independent variable is such that its manipulation could cause physical or mental harm to subjects, then that variable should not be controlled experimentally. For example, if we were interested in studying the effect of prenatal care on infant mortality, it would be unethical to provide such care to one group of pregnant women but totally deprive a second group. What we would need to do is locate a naturally occurring group of mothers-to-be who have not received prenatal care. The birth outcomes of these women could then be compared with those of a group of women who had received appropriate care. The problem, however, is that the two groups of women are likely to differ in terms of a number of other characteristics, such as age, education, nutrition, and health, any of which individually or in combination could have an impact on infant mortality, independent of the absence or presence of prenatal care. This is precisely why experimental designs are so strong in demonstrating cause-and-effect relationships.

Third, there are many research situations in which it is simply not practical to conduct a true experiment. Constraints might involve insufficient time, lack of administrative approval, excessive inconvenience to patients or staff, or lack of adequate funds.

Finally, there are many research questions for which an experimental design is not at all appropriate. This is especially true for descriptive studies and for most qualitative studies, which seek to capture what people think, feel, and do in their naturalistic environments. Because of this goal, researchers conducting in-depth qualitative studies typically want as little disturbance as possible to the people or groups they are studying. Manipulation is neither attempted nor considered desirable; the emphasis is on the natural everyday world of humans. Thus, although qualitative researchers sometimes focus on concepts that could be manipulated or could be affected by manipulation (e.g., dependency, coping, and decision making), they reject manipulation as a technique for studying certain problems.

Types of Nonexperimental Research

Essentially, there are two broad classes of nonexperimental research: correlational (ex post facto) and descriptive. The characteristics of each are discussed in this section.

EX POST FACTO OR CORRELATIONAL RESEARCH

The first broad class of nonexperimental research is *ex post facto research*. The literal translation of the Latin term ex post facto is "from after the fact." This expression is meant to indicate that the research in question has been conducted *after* the variations in the independent variable have occurred in the natural course of events. Ex post facto research attempts to understand relationships among phenomena as they naturally occur, without any researcher intervention.

Sometimes ex post facto research is referred to as correlational research.* The precise meaning of correlational will become clearer when we have covered some statistical concepts. Basically, a *correlation* is an interrelationship or association between two variables, that is, a tendency for variation in one variable to be related to variation in another. For example, in human adults, height and weight tend to be correlated because there is a tendency for taller people to weigh more than shorter people.

Ex post facto or correlational studies often share a number of structural and design characteristics with experimental, quasi-experimental, and pre-experimental research. If we use the notation scheme outlined in the previous section to represent symbolically the hypothetical study of the effects of widowhood, we find that it bears a strong resemblance to the nonequivalent control group posttest-only design. Both designs are presented in Figure 8-14. As these diagrams show, the pre-experimental design is distinguished from the ex post facto study only by the presence of an *X*, the manipulation of some experimental treatment by the researcher in the pre-experimental design.

The basic purpose of ex post facto research is essentially the same as experimental research: to understand relationships among

---

* The use of the terms *ex post facto* and *correlational* is not entirely consistent in the literature on research methods. Some authors use ex post facto to refer to all nonexperimental research that examines relationships among variables; others use the term correlational for this purpose. Still other researchers prefer to make a distinction between whether the intent of the study is causal and comparative (ex post facto) or merely descriptive of relationships (correlational). In general, the terms are used roughly equivalently in this chapter to designate studies of relationships among variables when the independent variable is not under the researcher's control.

GROUP A	X	O	Nonequivalent control group (pre-experimental) design
GROUP B		O	
GROUP A		O	Ex post facto design
GROUP B		O	

Figure 8-14. Schematic diagram comparing nonequivalent control group and ex post facto designs.

variables. The most important distinction between the two is the difficulty of inferring *causal* relationships in ex post facto studies because of the lack of manipulative control of the independent variables. In experiments, the investigator makes a prediction that a deliberate variation in *X*, the independent variable, will result in the occurrence of some event or behavior, *Y* (the dependent variable). For example, the researcher predicts that if some medication is administered, then patient improvement will ensue. The experimenter has direct control over the *X*: the experimental treatment can be administered to some and withheld from others, and subjects can be randomly assigned to an experimental group and a control group.

In ex post facto research, on the other hand, the investigator does not have control of the independent variable because it has already occurred. The examination of the independent variable—the presumed causative factor—is done after the fact. As a result, attempts to draw any cause-and-effect conclusions are often problematic. For example, we might hypothesize that there is a correlation between the number of cigarettes smoked and the incidence of lung cancer, and empirical data would most likely corroborate this expectation. The inference we would like to make based on observed relationships is that cigarette smoking *causes* cancer. This kind of inference, however, is a fallacy that has been called *post hoc ergo propter* ("after this, therefore caused by this"). The fallacy lies in the assumption that one thing has caused another merely because it occurred chronologically before the other.

To illustrate why such a cause-and-effect conclusion might not be warranted, let us assume (strictly for the sake of an example) that there is a preponderance of cigarette smokers in

urban areas, but people living in rural areas are largely nonsmokers. Let us further assume that bronchogenic carcinoma is actually caused by the poor environmental conditions typically associated with cities and industrial areas. Therefore, we would be incorrect to conclude that cigarette smoking causes lung cancer, despite the strong relationship that might be shown to exist between the two variables. This is because there is *also* a strong relationship between cigarette smoking and the "real" causative agent, living in a polluted environment. (Of course, the cigarette smoking and lung cancer studies in reality have been replicated in so many different places with so many different groups of people that causal inferences are increasingly justified.) This hypothetical example illustrates a famous research dictum: Correlation does not prove causation. That is, the mere existence of a relationship—even a strong one—between two variables is not enough to warrant the conclusion that one variable has caused the other.

Although correlational studies are inherently weaker than experimental studies in elucidating cause-and-effect relationships, different designs offer different degrees of supportive evidence. In the previous chapter, we discussed two types of ex post facto designs—retrospective and prospective. Prospective designs tend to be considerably stronger than retrospective designs with regard to causal inferences because the researcher does at least go forward in time from the independent to the dependent variable. However, the researcher can sometimes strengthen a retrospective design by taking certain steps. For example, one type of retrospective design, referred to as a *case-control design*, involves the comparison of cases or subjects with a certain illness or condition (e.g., lung cancer victims) with controls (e.g., people without lung cancer). To the degree that the researcher can demonstrate similarity between cases and controls with regard to extraneous traits, the inferences regarding the presumed cause of the disease are enhanced.

Researchers interested in testing theories of causation based on nonexperimental data are increasingly using a technique known as *path analysis*. Using sophisticated statistical procedures, the researcher tests a hypothesized causal chain among a set of independent variables, mediating variables, and a dependent variable. Path analytic procedures, which are described more fully in Chapter 19, allow researchers to test whether nonexperimental data conform sufficiently to the underlying model to justify causal inferences.

DESCRIPTIVE RESEARCH

The second broad class of nonexperimental studies is *descriptive research*. The purpose of descriptive studies is to observe, describe, and document aspects of a situation as it naturally occurs and sometimes to serve as a starting point for hypothesis generation or theory development.

Although there is considerable emphasis in scientific research on understanding what causes behaviors, conditions, and situations, researchers can often do little more than describe existing relationships without fully comprehending the complex causal pathways that exist. Thus, many of our research problems are often cast in noncausal terms. We ask, for example, whether men are less likely than women to achieve a bonding with their newborn infants, not whether a particular configuration of sex chromosomes has *caused* differences in parental attachment. As in the case of other types of ex post facto research, the investigator engaged in a *descriptive correlational study* has no control over the independent variables. That is, there is no experimental manipulation or random assignment to groups. However, unlike other types of ex post facto studies—such as the cigarette smoking and lung cancer investiga-

tions—the aim of descriptive correlational research is to describe the relationship among variables rather than to infer cause-and-effect relationships.

Other descriptive studies are undertaken to describe what exists in terms of frequency of occurrence (or its presence versus absence) rather than to describe the relationship between variables. For example, an investigator may wish to determine the health care and nutritional practices of pregnant teenagers. *Univariate descriptive studies* are not necessarily focused on only one variable. For example, a researcher might be interested in women's experiences during menopause. The investigation might describe the frequency with which various symptoms are reported, the average age at menopause, the percentage of women seeking formal health care, and the percentage of women using medications to alleviate symptoms. There are multiple variables in this study, but the primary purpose is to describe the status of each and not to relate them to one another.

Advantages and Disadvantages of Ex Post Facto or Correlational Research

As mentioned earlier, the quality of a study is not necessarily related to its approach; there are many excellent nonexperimental studies as well as seriously flawed experiments and quasi-experiments. Nevertheless, nonexperimental studies suffer from several drawbacks.

DISADVANTAGES OF EX POST FACTO OR CORRELATIONAL RESEARCH

As already noted, the major disadvantage of nonexperimental research is that, relative to experimental and quasi-experimental research, it is weak in its ability to reveal causal relationships. There is a continuum of design types in terms of capacity to reveal causal relationships. True experimental designs are at one end of that continuum, and retrospective correlational research is at the other, as shown in Figure 8-15; descriptive studies are not included on this continuum because they are not intended to elucidate cause-and-effect relations.

Ex post facto studies are in most instances susceptible to the possibility of faulty interpretation. This situation stems in large part from the fact that in ex post facto studies, the researcher works with preexisting groups that were not formed by a random process but rather by what might be termed a self-selecting process. Kerlinger (1986) offered the following description of *self-selection*:

> Self-selection occurs when the members of the groups being studied are in the groups, in part, because they differentially possess traits or characteristics extraneous to the research problem, characteristics that possibly influence or are otherwise related to the variables of the research problem. (p. 349)

As in the case of quasi-experimental or pre-experimental research, the researcher doing a correlational study cannot assume that the groups being compared were similar before the occurrence of the independent variable. Because of this fact, preexisting differences may be a plausible alternative explanation for any observed differences on the dependent variable of interest.

To illustrate this problem, let us consider a hypothetical study in which the researcher is interested in examining the relationship between type of nursing program (the independent variable) and job satisfaction after graduation. If the investigator finds that diploma school graduates are more satisfied with their work than baccalaureate graduates 1 year after graduation, the conclusion that the diploma school program provides better preparation for actual work situations and, hence, leads to increased satisfaction may or may not be accurate. The students in the two programs undoubtedly differed to begin with in terms of a number of important characteristics, such as personality, career goals, personal values, and so forth. That is, students self-selected themselves into one of the two programs; it may be the selection traits themselves that resulted in different job expectations and satisfactions.

The difficulty of interpreting correlational findings stems in large part from the fact that, in the real world, behaviors, states, attitudes, and characteristics are interrelated (correlated) in complex ways. An example might help to make this clear. Let us suppose we were interested in studying the differences between the postoperative convalescent behavior of patients who had undergone surgery for two different medical problems—hernia and ulcers. Our independent variable in this hypothetical study is the type of medical problem. We might use one or more of the following as measures of the dependent variable (postoperative convalescent behavior): ratings of nurses on the degree of cooperativeness of the patient, number of times the patient calls the nurse for help, the patient's self-ratings of distress, and the number of medications required to induce sleep or alleviate pain. Let us say that we find that the hernia patients receive a significantly lower rating by the nurses on degree of cooperation than the ulcer patients. We

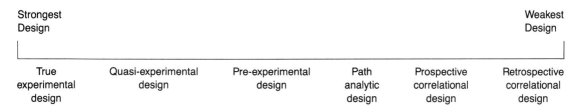

Figure 8-15. *Continuum of research designs with respect to power to elucidate causal relationships.*

could interpret this finding to mean that particular medical problems and their accompanying surgical treatment produce different patterns of cooperative behavior in individuals. This relationship is diagrammed in Figure 8-16(*A*).

For the sake of this discussion, let us examine some alternative explanations for the findings. Perhaps there is a third variable that influences *both* the degree of convalescent cooperativeness and the type of medical ailment, such as the degree of physical activity to which an individual is accustomed. That is, it may be that hernia patients are usually engaged in more physical activity than are ulcer patients, and this fact may be one of the causes of *both* the diagnosis and the inability to cope properly with the sedentary hospital routine. This set of relationships is diagrammed in Figure 8-16(*B*). A third possibility may be *reversed* causality, as shown in Figure 8-16(*C*). Willingness to cooperate in general may be thought of as one aspect of a person's personality, and it is possible that the dynamics of a person's psychological makeup result in the manifestation of different medical problems. In this interpretation, it is the person's disposition that causes the diagnosis and not vice versa. You may well be able to invent other explanations. The point is that interpretations of ex post facto results should generally be considered tentative, particularly if the research has no theoretical basis.

ADVANTAGES OF EX POST FACTO OR CORRELATIONAL RESEARCH

In an earlier section of this chapter, we discussed various constraints that limit the possibility of applying experimental designs to some research problems. Ex post facto or correlational research will continue to play a crucial role in nursing, medical, and social science research precisely because many of the interesting problems to be addressed in those fields are not amenable to experimentation.

Despite our emphasis on causality in relationships, it has already been noted that in some kinds of research, such as descriptive research, a full understanding of causal networks may not be important. Furthermore, if the study is testing a hypothesis that has been deduced from an established theory, determining the direction of causation may be relatively straightforward, especially if powerful techniques such as path analysis have been used.

Correlational research is often an efficient and effective means of collecting a large amount of data about a problem area. For example, it would be possible to collect extensive information about the health histories and eating habits of a large number of individuals. Researchers could then examine which health problems are correlated with which diets. Thus, they could discover a large number of interrela-

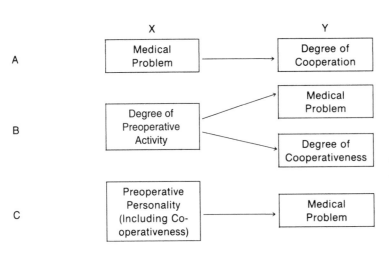

Figure 8-16. *Three possible explanations for relationship between medical diagnosis and degree of cooperativeness in patients. Arrow shows (as before) direction of influence; variable X is presumed to "cause" variable Y.*

tionships in a relatively short amount of time. By contrast, an experimenter usually looks at only a few variables at a time. For example, one experiment might be devoted to manipulating foods high in cholesterol to observe the effects on certain biophysiologic measures, another experiment could manipulate protein consumption, and so forth.

Finally, ex post facto research is often strong in realism and therefore has an intrinsic appeal for the solution of many practical problems. Unlike many experimental studies, ex post facto research is seldom criticized for its artificiality.

Research Example of Nonexperimental Research

We have used a number of hypothetical research problems to help explain many of the points made in this chapter. Table 8-6 presents a brief description of several actual nonexperimental studies that have been conducted by nurse researchers. An additional nonexperimental study is described in greater detail below.

Estok and her colleagues (1993) studied menstrual responses (e.g., duration and amount of menses) to women's running. Their sample consisted of 146 women aged

Table 8-6. *Examples of Nonexperimental Studies*

RESEARCH QUESTION	RESEARCH SUBJECTS
DESIGN: EX POST FACTO, RETROSPECTIVE	
Is there a relationship between a mother's time at first holding her infant and the development of feelings of maternal attachment? (Troy, 1993)	88 women recruited from pediatric treatment centers when their babies were 1–2 months old
DESIGN: EX POST FACTO, PROSPECTIVE	
What are the antecedent factors that best predict breastfeeding duration? (Duckett, Henly, & Garvis, 1993)	192 mothers followed up 12 months postpartum
DESIGN: CASE-CONTROL	
What are the prenatal, intrapartal, and/or postpartal factors that play a role in the etiology of cerebral palsy? (Polivka, Nickel, & Wilkins, 1993)	112 children with cerebral palsy (cases); 87 friend controls; 66 controls from birth certificates
DESIGN: PATH ANALYTIC	
What are the direct and indirect effects of family circumstances, maternal characteristics, and child temperament on the maladjustment of school-aged children? (McClowry, Giangrande, Tommasini, Clinton, Foreman, Lynch, & Ferketich, 1994)	89 mothers with children 8–11 years old
DESIGN: DESCRIPTIVE CORRELATIONAL	
Is ethnicity associated with insufficient milk supply among breastfeeding mothers? (Hill & Aldag, 1993)	42 black and 148 white breastfeeding mothers
DESIGN: UNIVARIATE DESCRIPTIVE	
What are the experiences associated with loss and dying among AIDS family caregivers? (Brown & Powell-Cope, 1993)	53 family caregivers of people with AIDS

20 to 36 years who were grouped according to their level of running intensity: group I, nonrunning women who did little exercise; group II, women who ran 1 to 14.9 miles per week; group III, women who ran 15 to 30 miles per week; and group IV, women who ran more than 30 miles per week. Menstrual and running data were recorded by the subjects in a Menstrual/Exercise Diary over 4 months or three menstrual cycles. The subjects also tested themselves for the presence of luteinizing hormone with the self-test, OvuQuick.

The four groups were found to be similar in terms of various background characteristics, such as age, height, weight, ethnicity, education, and age of menarche. The results indicated that the nonrunners had significantly more days of menses and larger amounts of menses than the two highest-intensity running groups. Women in all three running groups reported a shorter luteal phase than nonrunners and had significantly more ovulatory disturbances. Across groups, a history of menstrual irregularity before 18 years of age was a strong predictor of menstrual cycle characteristics.

❖ TIPS FOR DESIGNING EXPERIMENTAL AND NONEXPERIMENTAL STUDIES

Because research design has profound implications for the interpretability of study findings, we offer the following suggestions for strengthening designs along the experimental/nonexperimental continuum:

- It is usually advantageous to design a study with as many relevant comparisons as possible. Pre-experimental designs are weak in part because the comparative information they yield is weak. A one-group, before–after design is strengthened considerably by the addition of a second group. Sometimes having two or more comparison groups greatly enhances the value of a study. In an experimental context, for example, the comparison

of treatment A to treatment B yields much less information that the comparison of both treatments to no treatment (or to a placebo). In a nonexperimental context, having multiple comparison groups is often an effective way to address the problem of self-selection, especially if the comparison groups are selected to address competing biases. For example, in case-control studies of lung cancer, one comparison group could include people with a respiratory disease other than lung cancer and a second could include those with no respiratory disorder.

- Another way to maximize comparative possibilities is to design a study with more than one data collection point, as in before–after experimental designs. In such a design, the experimental and control groups can be compared not only with respect to differences in posttest status but also with respect to changes over time. Moreover, the availability of pretest data typically greatly enhances the precision of the statistical analyses. Data collection before the introduction of a treatment may be unwise when the researcher suspects that the data collection itself would have an effect on the dependent variable, but this is rarely the case. The major deterrents to the collection of pretest data are typically practical considerations such as time and cost.

- In general, it is wise to randomize whenever possible, to reduce the possibility of biases. In an experimental context, this means randomly assigning subjects to groups, groups to treatments, and conditions to subjects (in a repeated measures design). It also means looking for other opportunities to randomize whenever other conditions vary across subjects, such as randomly assigning patients to rooms or nursing staff to patients. In a nonexperimental context, there may also be opportunities to randomize, such as randomly assigning data collection staff to subjects, or subjects to different times for data collection (morning versus afternoon).

- When using an experimental design that involves the collection of data both before and after the intervention, it is considered good practice to collect the pretest data *before* randomization to groups. This ensures that subjects (and researchers) will not be biased in any way by knowledge of the group assignments.

❖ SUMMARY

Experiments are characterized by three fundamental properties: manipulation, control, and randomization. *Manipulation* involves doing something to or acting on at least some of the subjects in a research study. The experimenter manipulates, or varies, the independent variable (often referred to as the experimental *treatment* or *intervention*) to see if the manipulation has an effect on the dependent variable or variables of interest. True experiments always require the use of a *control group,* whose performance on the dependent (or *outcome*) measures is used as a basis for assessing the performance of the experimental group on the same measures. The third requirement for an experiment is that subjects be assigned to control and experimental groups by a process known as *randomization.* The random assignment procedure can be accomplished by any method that allows every subject an equal chance of being included in any group. Such methods include flipping a coin, drawing names from a hat, and using a *table of random numbers.* Randomization does not guarantee that all groups will be equal, but this technique is the most reliable method for equating groups on all possible characteristics that could affect the outcome of the study. Randomization usually involves the assignment of individual subjects to different conditions, but sometimes *cluster randomization,* which involves randomly assigning groups of subjects to conditions, is advantageous.

The most basic experimental design is the *after-only* or *posttest-only design,* which involves collecting data from subjects after the experimental treatment has been introduced. When data are also collected before treatment (i.e., at *baseline*), the design is a *before–after* or *pretest–posttest design.* If pretest sensitization may obscure the effect of the treatment, a *Solomon four-group design* may be needed. When a researcher manipulates more than one variable at a time, the design is known as a *factorial experiment.* Such a design is efficient in that it permits two simultaneous experiments with one sample of subjects. Furthermore, with factorial designs, we can test both *main effects* (effects resulting from the experimentally manipulated variables) and *interaction effects* (effects resulting from combining the treatments). In factorial designs, each independent variable is referred to as a *factor,* and each factor consists of two or more *levels* of the treatment. In *repeated measures (crossover) designs,* one group of subjects is exposed to two or more conditions in random order, thereby allowing subjects to serve as their own controls. When an experimental design is used to test the efficacy of a clinical treatment in a large, heterogeneous population, the study is often referred to as a *clinical trial.*

True experiments are considered by many as the ideal of science because experiments come closer than any other type of research approach to meeting the criteria for inferring causal relationships. On the other hand, there are many situations in which an experimental design is impossible, owing to ethical or practical considerations. Experiments have also been criticized because of their artificiality.

Quasi-experimental and pre-experimental designs involve manipulation but lack a comparison group or randomization. *Quasi-experimental designs* are designs in which efforts are made to introduce controls into the study to compensate in part for the absence of one or both of these important characteristics. In contrast, *pre-experimental designs* have no such safeguards and, therefore, are subject to ambiguity and multiple interpretations of results.

Several specific quasi-experimental designs were presented. The *nonequivalent control group design* involves the use of a control group (or *comparison group*) that is not designated by a randomization procedure. The problem with the use of such a comparison group is the possibility that the groups are initially different in ways that will affect the research outcomes, and so the collection of pretest data becomes an important means of assessing their initial equivalence. In studies in which there is no control group, a method for overcoming some of the difficulties in the interpretation of results is the collection of information over time before and after the treatment is instituted. Such a study is known as the *time series design*. An especially powerful design combines the features of the two most common quasi-experimental designs and is referred to as the *time series nonequivalent control group design*.

Despite some of the problems inherent in quasi-experimental designs, they may in some cases be more practical in the nursing field than the more rigorous experimental designs and, therefore, merit increased attention by nurse researchers. In evaluating the results of quasi-experiments, however, it is important to ask whether it is plausible that factors other than the experimental treatment caused or affected the obtained outcomes (i.e., whether there are *rival hypotheses* for explaining the results).

Basically, three types of constraints preclude experimentation and therefore make *nonexperimental research* useful or necessary. First, a number of independent variables, such as height, gender, and race, are human characteristics that are not amenable to control and randomization. Second, other independent variables are technically manipulable but are ethically inappropriate for experimental purposes with human subjects, as in the case of smoking versus not smoking cigarettes. Third, it may often be impractical or impossible to manipulate variables owing to insufficient time, inconvenience, administrative barriers, or prior manifestation of the phenomena of interest. Finally, researchers sometimes deliberately choose not to manipulate variables, to get a more realistic understanding of phenomena as they operate in naturalistic settings.

Nonexperimental research includes two broad categories: ex post facto or correlational research and descriptive research. *Ex post facto* or *correlational studies* are research investigations designed to examine the relationships among variables. Unlike experimental or quasi-experimental studies, however, ex post facto research lacks active manipulation of the independent variable. Because the investigation of the independent variable is done after the fact—that is, after it has occurred in the natural course of events—it becomes difficult to draw cause-and-effect conclusions. However, when there is a strong underlying theory or conceptual model, the technique of *path analysis* enhances the researcher's ability to test causal relationships using ex post facto data.

Descriptive research is designed to summarize the status of phenomena of interest as they currently exist. *Descriptive correlational studies* are less concerned with determining cause-and-effect relationships than with a description of how one phenomenon is related to another. *Univariate descriptive research* provides information on the occurrence, frequency of occurrence, or average value of the variables of interest without examining how variables are interrelated.

The primary weakness of ex post facto or correlational research is that the researcher lacks experimental control in terms of both inability to manipulate the independent variable and inability to randomly assign subjects to treatment groups, which can result in biases due to *self-selection* into groups. Because of this lack of control, ex post facto or correlational research is more likely to run the risk of erroneous interpretation of results than experimental research. On the other hand, because experimentation is often unfeasible or impractical in many research situations, ex post facto or correlational studies are important in nursing research. Correlational research is generally an efficient and useful method of collecting a large amount of data in a relatively short period. Finally, ex post facto studies are typically strong in terms of their realism.

❖ *STUDY SUGGESTIONS*

Chapter 8 of the accompanying *Study Guide for Nursing Research: Principles and Methods, 5th ed.*, offers various exercises and study suggestions for reinforcing the concepts presented in this chapter. Additionally, the following study questions can be addressed:

1. A researcher is interested in studying the effect of sensitivity training for nurses on their behavior in crisis intervention situations. Describe how you would set up an experiment to investigate this problem. Now describe two quasi-experimental or pre-experimental designs that could be used to study the same problem. Discuss what the weaknesses of each would be.
2. Assume that you have 10 individuals—Z, Y, X, W, V, U, T, S, R, and Q—who are going to participate in an experiment you are conducting. Using a table of random numbers, assign five individuals to group I and five to group II. Then randomly assign the groups to an experimental or control treatment.
3. Using the notation presented in Figures 8-4 to 8-13, diagram a few of the research examples described in the text that are not already shown.
4. A nurse researcher is interested in studying the success of several different approaches to feeding patients with dysphagia. Can the researcher use an ex post facto design to examine this problem? Why or why not? Could an experimental or quasi-experimental approach be used? How?
5. A nurse researcher is planning to investigate the relationship between the social class of hospitalized children and the frequency and content of children-initiated communications with the nursing staff. Which is the independent variable, and which is the dependent variable? Would you classify this research as basically experimental or correlational, or could both approaches be used?

❖ *SUGGESTED READINGS*

METHODOLOGICAL REFERENCES

Campbell, D. T., & Stanley, J. C. (1963). *Experimental and quasi-experimental designs for research.* Chicago: Rand McNally.

Christensen, L. M. (1991). *Experimental methodology.* (5th ed.). Boston: Allyn and Bacon.

Clinton, J., Beck, R., Radjenovic, D., Taylor, L., Westlake, S., & Wilson, S. E. (1986). Time series designs in clinical nursing research. *Nursing Research, 35,* 188–191.

Cook, T., & Campbell, D. T. (1979). *Quasi-experimental design and analysis issues for field settings.* Chicago: Rand McNally.

Fetter, M. S., Feetham, S. L., D'Apolito, K., Chaze, B. A., Fink, A., Frink, B., Hougart, M., & Rushton, C. (1989). Randomized clinical trials: Issues for researchers. *Nursing Research, 38,* 117–120.

Hauck, W. W., Gilliss, C. L., Donner, A., & Gortner, S. (1991). Randomization by cluster. *Nursing Research, 40,* 356–358.

Kerlinger, F. N. (1986). *Foundations of behavioral research* (3rd ed.). New York: Holt, Rinehart & Winston.

Kirchoff, K. T., & Dille, C. A. (1994). Issues in intervention research: Maintaining integrity. *Applied Nursing Research, 7,* 32–37.

Lazarsfeld, P. (1955). Foreword. In H. Hyman (Ed.), *Survey design and analysis.* New York: The Free Press.

SUBSTANTIVE REFERENCES

Badger, T. A., Mishel, M. H., Biocca, L. J., & Cardea, J. M. (1991). Depression assessment and management: Evaluating a community-based mental health training program for nurses. *Public Health Nursing, 8,* 170–175.

Brown, M. A., & Powell-Cope, G. (1993). Themes of loss and dying in caring for a family member with AIDS. *Research in Nursing and Health, 16,* 179–192.

Buckwalter, K. C., Cusack, D., Sidles, E., Wadle, K., & Beaver, M. (1989). Increasing communication ability in aphasic/dysarthric patients. *Western Journal of Nursing Research, 11,* 736–747.

Campbell, J. C., Poland, M. L., Waller, J. B., & Ager, J. (1992). Correlates of battering during pregnancy. *Research in Nursing and Health, 15,* 219–226.

Curley, M. A. (1988). Effects of the nursing mutual participation model of care on parental stress in the pediatric intensive care unit. *Heart and Lung, 17,* 682–688.

Duckett, L., Henly, S. J., & Garvis, M. (1993). Predicting breast-feeding duration during the postpartum hospitalization. *Western Journal of Nursing Research, 15,* 177–193.

Estok, P. J., Rudy, E. B., Kerr, M. E., & Menzel, L. (1993). Menstrual response to running: Nursing implications. *Nursing Research, 42,* 158–165.

Harrell, J. S., Champagne, M. T., Jarr, S., & Miyana, M. (1990). Heart sound simulation: How useful for critical care nurses? *Heart and Lung, 19,* 197–202

Hastings-Tolsma, M. T., Yucha, C. B., Tompkins, J., Robson, L., & Szeverenyi, N. (1993). Effect of warm and cold applications on the resolution of IV infiltrations. *Research in Nursing and Health, 16,* 171–178.

Hill, P. D., & Aldag, J. C. (1993). Insufficient milk supply among black and white breast-feeding mothers. *Research in Nursing and Health, 16,* 203–211.

Kaplow, R., & Bookbinder, M. (1994). A comparison of four endotracheal tube holders. *Heart and Lung, 23,* 59–66.

Kuhns-Hastings, J., Brakey, M. R., & Marshall, I. A. (1993). Effectiveness of a comprehensive breast cancer-screening class for women residing in rural areas. *Applied Nursing Research, 6,* 71–79.

McClowry, S. G., Giangrande, S. K., Tommasini, N. R., Clinton, W., Foreman, N. S., Lynch, K., & Ferketich, S. L. (1994). The effects of child temperament, maternal characteristics, and family circumstances on the maladjustment of school-age children. *Research in Nursing and Health, 17,* 25–35.

Melnyk, B. M. (1994). Coping with unplanned childhood hospitalization: Effects of informational interventions on mothers and children. *Nursing Research, 43,* 50–55.

Nyamathi, A. M., Leake, B., Flaskerud, J., Lewis, C., & Bennett, C. (1993). Outcomes of specialized and traditional AIDS counseling programs for impoverished women of color. *Research in Nursing and Health, 16,* 11–21.

Pickler, R. H., Higgins, K. E., & Crummette, B. D. (1993). The effect of nonnutritive sucking on bottle-feeding stress in preterm infants. *Journal of Obstetric, Gynecologic, and Neonatal Nursing, 22,* 230–234.

Polivka, B. J., Nickel, J. T., & Wilkins, J. R. III (1993). Cerebral palsy: Evaluation of a model of risk. *Research in Nursing and Health, 16,* 113–122.

Roberts, K. L., Brittin, M., Cook, M. A., & deClifford, J. (1994). Boomerang pillows and respiratory capacity. *Clinical Nursing Research, 3,* 157–165.

Rodrigues-Fisher, L., Bourguignon, C., & Good, B. V. (1993). Dietary fiber nursing intervention: Prevention of constipation in older adults. *Clinical Nursing Research, 2,* 464–477.

Schneider, J. K., Hornberger, S., Booker, J., Davis, A., & Kralicek, R. (1993). A medication discharge planning program: Measuring the effects on readmissions. *Clinical Nursing Research, 2,* 41–53.

Troy, N. W. (1993). Early contact and maternal attachment among women using public health care facilities. *Applied Nursing Research, 6,* 161–166.

Chapter 9

*A*DDITIONAL TYPES
OF RESEARCH

In Chapter 8, we explored research that varied along a single dimension: the investigator's control over the independent variable. All research studies can be categorized as either experimental, quasi-experimental or pre-experimental, or nonexperimental in design.

The discussion of experimental versus nonexperimental research, although useful in introducing some concepts of research design, fails to provide the beginning researcher with a sense of the full range of purposes of nursing research. This chapter is devoted to examining additional types of research not already discussed in previous chapters.* For ease of presentation, we have categorized these types into two broad groups, based on whether the research is primarily quantitative or qualitative.

---

* Because this chapter presents only an overview of many different types of research, the interested reader is urged to consult books cited under Methodological References at the end of the chapter for more detailed information on how to conduct the types of studies described here.

❖ *TYPES OF QUANTITATIVE RESEARCH*

Quantitative studies, as indicated in Chapter 1, tend to be highly structured investigations that yield numerical information amenable to statistical analysis. Most experimental and quasi-experimental research is quantitative, but many nonexperimental studies also use quantitative methods. This section describes several types of research that usually involve a quantitative approach, but it is important to note that for certain types of research described here (e.g., evaluation research), qualitative methods may also be used.

Survey Research

A *survey* is designed to obtain information from populations regarding the prevalence, distribution, and interrelations of variables within those populations. The decennial census of the U.S. population is one example of a survey. Political opinion polls, such as those conducted by

Polit DF, Hungler BP: NURSING RESEARCH: PRINCIPLES AND METHODS, 5th ed. © 1995 J. B. Lippincott Company.

Gallup or Harris, are other examples. When surveys use samples of individuals as subjects, as they usually do, they are often referred to as *sample surveys* (as opposed to a *census,* which covers the entire population). Surveys obtain information from a sample of people by means of *self-report*—that is, the subjects respond to a series of questions posed by the investigator. Surveys tend to collect data that are primarily quantitative. Surveys may be either cross-sectional or, as in the case of panel studies, longitudinal.

The content of a self-report survey is essentially limited only by the extent to which respondents are willing to report on the topic. Any information that can reliably be obtained by directly asking a person for that information is acceptable for inclusion in a survey. Often, a survey focuses on what people do: how or what they eat, how they care for their health needs, their compliance in taking medications, what kinds of family planning behaviors they engage in, and so forth. In some instances, particularly in political surveys, the emphasis is on what people plan to do—how they plan to vote, for example. Surveys also collect information on people's knowledge, opinions, attitudes, and values.

Survey data can be collected in a number of ways. The most respected method of securing survey information is through *personal interviews,* the method in which interviewers meet with individuals face to face and secure information from them. Generally, personal interviews are rather costly: they require considerable planning and interviewer training and tend to involve a lot of personnel time. Nevertheless, personal interviews are regarded as the most useful method of collecting survey data because of the quality of the information they yield. A further advantage of personal interviews is that relatively few people refuse to be interviewed in person.

Telephone interviews are a less costly, but often less effective, method of gathering survey information. When the interviewer is unknown, respondents may be uncooperative and unresponsive in a telephone situation, especially if the interview is long. However, telephoning can be a convenient method of collecting information quickly if the interview is short, specific, and not too personal, or if the researcher has had prior personal contact with the subjects.

Questionnaires differ from interviews primarily in that they are self-administered. That is, the respondent reads the questions on a form and gives an answer in writing. Since respondents differ considerably in their reading levels and in their ability to communicate in writing, questionnaires are *not* merely a printed form of an interview schedule. Great care must be taken in the development of a questionnaire to word questions clearly, simply, and unambiguously. Self-administered questionnaires are economical but are not appropriate for surveying certain populations (e.g., the elderly, children). In survey research, questionnaires are generally distributed through the mail.

The greatest advantage of survey research is its flexibility and broadness of scope. It can be applied to many populations, it can focus on a wide range of topics, and its information can be used for many purposes. However, the information obtained in most surveys tends to be relatively superficial: surveys rarely probe deeply into such complexities as contradictions of human behavior and feelings. Survey research is better suited to extensive rather than intensive analysis.

Nurse researchers have used the survey research approach to study a wide range of phenomena. For example, Martin and her colleagues (1993) surveyed employers using mailed questionnaires to determine their expectations for occupational health nurses. Stratton and co-researchers (1993) completed a telephone survey of directors of nursing in rural hospitals to examine barriers to recruiting nurses to rural practice settings. Brown and Marcy (1991) used personal interviews to survey members of a prepaid medical health plan regarding their use of botanical remedies for health problems.

Evaluation Research

Evaluation research is an applied form of research that involves finding out how well a program, practice, procedure, or policy* is working. Its goal is to assess or evaluate the success of a program. In evaluations, the research objective is utilitarian. The purpose of the evaluation is to answer the practical questions of people who must make decisions: Should the program be continued? Do current practices need to be modified, or should they be abandoned altogether? Do the costs of implementing the program outweigh the benefits?

Evaluation research has an important role to play both in localized settings and in programs at the national level. Evaluations are often the cornerstone of an area of research known as *policy research;* nurses have become increasingly aware of the potential contribution their research can make to the formulation of national and local health policies and thus are undertaking evaluations that have implications for such policies.

In doing an evaluation, the researcher often confronts a set of problems that are organizational, interpersonal, or political in nature. Evaluation research can be threatening to individuals. Even when the focus of an evaluation is on a nontangible entity, such as a program or procedure, it is *people* who developed and implemented it. People tend to think that they, or their work, are being evaluated and may in some cases feel that their job or reputation is at stake. Evaluation researchers, thus, need to have more than methodological skills: they need to be diplomats, adept in interpersonal dealings with people. If the people operating a program are defensive and noncooperative, the evaluation could be unproductive.

---

* For the most part, we use the term *program* throughout our discussion, but the reader should be aware that this term is meant to include practices, procedures, and policies as well.

EVALUATION RESEARCH MODELS

Various schools of thought have developed concerning the conduct of evaluation research. The traditional strategy for the conduct of evaluation research consists of four broad phases: determining the objectives of the program, developing a means of measuring the attainment of those objectives, collecting the data, and interpreting the data in terms of the objectives.

Often, the most difficult task is to spell out the program objectives. Typically, there are numerous objectives of a program, and these objectives may be vague. The term behavioral objective, frequently referred to in evaluation research literature, is a concept that has evolved as a means of coping with the broadness and fuzziness of program goals. A *behavioral objective* is the intended outcome of a program stated in terms of the behavior of those people at whom the program is aimed, that is, the behavior of the beneficiaries, rather than the agents, of the program. Thus, if the goal is to have patients ambulate after surgery, the behavioral objective might be stated as, "The patient will walk the length of the corridor within 5 days after surgery." The objective should *not* be stated as, "The nurse will *teach* the patient to walk the length of the corridor within 5 days after surgery." An emphasis on behavioral objectives can be taken to extremes. An evaluation may be concerned with psychological dimensions such as morale or an emotion (e.g., anxiety) that do not always manifest themselves in behavioral terms. However, the evaluator who tries to formulate program goals in terms of behavioral objectives will almost always find that the goals are less vague and diffuse than they might otherwise have been.

Once the program objectives have been delineated, the evaluation using a traditional approach can be designed much like other research studies. An evaluation can use either an experimental design (with subjects randomly assigned to either the program being evaluated or a control group), a quasi-experimental design, or a nonexperimental design. After developing a method to measure the behaviors under study, the researcher would then collect the data.

The traditional model of evaluation has sometimes been criticized for a certain narrowness of conceptualization. One alternative evaluation model is the so-called *goal-free approach*. Proponents of this model argue that programs may have a number of consequences besides accomplishing the official objectives of the program and that the classic model is handicapped by its inability to investigate these other effects. Goal-free evaluation represents an attempt to evaluate the outcomes of a program in the absence of information about intended outcomes. The job of the evaluator—a demanding one—is basically that of describing the repercussions of a program or practice on various components of the overall system. The goal-free model often may be a profitable approach, and it certainly leaves more room for creativity on the part of the evaluator. In many cases, however, the model may not be practical because there are seldom unlimited resources (personnel, time, or money) for the conduct of an evaluation. Decision makers may need to know whether objectives are being met so that immediate decisions can be made.

TYPES OF EVALUATIONS

Evaluations are undertaken to answer a variety of questions about a program or policy. This section briefly describes evaluations designed to address different types of questions. In evaluations of large-scale interventions (sometimes called *demonstrations* if they are implemented on a trial basis), the evaluator may well undertake all the evaluation activities discussed here.

PROCESS OR IMPLEMENTATION ANALYSIS. A *process* or *implementation analysis* is undertaken when there is a need for descriptive information about the process by which a program or procedure gets implemented and how it functions in actual operation. A process analysis is typically designed to address such questions as the following: Does the program function in the real world the way its designers intended it? What appear to be the strongest and weakest aspects of the program? What exactly *is* the treatment, and how does it differ (if at all) from traditional practices? What, if any, were the barriers to implementing the program successfully? A process analysis may be undertaken with the aim of improving a new or ongoing program; in such a situation, the evaluation may be referred to as a *formative evaluation.* In other situations, the purpose of the process analysis may be primarily to describe a program carefully so that it can be replicated by others. In either case, a process analysis typically involves an in-depth examination of the operation of a program, often involving the collection of both qualitative and quantitative data. As an example of an implementation analysis, Mitchell and colleagues (1989) studied the implementation of a special critical care nurses demonstration project with regard to nurse–physician collaboration, work and information flow, and staff morale.

OUTCOME ANALYSIS. Evaluations typically focus on whether a program or policy works, that is, whether it is effective in meeting its objectives. Evaluations that assess the worth of a program are sometimes referred to as *summative evaluations.* The intent of such evaluations is to help people decide whether the program should be discarded, replaced, modified, continued, or replicated. Some evaluation researchers distinguish between an outcome analysis and an impact analysis. An *outcome analysis* tends to be descriptive and does not use a rigorous design. Such an analysis simply documents the extent to which the goals of the program are attained, that is, the extent to which positive outcomes occur. For example, a program may be designed to encourage women in a poor rural community to obtain prenatal care. An outcome analysis would document outcomes without formal comparisons (for example, the percentage of women delivering babies in the community who had obtained prenatal care, the average month in which prenatal care was begun, and so on). As an actual example, Schirm (1993) evaluated a cholesterol screening program for older people to determine their cholesterol levels and their practices used to lower cholesterol levels.

IMPACT ANALYSIS.   An *impact analysis* attempts to identify the *net impacts* of an intervention, that is, the impacts that can be attributed exclusively to the intervention over and above the effects of other factors (such as the effect of the standard treatment). Impact analyses almost always use an experimental or quasi-experimental design because the aim of such evaluations is to attribute a causal influence to the special intervention. In the example cited earlier, let us suppose that the program to encourage prenatal care involved having nurses make home visits to women in the rural community to explain the benefits of early care during pregnancy. If the visits could be made to pregnant women on a random basis, the labor and delivery outcomes of the group of women receiving the home visits and of those not receiving them could be compared to determine the net impacts of the intervention, that is, the percentage increase in receipt of prenatal care among the experimental group relative to the control group. Most evaluations published in the nursing literature are impact analyses. In a double-blind experimental study, Kim and colleagues (1993) studied the effects of a 6-month muscle training program for patients with chronic obstructive pulmonary disease on inspiratory pressure and respiratory muscle endurance time. Becker and her colleagues (1993) evaluated the effectiveness of a staff training program focusing on developmental care with regard to the behavioral organization of very-low-birthweight infants.

COST–BENEFIT ANALYSIS.   New programs or policies are often expensive to implement. Therefore, evaluations sometimes include a *cost–benefit analysis* to determine whether the benefits of the program outweigh the costs, in terms of monetary value. Cost–benefit analyses are typically done in connection with impact analyses, that is, when there is solid evidence regarding the net impacts of an intervention. For example, in the example of home visitation, the evaluator would compare the total cost of operating the new program against the cost that could be incurred in its absence (e.g., for the treatment of low-birthweight infants in the control group). In the previously cited critical care nurses demonstration project (Mitchell, Armstrong, Simpson, & Lentz, 1989), the fiscal costs and benefits of the intervention were carefully assessed. Betz and her colleagues (1994) evaluated the cost-effectiveness of two intravenous additive systems, analyzing the effects of each system on nursing productivity.

Needs Assessment

Like evaluation research, a needs assessment represents an effort to provide a decision maker with information for action. As the name implies, a *needs assessment* is a study in which a researcher collects data for estimating the needs of a group, community, or organization. Thus, while an evaluation seeks to ascertain if a program is attaining its objectives, the aim of needs assessments is to determine if the objectives of a program are meeting the needs of the individuals who are supposed to benefit from it. Nursing educators may wish to assess the needs of their clients (students); hospital staff members may wish to learn the needs of those they serve (patients); a mental health outreach clinic may wish to gather information on the needs of some target population (e.g., adolescents in the community). Because resources are seldom limitless, information that can help in establishing priorities is almost always valuable.

There are various methods for doing a needs assessment; these methods are not necessarily mutually exclusive. The *key informant approach,* as the name implies, collects information concerning the needs of a group from people who are presumed to be in a key position to know those needs. These key informants could be community leaders, prominent health care workers, agency directors, or other knowledgeable individuals. Questionnaires or interviews are generally used to collect the data.

Another method is the *survey approach,* in which data are collected from a sample of the target group whose needs are being assessed. In a survey, there would be no attempt to question only people who are in positions of authority or who are knowledgeable. Any member of the group or community could be asked to give his or her viewpoint.

Another alternative is to use an *indicators approach,* which relies on inferences made from statistics available in existing reports or records. For example, a nurse-managed clinic that is interested in analyzing the needs of its clients could examine over a 5-year period the number of appointments that were kept, the employment rate of its clients, the changes in risk appraisal status, methods of payment, and so forth. The indicators approach is flexible and may also be economical because the data are generally available but need organization and interpretation.

Needs assessments almost always involve the development of recommendations. The role of the researcher conducting a needs assessment is often that of making judgments about priorities in light of considerations such as costs and feasibility and in advising on means by which the most highly prioritized needs can be addressed.

Nurse researchers have examined the needs of diverse groups. For example, Farran and her colleagues (1993) studied the needs of home-based people with dementia. Kleinpell and Powers (1992) studied the needs of family members of intensive care unit patients.

Secondary Analysis

Secondary analysis involves the use of data gathered in a previous study to test new hypotheses or explore new relationships. The amount of research conducted every year in such fields as nursing, medicine, the life sciences, and the social sciences is overwhelming. In a typical research project, more data are collected than the investigator actually analyzes. Secondary analysis is efficient and economical because data collection is typically the most time-consuming and expensive part of a research project.

A number of avenues are available for making use of an existing set of data:

1. Variables and relationships among variables that were previously unanalyzed can be examined (e.g., an independent variable in the original study could become the dependent variable in the secondary analysis).
2. The secondary analysis can focus on a particular subgroup rather than the full original sample (e.g., survey data about health habits from a national sample could be analyzed to study smoking among urban teenagers).
3. The unit of analysis can be changed (e.g., a study of individual nurses drawn from 25 hospitals could be converted to aggregated data about the hospitals).

In recent years, a number of groups such as university institutes and federal agencies have been attempting to organize data and make them available to researchers for secondary analysis. The policies regulating the public use of data vary from one organization to another, but it is not unusual for data to be provided to an interested researcher at about the cost of duplication plus handling. Thus, in some cases in which the gathering of the data involved an expenditure of hundreds of thousands of dollars, reproduced materials may be supplied for less than 1% of the initial costs. Many universities and research institutes within universities maintain libraries of data sets from large national surveys.

One source of secondary data for nurse researchers is the various surveys sponsored by the National Center for Health Statistics (NCHS).

For example, NCHS periodically conducts such national surveys as the National Health Interview Survey and the Health Promotion and Disease Prevention Survey, both of which gather health-related information from thousands of people all over the United States.

The use of available data makes it possible for the researcher to bypass time-consuming and costly steps in the research process, but there are some noteworthy disadvantages in working with existing data. In particular, if an investigator does not play a role in collecting the data, the chances are pretty high that the data set will be deficient or problematic in one or more ways, such as in the sample used, the variables measured, and so forth. The researcher may continuously face "if only" problems: if only they had asked a question about a certain topic or had measured a particular variable differently. Nevertheless, opportunities for secondary analysis are often worth exploring. Note that while most secondary analysis studies involve existing quantitative data sets, the approach can also be used with qualitative data.

Nurse researchers have used a secondary analysis approach with both large national data sets and with smaller, more localized ones. For example, Kocher and Thomas (1994) used data from Department of Defense surveys of military personnel in their study of factors that predicted retention among Army nurses. Long and Weinert (1992) used data from a survey of multiple sclerosis patients to study health perceptions in relation to urban versus rural residence.

Meta-Analysis

Chapter 4 described the function of a literature review as a preliminary step in a research project. However, there is growing recognition of the fact that the careful integration of knowledge on a topic in itself constitutes an important scholarly endeavor that can contribute new knowledge. The procedure known as *meta-analysis* represents an application of statistical procedures to findings from research reports. In essence, meta-analysis treats the findings from one study as a single piece of data. The findings from multiple studies on the same topic, therefore, can be combined to yield a data set that can be analyzed in a manner similar to that obtained from individual subjects.

The earliest form of nonnarrative research integration used what has been referred to as the *voting method*. This procedure involves tallying the outcomes of previous studies to determine what outcome has received the greatest empirical support. The voting method has since been superseded by methods of considerable sophistication and complexity. Because beginning researchers may have no statistical background, a discussion of actual statistical procedures cannot be included here. Suffice it to say that these methods, described in detail by Glass and colleagues (1981), generally involve the calculation of an index known as the *effect size,* which quantifies the strength of the relationship between the independent and dependent variables.

Traditional narrative reviews of the literature are handicapped by several factors uncharacteristic of meta-analysis. The first is that if the number of studies on a specific topic is large and if the results are inconsistent, then it is difficult to draw conclusions. Moreover, narrative reviews are often subject to potential biases. The researcher may unwittingly give more weight to findings that are congruent with his or her own viewpoints. Thus, meta-analytic procedures provide a convenient and objective method of integrating a large body of findings and of observing patterns and relationships that might otherwise have gone undetected. Furthermore, meta-analysis provides information about the magnitude of differences and relationships. Meta-analysis can thus serve as an important scholarly tool in theory development as well as in research utilization.

Meta-analysis has also been criticized on a number of grounds. One issue has been called the *fruit problem,* that is, the possibility of combining studies that conceptually do not belong with each other (apples and oranges). Another issue is that there is generally a bias in the studies appearing in published sources. Studies in which no differences or no relationships have been found are less likely to be published and, therefore, are less likely to be included in the meta-analysis. Narrative literature reviews are subject to the same two problems, but these problems may take on added significance in a meta-analysis because the quantitative results make the conclusions appear more concrete and absolute. Another problem is that a research report could provide general information about the study's findings but might not include sufficient quantitative information for computing an effect size. Despite these potential problems, careful and thorough meta-analyses represent an important advancement to the scientific community.

Delphi Surveys

Delphi surveys were developed as a tool for short-term forecasting. The technique involves a panel of experts who are asked to complete a series of questionnaires focusing on the experts' opinions, predictions, or judgment concerning a specific topic of interest.

The Delphi technique differs from other surveys in several respects. First, the Delphi technique consists of several rounds of questionnaires. Each of the cooperating experts is asked to complete at least two (and often more) questionnaires. This multiple iteration approach is used as a means of effecting group consensus of opinion, without the necessity of face-to-face committee work. A second feature is the use of feedback to members of the panel. Responses to each round of questionnaires are analyzed, summarized, and returned to the experts with a new questionnaire. The experts can then reformulate their opinions with the knowledge of the group's viewpoint in mind. The process of response–analysis–feedback–response usually is repeated three times until a general consensus is obtained.

The Delphi technique is a relatively efficient and effective method of combining the expertise of a large group of individuals to obtain information for planning and prediction purposes. The experts are spared the necessity of being brought together for a formal meeting, thus saving considerable time and expense for the panel members. Another advantage is that any one persuasive or prestigious expert cannot have an undue influence on the opinions of others, as could happen in a face-to-face situation. Each panel member is on an equal footing with all others. Anonymity probably encourages a greater frankness of opinion than might be expressed in a formal meeting. The feedback–response loops allow for multichanneled communication without any risk of the members being sidetracked from their mission.

At the same time, it must be conceded that the Delphi technique is both costly and time-consuming for the researcher. Experts must be solicited, questionnaires prepared and mailed, responses analyzed, results summarized, new questionnaires prepared, and so forth. The cooperation of the panel members may wane in later rounds of the questionnaire mailings. The problem of bias through attrition is a constant threat, though probably less severe than through ordinary questionnaire procedures. On the whole, the Delphi technique represents a significant methodological tool for solving problems, planning, and forecasting.

Methodological Research

Methodological research refers to controlled investigations of the ways of obtaining, organizing, and analyzing data. Methodological studies address the development, validation, and evaluation of research tools or techniques. Nurse researchers in recent years have become increasingly interested in methodological research. This is not surprising in light of growing demands for sound and reliable measures and for sophisticated procedures for obtaining and analyzing data.

The methodological researcher may, to take an example, concentrate on the development of an instrument that accurately measures patients' satisfaction with nursing care. The researcher in such a case is not interested in the level of patient satisfaction nor in how such satisfaction relates to characteristics of the nurses, the hospital, or the patients. The goals of the researcher are to develop an effective, serviceable, and trustworthy instrument that can be used by other researchers and to evaluate his or her success in accomplishing this goal.

Methodological research may appear less exciting and less rewarding than substantive research, but it is virtually impossible to conduct high-quality and useful research on a substantive topic with inadequate research tools. Studies of a methodological nature are indispensable in any scientific discipline, and perhaps especially so when a field is relatively new and deals with highly complex, intangible phenomena such as human behavior or welfare, as is the case in nursing research.

Content Analysis Studies

Content analysis involves the quantification of narrative, qualitative material. Although qualitative researchers who do not quantify their data sometimes refer to their analytic work as a content analysis, the term in its classic sense refers to "a research technique for the objective, systematic, and quantitative description of the manifest content of communication" (Berelson, 1971, p. 18).

Content analysis is applied to people's written and oral communications. It can be used with such materials as diaries, letters, speeches, books, articles, and other linguistic expressions. In traditional content analysis, the researcher enhances objectivity by proceeding on the basis of explicitly formulated rules. The rules serve as guidelines to enable two or more people analyzing the same materials to obtain the same results. The analysis is rendered systematic by the inclusion or exclusion of materials according to consistently applied selection criteria.

The most common applications of content analysis involve describing the characteristics of the content of the message (as opposed to its style, for example). The investigator must identify the variables to be recorded and the *unit of analysis* that will be used, that is, the unit that will be used to categorize the content into meaningful groupings. Individual *words*, which are easy to work with, are sometimes the unit. A *theme* is a larger and more inclusive unit of analysis. A theme may be a phrase, sentence, or paragraph embodying ideas or making an assertion about some topic. Some examples of themes that might emerge in patients' accounts of a long-term illness experience include coping with pain, fear of death, loneliness, and loss of motivation for recovery. These are illustrations of themes organized around the content of a message, but it is possible to detect stylistic themes such as different tones (proselytizing, admonishing, or informing), different grammatical structures, and so forth.

Another possible unit of analysis is the *item*. This unit refers to an entire message, document, or other production: a letter, editorial, diary entry, conference presentation, issue of a journal, and the like. The whole item can then be categorized in terms of one or more characteristics. For example, articles appearing in the journal *Nursing Research* can be classified according to whether the research problem was clinical in nature, and trends over time could then be analyzed. Finally, the unit may be a *space-and-time* measure. This type of unit consists of a physical measurement of content, such as the number of pages, number of words, number of speakers, amount of time spent in a discussion, and so forth. The units referred to here as item and theme are probably most useful for nurse researchers.

Once the researcher has established the unit of analysis, a method of categorizing the data must be developed. After the individual pieces of communication are sampled and categorized, analysis can proceed. The most common form of quantifying materials is the enumeration of recorded occurrences in each category. A second approach is to simply create a binary index (yes or no) of whether the concepts covered in the category scheme were present or absent in the materials. The ranking of materials according to prespecified criteria is a third possibility. Finally, rating scales can be used to assess various aspects of the communications.

Content analysis suffers from several disadvantages such as the risk of subjectivity and the amount of tedious work involved. However, this technique may be expedient and efficient in its use of available materials, and there may be several research problems for which there are no alternatives.

❖ TYPES OF QUALITATIVE RESEARCH

Nurse researchers are increasingly undertaking qualitative studies that involve an in-depth investigation of some phenomenon of interest. Qualitative studies are almost always nonexperimental, although sometimes qualitative studies are done as a separate substudy in conjunction with an experiment to enhance the interpretability of the quantitative findings. This section describes several types of research that typically use a qualitative approach.

Field Studies

Qualitative research that aims at describing and exploring phenomena in naturalistic settings is frequently referred to as field research. *Field studies* are naturalistic investigations that are done "in the field," in such social settings as nursing homes, housing projects, private residences, and so on. The purpose of field studies is to examine in an in-depth fashion the practices, behaviors, beliefs, and attitudes of individuals or groups as they normally function in real life. Unlike surveys, field studies are often intensive rather than extensive, and the data that are collected are usually narrative materials, based on researcher observation, conversations with those being studied, or available documents. The aim of the field researcher is to get close to the people under study to understand a problem or situation from their perspective.

In traditional scientific research, a heavy emphasis is placed on control and objectivity. In field research, the researcher continually uses subjective judgments about whom to interview, what to observe, what questions to ask, and so on. In field research, the main instrument of data collection is the researcher rather than technical apparatus or formal written tools. Field research is typically less linear than other types of research. That is, the steps do not necessarily follow a linear progression such as that suggested in Chapter 2. The field researcher may begin with only a general problem area or hypothesis to be explored, or hypotheses may be generated in the course of data collection and analysis and pursued more rigorously in subsequent data collection. Field researchers try to remain open and flexible about the research process in the hope that such flexibility will allow them to pursue the realities of the subjects' experience as that experience is lived.

Wilson (1989) identified the following five stages that are typically undertaken in field research:

Stage I: Identifying the setting in which the field work will take place and assessing the appropriateness of the setting for the problem of interest.

Stage II: Gaining access to the people or groups to be studied, including the development of strategies to use in approaching gatekeepers.

Stage III: Assuming an appropriate role (appropriate in terms of research aims or the demands and constraints of those under study) in the social setting, on a continuum ranging from full participant in the setting to complete observer.

Stage IV: Collecting, recording, analyzing, and interpreting data.

Stage V: Fulfilling commitments made to gain access to the social setting, and leaving the field.

Nurse researchers have undertaken field studies in a wide variety of settings. Leininger (1985) studied the health care values, beliefs, attitudes and general lifeways of black and white residents of a rural community in central Alabama. Grau and Wellin (1992) focused on the organizational cultures of nursing homes and their responses to external licensing and funding regulations. Kulig (1990) studied the child-bearing beliefs and knowledge of conception and fetal development among Cambodian refugee women living in Canada.

Field studies are strong on realism because they are done in natural settings without structure or controls imposed by the researcher. Because of the in-depth and flexible nature of field studies, they often provide a depth of understanding of social phenomena that is unattainable with more traditional methods of scientific research. Yet some of the very elements that make field research strong are potential problem areas. During data collection and analysis, the researcher is so thoroughly immersed in the phenomenon that the risk of bias may emerge. Moreover, field research can almost never be replicated because the methods evolve in situ. It is often difficult to evaluate whether two independent field researchers would come to different conclusions based on the same investigation.

Qualitative field studies share a number of similarities in terms of overall goals and techniques, but there are actually a variety of theoretical and philosophical traditions that fall within the broad umbrella of qualitative field research. These traditions vary in their conceptualization of what types of questions are important to ask in understanding the world in which we live. Below we briefly summarize some of those traditions and the terminology associated with them.

ETHNOGRAPHY

Ethnography, the approach used by anthropologists, focuses on the culture of a group of people. An underlying assumption of the ethnographer is that every human group eventually evolves a culture that guides the members' view of the world and the way they structure their experiences. Ethnographers almost invariably undertake extensive field work to learn about the cultural group in which they are interested.

The aim of the ethnographer is to learn from (rather than study) members of a cultural group—to understand their world view as they define it. Ethnographic researchers sometimes refer to emic and etic perspectives. An *emic* perspective refers to the way the members of the culture themselves envision their world—it is the insiders' view. The *etic* view, by contrast, is the outsiders' interpretation of the experiences of that culture. Ethnographers strive to acquire an emic perspective of a culture under study, generally through interviews and observations made while participating in the activities of the group under study.

Many nurse researchers have undertaken ethnographic studies. Indeed, Madeleine Leininger coined the phrase *ethnonursing research*, which she defines as "the study and analysis of the local or indigenous people's viewpoints, beliefs, and practices about nursing care behavior and processes of designated cultures" (Leininger, 1985, p. 38).

PHENOMENOLOGY

Phenomenology, rooted in a philosophical tradition developed by Husserl, is an approach to thinking about what the life experiences of people are like. The phenomenological researcher asks the question: What is the *essence* of this phenomenon as experienced by these people? The phenomenologist assumes there is an essence that can be understood, in much the same way that the ethnographer assumes that cultures exist.

The focus of phenomenological inquiry, then, is what people experience regarding some phenomena and how they interpret those experiences. For many phenomenological researchers, the inquiry includes not only learning about the experience by gathering information from those people under study (usually through in-depth interviews or diaries) but also efforts to actually experience the phenomenon in the same way, typically through participation, observation, and introspective reflection.

Phenomenological inquiry typically involves four basic steps: bracketing, intuiting, analyzing, and describing. *Bracketing* refers to the process of identifying and holding in abeyance any preconceived beliefs and opinions one may have about the phenomenon under investigation. The researcher brackets out the world and any presuppositions, in an effort to confront the data in pure form. *Intuiting* occurs when the researcher remains open to the meanings attributed to the phenomenon by those who have experienced it. Phenomenological researchers then proceed to the analysis phase (i.e., categorizing and making sense of the essential meanings of the phenomenon). Finally, the descriptive phase occurs when the researcher comes to understand and define the phenomenon.

ETHNOMETHODOLOGY

Just as ethnography has its roots in anthropology and phenomenology has its roots in philosophy, *ethnomethodology* is allied with the discipline of sociology. An ethnomethodological researcher seeks to discover how people make sense of their everyday activities and interpret their social worlds so as to behave in socially acceptable ways. Within this tradition, the focus is on the ordinary details of everyday life. Researchers attempt to understand a social group's norms and assumptions that are so deeply ingrained that the members no longer think about the underlying reasons for their behaviors. Ethnomethodologists often use similar processes to phenomenologists, such as bracketing.

Ethnomethodologists rely on observation and in-depth interviews as major sources of data. However, unlike most other qualitative researchers, they occasionally engage in *ethnomethodological experiments*. During these experiments, the researcher disrupts ordinary activity by doing something that violates the group's norms and assumptions. The researcher then observes what the group members do and how they try to make sense of what is happen-

ing. An example is going into the library and deliberately sitting next to someone at a table when there are plenty of empty tables, to observe how people make sense of and deal with this mild violation of social expectations about personal space.

Historical Research

Historical research is the systematic collection and critical evaluation of data relating to past occurrences. Generally, historical research is undertaken to answer questions concerning causes, effects, or trends relating to past events that may shed light on present behaviors or practices. An understanding of contemporary nursing theories, practices, or issues can often be enhanced by an investigation of a specified segment of the past. Historical data are typically qualitative, although in some cases quantitative data may be available.

Nurses have used historical research methods to examine a wide range of phenomena in both the recent and more distant past. Widerquist (1992) examined Florence Nightingale's spirituality and its influence on the development of early modern nursing. Stuart (1992) examined the ways in which gender became an important variable in the articulation of power among public health nurses in Ontario in the 1920s. King (1989) examined how solutions to past nursing shortages contributed to current nursing shortages.

The student should be careful not to confuse historical research with a review of the literature about historical events. Like other types of research, historical inquiry has as its goal the discovery of new knowledge, not the summary of existing knowledge. One important difference between historical research and a literature review is that a historical researcher is often guided by specific hypotheses or questions. The hypotheses represent attempts to explain and interpret the conditions, events, or phenomena under investigation. Hypotheses in historical research are not usually tested in a statistical sense. They are broadly stated conjectures about relationships among historical events, trends, and phenomena. For example, it might be hypothesized that a relationship exists between the presence or absence of war on the one hand and the amount of scientific nursing knowledge generated on the other. This hypothesis could be tested by analyzing research trends in nursing in relation to political conflicts.

The steps involved in performing historical research are similar to those for other types of research: the historical researcher defines a problem area, develops specific questions, collects data according to a systematic framework, analyzes the data, and interprets the findings. However, historical researchers typically need to devote considerable effort to identifying and evaluating data sources on events, situations, and human behavior that occurred in the past.

COLLECTION OF HISTORICAL DATA

Data for historical research are usually in the form of written records of the past: periodicals, diaries, books, letters, newspapers, minutes of meetings, legal documents, and so forth. However, a number of nonwritten materials may also be of interest. For example, physical remains and objects are potential sources of information. Visual materials such as photographs and films are forms of data, as are audio materials such as records and tapes.

Many of these materials may be difficult to obtain—even written materials are not always conveniently indexed by subject, author, or title. The identification of appropriate historical materials may require a considerable amount of time, effort, and detective work. Fortunately, there are several archives of historical nursing documents, such as the collections at several universities (e.g., Boston University, Columbia University) as well as collections at the National Library of Medicine, the Nursing Museum in Philadelphia, the American Journal of Nursing Company, and the National League for Nursing. Fairman (1987) identified additional sources for those interested in nursing history.

Historical materials generally are classified as either primary or secondary sources. A *primary source* is first-hand information, such as original documents, relics, or artifacts. Examples are Louisa May Alcott's book *Hospital Sketches,* minutes of early American Nurses Association meetings, hospital records, and so forth. Primary sources represent the most direct link with historical events or situations: only the narrator (in the case of written materials) intrudes between original events and the historical researcher.

Secondary sources are second- or third-hand accounts of historical events or experiences. For example, textbooks, encyclopedias, or other reference books are generally secondary sources. Secondary sources, in other words, are discussions of events written by individuals who are summarizing or interpreting primary source materials. Primary sources should be used whenever possible in historical research. The further removed from the historical event the information is, the less reliable, objective, and comprehensive the data are likely to be.

EVALUATION OF HISTORICAL DATA

Historical evidence usually is subjected to two types of evaluation, which historians refer to as external and internal criticism. *External criticism* is concerned basically with the authenticity and genuineness of the data. For example, a nursing historian might have a diary presumed to be written by Dorothea Dix. External criticism would involve asking such questions as: Is this the handwriting of Ms. Dix? Is the paper on which the diary is written of the right age? Are the writing style and ideas expressed consistent with her other writings? There are various scientific techniques available to determine the age of materials, such as x-ray and radioactive procedures. However, other flaws may be less easy to detect. For example, there is the possibility that material of interest may have been written by a ghost writer, that is, by someone other than the person in whom we are really interested. There is also the potential problem of mechanical errors associated with transcriptions, translations, or typed versions of historical materials.

Internal criticism of historical data refers to the evaluation of the worth of the evidence. The focus of internal criticism is not so much on the physical aspects of the materials but rather on their content. An important issue here is the accuracy or truth of the data. For example, the historical researcher must question whether a writer's representations of historical events are unbiased. It may also be appropriate to ask if the author of a document was in a position to make a valid report of an event or occurrence, or whether the writer was competent as a recorder of fact. Evidence bearing on the accuracy of historical data might include comparisons with other people's accounts of the same event to determine the degree of agreement; knowledge of the time at which the document was produced (reports of events or situations tend to be more accurate if they are written immediately after the event); knowledge of the point of view or biases of the writer; and knowledge of the degree of competence of the writer to record events authoritatively and accurately.

Case Studies

Case studies are in-depth investigations of an individual, group, institution, or other social unit. The researcher conducting a case study attempts to analyze and understand the variables that are important to the history, development, or care of the subject or the subject's problems. As befits an intensive analysis, the focus of case studies is typically on determining the dynamics of *why* the subject of the investigation thinks, behaves, or develops in a particular manner rather than *what* his or her status, progress, actions, or thoughts are. It is not unusual for probing research of this type to require a detailed study over a considerable period. Data are often collected that relate not only to the subject's present state but also to past experiences and situational and environmental factors relevant to the problem being examined. Data are often (but not always) qualitative.

Case studies are a useful way to explore phenomena that have not been rigorously researched. The information obtained in case studies can be extremely useful in the production of hypotheses to be tested more rigorously in subsequent research. The intensive probing that characterizes case studies often leads to insights concerning previously unsuspected relationships. Furthermore, in-depth case studies may serve the important role of clarifying concepts and variables or of elucidating ways to measure them.

Case studies sometimes are used in conjunction with large-scale research projects to serve in an illustrative capacity. Research reports that are filled with extensive statistical information often fail to convey some of the richness of the real-life subject matter. Qualitative case materials presented in such a context can be extremely effective in elucidating certain points or in imparting a more realistic impression to data that might otherwise appear overly abstract.

Most case studies are nonexperimental; in such studies, the researcher obtains a wealth of descriptive information and may examine relationships among different variables, or may examine trends over time. Some case studies, however, involve the administration of a treatment and an analysis of ensuing consequences on the individual. Such studies are sometimes referred to as *single-subject experiments*. Time series designs are often especially appropriate in such situations (i.e., repeated observations before and after the initiation of an intervention).

The greatest advantage of case studies is the depth that is possible when a limited number of individuals, institutions, or groups is being investigated. A common complaint leveled at other types of research is that the data tend to be superficial. Case studies provide the researcher with the opportunity of having an intimate knowledge of the subject's condition, thoughts, feelings, actions (past and present), intentions, and environment. On the other hand, this same strength is a potential weakness because the familiarity of the researcher with the subject may make objectivity more difficult—especially if the data are collected by observational techniques for which the researcher is the main (or only) observer. Perhaps the most serious disadvantage of the case study method is its lack of generalizability. That is, if the researcher reveals the existence of important relationships, it is generally difficult to know whether the same relationships would manifest themselves in other subjects (or in other institutions). However, it may be perfectly reasonable to predict the future behavior of an individual who is the subject of the case study based on events or relationships experienced by the person in the past.

❖ RESEARCH EXAMPLES

Nurse researchers are undertaking a wide variety of studies designed to address a broad range of problems. All the types of research described in this chapter have been reported on in the nursing research literature.

Examples of Various Types of Quantitative Studies

Table 9-1 presents a brief description of nursing studies corresponding to each of the types of quantitative research described in this chapter. Two quantitative studies are described in greater detail next.

EXAMPLE OF A SURVEY

Pollow, Stoller, Forster, and Duniho (1994) conducted a survey of elderly people living in community settings and managing their own health, to examine their use of over-the-counter (OTC) medications and their consumption of alcohol. A major purpose of the study was to document drug utilization patterns among community-dwelling elders and their risk of adverse drug reactions.

Data were collected from a sample of 667 people living in community settings in northeastern New York, all of whom were 65 years of age or older. Of the people who were approached for the study, 79% agreed to participate.

Data were gathered through personal interviews in the respondents' homes. The interview covered a wide range of topics, including the respondents' health and disabilities, use of prescription and OTC medications, consumption of alcohol, and other health-related behaviors (e.g., smoking, exercise, eating patterns). Respondents who had difficulty remembering the names or therapeutic intent of any medications were asked to show the medicine to the interviewers, who recorded the names of the medications.

The findings indicated that almost two-thirds of the respondents reported one or more drug–drug or drug–alcohol combination associated with a possible adverse reaction. The potential for risk was highest among people taking psychoactive drugs, antidiabetic agents, anticoagulants, and ulcer medications. The results suggest the need for health care practitioners to obtain more detailed drug histories when treating elderly clients who are taking certain categories of medications.

EXAMPLE OF AN EVALUATION

Gardner (1991) used a quasi-experimental design to evaluate primary versus team nursing in a large urban tertiary care hospital. The two modes of nursing care delivery were compared in terms of quality of nursing care, nurse retention, stress among nurses, and costs over a 5-year period.

The study data were collected in three phases—a preintervention phase and two postintervention phases. During the preintervention phase, the medical units involved in the study used a functional/team nursing model. The intervention involved the implementation of primary nursing in several units, while several other units continued to use team nursing. The implementation of primary nursing was monitored on a yearly basis. The first postintervention data phase involved collection of data 12 months after implementing primary nursing, and the second involved data collection 20 months after

Table 9-1.   *Examples of Different Types of Quantitative Studies*

RESEARCH QUESTION	TYPE OF STUDY
What are nurses' experiences with working with an impaired nurse coworker, and how did the nurse become aware of the impairment? (Damrosch & Scholler-Jaquish, 1993)	Survey
How effective is an art future-image intervention in increasing the self-esteem and decreasing depression among hospitalized suicidal adolescents? (Walsh, 1993)	Evaluation
What are the informational needs of patients undergoing surgical procedures performed on an outpatient basis? (Oberle, Allen, & Lynkowski, 1993)	Needs assessment
Do nurses and clients have different perceptions about the meaning of the American Association of Colleges of Nursing values for professional nursing practice? (Tompkins, 1993)	Secondary analysis
What are the effects of hospital intervention programs on the physiological development of premature infants? (Krywanio, 1994)	Meta-analysis
Are the definition and defining characteristics of the nursing diagnosis of ineffective breastfeeding valid? (Lethbridge, McClurg, Henrikson, & Wall, 1993)	Delphi survey
Does a shortened form of the Oucher Scale (a tool for pain assessment in children) yield equally accurate measures as the original form, and do differences vary according to the gender, ethnicity, or age of the child? (Jordan-Marsh, Yoder, Hall, & Watson, 1994)	Methodological study
What are the characteristics of group processes that are personally most important to in-patients with bipolar disorder in group therapy? (Pollack, 1993)	Content analysis

implementation. Throughout the study, all units had similar staffing mix and nursing competency and comparable patient population and bed occupancy.

Data relating to the effectiveness of the intervention were obtained through observation of the nurses' care by trained nurse raters; patients' ratings of the nurses' supportive behaviors; and nurses' ratings of their own stress. Administrative records provided information regarding staff retention and costs, which were calculated as the cost of nursing personnel per patient day. The analysis of the postintervention data revealed that primary nursing resulted in a higher quality of nursing care than team nursing and that nurse retention was substantially better in primary nursing. In addition, cost per patient day was significantly lower for primary nursing.

Examples of Various Types of Qualitative Studies

Table 9-2 presents a brief description of nursing studies corresponding to the types of

Table 9-2.   *Examples of Different Types of Qualitative Studies*

RESEARCH QUESTION	TYPE OF STUDY
What are the differences between official and lay definitions of maternal and child health needs in Northern Ireland and Jamaica? (Mason, 1994)	Field study: ethnonursing
What is the essential meaning of stressful life experiences in 9- to 11-year-old children? (Jacobsen, 1994)	Field study: phenomenological
What is the structure and function of gift-giving in the patient-nurse relationship? (Morse, 1991)	Field study: ethnomethodological
What was the process by which racial concerns in a race- and class-conscious society become superceded by the concerns of caring for the sick? (Buhler-Wilkerson, 1992)	Historical study
What are the communication strategies used by an expert nurse in individualizing care? (Brown, 1994)	Case study

qualitative research described in this chapter. Two qualitative studies are described in greater detail next.

EXAMPLE OF A FIELD STUDY

Dreher and Hayes (1993) spent 6 years in the field studying marijuana use among pregnant Jamaican women and subsequent effects on the offspring. The researchers combined two types of investigations: an ethnographic study of perinatal use of marijuana in rural Jamaican communities, and a clinical study of a sample of women (including both users and nonusers of marijuana) and their children. The field researchers lived in a rural parish for most of the 6-year period and had regular contact with each of the families in the study.

The ethnographic portion of the study involved general observations and interviews related to perinatal use of marijuana (called *ganja* in Jamaica). The researchers found that most female users prepared and consumed ganja for themselves and their families in the form of teas and tonics for medicinal or health-rendering purposes. Ganja

smoking was less common among Jamaican women than Jamaican men, although the researchers found that smoking increased among women over the course of the field work. Women who smoked ganja often smoked throughout pregnancy, during labor, and into the breastfeeding period.

In the clinical portion of the study, the researchers compared the offspring of 30 ganja users and 30 nonusers using standardized measures of development (e.g., the Bayley Scales of Infant Development). The ethnographic work proved to be critical in suggesting adaptations that made these instruments appropriate for a different culture.

EXAMPLE OF A CASE STUDY

Price (1992) undertook a series of case studies in highland Ecuador to analyze the processes by which people cope with serious illness. The case studies were used as a vehicle for illuminating psychological coping mechanisms within family and sociocultural contexts.

Price conducted eight in-depth case studies of families who were involved in a serious illness over a 2-year period. Data were gathered by observation and in-depth interviewing. A complete story of the illness was obtained from individuals with caretaking responsibility and from others associated with the family. Price also used interviews to address specific questions on coping, interactions with health specialists, and illness meanings. Two case study examples were described in Price's report. The following is a summary of the first case study:

> Susana was a 6-year-old who suffered from severe hip malformation. The first symptoms appeared when she was 1 year old after she had been hospitalized for an acute intestinal infection. The family consulted many different health care specialists and tried many therapies to prevent total disability. Ultimately, Susana underwent surgery in the public children's hospital, then physical therapy in the same hospital; finally, she received treatment from a spiritualist healer, including a spiritualist operation performed from a distance.

Price noted that Susana's mother, Maria, was able to cope effectively with her daughter's illness because she took steps to preserve her self-esteem and sense of participation, both of which were undermined by the traditional health care practitioners at the hospital. The researcher concluded that Maria achieved a renewal of faith in herself as caretaker, which allowed the family to transform the experience of illness.

Based on the case analyses, Price concluded that two mechanisms are critical in constructive psychological coping in an illness situation. First, coping functions by preserving and strengthening self-esteem. And second, patients and their caretakers must maintain a sense of participation in shaping the outcome of events.

❖ *SUMMARY*

This chapter presents an overview of different types of research that nurse researchers have used to address a variety of problems. These types include studies that are typically quantitative and others that are typically qualitative.

Survey research is the branch of research that examines the characteristics, behaviors, attitudes, and intentions of a group of people by asking individuals belonging to that group to answer a series of questions. The preferred method of collecting survey information is through *personal interviews*, in which interviewers meet with participants in a face-to-face situation and question them directly. This method has the advantage of encouraging cooperation, which results in higher response rates and a better quality of data. *Telephone interviews* are convenient and economical, but they are not recommended when the interview is long or detailed or when the questions are sensitive or highly personal. *Questionnaires* are self-administered; that is, questions are read by the respondent, who then gives a written response.

Evaluation research assesses the effectiveness of a program, policy, or procedure to assist decision makers in choosing a course of action. Various evaluation models have been developed. The *classic approach* evaluates the congruence between the goals of the program and actual outcomes. Goals are typically phrased in the form of *behavioral objectives,* which delineate the intended outcomes of a program in terms of the behaviors of the program's beneficiaries. The *goal-free approach* attempts to understand all the effects of a program, whether or not they were intended. Evaluations can answer a variety of questions. *Process* or *implementation analyses* are undertaken to describe the process by which a program gets implemented and how it is functioning in practice. *Outcome analyses* basically describe the status of some condition after the introduction of an intervention. *Impact analyses,* which typically use rigorous comparative designs, test whether an intervention caused any *net impacts. Cost–benefit analyses* attempt to answer the question of whether the monetary costs of a program are outweighed by the monetary benefits.

Needs assessments are investigations of the needs of a group, community, or organization for certain types of services or policies. Needs assessments are thus another type of applied research aimed at providing useful information for planners and decision makers. Several techniques or approaches are used in the conduct of needs assessments, notably the *key informant, survey,* or *indicator* approaches.

Secondary analysis refers to research projects in which the investigator analyzes previously collected data. The secondary analyst may examine unanalyzed variables, test unexplored relationships, focus on a particular subsample, or change the *unit of analysis.* The use of existing data offers the potential of saving time and resources, but the researcher pays for this efficiency by the inability to gather *exactly* the kinds of data that he or she needs.

Meta-analysis is a method of integrating the findings of prior research using statistical procedures. Meta-analyses typically involve the calculation of an *effect size* that quantifies relationships between variables. Effect sizes from numerous studies can then be averaged to provide a numerical estimate of the magnitude of relationships. Although meta-analytic procedures are subject to some constraints and problems, they represent an important avenue of knowledge integration.

The *Delphi technique* is a method in which several rounds of questionnaires are mailed to a panel of experts. Feedback from previous questionnaires is provided with each new questionnaire so that the experts can converge on a consensus opinion in subsequent rounds. Delphi studies are used for problem solving, planning, and forecasting.

In *methodological research,* the investigator is concerned with the development, validation, and assessment of methodological tools or strategies. The researcher conducting a methodological study focuses primarily on increasing knowledge with respect to the methods used in performing scientific research rather than contributing to some substantive area.

Content analysis is a method for quantifying the content of narrative communications in a systematic and objective fashion. Communications include diaries, speeches, letters, and other verbal expressions. A variety of units of analysis exist for verbal expressions. The most useful unit for nurse researchers are *themes,* which embody ideas or concepts, and *items,* which refer to the entire message.

Field studies are in-depth qualitative studies of people or groups conducted in naturalistic settings, that is, in the field. The aim of the researcher is to get close to some phenomenon as it evolves in real life (i.e., to obtain first-hand information about how people think, act, and feel relative to the phenomenon of interest). Field research generally involves the simultaneous collection and analysis of narrative, qualitative materials that may be collected through in-depth interviews, observations of naturally occurring events and behavior, and examination of available documents.

A variety of disciplinary traditions fall within the broad umbrella of qualitative field research. *Ethnography* focuses on the culture of a group of people. The ethnographer strives to acquire an *emic* (insider's) perspective of the culture under study; the outsider's perspective is known as *etic. Phenomenology* strives to discover the essence of a phenomenon as it is experienced by some people. The phenomenological researcher strives to *bracket* out any preconceived views so that the data can be confronted in pure form, and to *intuit* the essence of the phenomenon by remaining open to the meanings attributed to it by those who have experienced it. *Ethnomethodology* is a qualitative tradition that has its roots in sociology. An ethnomethodological researcher seeks to discover how people make sense of their everyday activities and come to behave in socially acceptable ways. Researchers sometimes undertake *ethnomethodological experiments* by doing something to violate the norms of a social situation and then observing what the group members do.

Historical research is the systematic attempt to establish facts and relationships concerning past events. The historical researcher uses the scientific method insofar as possible to answer questions or test hypotheses by objectively evaluating and interpreting available historical evidence. Historical data are normally subjected to two forms of evaluation: *external criticism,* which is concerned with the authenticity of the source, and *internal criticism,* which assesses the worth of the evidence.

Case studies are intensive investigations of a single entity or a small number of entities. Typically, that entity is a human, but groups, organizations, families, or communities may sometimes be the focus of concern. When an intervention is being tested, it may be possible to conduct a *single-subject experiment.* Such studies generally involve collecting data over an extended period using a time series design. The case study offers the potential of great depth but runs the risk of subjectivity and limited generalizability.

❖ STUDY SUGGESTIONS

Chapter 9 of the accompanying *Study Guide for Nursing Research: Principles and Methods, 5th ed.*, offers various exercises and study suggestions for reinforcing the concepts presented in this chapter. Additionally, the following study questions can be addressed:

1. Suppose you were interested in studying the attitude of nurses toward caring for cancer patients. Would you use a survey or a field study? If you prefer a survey, would you use a personal interview, telephone interview, or questionnaire to collect your data? Defend your decisions.

2. A psychiatric nurse therapist working with emotionally disturbed children is interested in evaluating a program of play therapy. Explain how you might proceed if you were to use (a) the classic evaluation model and (b) a goal-free approach. Which approach do you think would be more useful, and why?

3. Explain how you would use the key informant, survey, and indicator approaches to assess the need to teach Spanish to nurses in a given community.

4. What units of analysis might be especially appropriate for performing a content analysis of the following materials: letters from nurses stationed in Europe during World War II, the diary of an adolescent dying from leukemia, the minutes of meetings from a state nurses' association, and the articles appearing in the *American Journal of Nursing*?

5. An investigator is interested in doing a field study that focuses on efforts of drug addicts to shake their addiction. Where might such a field study take place? How might the researcher gain entry into an appropriate setting?

❖ SUGGESTED READINGS

METHODOLOGICAL REFERENCES

Quantitative Methodological References

Berelson, B. (1971). *Content analysis in communication research.* New York: Free Press.

Brown, J. S., & Semradek, J. (1992). Secondary data on health-related subjects: Major sources, uses, and limitations. *Public Health Nursing, 3,* 162–171.

Brown, S. A. (1991). Measurement of quality of primary studies for meta-analysis. *Nursing Research, 40,* 352–355.

Dillman, D. (1978). *Mail and telephone surveys: The Total Design Method.* New York: John Wiley and Sons.

Fink, A., & Kosecoff, J. (1985). *How to conduct surveys: A step-by-step guide.* Thousand Oaks, CA: Sage.

Fowler, F. J. (1993). *Survey research methods* (2nd ed.). Beverly Hills, CA: Sage.

Glass, G. V., McGaw, B., & Smith, M. L. (1981). *Meta-analysis of social research.* Beverly Hills: Sage.

Hedges, L. V., & Olkin, I. (1985). *Statistical methods for meta-analysis.* Orlando, FL: Academic Press.

Herman, J. L., Morris, L. L., & Fitz-Gibbon, C. T. (1987). *Evaluator's handbook.* Newbury Park, CA: Sage.

Jacobson, A. F., Hamilton, P., & Galloway, J. (1993). Obtaining and evaluating data sets for secondary analysis in nursing research. *Western Journal of Nursing Research, 15,* 483–494.

Krippendorff, K. (1980). *Content analysis: An introduction to its methodology.* Beverly Hills, CA: Sage.

Lavrakas, P. J. (1993). *Telephone survey methods.* Thousand Oaks, CA: Sage.

McCain, N. L., Smith, M. C., & Abraham, I. L. (1986). Meta-analysis of nursing interventions. *Western Journal of Nursing Research, 8,* 155–167.

McKillip, J. (1986). *Needs analysis: Tools for the human services and education.* Beverly Hills, CA: Sage.

Patton, M. Q. (1986). *Utilization-focused evaluation.* (2nd ed.). Newbury Park, CA: Sage.

Reynolds, N. R., Timmerman, G., Anderson, J., & Stevenson, J. S. (1992). Meta-analysis for descriptive research. *Research in Nursing and Health, 15,* 467–475.

Rossi, P. H., & Freeman, H. E. (1993). *Evaluation: A systematic approach.* (5th ed.). Beverly Hills: Sage.

Stewart, D. W., & Kamins, M. A. (1993). *Secondary research: Information sources and methods.* (2nd ed.). Thousand Oaks, CA: Sage.

Warheit, G. J., Bell, R. A., & Schwab, J. J. (1975). *Planning for change: Needs assessment approaches.* Washington, DC: National Institute of Mental Health.

Qualitative Methodological References

Christy, T. E. (1975). The methodology of historical research. *Nursing Research, 24,* 189–192.

Denzin, N. K. (1994). *Handbook of qualitative research.* Thousand Oaks, CA: Sage.

Fairman, J. A. (1987). Sources and references for research in nursing history. *Nursing Research, 36,* 56–59.

Hamel, J. (1993). *Case study methods.* Thousand Oaks, CA: Sage.

Leininger, M. (Ed.). (1985). *Qualitative research methods in nursing.* New York: Grune & Stratton.

Meier, P., & Pugh, E. J. (1986). The case study: A viable approach to clinical research. *Research in Nursing and Health, 9,* 195–202.

Morse, J. M. (1991). *Qualitative nursing research: A contemporary dialogue.* Newbury Park, CA: Sage.

Pallikkathayil, L., & Morgan, S. A. (1991). Phenomenology as a method for conducting clinical research. *Applied Nursing Research, 4,* 195–200.

Rose, D. (1990). *Living the ethnographic life.* Newbury Park, CA: Sage.

Sorenson, E. S. (1988). Historiography: Archives as sources of treasure in historical research. *Western Journal of Nursing Research, 10,* 666–670.

Wilson, H. S. (1989). *Research in nursing* (2nd ed.). Menlo Park, CA: Addison-Wesley.

Yin, R. K. (1989). *Case study research* (rev. ed.). Beverly Hills, CA: Sage.

SUBSTANTIVE REFERENCES

Becker, P. T., Grunwald, P. C., Moorman, J., & Stuhr, S. (1993). Effects of developmental care on behavioral organization in very-low-birth-weight infants. *Nursing Research, 42,* 214–220.

Betz, M. L., Traw, B., & Bostrom, J. (1994). The cost-effectiveness of two intravenous additive systems. *Applied Nursing Research, 7,* 59–66.

Brown, J. S., & Marcy, S. A. (1991). The use of botanicals for health purposes by members of a prepaid health plan. *Research in Nursing and Health, 14,* 339–349.

Brown, S. J. (1994). Communication strategies used by an expert nurse. *Clinical Nursing Research, 3,* 43–56.

Buhler-Wilkerson, K. (1992). Caring in its "proper place": Race and benevolence in Charleston, SC, 1813–1930. *Nursing Research, 41,* 14–20.

Damrosch, S., & Scholler-Jaquish, A. (1993). Nurses' experiences with impaired nurse coworkers. *Applied Nursing Research, 6,* 154–160.

Dreher, M. C., & Hayes, J. S. (1993). Triangulation in cross-cultural research of child development in Jamaica. *Western Journal of Nursing Research, 15,* 216–229.

Farran, C. J., Keane-Hagerty, E., Tatarowicz, L., & Scorza, E. (1993). Dementia care-receiver needs and their impact on caregivers. *Clinical Nursing Research, 2,* 86–97.

Gardner, K. (1991). A summary of findings of a five-year comparison study of primary and team nursing. *Nursing Research, 40,* 113–116.

Grau, L., & Wellin, E. (1992). The organizational cultures of nursing homes: Influences on responses to external regulatory controls. *Qualitative Health Research, 2,* 42–60.

Jacobson, G. (1994). The meaning of stressful life experiences in nine- to eleven-year-old children: A phenomenological study. *Nursing Research, 43,* 95–99.

Jordan-Marsh, M., Yoder, L., Hall, D., & Watson, R.

(1994). Alternate Oucher form testing: Gender, ethnicity, and age variations. *Research in Nursing and Health, 17,* 111–118.

Kim, M. J., Larson, J. L., Covey, M. K., Vitalo, C. A., Alex, C. G., & Patel, M. (1993). Inspiratory muscle training in patients with chronic obstructive pulmonary disease. *Nursing Research, 42,* 356–362.

King, M. G. (1989). Nursing shortage, circa 1915. *Image: Journal of Nursing Scholarship, 21,* 124–127.

Kleinpell, R. M., & Powers, M. J. (1992). Needs of family members of intensive care unit patients. *Applied Nursing Research, 5,* 2–8.

Kocher, K. M., & Thomas, G. W. (1994). Retaining Army nurses: A longitudinal model. *Research in Nursing and Health, 17,* 59–65.

Krywanio, M. L. (1994). Meta-analysis of physiological outcomes of hospital-based infant intervention programs. *Nursing Research, 43,* 133–137.

Kulig, J. C. (1990). Childbearing beliefs among Cambodian refugee women. *Western Journal of Nursing Research, 12,* 108–118.

Leininger, M. M. (1985). Southern rural black and white American lifeways with a focus on care and health phenomena. In M. M. Leininger (Ed.), *Qualitative research methods in nursing.* New York: Grune & Stratton.

Lethbridge, D. J., McClurg, V., Henrikson, M., & Wall, G. (1993). Validation of the nursing diagnosis of ineffective breastfeeding. *Journal of Obstetric, Gynecologic, and Neonatal Nursing, 22,* 57–63.

Long, K. A., & Weinert, C. (1992). Descriptions and perceptions of health among rural and urban adults with multiple sclerosis. *Research in Nursing and Health, 15,* 335–342.

Martin, K. J., Shortridge, L. A., Dyehouse, J. M., & Migliozzi, A. N. (1993). Corporate perspective of the role of the occupational health nurse. *Research in Nursing and Health, 16,* 305–311.

Mason, C. (1994). Maternal and child health needs in Northern Ireland and Jamaica: Official and lay perspectives. *Qualitative Health Research, 4,* 74–93.

Mitchell, P. H., Armstrong, S., Simpson, T. F., & Lentz, M. (1989). American Association of Critical-Care Nurses Demonstration Project: Profile of excellence in critical care nursing. *Heart and Lung, 18,* 219–237.

Morse, J. M. (1991). The structure and function of gift giving in the patient-nurse relationship. *Western Journal of Nursing Research, 13,* 597–615.

Oberle, K., Allen, M., & Lynkowski, P. (1993). Submucous resection: Is it a simple procedure? *Clinical Nursing Research, 2,* 54–66.

Pollack, L. E. (1993). Content analysis of groups for inpatients with bipolar disorder. *Applied Nursing Research, 6,* 19–27.

Pollow, R. L., Stoller, E. P., Forster, L. E., & Duniho, T. S. (1994). Drug combinations and potential for risk of adverse drug reaction among community-dwelling elderly. *Nursing Research, 43,* 44–49.

Price, L. J. (1992). Metalogue on coping with illness: Cases from Ecuador. *Qualitative Health Research, 2,* 135–158.

Schirm, V. (1993). Cholesterol screening of older persons: Focusing on health education. *Applied Nursing Research, 6,* 119–124.

Stratton, T. D., Dunkin, J. W., Juhl, N., & Geller, J. M. (1993). Recruiting registered nurses to rural practice settings. *Applied Nursing Research, 6,* 64–70.

Stuart, M. (1992). "Half a loaf is better than no bread": Public health nurses and physicians in Ontario, 1920–1925. *Nursing Research, 41,* 21–27.

Tompkins, E. S. (1993). Nurses and client perceptions of the American Association of Colleges of Nursing values. *Western Journal of Nursing Research, 15,* 363–372.

Walsh, S. M. (1993). Future images: An art intervention with suicidal adolescents. *Applied Nursing Research, 6,* 111–118.

Widerquist, J. G. (1992). The spirituality of Florence Nightingale. *Nursing Research, 41,* 49–55.

Chapter 10

RESEARCH CONTROL

Chapters 7 through 9 introduced a wide variety of research approaches and designs. A major function of research design for most research questions—especially those addressed through structured, quantitative procedures—is to maximize the amount of control that an investigator has over the research situation and variables. As discussed in Chapter 7, the researcher strives to control extraneous variables to determine the true nature of the relationship between the independent and dependent variables under investigation. Extraneous variables are variables that have an irrelevant association with the dependent variable and that can confound the testing of the research hypothesis. This chapter discusses various methods of controlling extraneous variables.*

There are two basic types of extraneous variables: those that are intrinsic to the subjects

---

* Many of the control techniques outlined in this chapter are not normally used in qualitative studies, in which the aim is for the research setting to be as natural as possible. The qualitative researcher often wants to study, rather than control, extraneous variables to understand better the context of the phenomena under investigation.

of the study and those that are external factors stemming from the research situation. We begin with a discussion of methods of controlling external factors.

❖ CONTROLLING EXTERNAL FACTORS

In quantitative studies, the researcher often takes a number of steps to minimize situational contaminants. It is generally good practice to make the conditions under which the data are collected as similar as possible for every participant in the study. The control that a researcher imposes on a study by attempting to maintain *constancy of conditions* probably represents one of the earliest forms of scientific control.

The environment has been found to exert a powerful influence on people's emotions and behavior. In designing research, therefore, the investigator needs to pay attention to the environmental context within which the study is to be conducted. Control over the environment is most easily achieved in laboratory experiments in which all subjects are brought into an environment that the experimenter is in a position to arrange. Researchers have much less freedom in controlling the environment in studies that occur in natural settings. This does not mean that the researcher should abandon all efforts to make the environments as similar as possible. For example, in conducting a survey in which the information is to be gathered by means of an interview, the researcher should attempt to conduct all interviews in basically the same kind of environment. That is, it would not be desirable to interview some of the respondents in their own homes, some in their places of work, some in the researcher's office, and so forth. In each of these settings, the participant normally assumes different roles (e.g., wife, husband, parent; employee; and client or patient), and responses to questions may be influenced to some degree by the role in which the respondent is operating.

One of the advantages of conducting a study in an artificial setting such as a laboratory is that the researcher has greater confidence of having control over the independent and extraneous variables. In real-life settings, even when subjects are randomly assigned to groups, the differentiation between groups may be difficult to control. Let us look at another example to see why this is so. Suppose we are planning to teach nursing students a unit on dyspnea, and we have used a lecture-type approach in the past. If we are interested in trying an individualized, autotutorial approach to cover the same material and want to evaluate the effectiveness of this method before adopting it for all students, we might randomly assign students to one of the two methods. Scores on a test covering the content of the unit could be used as the dependent or criterion variable. But now, suppose the students in the two groups talk to one another about their learning experiences. Some of the lecture-group students might go through parts of the programmed text. Perhaps some of the students in the autotutorial group will sit in on some of the lectures. In short, field experiments are often subject to the problem of *contamination of treatments*. In the same study, it would also be difficult to control other variables, such as the time or place in which the learning occurs for the individualized group.

Another external factor that is often controlled is the time factor. Depending on the topic of the study, the dependent variable may be influenced by the time of day or time of year in which the data are collected, or both. It would, in such cases, be desirable for the researcher to strive for constancy of times across subjects. If an investigator were studying fatigue or perceptions of physical well-being, it would probably matter a great deal whether the data were gathered in the morning, afternoon, or evening, or in the summer as opposed to the winter. Although time constancy is not always critical, it is often relatively easy for the researcher to control and should, therefore, be sought whenever possible.

Another aspect of maintaining constancy of conditions concerns constancy in the communications to the subjects and in the treatment itself in the case of experiments or quasi-experiments. In most research efforts, the researcher informs participants about the purpose of the study, what use will be made of the data, under whose auspices the study is being conducted, and so forth. This information generally should be prepared ahead of time, and the same message should be delivered to all subjects. In most research situations, there should be as little ad-libbing as possible.

In studies involving the implementation of a treatment, care should be taken to adhere to the specifications (often referred to as *research protocols*) for that treatment. For example, in experiments to test the effectiveness of a new drug to cure a medical problem, the researcher would have to take great care to ensure that the subjects in the experimental group received the same chemical substance and the same dosage, that the substance was administered in the same way, and so forth. Some treatments are much "fuzzier" than in the case of administering a drug, as is the case for most nursing interventions. In such a situation, the investigator should spell out in detail the exact behaviors required of the personnel responsible for delivering or administering the treatment.

One of the features that distinguishes non-experimental research from experimental and quasi-experimental studies is that if the researcher has not manipulated the independent variable, then there is no means of ensuring constancy of conditions. Let us take as an example an ex post facto study that attempts to determine if there is a relationship between a person's knowledge of nutrition and his or her own eating habits. Suppose the investigator finds no relationship between nutritional knowledge and eating patterns. That is, the investigator finds that people who are well-informed about nutrition are just as likely as uninformed people to maintain inadequate diets. In this case, however, the researcher has had no control over the source of a person's nutritional knowledge (the independent variable). This knowledge was measured after the fact (post facto), and the conditions under which the information was obtained cannot be assumed to be constant or even similar. The researcher may conclude from the study that it is useless to teach nutrition to people because knowledge has no impact on their eating behavior. It may be, however, that different methods of providing nutritional information vary in their ability to motivate people to alter their nutritional habits. Thus, the ability of the investigator to control or manipulate the independent variable of interest may be extremely important in understanding the relationships between variables, or the absence of relationships.

❖ CONTROLLING INTRINSIC FACTORS

Characteristics of the participants in a quantitative scientific study almost always need to be controlled for the findings to be interpretable. The control of intrinsic extraneous variables is especially important when the dependent variable is psychosocial rather than biophysiologic in nature. That is because psychosocial variables (e.g., stress) are more susceptible than physiologic ones (e.g., heart rate) to the influence of individual characteristics (e.g., gender, marital status). This section describes six specific ways of controlling extraneous variables associated with subject characteristics.

Randomization

We have already discussed the most effective method of controlling individual extraneous variables—randomization. The primary function of randomization is to secure comparable groups, that is, to equalize the groups with respect to the extraneous variables. A distinct advantage of random assignment, compared with other methods of controlling extraneous variables, is that randomization controls *all* possible sources of extraneous variation, without any conscious decision on the researcher's part about which variables need to be controlled.

Suppose, for example, that we were interested in assessing the effect of a physical training program on cardiovascular functioning among nursing home residents. Characteristics such as the individual's age, gender, prior occupation, history of smoking, and length of stay in the nursing home could all affect the patient's cardiovascular system, independently of the physical training program. The effects of these other variables are extraneous to the research problem and should be controlled. Through randomization, we could expect that an experimental group (receiving the physical training program) and control group (not receiving the program) would be comparable in terms of these as well as any other factors that influence cardiovascular functioning.

Repeated Measures

Randomization within the context of a repeated measures design is an especially powerful method of ensuring equivalence between groups being compared, that is, of controlling all extraneous subject characteristics. However, such a design is not appropriate for all studies because of the problem of carry-over effects. When subjects are exposed to two different treatments or conditions, they may be influenced in the second condition by their experience in the first condition. In our example of the physical training program, for instance, a repeated measures design is unsuitable because the no-program-followed-by-program condition would not be the same as the program-followed-by-no-program condition: those subjects who were in the program in the first condition might independently decide to exercise more during the time they are not in the program.

Thus, because the two (or more) treatments are not applied simultaneously in repeated measures designs, the order of the treatment may be important in affecting the subject's performance. The best approach is to use randomization to determine the ordering. When there are only two conditions in a repeated measures design, the researcher simply designates that half the subjects, at random, will receive treatment A first, and the other half will receive treatment B first. When there are three or more conditions to which each subject will be exposed, the procedure of *counterbalancing* is frequently used to minimize the impact of ordering effects. For example, if there were three conditions (A,B,C), subjects would be randomly assigned to six different orderings in a counterbalanced scheme:

A, B, C	A, C, B
B, C, A	B, A, C
C, A, B	C, B, A

Note that, in addition to their potential for excellent control over extraneous subject characteristics, repeated measures designs offer another important advantage: fewer research subjects are needed. Fifty subjects exposed to two treatments in random order yield 100 pieces of data (50 × 2); 50 subjects randomly assigned to two different treatment groups yield only 50 pieces of data (25 × 2).

In sum, repeated measures can be a useful, rigorous, and efficient design for eliminating extraneous variables. However, when carryover effects from one condition to another are anticipated, as might be the case in many medical or nursing interventions, the researcher will need to seek other designs.

Homogeneity

When randomization and repeated measures are not feasible, there are alternative methods of controlling intrinsic subject characteristics that could contaminate the relationships under investigation. One such method is to use only subjects who are homogeneous with respect to those variables that are considered extraneous. The extraneous variables, in this case, are not allowed to vary. In the example of the physical training program, if gender were considered to be an important confounding variable, the researcher might wish to use only men (or only women) as subjects. Similarly, if the researcher were concerned about the effects of the subjects' age on cardiovascular functioning, participation in the study could be limited to those within a specified age range.

This method of utilizing a homogeneous subject pool is fairly easy and offers considerable control. However, the limitation of this approach lies in the fact that the research findings can only be generalized to the type of subjects who participated in the study. If the physical training program were found to have beneficial effects on the cardiovascular status of a sample of men 65 to 75 years of age, its usefulness for improving the cardiovascular status of women in their 80s would be strictly a matter of conjecture.

Blocking

A fourth approach to controlling extraneous variables is to include them in the design of a study as independent variables. To pursue our example of the physical training program, if gender were thought to be a confounding variable, it could be built into the study design, as illustrated in Figure 10-1. This procedure would allow us to make an assessment of the impact of

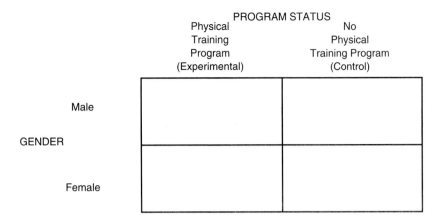

Figure 10-1*. Schematic diagram of a 2 × 2 randomized block design.*

our training program on the cardiovascular functioning of both elderly men and women. Furthermore, this approach has the advantage of adding greater precision and enhancing the likelihood of detecting differences between our experimental and control groups because the effect of the extraneous variable on the dependent variable can be assessed.

Let us consider this third approach in greater detail. We refer to the design shown in Figure 10-1 as a *randomized block design.** The variable gender, which cannot be manipulated by the researcher, is known as a *blocking variable*. In an experiment to test the effectiveness of the physical training program, the experimenter obviously could not randomly assign subjects to one of four cells, as in a factorial experiment: the gender of the subjects is a given. However, the experimenter can randomly assign men and women separately to the experimental and control conditions. Let us say that there are 40 men and 40 women available for the randomized block study. The researcher would not take the 80 subjects and assign half to

the physical training program group and the other half to the control group. Rather, the randomization procedure would be performed separately for men and women, thereby guaranteeing 20 subjects in each cell of the four-cell design.

The design can be extended to include more than one blocking variable, as shown in Figure 10-2. In this design, the age of the subject has been included to control for this second extraneous variable. Once again, the experimenter would randomly assign subjects from each block to either the experimental or control conditions. In other words, half the men 66 to 70 years of age would randomly be assigned to the program, as would half the men 71 to 75 years of age, and so forth. Although in theory the number of blocks that could be added is unlimited, practical concerns usually dictate a relatively small number of blocks (and, hence, a small number of extraneous variables that can be controlled). Expansion of the design usually requires that a larger subject pool be used. As a general rule of thumb, a minimum of 20 to 30 subjects per cell is often recommended. This means that, whereas a minimum of 80 subjects would be needed for the design in Figure 10-1, 240 subjects would be needed for the design in Figure 10-2. This suggests that, if a decision is made to introduce extraneous variables into the

* The terminology for this design varies from text to text. Some authors refer to this as a factorial design; others call it a levels-by-treatment design. We have chosen not to use the term factorial because gender is not under experimental control, and hence, complete randomization is impossible.

Program Status

Gender	Age Group	Physical Training Program (Experimental)	No Physical Training Program (Control)
Male			
	66–70		
	71–75		
	76–80		
Female			
	66–70		
	71–75		
	76–80		

Figure 10-2. *Schematic diagram of a 2 × 2 × 3 randomized block design.*

design of a study, great care should be taken to choose the most relevant subject characteristics as the blocking variables.

Strictly speaking, the type of design we have discussed is appropriate only in experimental studies, but, in reality, it is used commonly in quasi-experimental and ex post facto studies as well. If an investigator were studying the effects of a physical training program on cardiovascular functioning after the fact (i.e., subjects self-selected themselves into one of the two groups and the researcher had no control over who was included in each group), the investigator might want to set up the analysis in such a way that differential effects for men and women would be analyzed. The design structure would look the same as the one presented in Figure 10-1, although the implications and conclusions that could be drawn from the results would be different than if the researcher had been in control of the manipulation and randomization procedures.

Matching

A fifth method of dealing with extraneous variables is known as matching. *Matching* (also referred to as *pair matching*) involves using knowledge of subject characteristics to form comparison groups. If a matching procedure were to be adopted for our physical training program example, and age and gender were the extraneous variables of interest, we would need to match each subject in the experimental group with one in the control group with respect to age and gender. If the subjects could be assigned on a random basis, we would actually have a special type of randomized block design with one subject per cell.

Pair matching, however, is usually a post hoc attempt to approximate this experimental blocking design. That is, the researcher may begin with 20 subjects who participate in the training program and then create a control group by matching, one by one, individuals from the general population in terms of age and gender of the experimental subjects. This design is common in epidemiological research.

Despite the intuitive appeal of such a design, there are reasons why matching is problematic. First, to match effectively, the researcher must know in advance what the relevant extraneous variables are. Second, after two or three variables, it often becomes impossible to pair match adequately. Let us say that we are interested in controlling for the age, gender, race, and length of nursing home stay of the subjects. Thus, if subject 1 in the physical training program were an African American woman, aged 80 years, whose length of stay is 5 years, the researcher would need to seek another woman with these same or similar characteristics as a comparison group counterpart. With more than three variables, the matching procedure becomes extremely cumbersome, if not impossible. For these reasons, matching as a technique for controlling extraneous variables should, in general, be used only when other, more powerful procedures are not feasible, as might be the case for some ex post facto studies.

Sometimes as an alternative to pair matching (in which subjects are matched on a one-to-one basis for every matching variable), researchers choose to have a *balanced design* with regard to key extraneous variables. In such situations, the researcher attempts only to ensure that the composition of the groups being compared have proportional representation with regard to variables believed to be correlated with the dependent variable. For example, if gender and race were the two extraneous variables of interest in our example of the physical training program, the researcher adopting a balanced design would strive to ensure that the same percentage of men and women (and the same percentage of white and African American subjects) were in the group participating in the physical training program as in a comparison group of nonparticipants. Such an approach is much less cumbersome than pair matching, but it also has similar limitations. Nevertheless, both pair matching and balancing are preferable to

failing to control for intrinsic subject characteristics at all.

Analysis of Covariance

A sixth method of controlling unwanted variables is through statistical procedures. We recognize that, at this point, many readers may be unfamiliar with basic statistical procedures, let alone the sophisticated techniques referred to here. Therefore, a detailed description of a powerful statistical control mechanism, known as *analysis of covariance,* will not be attempted. The interested reader with a background in statistics should consult Chapter 19 or a textbook on advanced statistics for fuller coverage of this topic. However, because the possibility of statistical control may mystify readers, we explain the underlying principle next with a simple illustration.

Returning to the physical training program example, suppose we have a group that is undergoing a physical training program and another group that is not. The groups represent intact groups (e.g., residents of two different nursing homes, only one of which is offering the physical training program), and therefore randomization is impossible. As our measures of cardiovascular functioning, suppose we use maximal oxygen consumption and resting heart rate. As with most things in life, there undoubtedly will be individual differences on these two measures. The research question is, can some of the individual differences be attributed to a person's participation in the physical training program? Unfortunately, the individual differences in cardiovascular functioning are also related to other, extraneous characteristics of the subjects, such as age. The large circles in Figure 10-3 may be taken to represent the total variability (extent of individual differences) for both groups on, say, resting heart rate. A certain amount of that total variability can be explained simply by virtue of the subject's age, which is schematized in the figure as the small circle on the left in Figure 10-3(*A*). Another part of the variability can be explained by the subject's participation or

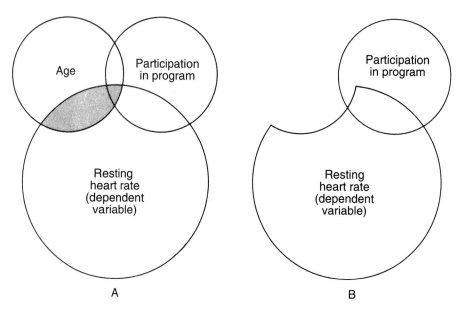

Figure 10-3.   *Schematic diagram illustrating the principle of analysis of covariance.*

nonparticipation in the physical training program, represented as the small circle on the right in (*A*). In (*A*), the fact that the two small circles (age and participation in program) overlap indicates that there is a relationship between those two variables. In other words, subjects in the group receiving the physical training program are, on average, either older or younger than members of the comparison group. Therefore, age should be controlled. Otherwise, it will be impossible to determine whether differences in resting heart rate should be attributed to age differences or to differences in program participation.

Analysis of covariance can accomplish this control function by statistically removing the effect of the extraneous variable on the dependent variable. In the illustration, that portion of heart rate variability that is attributable to age could be removed through the analysis of covariance technique. This is designated in Figure 10-3(*A*) by the darkened area in the large circle; (*B*) illustrates that the final analysis would examine the effect of program participation on heart rate after removing the effect of age.

With the variability of heart rate resulting from age controlled, we can have a much more precise estimate of the effect of the training program on heart rate. Note that even after removing the variability resulting from age, there is still individual variability not associated with the program treatment—the bottom half of the large circle in (*B*). This means that the precision of the study can probably be further enhanced by controlling additional extraneous variables, such as gender, type of previous occupation, and so forth. The analysis of covariance procedure can accommodate multiple extraneous variables.

When pretest measures of the dependent variables have been obtained, these are often controlled statistically through analysis of covariance—a procedure that greatly enhances the precision of the estimates of the effect of an intervention. In our example here, controlling pretest measures of cardiovascular functioning through analysis of covariance would be especially powerful because it would remove the effect of most individual variation stemming from a host of other extraneous factors.

Evaluation of Control Methods

Overall, the random assignment of subjects to groups is the most effective approach of managing extraneous variables because randomization tends to cancel out individual variation on all possible extraneous variables. Repeated measures designs, although extremely useful in controlling all possible sources of extraneous variation, cannot be applied to most nursing research problems. The remaining alternatives to randomization—homogeneity, blocking, matching, and analysis of covariance—have one disadvantage in common: the researcher must know or predict in advance the relevant extraneous variables. To select homogeneous samples, develop a blocking design, match, or perform an analysis of covariance, the researcher must make a decision about what variables need to be measured and controlled. This constraint may pose severe limitations on the degree of control that is possible, particularly because the researcher can seldom deal explicitly with more than two or three extraneous variables at one time (except in the case of analysis of covariance).

Although we have repeatedly hailed randomization as the ideal mechanism for controlling extraneous subject characteristics, it is clear that randomization is not always possible. For example, if the independent variable cannot be manipulated, then other techniques must be used. In ex post facto and quasi-experimental studies, the control options available to researchers include homogeneity, blocking, matching, and analysis of covariance. In quantitative research, the use of any of the control procedures discussed here is far preferable to the absence of any attempt to control intrinsic extraneous variables.

❖ *INTERNAL VALIDITY*

One method of evaluating the adequacy of research control mechanisms and overall research design is to assess its internal and external validity. *Internal validity* is attained in a study when the findings can be shown to result only from the effect of the independent variable of interest and cannot be interpreted as reflecting the effects of extraneous variables. *External validity*, which is discussed in the next section, is achieved when the results can confidently be generalized to situations outside the specific research setting.

The control mechanisms reviewed in the previous sections are all strategies for improving the internal validity of research studies. If the researcher is not careful in managing extraneous variables and in other ways controlling the design of the study, there may be reason to challenge the conclusion that the subjects' performance on the dependent measure resulted from the effect of the independent variable.

Threats to Internal Validity

True experiments possess a high degree of internal validity because the use of control procedures (manipulation and randomization) enables the researcher to rule out most alternative explanations for the results. With quasi-experimental, pre-experimental, or ex post facto designs, the investigator must always contend with competing explanations for the obtained results. These competing explanations, referred to as *threats to internal validity,* have been grouped into several classes, a few of which are examined here.

HISTORY

The threat of *history* refers to the occurrence of external events that take place concurrently with the independent variable that can affect the dependent variables of interest. For example, suppose we were studying the effectiveness of a county-wide nurse outreach program designed to encourage pregnant women in rural areas to improve their health-related practices before delivery (e.g., better nutritional practices, cessation of smoking and drinking, and earlier prenatal care). The program might be evaluated by comparing the average birthweight of infants in the 12 months before the outreach program with the average birthweight of those born in the 12 months after the program was introduced. However, suppose that 1 month after the new program was launched, a highly publicized docudrama regarding the inadequacies of prenatal care for poor women was aired on national television. Our dependent variable in this case, infants' birthweight, might now be affected by both the intervention and the messages in the docudrama, and it becomes impossible for us to disentangle the two effects.

In a true experiment, history generally is not a threat to the internal validity of a study because we can often assume that external events are as likely to affect the experimental as the control group. When this is the case, any group differences that emerge at the end of the study represent effects over and above those created by external factors. An exception, however, is when a repeated measures design is used. If an external event that has an effect on the dependent variable occurs during the first half (or second half) of the experiment, then the treatments would be contaminated by the effect of that event. That is, some people would receive treatment A with the event and others would receive treatment A without it, and the same would be true for treatment B.

SELECTION

The term *selection* encompasses biases resulting from pre-existing differences between groups. When individuals are not assigned randomly to groups, we must always be alert to the possibility that the groups are nonequivalent. They may differ, in fact, in ways that are subtle and difficult to detect. If the groups are nonequivalent, the researcher is faced with the possibility that any group difference on the dependent variable is the result of initial differences rather than the effect of the independent variable. For example, if a researcher found that women with a fertility problem were more

likely to be depressed than women who were mothers, it would be impossible to conclude that the two groups differed in terms of depression *because* of their differences in reproductive statuses; the women in the two groups might have been different in terms of psychological adjustment to begin with. The problem of selection is clearly reduced when the researcher can collect data regarding the characteristics of the subjects before the occurrence of the independent variable, but this is often difficult to accomplish. In the example relating to the fertility problem, the best design would involve the collection of information on the women's level of depression even before their attempts to become pregnant. Selection bias is one of the most problematic and frequently encountered threats to the internal validity of studies not using an experimental design.

Selection biases also often interact with other biases to compound the threat to the internal validity of the study. For example, if the comparison group is different from the experimental group or main group of interest, then the characteristics of the members of the comparison group could lead them to have different intervening experiences, thereby introducing both history and selection biases into the design.

MATURATION

In a research context, *maturation* refers to processes occurring within the subjects during the course of the study as a result of the passage of time rather than as a result of a treatment or independent variable. Examples of such processes include physical growth, emotional maturity, fatigue, and the like. For example, if we wanted to evaluate the effects of a special sensorimotor development program for developmentally retarded children, we would have to consider that progress does occur in these children even without special assistance. A design such as a one group pretest–posttest design (see Figure 8-7 in Chapter 8), for example, would be highly susceptible to this threat to internal validity.

Maturation would be a relevant consideration in many areas of nursing research. Remember that maturation here does not refer to aging or developmental changes exclusively but rather to any kind of change that occurs with the individual as a function of time. Thus, wound-healing, postoperative recovery, and many other bodily changes that can occur with little or no nursing or medical intervention must be considered as an explanation for outcomes to subjects that rivals an explanation based on the effects of the independent variable.

TESTING

The effects of taking a pretest on the scores of a posttest are known as *testing* effects. It has been documented in numerous studies, particularly in those dealing with opinions and attitudes, that the mere act of collecting information from people changes them. Let us say that we administer to a group of nursing students a questionnaire dealing with their attitudes toward euthanasia. We then proceed to acquaint the students with various arguments that have been made for and against euthanasia, outcomes of court cases, and the like. At the end of instruction, we give them the same attitude measure as before and observe whether their attitudes have changed as a function of the instruction. The problem here is that the first administration of the questionnaire might sensitize the students to issues that they had not contemplated before. The sensitization may, in fact, result in attitude changes regardless of whether instruction follows. If a comparison group is not used in the study, it becomes impossible to segregate the effects of the instruction from the effects of having taken the pretest (as well as from the effects of history, maturation, and so forth). In true experiments, testing may not be a problem because its effects would be expected to be about equal in all groups, but the Solomon four-group design (discussed in Chapter 8) could be used if the researcher wanted to segregate the effects of the intervention from those of the pretest.

Sensitization, or testing, problems are typically much more likely to occur when the pretest involves information that subjects provide through self-report (e.g., in a questionnaire), especially if we are exposing the subjects to controversial or novel material. For many nursing studies (e.g., those that involve the collection of biophysiologic information), testing effects are not a major concern.

INSTRUMENTATION

Another threat that is related to the researcher's measurements is referred to as the threat of *instrumentation*. This bias reflects changes in the researcher's measuring instruments between an initial point of data collection and a subsequent point. For example, if the researcher uses one measure of stress at baseline and a different measure at follow-up, then any changes might reflect changes in the measuring tool rather than the effects of the independent variable.

Instrumentation effects can occur even if the same measure is used. For example, if the measuring tool yields more accurate measures on the second administration (e.g., if the people collecting the data are more experienced) or less accurate measures the second time (e.g., if the subjects become bored or fatigued), then these differences could bias the results.

MORTALITY

Mortality refers to the threat that arises from differential attrition from the groups being compared. The loss of subjects during the course of a study may differ from one group to another because of a priori differences in interest, motivation, health, and so on. For example, suppose we used a nonequivalent control group design to assess the morale of the nursing personnel from two different hospitals, one of which was initiating primary nursing. The dependent variable, nursing staff morale, is measured in both hospitals before and after the intervention. Comparison group members, who may have no particular commitment to the study, may decline to complete a posttest questionnaire because of lack of incentive. Those who do fill it out may be unrepresentative of the group as a whole—they may be those who are most enthusiastic about their work environment, for example. If this were the case, it might appear that the morale of the nurses in the comparison hospital had improved over time, but this improvement might only be an artifact of the mortality from the study of a biased segment of this group.

The threat of attrition is apt to be especially high when the length of time between points of data collection is long. A 12-month follow-up of subjects, for example, is likely to produce higher rates of attrition than a 1-month follow-up. In clinical nursing studies, the problem of attrition may be especially acute because of patient death or disability.

Note that if attrition is random (i.e., those dropping out of the study are highly similar to those remaining in the study with respect to characteristics that are related to the dependent variable), then the risk of mortality biases are low. However, attrition is rarely totally random. In general, the higher the rate of attrition, the greater the likelihood of bias. Although there is no absolute standard for acceptable attrition rates, biases are generally of concern if the rate exceeds 20%.

Internal Validity
and Research Design

Quasi-experimental and ex post facto studies are especially susceptible to threats to internal validity. The threats just described (as well as others, which are less frequently of concern to nurse researchers) represent alternative explanations that compete with the independent variable as a cause of the dependent variable. The aim of a good research design is to rule out these competing explanations.

A good experimental design normally controls for these factors, but it must not be assumed that in a true experiment the researcher

need not worry about them. For example, if constancy of conditions is not maintained for experimental and control groups, then history might be a rival explanation for any group differences. Mortality is, in particular, a salient threat in true experiments. Because the experimenter does things differently with the experimental and control groups, subjects in the groups may drop out of the study differentially. This is particularly apt to happen if the experimental treatment is painful, inconvenient, or time-consuming, or if the control condition is boring or considered a nuisance. When this happens, the subjects remaining in the study may differ from those who left in important ways, thereby nullifying the initial equivalence of the groups.

Internal Validity
and Data Analysis

A researcher's best strategy for enhancing the internal validity of a study is to use a strong research design that includes the use of the control mechanisms discussed earlier in this chapter. Even when this is possible (and, certainly, when this is *not* possible), it is highly advisable to analyze the data to determine the nature and extent of any biases. When biases are detected, the information can be used to interpret the results of the substantive analyses, and in some cases, the biases can be statistically controlled.

The researcher must essentially be a self-critic and consider the types of biases that could have arisen within the context of the chosen design—and then systematically search for evidence of their existence (while hoping, of course, that no evidence can be found). A few examples should illustrate how the researcher should proceed.

Selection biases are the most prevalent of the threats to internal validity and should be examined whenever possible. Typically, this involves the comparison of subjects on pretest measures, when pretest data have been collected. For example, if we were studying depression in women who delivered a baby by cesarean section versus those who delivered vaginally, an ideal way to evaluate selection bias would be to compare the level of depression in these two groups during the pregnancy. If there are significant predelivery differences, then postdelivery differences would have to be interpreted with these initial differences in mind (or with these differences controlled). In after-only designs or in cross-sectional ex post facto studies in which there is no pretest information on the dependent variable, the researcher should nevertheless search for selection biases by comparing groups with respect to important background variables such as age, gender, ethnicity, social class, health status, and so on. When group differences are detected, they should be controlled if possible (through analysis of covariance) or at least taken into account in the interpretation of the findings. Selection biases should be analyzed even when random assignment has been used to form groups because there is no absolute guarantee that randomization will yield perfectly comparable groups.

Whenever the research design involves multiple points of data collection, the researcher should analyze attrition biases. This is typically achieved through a comparison of those who did and did not complete the study with regard to initial measures of the dependent variable or other characteristics measured at the first point of data collection.

In a repeated measures design, history is a potential threat both because an external event could differentially affect subjects in different treatment orderings and because the different orderings are in themselves a kind of differential history. The substantive analysis of the data would involve a comparison of the dependent variable under treatment A versus treatment B. The analysis for evidence of bias, by contrast, would involve a comparison of subjects in the different orderings (e.g., A then B versus B then A). If there are significant differences between the two orderings, then the researcher would have evidence of an ordering bias.

In summary, efforts to enhance the internal validity of a study should not end once the

design strategy has been put in place. The researcher should seek additional opportunities to understand (and possibly to correct) the various threats to internal validity that can arise.

❖ EXTERNAL VALIDITY

External validity refers to the generalizability of the research findings to other settings or samples. Research is almost never conducted with the intention of discovering relationships among variables for one group of people at one point in time. The aim of research is typically to reveal enduring relationships, the understanding of which can be used to improve the human condition. If a nursing intervention under investigation is found to be successful, others will want to adopt the procedure. Therefore, an important question is whether the intervention will work in another setting and with different patients. Researchers should routinely ask themselves: To what populations, environments, and conditions can the results of the study be applied?

External Validity and Sampling

Strictly speaking, the findings of a study can only be generalized to the population of subjects from which a study sample has been randomly selected. If an investigator were studying the effects of a newly developed therapeutic treatment for heroin addicts, then the researcher might begin with a population of addicts in a particular clinic or drug treatment center. From this population, a random sample of drug users could be selected for participation in the study. Individuals from the sample would then be randomly assigned to one of two or more conditions, assuming that an experiment were possible. If the results revealed that the new therapeutic treatment was highly effective in reducing recidivism among the sample of addicts, can it be concluded that all addicts in the United States would benefit from the treatment? Unfortunately, no. The population of heroin addicts undergoing treatment in one particular facility may not be representative of all addicts. For example, the facility in question may attract drug users from certain ethnic, socioeconomic, or age groups. Perhaps the new treatment is only effective with individuals from such groups.

Of relevance here is Kempthorne's (1961) distinction between accessible populations and target populations. The *accessible population* is the population of subjects available for a particular study. In our drug treatment example, all the heroin addicts in treatment at a particular treatment center would constitute the accessible population. When random procedures have been used to select a sample from an accessible population, there is no difficulty in generalizing the results to that group.

The *target population* is the total group of subjects about whom the investigator is interested and to whom the results could reasonably be generalized. This second type of generalization is considerably more risky than the first and cannot be done with as much confidence as in the case of generalizations to the accessible population. The adequacy and utility of this type of inference hinges strongly on the similarity of the characteristics of the two populations. Thus, the researcher must be aware of the characteristics of the accessible population and, in turn, define the target population to be like the accessible population. In the drug treatment example, the accessible population might predominantly comprise voluntarily admitted white men in their 20s living in New York City. Although we might ideally like to generalize our results to all drug addicts, we would be on much safer ground if we defined our target population as young, urban, white men who present themselves for treatment.

Threats to External Validity

In addition to characteristics of the sample that limit the generalizability of research findings, there are various characteristics of the environment or research situation that affect the study's representativeness and, hence, its external validity. These characteristics should be taken into consideration in developing a research design and in interpreting results once the data have been collected. Among the most noteworthy threats to the external validity of studies are the following five effects:

1. *The Hawthorne effect.* Subjects in an investigation may behave in a particular manner largely because they are aware of their participation in a study. If a certain type of behavior or performance is elicited only in a research context, then the results cannot be generalized to more natural settings. This threat to external validity was discussed at greater length in Chapter 8.

2. *Novelty effects.* When a treatment is new, subjects and research agents alike might alter their behavior in a variety of ways. People may be either enthusiastic or skeptical about new methods of doing things. The results may reflect these reactions to the novelty; once the treatment is more familiar, the same results may fail to appear.

3. *Interaction of history and treatment effect.* The results may reflect the impact of the treatment *and* some other events external to the study. When the treatment is implemented again in the absence of the other events, different results may be obtained. For example, if a dietary intervention for people with high cholesterol levels was being evaluated shortly after extensive media coverage of research demonstrating a link between consumption of oat bran and reduction in cholesterol levels, it would be difficult to know whether any observed effects would be observed again if the intervention were implemented several months later with a new group of people.

4. *Experimenter effects.* The performance of the subjects may be affected by characteristics of the researchers. The investigators often have an emotional or intellectual investment in demonstrating that their hypotheses are correct and may unconsciously communicate their expectations

to the subjects, or they may be somewhat biased in their observations. If this is the case, any observed relationships in the original study might be difficult to replicate in a more neutral situation.

5. *Measurement effects.* In research studies, the investigators collect a considerable amount of data, such as pretest information, background data, and so forth. The results may not apply to another group of people who are not also exposed to the same data collection procedures.

❖ EXTERNAL VERSUS INTERNAL VALIDITY

Ideally, the researcher strives to design studies that are strong with respect to both internal and external validity. In some instances, however, the requirements for ensuring one type of validity may interfere with the possibility of achieving the second.

As one example of why this is so, consider a researcher who uses the principle of homogeneity to enhance the internal validity of a study. By controlling extraneous variables through the selection of a homogeneous sample with respect to those variables, the researcher has limited his or her ability to generalize the study results to the entire population of interest.

As another example of the conflict between internal and external validity, if the researcher exerts a high degree of control over a study through constancy of conditions in an effort to maximize internal validity, the setting may become highly artificial and pose a threat to the generalizability of the findings to more naturalistic environments. Thus, it is often necessary to reach a compromise by introducing sufficient controls while maintaining some semblance of realism.

When there is a conflict between internal and external validity, it is often preferable to opt for stronger internal validity. Indeed, it has been argued that if the findings are not internally valid, they cannot possibly be externally valid.

That is, it makes little sense to generalize the findings when the findings are themselves uninterpretable. Whenever a compromise is necessary, the concept of replication, or the repeating of a study in a new setting with new subjects, is an extremely important one. Much greater confidence can be placed in the findings of a study if it can be demonstrated that the results can be replicated in other settings and with new subjects.

❖ TIPS FOR ENHANCING RESEARCH CONTROL

In most quantitative studies, it is extremely important to control for the effects of extraneous variables. When external factors or intrinsic subject characteristics confound the relationship between the independent and dependent variables, the results of the study are likely to be ambiguous. We offer the following suggestions for enhancing research control:

- Whenever constancy of research conditions cannot be achieved, the researcher should consider controlling external factors by using some of the same strategies we suggested for controlling intrinsic subject characteristics. For example, if the researcher suspects that the time of day may influence measurement of the dependent variable but cannot collect all the data at the same time of day, perhaps it is possible to assign subjects randomly to morning versus afternoon sessions.
- Achieving constancy of conditions is not always easy, especially in clinical studies, but various steps can be taken. For example, in addition to having standard protocols, it is critical to thoroughly train the people who will be collecting the data and, in the case of an experiment or quasi-experiment, the personnel responsible for implementing the intervention. The extent to which the protocols are followed should also be monitored.
- This chapter offered various strategies for controlling the most important source of ex-

traneous variation: the subjects themselves. These alternative strategies are not mutually exclusive; whenever possible, multiple methods should be used. For example, statistical methods of control, such as analysis of covariance, can be used in conjunction with blocking or matching. Even when randomization has been used, analysis of covariance increases the precision of the design.

- The first and best defense against threats to internal validity is a strong research design. As noted earlier, the next line of defense is through analysis. The researcher must, therefore, plan the study in such a way that opportunities to analyze bias are possible. This means giving careful consideration to variables that should be measured. Information on characteristics of the subjects that are likely to have a strong effect on the dependent variable should be collected whenever possible. In a longitudinal study, variables that are likely to be related to attrition should also be measured.

- The extraneous variables that need to be controlled obviously vary from one study to another, but we can nevertheless offer some guidance in identifying variables that should be measured. The single best variable to measure and control is the dependent variable itself, before the introduction of the independent variable. Major demographic variables—age, ethnicity, gender, educational attainment, income level, marital status—should almost always be measured because these variables are related to many other variables of a social or psychological nature (including willingness to participate and remain in a scientific study). When the dependent variable is biophysiologic, measures of health status, medication, hospitalization history, and so on are likely to be important. Idiosyncratic extraneous variables should be identified through the review of the research literature.

- In longitudinal studies, the best method of avoiding attrition is to implement procedures to re-locate subjects. Attrition typically occurs because of the researcher's inability to find subjects, not because of refusals on the part of subjects to continue in the study. There are many sophisticated (and costly) methods of tracing subjects, but the simplest and most effective is to obtain *contact information* from subjects at each major point of data collection. Contact information includes, at a minimum, the names, addresses, and telephone numbers of two or three people with whom the subject is close (e.g., his or her mother, father, siblings, or good friends)—people who would be likely to know how to contact the subject if he or she moved between points of data collection.

❖ RESEARCH EXAMPLES

All the control techniques discussed in this chapter have been profitably used by nurse researchers. Table 10-1 presents some research examples of the use of these procedures. We conclude this chapter with a more detailed example of a study that was especially careful in exercising research control.

> Gilliss and a team of colleagues (1993) undertook a randomized clinical trial in two hospitals. The researchers were testing the effect of a psychoeducational nursing intervention on several posthospital recovery outcomes (e.g., self-efficacy expectations, mood, quality of life) after cardiac surgery. To avoid contamination of treatments, the subjects were randomly assigned to the experimental or control group using cluster randomization, in groups of 8 to 10 patients. For patients in the experimental group, standard care was supplemented with in-hospital education on emotional reactions to surgery and follow-up telephone contact for 2 months.
>
> The subjects were English-speaking cardiac patients between the ages of 25 and 75 years. Patients with certain conditions (e.g., aneurysms, aortic arch repairs, chronic ventricular arrhythmia) were excluded from the sample. A total of 91% of the subjects origi-

Table 10-1.   *Examples of Studies Using Various Techniques To Control Intrinsic Subject Characteristics*

RESEARCH QUESTION	CONTROL TECHNIQUE	EXTRANEOUS CHARACTERISTICS CONTROLLED
Is an intravenous infusion of meperidine with caregiver-controlled boluses more effective in alleviating pain in laboring women than intermittent intramuscular injections of meperidine? (Isenor & Penny-MacGillivray, 1993)	Randomization	All characteristics
What is the relative effectiveness of prochlorperazine (Compazine) and lorazepam (Ativan) in the management of postchemotherapy symptoms? (Simms, Rhodes, & Madsen, 1993)	Repeated measures	All characteristics
How effective are various comfort measures in alleviating nipple soreness in breastfeeding women? (Buchko, Pugh, Bishop, Cochran, Smith, & Lerew, 1994)	Homogeneity	Parity, riskiness of pregnancy, method of delivery, infant's gestational age
Is massage an effective intervention for alleviating pain in cancer patients? (Weinrich & Weinrich, 1990)	Blocking Randomization	Patients' gender All others
What are the differences in parental perception of vulnerability and child temperament between very-low-birthweight and normal-birthweight children at age seven years? (Schraeder, Heverly, O'Brien, & McEvoy-Shields, 1992)	Matching	Grade in school, gender, race, maternal education, birth order, social class
Do women who receive different treatments for breast cancer (mastectomy, mastectomy with delayed reconstruction, mastectomy with immediate reconstruction, and conservative surgery) differ with respect to body image? (Mock, 1993)	Analysis of covariance	Age

nally recruited into the study were retained through the in-hospital treatment period, and of these, 95% remained in the study for the 6-month period of follow-up. The instruments used to measure patient outcomes were administered at baseline (before the intervention) and again at 4, 12, and 24 weeks after discharge. The follow-up data were analyzed through a statistical procedure that took the baseline measures into account.

The data analysis revealed that the experimental and control groups were comparable with respect to age, gender, history of previous myocardial infarction, functional status, surgery type, and education. They were also comparable with respect to baseline measures of the dependent variables. The results indicated that the subjects in the experimental group reported greater expectations regarding their self-efficacy for walking, and also in actual walking behavior after surgery.

❖ SUMMARY

A major function of most research designs—especially highly structured ones—is to control extraneous variables, that is, the variables irrelevant to the study that could affect the dependent variable. Extraneous variables include both factors in the research setting and characteristics of the study participants.

One important type of control relates to the *constancy of conditions* under which a study is performed, as a means of controlling external factors. A number of aspects of the study, such as the environment, timing, communications, and the implementation of treatment, should be held constant or kept as similar as possible for each participant.

The most problematic and pervasive extraneous variables are intrinsic characteristics of the subjects. Several techniques are available to control such characteristics. First, the ideal method of control is through the random assignment of subjects to groups, which effectively controls for all possible extraneous variables. Second, in some types of studies, subjects can be exposed to more than one level of a treatment and thus serve as their own controls, although such repeated measures designs may be unsuitable because of the potential problem of carry-over effects. Third, a homogeneous sample of subjects can be used such that there is no variability relating to characteristics that could affect the outcome of a study. Fourth, the extraneous variables can be built into the design of a study, as in the case of a *randomized block design*. The fifth approach, *matching*, is essentially an after-the-fact attempt to approximate a randomized block design. This procedure matches subjects (either through *pair-matching* or *balancing* groups) on the basis of one or more extraneous variables in an attempt to secure comparable groups. Finally, another technique is to control extraneous variables by means of a statistical procedure known as *analysis of covariance*. Four of the procedures for controlling extraneous individual characteristics—homogeneity, blocking, matching, and analysis of covariance—share one disadvantage, and that is that the researcher must know which variables need to be controlled.

The control mechanisms reviewed here help to improve the *internal validity* of studies. Internal validity is concerned with the question of whether the results of a project are attributable to the independent variable of interest or to other, extraneous factors. *Threats to the internal validity* of a study, which represent rival hypotheses, include *history, selection, maturation, testing, instrumentation,* and *mortality.*

External validity refers to the generalizability of the research findings to other individuals and other settings. A research study possesses external validity to the extent that the sample is representative of the broader population and to the extent that the study setting and experimental arrangements are representative of other environments. A useful distinction can be made between the *accessible population,* the population from which a sample is drawn, and the *target population,* which represents a larger group of individuals in whom the investigator is interested. The researcher should define the target population in terms of those characteristics that are present in the accessible population. A research design must balance the need for internal and external validity to produce useful scientific results.

❖ STUDY SUGGESTIONS

Chapter 10 of the accompanying *Study Guide for Nursing Research: Principles and Methods, 5th ed.,* offers various exercises and study suggestions for reinforcing the concepts presented in this chapter. Additionally, the following study questions can be addressed:

1. How do you suppose the use of identical twins in a research study can enhance control?
2. Read a research report suggested under Substantive References in Chapters 7

through 9. Assess the adequacy of the control mechanisms used by the investigator and recommend additional ones if appropriate.

3.   For each of the examples below, indicate the types of research approach that could be used to study the problem (e.g., experimental, quasi-experimental, and so forth); the type of approach you would recommend using; and how you would go about controlling extraneous variables.

a.   What effect does the presence of the newborn's father in the delivery room have on the mother's subjective report of pain?

b.   What is the effect of different types of bowel evacuation regimes on quadriplegics?

c.   Does the reinforcement of intensive care unit nonsmoking behavior in smokers affect postintensive care unit behaviors?

d.   Is the degree of change in body image of surgical patients related to their need for touch?

❖ SUGGESTED READINGS

METHODOLOGICAL REFERENCES

Beck, S. L. (1989). The crossover design in clinical nursing research. *Nursing Research, 38,* 291–293.

Braucht, G. H., & Glass, G. V. (1968). The external validity of experiments. *American Educational Research Journal, 5,* 437–473.

Campbell, D. T., & Stanley, J. C. (1963). *Experimental and quasi-experimental designs for research.* Chicago: Rand McNally.

Conlon, M., & Anderson, G. C. (1991). Three methods of random assignment: Comparison of balance achieved on potentially confounding variables. *Nursing Research, 39,* 376–378.

Gilliss, C. L., & Kulkin, I. L. (1991). Technical notes: Monitoring nursing interventions and data collection in a randomized clinical trial. *Western Journal of Nursing Research, 13,* 416–422.

Kempthorne, O. (1961). The design and analysis of experiments with some reference to educational research. In R. O. Collier & S. M. Elan (Eds.), *Research design and analysis* (pp. 97–126). Bloomington, IN: Phi Delta Kappa.

Kerlinger, F. N. (1986). *Foundations of behavioral research* (3rd ed.). New York: Holt, Rinehart & Winston.

Kirk, R. E. (1982). *Experimental design: Procedures for the behavioral sciences* (2nd ed.). Belmont, CA: Wadsworth.

Lipsey, M. W. (1990). *Design sensitivity: Statistical power for experimental research.* Newbury Park, CA: Sage.

Rosenthal, R. (1976). *Experimenter effects in behavioral research.* New York: Halsted Press.

SUBSTANTIVE REFERENCES

Buchko, B. L., Pugh, L. C., Bishop, B. A., Cochran, J. F., Smith, L. R., & Lerew, D. J. (1994). Comfort measures in breastfeeding, primiparous women. *Journal of Obstetric, Gynecologic & Neonatal Nursing, 23,* 46–52.

Gilliss, C. L., Gortner, S. R., Hauck, W. W., Shinn, J. A., Sparacino, P. A., & Tompkins, C. (1993). A randomized clinical trial of nursing care for recovery from cardiac surgery. *Heart and Lung, 22,* 125–133.

Kelley, S. J. (1990). Parental stress response to sexual abuse and ritualistic abuse of children in daycare centers. *Nursing Research, 39,* 25–29.

Isenor, L., & Penny-MacGillivray, T. (1993). Intravenous meperidine infusion for obstetric analgesia. *Journal of Obstetric, Gynecologic, and Neonatal Nursing, 22,* 349–356.

Mock, V. (1993). Body image in women treated for breast cancer. *Nursing Research, 42,* 153–157.

Schraeder, B. D., Heverly, M. A., O'Brien, C., & McEvoy-Shields, K. (1992). Vulnerability and temperament in very low birth weight school-aged children. *Nursing Research, 41,* 161–165.

Simms, S. G., Rhodes, V. A., & Madsen, R. W. (1993). Comparison of prochlorperazine and lorazepam antiemetic regimens in the control of postchemotherapy symptoms. *Nursing Research, 42,* 234–239.

Weinrich, S. P., & Weinrich, M. C. (1990). The effect of massage on pain in cancer patients. *Applied Nursing Research, 3,* 140–145.

Chapter 11

SAMPLING DESIGNS

Sampling is a complex and technical topic to which entire texts have been devoted. At the same time, it is a topic whose basic features are familiar to us all. In the course of our daily activities, we gather knowledge, make decisions, and make predictions through sampling. A nursing student may decide on an elective course for a semester by sampling two or three classes on the first day of the semester. Patients may generalize about nurses' competence and empathy as a result of their exposure to a sample of nurses during a 1-week hospital stay. We all come to conclusions about phenomena based on exposure to a limited portion of those phenomena.

The scientist, too, generally derives knowledge from samples. For example, in testing the efficacy of a medication for asthma patients, a scientific researcher must reach a conclusion without administering the drug to every asthmatic. However, the scientist can rarely afford to draw conclusions based on a sample of only three or four subjects. Research methodologists have devoted considerable attention to the development of sampling plans that produce accurate and meaningful information. In this chapter, we review some of these plans.

❖ BASIC SAMPLING CONCEPTS

Sampling is an indispensable step in the research process, and a step to which too little attention is typically paid. Before discussing applications, let us first review some terms associated with sampling.

Populations

A *population* is the entire aggregation of cases that meet a designated set of criteria. For instance, if a nurse researcher were studying American nurses with doctoral degrees, the population could be defined as all United States citizens who are registered nurses (RNs) and who have acquired a Ph.D., D.Sc.N., D.Ed., or other doctoral-level degree. Other possible populations might be all the male patients who underwent cardiac surgery in St. Peter's Hospital during 1993, all the women living in a nursing home in Ohio, or all the children in the United States with cystic fibrosis. As this list illustrates, a population may be broadly defined, involving millions of individuals, or may be narrowly specified to include only several hundred people.

The definition of population by no means restricts populations to human subjects. A population might consist of all the hospital records on file in a particular hospital, all the blood samples taken from clients of a health maintenance organization, or all the correspondence of Florence Nightingale. Whatever the basic unit, the population always comprises the entire aggregate of elements in which the researcher is interested.

In identifying a population, the researcher should be specific about the inclusion criteria. Consider the population of American nursing students. Does this population include students in all types of basic nursing programs? Are part-time students included? How about RNs returning to school for a bachelor's degree? Or students who dropped out of school for a semester? Do foreign students enrolled in American nursing programs qualify? Insofar as possible, the researcher must consider the exact criteria by which it could be decided whether an individual would or would not be classified as a member of the population in question. These criteria are sometimes referred to as *eligibility criteria*. The eligibility criteria specified in one nursing study are presented in Table 11-1.

As noted in Chapter 10, it is often useful to make a distinction between target and accessible populations. The *accessible population* is the aggregate of cases that conform to the designated criteria *and* that are accessible to the researcher as a pool of subjects for a study. The *target population* is the aggregate of cases about which the researcher would like to make generalizations. A target population might consist of all diabetics in the United States, but the more modest accessible population might consist of all diabetics who are members of a particular health plan. Researchers usually sample from an accessible population and hope to generalize to a target population.

Samples and Sampling

Sampling refers to the process of selecting a portion of the population to represent the entire population. A *sample*, then, consists of a subset of the units that compose the population. In sampling terminology, the units that make up the samples and populations are referred to as elements. The *element* is the most basic unit about which information is collected. In nursing research, the elements are usually humans.

Samples and sampling plans vary considerably in quality. The overriding consideration in assessing a sample is its *representativeness*. A representative sample is one whose key characteristics closely approximate those of the population. If a population in a study of family plan-

Table 11-1. *Eligibility Criteria Specified in a Nursing Study**

RESEARCH QUESTION	ELIGIBILITY CRITERIA
What are the types and amounts of narcotic analgesics administerd to postoperative patients by nurses? (McDonald, 1993)	To be eligible for the study, the patient must: • Have a diagnosis of nonperforated appendicitis with subsequent uncomplicated appendectomy as documented by the diagnostic-related grouping codes • Be between the ages of 18 and 64 years • Have no concurrent medical problem documented on the history and physical examination • Not be participating in patient-controlled analgesia • Be admitted for an appendectomy between 1988 and 1990

*The final sample consisted of 180 patients meeting the eligibility criteria from three large New England hospitals.

ning practices consists of women 15 to 44 years of age, 40% of whom were using oral contraception and 10% of whom were using Norplant, then a representative sample would reflect these attributes in similar proportions.

Unfortunately, there is no method for making certain that a sample is representative without obtaining the information from the entire population. Certain sampling procedures are less likely to result in biased samples than others, but there is never any guarantee of a representative sample. This may sound somewhat discouraging, but it must be remembered that the scientist always operates under conditions in which error is possible. An important role of the scientist is to minimize or control those errors and, if possible, to estimate the magnitude of their effects. With certain types of sampling plans, it is possible to estimate through statistical procedures the *margin of error* in the data obtained from samples. Advanced textbooks on sampling elaborate on the procedures for making such estimates.

Sampling plans can be grouped into two categories: probability sampling and nonprobability sampling. *Probability sampling* involves some form of random selection in choosing the elements. The hallmark of a probability sample is that a researcher is in a position to specify the probability that each element of the population will be included in the sample. Probability sampling is the more respected of the two approaches because greater confidence can be placed in the representativeness of probability samples. In *nonprobability samples,* elements are selected by nonrandom methods. There is no way to estimate the probability that each element has of being included in a nonprobability sample, and every element usually does *not* have a chance for inclusion.

Strata

Sometimes it is useful to think of populations as consisting of two or more subpopulations or strata. A *stratum* refers to a mutually exclusive segment of a population established

by one or more characteristics. For instance, suppose our population consisted of all RNs currently employed in the United States. This population could be divided into two strata based on the gender of the nurse. Alternatively, we could specify three strata consisting of nurses younger than 30 years of age, nurses aged 30 to 45 years, and nurses 46 years of age or older. Strata are often identified and used in the sample selection process to enhance the representativeness of the sample.

Sampling Bias

Scientists work with samples rather than with populations because it is more economical and efficient to do so. The typical researcher has neither the time nor the resources to study all possible members of a population. Furthermore, it is usually unnecessary to gather data on some phenomenon from an entire population—it is almost always possible to obtain a reasonably accurate understanding of the phenomenon by securing information from a sample. Samples, thus, are practical and efficient means of collecting data.

Still, the data obtained from samples *can* lead to erroneous conclusions. Finding 100 willing subjects to participate in a research project seldom poses difficulty, even to a novice researcher. It is considerably more problematic to select 100 subjects who are not a biased subset of the population. *Sampling bias* refers to the systematic overrepresentation or underrepresentation of some segment of the population in terms of a characteristic relevant to the research question.

As an example of consciously biased selection, suppose a nurse researcher is investigating patients' responsiveness to touch by nurses and decides to use as a sample the first 50 patients meeting certain criteria who are admitted to a specific hospital unit. The researcher decides to omit Mr. Z from the sample because of his hostility to nurses. Mrs. X, who has just lost a spouse, is also excluded from the study out of consideration for her psychological discomfort.

The researcher has made conscious decisions to exclude certain types of individuals, and the decisions do not reflect bona fide criteria for selection. This can lead to bias because responsiveness to touch by nurses (the dependent variable) may be affected by a patient's feelings about nurses or psychological state.

Sampling bias is more likely to occur unconsciously than consciously, however. If a researcher studying nursing students systematically interviews every 10th student who enters the nursing school library, the sample of students will be biased in favor of library-goers, even if the researcher exerted a conscientious effort to include every 10th entrant irrespective of the person's appearance, gender, or other characteristics.

The extent to which sampling bias is likely to cause concern is a function of the homogeneity of the population with respect to the attributes under investigation. If the elements in a population were all identical with respect to the critical attributes, then any sample would be as good as any other. Indeed, if the population were completely homogeneous, that is, exhibited no variability at all, then a single element would constitute a sufficient sample for drawing conclusions about the population. With regard to many physical or physiologic attributes, it may be safe to assume a reasonably high degree of homogeneity and to proceed in selecting a sample on the basis of this assumption. For example, the blood in a person's veins is relatively homogeneous. A single blood sample chosen haphazardly is usually adequate for clinical purposes. As another illustration, the physiology of laboratory rats is sufficiently similar that elaborate sampling procedures are unnecessary when testing physiologic processes with a sample of rats. For most human attributes, however, homogeneity is the exception rather than the rule. Variables, after all, derive their name from the fact that traits vary from one individual to the next. Age, income, health condition, stress, attitudes, needs, habits—all these attributes reflect the heterogeneity of humans. The researcher must be concerned with the problem of sampling bias to the degree that a population is heterogeneous on key variables. Whenever variation occurs in the population, then the same variation should be reflected in a sample.

❖ NONPROBABILITY SAMPLING

Nonprobability sampling is less likely than probability sampling to produce accurate and representative samples. Despite this fact, most research samples in most disciplines, including nursing, are nonprobability samples. There are three primary methods of nonprobability sampling: convenience, quota, and purposive.

Convenience Sampling

Convenience sampling entails the use of the most conveniently available people or objects for use as subjects in a study. The faculty member who distributes questionnaires to the nursing students in her or his class is using a convenience sample, or an *accidental sample,* as it is sometimes called. The nurse who conducts an observational study of husbands whose wives are delivering a baby at the local hospital is also relying on a convenience sample. The problem with convenience sampling is that available subjects might be atypical of the population with regard to the critical variables being measured.

Convenience samples do not necessarily comprise individuals known to the researchers. Stopping people at a street corner to conduct an interview is sampling by convenience. Sometimes a researcher seeking individuals with certain characteristics will place an advertisement in a newspaper or place signs in clinics, supermarkets, or community centers. These approaches are subject to problems of bias because people self-select themselves as pedestrians on certain streets or as volunteers in response to public notices.

Another type of convenience sampling is known as *snowball sampling* or *network sampling*. With this approach, early sample members are asked to identify and refer other people who meet the eligibility criteria. This method of sampling is most likely to be used when the research population consists of people with specific traits who might otherwise be difficult to identify (e.g., women who stopped breastfeeding within 1 month of delivery; people who are afraid of hospitals). The snowballing process begins with a few eligible subjects and then continues on the basis of subject referrals until the desired sample size has been obtained. Like other types of convenience sampling, snowball sampling is often expedient but runs the risk of sampling bias.

Convenience sampling is the weakest form of sampling. It is also the most commonly used sampling method in nursing studies. In cases in which the phenomena under investigation are fairly homogeneous within the population, the risks of bias may be minimal. In heterogeneous populations, there is no other sampling approach in which the risk of bias is greater.

Quota Sampling

Quota sampling is another form of nonprobability sampling. The *quota sample* is one in which the researcher identifies strata of the population and determines the proportions of elements needed from the various segments of the population. By using information about the composition of a population, the investigator can ensure that diverse segments are represented in the sample in the proportions in which they occur in the population. Quota sampling gets its name from the procedure of establishing quotas for the various strata from which data are to be collected.

Let us consider the example of a researcher interested in studying the attitudes of undergraduate nursing students toward working with AIDS patients. The accessible population is a single school of nursing that has an undergraduate enrollment of 1000 students. A sample size of 200 students is desired. The easiest procedure would be to use a convenience sample by distributing questionnaires in classrooms or catching students as they enter or leave the library. Suppose, however, that the researcher suspects that male and female students, as well as members of the four classes, have different attitudes toward working with AIDS victims. A convenience sample could easily sample too many or too few students from these subgroups. Table 11-2 presents some fictitious data showing the proportions of each stratum for the population and for a convenience sample. As this table

Table 11-2. *Numbers and Percentages of Students in Strata of a Population, Convenience Sample, and Quota Sample*

GROUP	*GENDER*	*FRESHMEN*	*SOPHOMORES*	*JUNIORS*	*SENIORS*	*TOTAL*
Population	Males	25 (2.5%)	25 (2.5%)	25 (2.5%)	25 (2.5%)	100 (10%)
	Females	225 (22.5%)	225 (22.5%)	225 (22.5%)	225 (22.5%)	900 (90%)
	Total	250 (25%)	250 (25%)	250 (25%)	250 (25%)	1000 (100%)
Convenience sample	Males	2 (1%)	4 (2%)	3 (1.5%)	1 (.5%)	10 (5%)
	Females	98 (49%)	36 (18%)	37 (18.5%)	19 (9.5%)	190 (95%)
	Total	100 (50%)	40 (20%)	40 (20%)	20 (10%)	200 (100%)
Quota sample	Males	5 (2.5%)	5 (2.5%)	5 (2.5%)	5 (2.5%)	20 (10%)
	Females	45 (22.5%)	45 (22.5%)	45 (22.5%)	45 (22.5%)	180 (90%)
	TOTAL	50 (25%)	50 (25%)	50 (25%)	50 (25%)	200 (100%)

shows, the convenience sample seriously over-represents freshmen and women, and under-represents males and members of the sopho-more, junior, and senior classes. In anticipation of a problem of this type, the researcher can guide the selection of subjects such that the final sample includes the correct number of cases from each stratum. The bottom panel of Table 11-2 shows the number of cases that would be required for each stratum in a quota sample for this example.

If we pursue this same example a bit fur-ther, the reader may perhaps better appreciate the dangers of inadequate representation of the various strata. Suppose that one of the key ques-tions in this study was: Would you be willing to work on a unit that cared exclusively for AIDS patients? The percentage of students in the pop-ulation who would respond "yes" to this inquiry is shown in the first column of Table 11-3. Of course, these values would not be known by the researcher; they are displayed to illustrate a point. Within the population, males and older students are more likely than females and younger students to express willingness to work on a unit with AIDS patients, yet these are the very groups that are underrepresented in the convenience sample. As a result, there is a siz-able discrepancy between the population and sample values: nearly twice as many students

are favorable toward working with AIDS victims (12.5%) than one would suspect based on the results obtained from the convenience sample (6.5%). The quota sample, on the other hand, does a reasonably good job of mirroring the viewpoint of the population. In actual research situations, the distortions introduced by conve-nience sampling may be much smaller than in this fictitious example but, conceivably, could be larger as well.

Quota sampling does not require sophisti-cated skills or an inordinate amount of time or effort. Many researchers who claim that the use of a convenience sample is unavoidable for their projects could probably design a quota sampling plan, and it would be to their advan-tage to do so. The characteristics chosen to form the strata are necessarily selected according to the researcher's judgment. The basis of stratifi-cation should be some variable that, in the esti-mation of the investigator, would reflect impor-tant differences in the dependent variable under investigation. Such variables as age, gender, ethnicity, educational attainment, and medical diagnosis are often good stratifying variables in nursing research investigations.

Except for the identification of the strata and the proportional representation for each, quota sampling is procedurally similar to conve-nience sampling. The subjects in any particular

Table 11-3.   *Students Willing To Work on an AIDS Unit*

SAMPLE	NUMBER IN POPULATION	NUMBER IN CONVENIENCE SAMPLE	NUMBER IN QUOTA SAMPLE
Freshmen males	2	0	0
Sophomore males	6	1	1
Junior males	8	1	2
Senior males	12	0	3
Freshmen females	6	2	1
Sophomore females	16	2	3
Junior females	30	4	7
Senior females	45	3	9
Number of willing students	125	13	26
Total number of students	1000	200	200
PERCENTAGE	12.5%	6.5%	13.0%

cell constitute, in essence, a convenience sample from that stratum of the population. Referring back to the example in Table 11-2, the initial sample of 200 students constituted a sample chosen by convenience from the population of 1000. In the quota sample, the 45 female seniors would constitute a convenience sample of the 225 female seniors in the population. Because of this fact, quota sampling shares many of the same weaknesses as convenience sampling. For instance, if a researcher is required by a quota sampling plan to interview 10 men between the ages of 65 and 80 years, a trip to a nursing home might be the most convenient method of obtaining those subjects. Yet this approach would fail to give any representation to those many senior citizens who are living independently in the community. Despite its problems, quota sampling represents an important improvement over convenience sampling and should be considered by any researcher whose resources prevent the utilization of a probability sampling plan.

Purposive and Theoretical Sampling

Purposive or *judgmental sampling* is based on the belief that a researcher's knowledge about the population can be used to hand pick the cases to be included in the sample. The researcher might decide purposely to select the widest possible variety of respondents or might choose subjects who are judged to be typical of the population in question or particularly knowledgeable about the issues under study. Sampling in this subjective manner, however, provides no external, objective method for assessing the typicalness of the selected subjects. Nevertheless, this method can be used to advantage in certain situations. Newly developed instruments can be effectively pretested and evaluated with a purposive sample of diverse types of people. Purposive sampling is often used when the researcher wants a sample of experts, as in the case of a needs assessment using the key informant approach or in Delphi surveys.

A special type of purposive sampling, referred to as *theoretical sampling*, is often used in in-depth qualitative studies. Theoretical sampling involves the selection of sample members based on emerging findings as the study progresses, to ensure the adequate representation of important themes and to ensure that the best informants are selected to meet the information needs of the study. For example, a researcher studying reactions to a natural disaster such as a flood or hurricane may find during the course of the study that people's reactions are influenced by how long they and their families have lived in the area. This might lead the researcher to select people with a range of ties to the affected communities so that the full scope of reactions can be captured. Such sampling is often well suited to the study goals because in-depth qualitative research generally is more concerned with describing the full nature of a phenomenon than with developing a precise estimate of what percentage of people behaved or felt in a certain way. In other words, the qualitative researcher is more concerned with good representation of the theoretical constructs rather than with proper representation of the people under study.

Evaluation of Nonprobability Sampling

Although a nonprobability sample is often acceptable for pilot, exploratory, or in-depth qualitative research, for most studies, the use of nonprobability samples is problematic. Nonprobability samples are rarely representative of the researcher's target population. The difficulty stems from the fact that not every element in the population has a chance of being included in the sample. Therefore, it is likely that some segment of the population will be systematically underrepresented. If the population is homogeneous on the critical attributes, then biases may be negligible. However, only a small fraction of the characteristics in which nurse researchers are interested are sufficiently homogeneous to render sampling bias an irrelevant consideration.

Why, then, are nonprobability samples used in most nursing studies? Clearly, the advantage of these sampling designs lies in their convenience and economy. Probability sampling, which is discussed in the next section, requires skill, resources, time, and opportunity. There is often no option but to use a nonprobability approach or to abandon the project altogether. Even hard-nosed research methodologists would hesitate to advocate a total abandonment of one's ideas in the absence of a random sample. The researcher using a nonprobability sample out of necessity must be cautious about the inferences and conclusions drawn from the data. With care in the selection of the sample, a conservative interpretation of the results, and replication of the study with new samples, the researcher may find that nonprobability samples work reasonably well.

❖ PROBABILITY SAMPLING

The hallmark of probability sampling is the random selection of elements from the population. Random selection should not be confused with random assignment, which was described in connection with experimental research in Chapter 8. Random assignment refers to the process of allocating subjects to different experimental conditions on a random basis. Random assignment has no bearing on how the subjects participating in an experiment are selected in the first place. A *random selection process* is one in which each element in the population has an equal, independent chance of being selected. The four most commonly used probability sampling methods are simple random, stratified random, cluster, and systematic sampling.

Simple Random Sampling

Simple random sampling is the most basic of the probability sampling designs. Because the more complex probability sampling designs incorporate the features of simple random sampling, the procedures involved are described here in some detail.

In simple random sampling, the researcher establishes what is known as a sampling frame. The term *sampling frame* is the technical name for the actual list of the sampling units or elements from which the sample will be chosen. If nursing students attending Wayne State University constituted the accessible population, then a roster of those students would be the sampling frame. If the sampling unit were 400-bed (or larger) general hospitals in the United States, then a list of all such hospitals would be the sampling frame. In actual practice, a population may be defined in terms of an existing sampling frame rather than starting with a population and then developing a list of elements. For example, if we wanted to use a telephone directory as a sampling frame, we would have to define the population as the residents of a certain community who are clients of the telephone company and who have a listed number. Because not all members of a community own a telephone and others fail to have their numbers listed, it would be inappropriate to consider a telephone directory to be the sampling frame for the entire community population.

Once a listing of the population elements has been developed or located, the elements must be numbered consecutively. A table of random numbers would then be used to draw a sample of the desired size. An example of a sampling frame with 50 individuals is presented in Table 11-4. Let us assume that a sample of 20 people is sufficient for our purposes. As in the case of random assignment, we would find a starting place in a table of random numbers by blindly placing our finger at some point on the page. To include all numbers between 1 and 50, two-digit combinations would be read. Suppose, for the sake of the example, that we began the random selection with the very first number in the random number table of Table 8-1 (in Chapter 8), which is 46. The person corresponding to the number, D. Abraham, is the first subject selected to participate in the study. Number 05, C. Eldred, is the second selection, and number 23, D. Young, is the third. This process would continue until the 20 subjects

Table 11-4. *Sampling Frame for Simple Random Sampling Example*

(1.) N. Alexander	(26.) G. Berlin
2. H. Bos	27. G. Cave
3. M. Coiro	28. R. Donofrio
4. F. Doolittle	29. D. Edelstein
(5.) C. Eldred	(30.) D. Friedlander
(6.) R. Fellerath	(31.) J. Gueron
7. B. Granger	32. J. Healy
8. G. Hamilton	(33.) S. James
9. R. Ivry	(34.) J. Kemple
10. D. Jamison	35. D. Long
11. H. Kopp	36. K. Martinson
12. M. Little	37. D. Navarro
(13.) P. Miles	(38.) J. O'Hara
(14.) S. Nelson	39. K. Paget
15. G. Oliver	40. J. Quint
16. M. Price	41. J. Riccio
(17.) D. Queenan	42. A. Starr
(18.) S. Rowser	(43.) L. Traeger
19. K. Sherwood	44. E. Vallejo
20. K. Trister	(45.) J. Wallace
(21.) J. Vega	(46.) D. Abraham
22. J. Walter	47. P. Buffum
(23.) D. Young	48. L. Curtin
(24.) M. Zaslow	49. F. Derocher
25. M. Agudelo	(50.) J. Edison

were chosen. The selected elements are circled in Table 11-4.

It should be clear that a sample selected randomly in this fashion is not subject to the biases of the researcher. There is no chance for the operation of personal preferences. Although there is no guarantee that a randomly drawn sample will be representative, random selection does ensure that differences in the attributes of the sample and the population are purely a function of chance. The probability of selecting a markedly deviant sample is low, and this probability decreases as the size of the sample increases.

Simple random sampling tends to be a laborious process. The development of the sampling frame, enumeration of all the elements, and selection of the sample elements are time-consuming chores, particularly if the population is large. Imagine enumerating all the telephone subscribers listed in the New York City telephone directory! If the elements can be arranged in computer-readable form, then the computer can be programmed to automatically select the sample. In actual practice, simple random sampling is not used frequently because it is a relatively inefficient procedure. Furthermore, it is often impossible to get a complete listing of every element in the population, so other methods may be required.

Stratified Random Sampling

Stratified random sampling is a variant of simple random sampling in which the population is first divided into two or more strata or subgroups. As in the case of quota sampling, the aim of stratified sampling is to obtain a greater degree of representativeness. Stratified sampling designs subdivide the population into homogeneous subsets from which an appropriate number of elements can be selected at random.

The stratification may be based on a wide variety of attributes, such as age, gender, occupation, and so forth. The chosen variable should be one that will result in internally homogeneous strata on the attributes about which information is being sought. The difficulty lies in the fact that the attributes of interest may not be readily discernible or available for stratification purposes. If one is working with a telephone directory, it would be risky to make decisions about a person's gender, and certainly age, ethnicity, or other personal information that is not listed. Patient listings, student rosters, or organizational directories might contain the information needed for a meaningful stratification. Quota sampling does not have the same problem because the researcher can ask the prospective subject questions that determine his or her eligibility for a particular stratum. In stratified sampling, however, decisions about a person's status in a stratum are made before a sample is chosen.

Various procedures for drawing a stratified sample have been used. The most common is to group together those elements that belong to a stratum and to select randomly the desired number of elements. The researcher either may take an equal number of elements from each stratum or may decide to select unequal numbers, for reasons discussed later in this section. To illustrate the procedure used in the simplest case, suppose that the list in Table 11-4 consisted of 25 males (numbers 1 through 25) and 25 females (numbers 26 through 50). Using gender as the stratifying variable, we could guarantee a sample of 10 males and 10 females by randomly sampling 10 numbers from the first half of the list and 10 from the second half. As it turns out, our simple random sampling did result in 10 elements being chosen from each half of the list, but this was purely by chance. It would not have been unusual to draw, say, 8 names from one half and 12 from the other. Stratified sampling can guarantee the appropriate representation of different segments of the population.

In many cases, the stratifying variables divide the population into unequal subpopulations. For example, if the person's race were used to stratify the population of U.S. citizens, the subpopulation of white people would be larger than that of African American and other nonwhite people. In such a situation, the researcher might decide to select subjects in proportion to the size of the stratum in the population. This procedure is referred to as *proportionate stratified sampling*. If an undergraduate population in a school of nursing consisted of 10% African American students, 5% Hispanic students, and 85% white students, then a proportionate stratified sample of 100 students, with racial/ethnic background as the stratifying variable, would consist of 10, 5, and 85 students from the respective subpopulations.

When the researcher is interested in understanding differences among the strata, proportionate sampling may result in an insufficient base for making comparisons. In the previous example, would the researcher be justified in coming to conclusions about the characteristics

of Hispanic nursing students based on only five cases? It would be extremely unwise to do so in most types of research. When random selection procedures are used, the probability of obtaining a representative sample increases as the sample size increases. For this reason, researchers often adopt a *disproportionate sampling design* whenever interstratum comparisons are sought between strata of greatly unequal membership size. In the example, the sampling proportions might be altered to select 20 African American students, 20 Hispanic students, and 60 white students. This design would ensure a more adequate representation of the viewpoints of the two racial/ethnic minorities. When disproportionate sampling is used, however, it is necessary to make an adjustment to the data to arrive at the best estimate of overall population values. This adjustment process, known as *weighting*, is a simple mathematical computation that is described in detail in most texts on sampling.

Stratified random sampling offers the researcher the opportunity to sharpen the precision and representativeness of the final sample. When it is desirable to obtain reliable information about subpopulations whose membership is relatively small, stratification provides a means of including a sufficient number of cases in the sample by oversampling for that stratum. Stratified sampling, however, may be impossible if information on the critical variables is unavailable. Furthermore, a stratified sample requires even more labor and effort than simple random sampling because the sample must be drawn from multiple enumerated listings.

Cluster Sampling

For many populations, it is simply impossible to obtain a listing of all the elements. For example, the population consisting of all full-time nursing students in the United States would be difficult to list and enumerate for the purpose of drawing a simple or stratified random sample. In addition, it would often be prohibitively expensive to sample nursing students in this way because the resulting sample would include no more than one or two students per institution. If interviews were involved, the interviewers would have to travel to individuals scattered throughout the country. Because of these considerations, large-scale studies almost never use simple or stratified random sampling. The most common procedure for large-scale surveys is cluster sampling.

In *cluster sampling,* there is a successive random sampling of units. The first unit to be sampled is large groupings, or clusters. In drawing a sample of nursing students, the researcher might first draw a random sample of nursing schools and then draw a sample of students from the selected schools. The usual procedure for selecting a general sample of citizens is to sample successively such administrative units as states, cities, districts, blocks, and then households. Because of the successive stages in cluster sampling, this approach is often referred to as *multi-stage sampling.*

The clusters can be selected either by simple or stratified methods. For instance, in selecting clusters of nursing schools, it may be advisable to stratify on program type. The final selection from within a cluster may also be performed by simple or stratified random sampling.

For a specified number of cases, cluster sampling tends to contain more sampling errors than simple or stratified random sampling. Despite these disadvantages, cluster sampling is considerably more economical and practical than other types of probability sampling, particularly when the population is large and widely dispersed.

Systematic Sampling

The final type of sampling design to be discussed can be classified as either a probability or nonprobability sampling approach, depending on the exact procedure used. *Systematic sampling* involves the selection of every *k*th case from some list or group, such as every 10th person on a patient list or every 100th person listed in a directory of American Nurses' Associ-

ation members. Systematic sampling is sometimes used to sample every *k*th person entering a bookstore, or passing down the street, or leaving a hospital, and so forth. In such situations, unless the population is narrowly defined as consisting of all those people entering, passing by, or leaving, the sampling is nonprobability in nature.

Systematic sampling designs can be applied in such a way that an essentially random sample is drawn. If the researcher has a list, or sampling frame, the following procedure can be adopted. The desired sample size is established at some number (n). The size of the population must be known or estimated (N). By dividing N by n, the sampling interval width (k) is established. The *sampling interval* is the standard distance between the elements chosen for the sample. For instance, if we were seeking a sample of 200 from a population of 40,000, then our sampling interval would be as follows:

$$k = \frac{40,000}{200} = 200$$

In other words, every 200th element on the list would be sampled. The first element should be selected randomly, using a table of random numbers. Let us say that we randomly selected number 73 from a table. The people corresponding to numbers 73, 273, 473, 673, and so forth would be included in the sample.

In actual practice, systematic sampling conducted in this manner is essentially identical to simple random sampling. Problems may arise if the list is arranged in such a way that a certain type of element is listed at intervals coinciding with the sampling interval. For instance, if every 10th nurse listed in a nursing personnel roster were a head nurse and the sampling interval was 10, then head nurses would either always or never be included in the sample. Problems of this type are not too common, fortunately. In most cases, systematic sampling is preferable to simple random sampling because the same results are obtained in a more convenient and efficient manner. Systematic sampling procedures can also be applied to lists that have been stratified.

Evaluation of Probability Sampling

Probability sampling is really the only viable method of obtaining representative samples. If all the elements in the population have an equal probability of being selected, then the likelihood is high that the resulting sample will do a good job of representing the population. A further advantage is that probability sampling allows the researcher to estimate the magnitude of sampling error. *Sampling error* refers to differences between population values (such as the average age of the population) and sample values (such as the average age of the sample). It is a rare sample that is perfectly representative of a population and contains no sampling error on any of the attributes under investigation. Probability sampling does, however, permit estimates of the degree of expected error.*

The great drawback of probability sampling is its expense and inconvenience. Unless the population is narrowly defined, it is usually beyond the scope of most research projects to sample using a probability design. A researcher using nonprobability sampling might well be able to argue that the homogeneity of the attribute under consideration makes an elaborate sampling scheme unnecessary. This justification will probably be implausible, however, if psychological, social, or economic attributes are being studied.

In sum, probability sampling is the preferred and most respected method of obtaining sample elements, but it may in some cases be impractical or unnecessary.

---

* Probability sampling is at the heart of most statistical testing. Strictly speaking, it is inappropriate to apply inferential statistics to data obtained from nonprobability samples, although most researchers ignore this issue in their treatment of data.

❖ SAMPLE SIZE

A major concern to beginning researchers is the number of subjects needed in a sample. There are some sophisticated methods for developing sample size estimates using a procedure known as *power analysis,* but some statistical knowledge is needed before this procedure can be explained. Below we offer guidelines to beginning researchers; the advanced student should review the discussion of power analysis in Chapter 19 or consult an advanced sampling or statistical text.

Although there are no simple formulas that indicate how large a sample is needed in a given study, we can offer a simple piece of advice: you generally should use the largest sample possible. The larger the sample, the more representative of the population it is likely to be. Every time a researcher calculates a percentage or an average based on sample data, the purpose is to estimate a population value. Smaller samples tend to produce less accurate estimates than larger samples. In other words, the larger the sample, the smaller is the sampling error.

Let us illustrate this notion with a simple example of, say, monthly aspirin consumption in a nursing home facility, as shown in Table 11-5. The population consists of 15 residents whose aspirin consumption averages 16 aspirins per month. Two simple random samples with sample sizes of 2, 3, 5, and 10 each have been drawn. Each sample average represents an estimate of the population, which is 16. Under ordinary circumstances, the population value would be unknown to us, and we would draw only one sample. With a sample size of two, our estimate might have been wrong by as many as eight aspirins in sample 1B—a 50% error. As the sample size increases, the averages not only get closer to the true population value, but the differences in the estimates between samples A and B get smaller as well. As the sample size increases, the probability of getting a markedly deviant sample diminishes. Large

Table 11-5. *Comparison of Population and Sample Values and Averages*

NUMBER IN GROUP	GROUP	VALUES (MONTHLY NUMBER OF ASPIRINS CONSUMED)	AVERAGE
15	Population	2, 4, 6, 8, 10, 12, 14, 16, 18, 20, 22, 24, 26, 28, 30	16.0
2	Sample 1A	6, 14	10.0
2	Sample 1B	20, 28	24.0
3	Sample 2A	16, 18, 8	14.0
3	Sample 2B	20, 14, 26	20.0
5	Sample 3A	26, 14, 18, 2, 28	17.6
5	Sample 3B	30, 2, 26, 10, 4	14.4
10	Sample 4A	22, 16, 24, 22, 2, 8, 14, 28, 20, 2	15.8
10	Sample 4B	14, 18, 12, 20, 6, 14, 28, 12, 24, 16	16.4

samples provide an opportunity to counterbalance atypical values. The safest procedure in most circumstances is to obtain data from as large a sample as is economically and practically feasible.

Large samples are no assurance of accuracy, however. When nonprobability sampling methods are used, even a large sample can harbor extensive bias. The famous example illustrating this point is the 1936 presidential poll conducted by the magazine *Literary Digest,* which predicted that Alfred M. Landon would defeat Franklin D. Roosevelt by a landslide. About 2.5 million individuals participated in this poll—a substantial sample. Biases resulted from the fact that the sample was drawn from telephone directories and automobile registrations during a depression year when only the well-to-do had a car or telephone. Thus, a large sample cannot correct for a faulty sampling design. The researcher should make decisions about the sample size and design based primarily on how representative of the population the sample is likely to be.

Because practical constraints such as time, availability of subjects, and resources often limit the number of subjects included in nursing studies, many are based on relatively small samples. In a survey of nursing studies published over four decades (the 1950s to the 1980s), Brown and her colleagues (1984) found that the average sample size was under 100 subjects in all four decades, and similar results were reported in a more recent analysis (Moody, Wilson, Smyth, Schwartz, Tittle, & VanCott, 1988). In many cases, a small sample is inappropriate and can lead to misleading results. In some cases, however, a small sample size may be justifiable. Below we discuss some considerations that affect sample size decisions.

Nature of the Investigation

When a researcher undertakes an in-depth, qualitative study, the sample is typically small—usually well under 100 subjects. This is because the qualitative researcher is interested in studying some phenomenon intensively rather than extensively. Such studies are often descriptive and serve to generate hypotheses and theory rather than to test them. Small samples are usually adequate to capture a full range of themes emerging in relation to the phenomenon of interest, especially if theoretical sampling has been used judiciously. Moreover, qualitative analysis is typically a time-consuming procedure that would become unwieldy with very large samples.

In quantitative studies, the researcher generally tests hypotheses using formal statistical procedures. Small samples are generally insufficiently powerful to provide a meaningful statistical test (and hence the use of power analysis to estimate sample size needs). Thus, whenever hypotheses are being tested, or when the researcher is interested in describing the extensiveness of some phenomenon (as is often the case in survey research), fairly large samples of subjects are generally needed.

Homogeneity of the Population

When the researcher has reason to believe that the population is relatively homogeneous with respect to the variables of interest, then a small sample may be adequate for research purposes. Let us demonstrate that this is so. The top half of Table 11-6 presents hypothetical population values for three different populations, with only 10 people in each population. These values could reflect, for example, scores on a measure of anxiety. In all the populations, the average anxiety score is 100. In population A, however, the individuals have fairly similar anxiety scores: the scores range in value from a low of 90 to a high of 110. In population B, the scores are more variable, and in population C, the scores are more variable still: the scores range from 70 to 130.

The second half of Table 11-6 presents three sample values from the three populations. In the most homogeneous population (A), the average anxiety score for the sample is 98.33, which is close to the population value of 100. As the population becomes less homogeneous with regard to anxiety scores, the average sample values less accurately reflect the population values. In other words, there is greater sampling error when the population is heterogeneous on the key variable. By increasing the sample size, the risk of sampling error would be reduced. For example, if sample C consisted of five values rather than three (say, all the even-numbered values), then the average would be closer to the population value (i.e., 102.0 rather than 91.67).

For clinical studies that deal with biophysiologic processes in which variation is limited, a small sample may adequately represent the population. For most nursing studies, however, it is probably safer to assume a fair degree of heterogeneity, unless there is evidence from prior research or from experience to the contrary.

Effect Size

Power analysis builds on the concept of effect size, a term that we mentioned briefly in connection with meta-analyses. *Effect size* is

Table 11-6.   *Three Populations of Different Homogeneity*

POPULATION	POPULATION VALUES	POPULATION AVERAGE
A	100 110 105 95 90 110 105 95 90 100	100
B	100 120 115 85 80 120 115 85 80 100	100
C	100 130 125 75 70 130 125 75 70 100	100

SAMPLE	SAMPLE VALUES	SAMPLE AVERAGE
A	110 90 95	98.33
B	120 80 85	95.00
C	130 70 75	91.67

concerned with the strength of the relationship among research variables. If the researcher has reason to believe that the independent and dependent variables are strongly interrelated, then a relatively small sample is generally adequate to demonstrate the relationship statistically. For example, if a researcher were testing a powerful new drug to treat AIDS, it might be possible to demonstrate the drug's effectiveness with a small number of subjects. Typically, however, interventions have modest effects, and variables are usually only moderately correlated with one another. When the researcher has no a priori reason for believing that relationships will be strong (i.e., when the effect size is expected to be modest), then small samples are risky.

Attrition

In many situations, the number of subjects recruited to participate in a study declines during the course of the project. This is most likely to occur in longitudinal studies, especially if the time lag between data collection points is great; if the population is a mobile or a hard-to-locate one; or if the population is a high-risk, vulnerable one at risk of death or disability. If resources are devoted to tracing subjects in longitudinal studies, or if the researcher has an ongoing relationship with subjects (as might be true in many clinical studies), then the rate of attrition might be low. However, it is the rare longitudinal study that maintains the entire research sample. Therefore, in estimating sample size needs, the researcher should factor in anticipated loss of subjects from the sample.

Attrition problems are not restricted to longitudinal studies. Subjects who agree to cooperate in a study may be subsequently unable or unwilling to participate for a number of reasons, such as death, deteriorating health, early discharge, discontinued need for a particular intervention, or simply a change of heart. Researchers should attempt to anticipate a certain amount of subject loss and to recruit subjects accordingly.

Other Considerations

Several other factors should be considered in deciding how large the research sample should be. These include the following:

Number of variables. In general, the greater the number of independent and extraneous variables, the larger the sample should be. If the research design can be laid out such that the number of "cells" can be determined, then the study should aim to have at least 20 to 30 subjects for each cell of the design. For example, a study of the effects of gender (male/female); race/ethnicity (white, African American, Hispanic); and marital status (married/not married)—$2 \times 3 \times 2$—on success in an alcohol treatment program should ideally have at least 140 to 210 subjects. This requirement enhances the likelihood of obtaining a stable estimate for each cell but does not ensure that relationships between variables will be detected. A power analysis may indicate that even more subjects should be included.

Subgroup analyses. A related point is that a researcher is sometimes interested in testing hypotheses not only for an entire population of subjects but also for specific subgroups. For example, a researcher might be interested in determining whether a structured exercise program is effective in improving infants' motor skills. After the researcher has tested this general hypothesis with a sample of infants, it might be useful to test whether the intervention is more effective for certain types of infants (e.g., very-low-birthweight infants) than for others. When a sample is divided to test for effects in specific subgroups, the sample must be large enough to support these divisions of the sample.

Sensitivity of the measures. Different measures vary in their ability to measure precisely the concepts under study. Biophysiologic measures are generally very sensitive—they measure phenomena accurately, and they can often make fine discriminations in values. Measures that are psychological in nature often contain a fair amount of error and are typically not precise. In general, when the measuring tool is imprecise and susceptible to errors, larger samples are needed to test hypotheses adequately.

❖ STEPS IN SAMPLING

The steps to be undertaken in drawing a sample vary somewhat from one sampling design to the next. Moreover, in in-depth, qualitative studies, the sampling plan often evolves as the study progresses. However, a general outline of procedures for most studies can be described.

1. *Identify the target population.* The first phase of the sampling process involves the identification of the target population. This is the group to which you want to be able to generalize your results. For example, the target population could consist of all RNs currently unemployed in the United States, or all diabetics, or all women who have had a miscarriage.

2. *Identify the accessible population.* Unless you have extensive resources at your disposal, you are unlikely to have access to the entire target population. Therefore, you should identify the portion of the target population that is accessible to you. In essence, an accessible population is a sample from the larger target population. An accessible population might consist of unemployed RNs in metropolitan Atlanta, or all diabetics under the care of a specific health maintenance organization, or women who had a miscarriage in a particular hospital in the past year.

3. *Specify the eligibility criteria.* The criteria for eligibility in the sample should then be spelled out, preferably in writing. The criteria should be as specific as possible with respect to characteristics that might exclude potential subjects (e.g., extremes of poor health, inability to read English, and so on).

4. *Specify the sampling plan.* Once the accessible population has been identified, you must decide how the sample will be chosen and how large it will be. The sample size specification should consider the various aspects of the study that were discussed in the previous section. If you can perform a power analysis to determine the desired number of subjects, it is highly recommended that you do so. Similarly, if probability sampling is an option, that option should generally be exercised. The typical nurse researcher is not in a position to do either. In such a situation, we recommend using as large a sample as possible and taking steps to build representativeness into the design (e.g., by using quota sampling).

5. *Recruit the sample.* Once the sampling design has been specified, the next step is to recruit the subjects according to the designated plan (after any needed institutional permissions have been obtained) and ask them for their cooperation. In many studies, it is necessary to develop a *screening instrument*, which is a brief interview or form that allows the researcher to determine whether a prospective subject meets all the eligibility criteria for the study.

One final point concerns the interpretation of results. Ideally, the sample is representative of the accessible population, and the accessible population is representative of the target population. By using an appropriate sample size and sampling plan, the researcher can be reasonably confident that the first part of this ideal has been realized. A greater risk is involved in assuming that the second part of the ideal is also realized. Are the unemployed nurses in Atlanta representative of all unemployed nurses in the United States? One can never be sure. The researcher must exercise judgment in assessing the degree of similarity. The best advice is to be realistic and somewhat conservative. The researcher should interpret the findings and come to conclusions after asking: Is it reasonable to assume that the accessible population is representative of the target population? In what ways might they be expected to differ? How would such differences affect the conclusions? If the researcher decides that the differences in the two populations are too great, it would be prudent to identify a more restricted target population to which the findings could be meaningfully generalized.

❖ *TIPS FOR SAMPLING*

Many nursing studies use less-than-optimal sampling plans that run the risk of yielding erroneous or inconclusive results. We offer below some suggestions on how to strengthen a study's sampling design.

- If, in conducting a research study, you decide that there is no alternative to convenience sampling, you should take several steps to enhance the likelihood of achieving a representative sample. First, identify important extraneous variables. That is, identify the factors that influence the heterogeneity of the population with respect to the dependent variable. For example, in a study of the relationship between stress and health, a person's socioeconomic status is likely to be an important extraneous variable because poor people are likely to be less healthy and more stressed than more affluent ones. Then, decide how to account for this source of variation in the sampling design. One solution is to define the population such that variation resulting from extraneous variables is minimized, as discussed in Chapter 10. In the stress and health example, we might, for instance, restrict the population to middle-class people. Alternatively, we could select the sample from communities known to differ in socioeconomic characteristics so that our sample would be known to reflect the experiences of both lower- and middle-class subjects. This approaches using a quota sampling method. In other words, if the popula-

tion is known to be heterogeneous, we should take steps to either make it more homogeneous or to capture the full variation in the sample.

- One fairly simple way to increase the generalizability of a study is to select subjects from two or more sites, such as from different hospitals, nursing homes, communities, and so on. Ideally, the two different sites would be sufficiently divergent that broader representation of the population would be obtained (e.g., in a study of compliance with a medication regimen, using patients from an inner-city health clinic and a suburban health maintenance organization). The major issue in using multiple sites is taking steps to ensure that constancy of conditions is maintained across sites insofar as possible.

- Regardless of the type of sampling plan used, it is important to understand and document who the subjects are so that biases can be identified and taken into consideration in interpreting the results and developing recommendations. It is particularly helpful to compare sample characteristics to population characteristics whenever possible. Published information about the characteristics of many groups of interest to nurses is usually available to help provide an important context for evaluating sampling bias. For example, if you are studying teenaged mothers, obtain information in the library about the characteristics of the population of teenaged mothers—for example, their marital status, family income, ethnic distribution, and so on. This information can then be compared with sample characteristics, and differences can be taken into account in interpreting the findings.

- As you proceed in recruiting your sample, it is wise to document thoroughly. The more information you have about who the sample is and who it is not, the better able you will be to identify potential biases. Biases can occur even in probability sampling because the *selection* of elements that are representative of the population does not guarantee the participation of all those elements, and refusals to participate in a study are rarely random. Thus, you should calculate a *response rate* (the number of people participating in the study relative to the number of people sampled) and document, to the extent possible, the characteristics of people who were asked to participate in the study. Then you can compare those who agreed with those who refused. Also, those who remain in a study should be compared with those who drop out to detect possible attrition biases.

- Subject recruitment often proceeds at a slower pace than researchers anticipate, in part because not everybody who is approached agrees to cooperate. Once you have determined your sample size needs, it is often wise to develop contingency plans for recruiting more subjects, should the initial plan prove overly optimistic. For example, a contingency plan might involve relaxation of some of the eligibility criteria, the identification of another institution through which subjects could be recruited, the payment of a subject stipend to make participation in the study more attractive, or the lengthening of the time for recruitment into the study. When contingency plans are developed at the outset, it reduces the likelihood that you will have to settle for a less-than-desirable sample size.

❖ RESEARCH EXAMPLES

Most nursing studies use convenience samples. However, an increasing number of investigations are using sophisticated sampling designs, including probability sampling. Table 11-7 presents some examples of nursing studies that used various methods of sampling. Below we describe a sampling plan of two nursing studies in greater detail.

Example of Probability Sampling

Ferrans and Powers (1992) conducted a methodological study to appraise a data collection instrument known as the Quality of Life Index (QLI), which measures people's satisfaction with various domains of life. The study involved administering the QLI to a sample of subjects and analyzing the results to determine if the QLI is a good measure of a person's overall quality of life so that the instrument could be used by other researchers interested in the quality of life construct. A description of their sampling plan for this study follows.

The sample for the methodological study consisted of 800 subjects randomly selected from an accessible population of nearly 3000 adult, in-unit hemodialysis patients. The population represented all in-unit hemodialysis patients from 93% of the counties in Illinois, excluding patients undergoing treatment in Veterans Administration hospitals.

Of the 800 sampled patients, 36 had died or had a kidney transplantation. Of the 764 remaining subjects, 57% (434) returned a questionnaire. Eighty-five subjects were dropped from the study because they left too many questions blank. The final sample consisted of 349 subjects, which represented a 46% response rate (i.e., 349/764).

The representativeness of the research sample was evaluated by comparing the sample and the population in terms of a number of characteristics about which information was available: gender, number of months on dialysis, presence of diabetes mellitus, primary cause of renal failure, age, and race. The sample and population were comparable with respect to the first four characteristics. However, the sample had a higher proportion of white patients and older patients than the population, although the differences were relatively small. Ferrans and Powers concluded that the sample was adequately representative of the population for the purposes of their study.

Example of Theoretical Sampling

Quinn (1993) conducted an in-depth study to examine how nurses explained their use of physical restraints with elderly patients and the extent to which the nurses perceived the re-

Table 11-7.   *Examples of Sampling Designs Used in Nursing Studies*

RESEARCH PROBLEM	TYPE OF SAMPLING	DESCRIPTION OF SAMPLE
What are the effects of age, gender, and analgesic administration on the magnitude of pain experienced by critically ill cardiovascular surgical patients? (Puntillo & Weiss, 1994)	Convenience	74 cardiovascular surgical patients from a 500-bed metropolitan teaching hospital
What are the health complaints of remarried men versus remarried women? (Ganong & Coleman, 1991)	Snowball	205 remarried men and women
What is the nature of the reminiscences of elderly women? (Kovach, 1991)	Quota	21 elderly women—7 in each of 3 age groups: 65–74, 75–84, and 85–95 years
What are family caregivers' perceptions and interpretations of dementia-related problems? (Harvath, 1994)	Purposive	10 family caregivers of people with multi-infarct dementia— 5 with low stress and 5 with very high stress
What is the role of social networks in influencing individual wellness motivation in the context of cardiac rehabilitation? (Fleury, 1993)	Theoretical	24 patients participating in an outpatient cardiac rehabilitation program
What is the relationship between current life events and personal hardiness on the one hand and perceptions of health on the other among rural adults? (Lee, 1991)	Simple random	Random sample of 300 out of 3000 members of a state agricultural organization (162 people responded)
What level of confidence do nurse practitioners have regarding their practice skills and knowledge? (Thibodeau & Hawkins, 1994)	Stratified random	National sample of 900 nurse practitioners, stratified by specialty area (482 nurses responded)
What are the work situation characteristics, levels of satisfaction, and individual characteristics of ICU and non-ICU nurses? (Boumans & Landeweerd, 1994)	Multi-stage	Nurses in randomly selected ICU and non-ICU units from 16 randomly selected general hospitals in The Netherlands
What is the extent to which nurses in a wide variety of practice settings discuss sexual concerns with their patients? (Matocha & Waterhouse, 1993)	Systematic	Systematic sample of 500 nurses: every 17th nurse listed by a state Board of Nursing in a South Atlantic state (155 nurses responded)

straint decision as a moral problem. A description of their sampling plan follows.

> A sample of nurses was recruited from the medical-surgical unit of a hospital. Nurses were eligible to participate in Quinn's study if they were women, were direct caregivers on the medical-surgical unit, and had cared for a restrained elderly patient (65 years old or older) within the previous 48 hours.
>
> After the first few interviews were completed, theoretical sampling was used to guide the recruitment of subsequent respondents. For example, analysis of the early interviews revealed that nurses made a distinction between initiating physical restraint and continuing restraint that had been initiated by a previous caregiver. Thus, the researcher took care to include respondents with sufficient experience with both types of restraint. As another example, it was noted early in the study that respondents identified time of day as a factor in the use of restraint. Thereafter, Quinn made sure her sample included nurses who cared for restrained patients during all three tours of duty. The final sample consisted of 20 nurses ranging in age from 21 to 58 years, representing a wide range of nursing experience and educational preparation.

❖ SUMMARY

Sampling is the process of selecting a portion of the population to represent the entire population. A *population,* in turn, is the entire aggregate of cases that meet a designated set of *eligibility criteria*. In a sampling context, an *element* is the most basic unit about which information is collected.

The overriding consideration in assessing the adequacy of any sample is the degree to which it is representative of the population. Sampling plans vary in their ability to reflect adequately the population from which the sample was drawn. *Sampling bias* refers to the systematic overrepresentation or underrepresentation of some segment of the population. The greater the heterogeneity of the population with respect to the critical attributes, the greater is the risk of sampling bias.

Sampling plans may be classified as either nonprobability or probability sampling. In *nonprobability sampling,* elements are selected by nonrandom methods. Convenience, quota, and purposive sampling are the principal nonprobability methods. *Convenience sampling* (sometimes called *accidental sampling*) involves using the most readily available or most convenient group of subjects for the sample. A form of convenience sampling is *snowball* or *network sampling,* in which early sample members are asked to identify other potential subjects meeting the eligibility criteria. *Quota sampling* divides the population into homogeneous *strata* or subpopulations to promote representation of the various strata in the sample. Within each stratum, the researcher selects subjects by convenience sampling. In *purposive sampling* (also referred to as *judgmental sampling*), subjects or objects are handpicked to be included in the sample, based on the researcher's knowledge about the population. A special type of purposive sampling known as *theoretical sampling* is often used in in-depth qualitative research to ensure the adequate representation of themes relating to the phenomenon under study. Nonprobability sampling designs have the advantage of being convenient and economical. The major disadvantage of nonprobability sampling designs is their potential for serious biases.

Probability sampling designs involve the random selection of elements from the population. A *simple random sample* involves the selection of elements on a random basis from a *sampling frame* that enumerates all the elements. A *stratified random sample* divides the population into homogeneous subgroups from which elements are selected at random. *Cluster sampling* (also called *multi-stage sampling*) involves the successive selection of random samples from larger to smaller units by either simple random or stratified random methods. *Systematic sampling* is the selection of every *k*th case from some list or group. By dividing the population size by the desired sample size, the researcher is able to establish the *sampling interval,* which is the standard distance between the elements chosen for the systematic sample. Probability sampling designs are generally preferred to nonprobability methods because probability sampling designs tend to result in more representative samples and because they permit the researcher to estimate the magnitude of sampling error. Probability samples, however, are time-consuming, expensive, inconvenient, and, in some cases, impossible to obtain.

No simple equation can be used to determine how large a sample is needed for a particular research project. If researchers cannot use *power analysis* to estimate the number of subjects needed for a study, they should use as large a sample as is possible and practical, considering such factors as the nature of the study, the homogeneity of the population with respect to key variables, the risk of subject loss, and the anticipated magnitude of the relationships among key variables (i.e., the *effect size*). In general, the larger the sample, the more representative of the population it is likely to be. Even a very large sample, however, does not guarantee representativeness if nonprobability sampling methods are used.

❖ *STUDY SUGGESTIONS*

Chapter 11 of the accompanying *Study Guide for Nursing Research: Principles and Methods, 5th ed.,* offers various exercises and study suggestions for reinforcing the concepts presented in this chapter. Additionally, the following study questions can be addressed:

1. Draw a simple random sample of 15 people from the sampling frame of Table 11-4, using the table of random numbers that appears in Table 8-1 in Chapter 8. Begin your selection by blindly placing your finger at some point on the table.
2. Suppose you have decided to use a systematic sampling design for a research project. The known population size is 5000,

and the sample size desired is 250. What is the sampling interval? If the first element selected is 23, what would be the second, third, and fourth elements to be selected?
3. Suppose a researcher is interested in studying the attitude of clinical specialists toward autonomy in the work situation. Suggest a possible target and accessible population. What strata might be identified by the researcher if quota sampling were used?
4. What type of sampling design was used to obtain the following samples?
    a. 25 experts in critical care nursing
    b. 60 couples attending a particular prenatal class
    c. 100 nurses from a list of nurses registered in the state of Pennsylvania, using a table of random numbers
    d. 20 adult patients randomly selected from a random selection of 10 hospitals located in one state
    e. Every fifth article published in *Nursing Research* during the 1980s, beginning with the first article

❖ *SUGGESTED READINGS*

METHODOLOGICAL REFERENCES

Babbie, E. (1990). *Survey research methods.* (2nd ed.). Belmont, CA: Wadsworth.

Brown, J. S., Tanner, C. A., & Padrick, K. P. (1984). Nursing's search for scientific knowledge. *Nursing Research, 33,* 26–32.

Cochran, W. G. (1977). *Sampling techniques* (3rd ed.). New York: John Wiley and Sons.

Cohen, J. (1977). *Statistical power analysis for the behavioral sciences* (rev. ed.). New York: Academic Press.

Diekmann, J. M., & Smith, J. M. (1989). Strategies for accessment and recruitment of subjects for nursing research. *Western Journal of Nursing Research, 11,* 418–430.

Kish, L. (1965). *Survey sampling.* New York: John Wiley and Sons.

Levey, P. S., & Lemeshow, S. (1980). *Sampling for health professionals.* New York: Lifetime Learning.

Moody, L. E., Wilson, M. E., Smyth, K., Schwartz, R., Tittle, M., & VanCott, M. L. (1988). Analysis of a decade of nursing practice research: 1977–1986. *Nursing Research, 37,* 374–379.

Morse, J. M. (1991). Strategies for sampling. In J. M. Morse (Ed.), *Qualitative nursing research: A contemporary dialogue.* Newbury Park, CA: Sage.

Polit, D. F., & Sherman, R. (1990). Statistical power analysis in nursing research. *Nursing Research, 39,* 365–369.

Sudman, S. (1976). *Applied sampling.* New York: Academic Press.

Williams, B. (1978). *A sampler on sampling.* New York: John Wiley and Sons.

SUBSTANTIVE REFERENCES

Belec, R. H. (1992). Quality of life: Perceptions of long-term survivors of bone marrow transplantation. *Oncology Nursing Forum, 19,* 31–37.

Boumans, N. P. G., & Landeweerd, J. A. (1994). Working in an intensive or non-intensive care unit: Does it make any difference? *Heart and Lung, 23,* 71–79.

Ferrans, C. E., & Powers, M. J. (1992). Psychometric assessment of the Quality of Life Index. *Research in Nursing and Health, 15,* 29–38.

Fleury, J. (1993). An exploration of the role of social networks in cardiovascular risk reduction. *Heart and Lung, 22,* 134–144.

Ganong, L. H., & Coleman, M. (1991). Remarriage and health. *Research in Nursing and Health, 14,* 205–211.

Harvath, T. A. (1994). Interpretation and management of dementia-related behavior problems. *Clinical Nursing Research, 3,* 7–26.

Kovach, C. R. (1991). Content analysis of reminiscences of elderly women. *Research in Nursing and Health, 14,* 287–295.

Lee, H. J. (1991). Relationship of hardiness and current life events to perceived health in rural adults. *Research in Nursing and Health, 14,* 351–358.

Matocha, L. K., Waterhouse, J. K. (1993). Current nursing practice related to sexuality. *Research in Nursing and Health, 16,* 371–378.

McDonald, D. D. (1993). Postoperative narcotic analgesic administration. *Applied Nursing Research, 6,* 106–110.

Puntillo, K., & Weiss, S. J. (1994). Pain: Its mediators and associated morbidity in critically ill cardiovascular surgical patients. *Nursing Research, 43,* 31–36.

Quinn, C. A. (1993). Nurses' perceptions about physical restraints. *Western Journal of Nursing Research, 15,* 148–158.

Thibodeau, J. A., & Hawkins, J. W., (1994). Moving toward a nursing model in advanced practice. *Western Journal of Nursing Research, 16,* 205–218.

Part IV

MEASUREMENT AND DATA COLLECTION

Chapter 12

DESIGNING AND IMPLEMENTING A DATA COLLECTION PLAN

The concepts in which a researcher is interested must ultimately be translated into variables that can be observed and recorded. The tasks of defining the research variables and selecting or developing appropriate methods for collecting data are among the most challenging in the research process. Without high-quality data collection methods, the accuracy and robustness of the conclusions are always subject to challenge. As in the case of research designs and sampling plans, the researcher must often choose from an array of alternatives in deciding how to collect data. This chapter provides an overview of various alternative methods of data collection and discusses the development of a *data collection plan.*

❖ DIMENSIONS OF DATA COLLECTION APPROACHES

Many methods of collecting data are used for nursing studies. For example, subjects can be interviewed, observed by the researcher, or tested with measures of physiologic functioning. Re-gardless of what specific approach is used, data collection methods vary along four important dimensions: structure, quantifiability, researcher obtrusiveness, and objectivity.

Structure

Research data are often collected according to a highly structured plan that indicates what information is to be gathered and exactly how to gather it. For example, most self-administered questionnaires are highly structured: they include a fixed set of questions that are generally answered in a specified sequence and with predesignated response options (e.g., yes or no). In highly structured methods, there is little opportunity for subjects to qualify their answers or to explain the underlying meaning of their responses.

In some studies, however, it is more appropriate to impose a minimum of structure and to provide subjects with opportunities to reveal relevant information in a naturalistic way. Most qualitative studies rely heavily on unstructured or loosely structured methods of data collection.

Polit DF, Hungler BP: NURSING RESEARCH: PRINCIPLES AND METHODS, 5th ed. © 1995 J. B. Lippincott Company.

There are advantages and disadvantages to both structured and unstructured approaches. Structured methods often take considerable effort to develop and refine, but they yield data that are relatively easy to analyze. Structured methods are seldom appropriate for an in-depth examination of a phenomenon, however. Consider the following two methods of asking subjects about their feelings of depression:

Structured: During the past week, would you say you felt depressed:
1. Rarely or none of the time
2. Some or a little of the time
3. Occasionally or a moderate amount of the time
4. Most or all of the time

Unstructured: How sad or depressed have you been this past week? Tell me how you've been feeling.

The structured approach would allow the researcher to compute exactly what percentage of respondents felt depressed most of the time but would provide no information about the intensity, cause, or circumstances of the depression. The unstructured question, while allowing for deeper and more thoughtful responses, may pose difficulties for people who are not good at expressing themselves verbally. Moreover, the unstructured question is likely to yield data that are considerably more difficult to analyze.

When data are collected in a highly structured fashion, the researcher must develop (or borrow) what is referred to as the data collection *instrument* (or *tool*), which is the formal document used to collect and record information, such as a questionnaire. When unstructured methods are used, there is typically no formal instrument, although there may be a list of the types of information that are needed.

Quantifiability

Data that will be subjected to statistical analysis must be gathered in such a way that they can be quantified. For statistical analysis, all variables must be quantitatively measured—

even though the variables are abstract and intangible phenomena that represent *qualities* of humans, such as hope, loneliness, pain, and body image. Data that are to be analyzed qualitatively are typically collected in narrative form.

Structured data collection approaches generally yield data that are easily quantified. It is often possible (and it is sometimes useful), however, to quantify unstructured information as well. For example, responses to the unstructured question concerning depression could be categorized after the fact according to the four levels of depression indicated in the structured question. Whether it is *wise* to do so depends on the nature of the research problem, the philosophical orientation of the researcher, and the nature of the responses.

Researcher Obtrusiveness

Data collection methods differ in terms of the degree to which subjects are aware of their subject status. If subjects are fully aware of their role in a study, their behavior and responses may not be normal. When subjects distort the data, the entire value of the research can be undermined. When data are collected unobtrusively, however, ethical problems may emerge, as discussed in Chapter 6.

Subjects are most likely to distort their behavior and their responses to questions under certain circumstances. In particular, researcher obtrusiveness is likely to be most problematic when: a program is being evaluated and subjects have a vested interest in the evaluation outcome; the subjects are engaged in socially unacceptable or atypical behavior; the subjects have not complied with medical and nursing instructions; and the subjects are the type of people who have a strong need to "look good." When researcher obtrusiveness is unavoidable under any of these circumstances, the researcher should make a strong effort to put subjects at ease, to stress the importance of candor and naturalistic behavior, and to use research personnel trained to convey a neutral and nonjudgmental demeanor.

Objectivity

Objectivity refers to the degree to which two independent researchers can arrive at similar "scores" or make similar observations regarding the variables of interest, that is, make judgments regarding subjects' attributes or behavior that are not biased by personal feelings or beliefs. Some data collection approaches require more subjective judgment than others, and some research problems require a higher degree of objectivity than others.

Scientists generally strive for a reasonable amount of objectivity. Clearly, data that are strongly biased by the subjective feelings of the researcher are unlikely to be useful. However, in some research (especially, phenomenologically based research), the subjective judgment of the investigator is considered a valuable component of data collection because subjectivity is thought to be essential for the understanding of human experiences.

❖ MAJOR TYPES OF DATA COLLECTION METHODS

In addition to making decisions regarding these four dimensions, nurse researchers must select the form of data collection to use. Three types of approach have been used most frequently by nurse researchers: self-reports, observation, and biophysiologic measures. This section presents an overview of these methods, and subsequent chapters provide more in-depth guidance.

Self-Reports

In the human sciences, a good deal of information can be gathered by questioning people directly, a method known as *self-report.* If, for example, we are interested in learning about patients' perceptions of hospital care, patients' preoperative fears, or nursing students' attitudes toward gerontologic nursing, then we are likely to try to find answers by questioning a group of relevant people. For some research variables, alternatives to direct questions exist. However, the unique ability of humans to communicate verbally on a sophisticated level makes it unlikely that systematic questioning will ever be eliminated from the repertoire of data collection techniques. An analysis of published nursing studies spanning four decades revealed that most nursing investigations involve data collected by means of self-reports (Brown, Tanner, & Padrick, 1984).

The self-report method is strong with respect to its directness and versatility. If we want to know what people think, feel, or believe, the most direct means of gathering the information is to ask them about it. Perhaps the strongest argument that can be made for the self-report method is that it frequently yields information that would be difficult, if not impossible, to gather by any other means. Current behaviors can be directly observed, but only if the subject is willing to manifest them publicly. For example, it may be impossible for a researcher to observe such behaviors as child abuse, contraceptive practices, or drug usage. Furthermore, observers can only observe behaviors occurring at the time of the study; self-report instruments can gather retrospective data about activities and events occurring in the past or gather projections about behaviors in which subjects plan to engage in the future. Information about feelings, values, opinions, and motives can sometimes be inferred through observation, but behaviors and feelings do not always correspond exactly. People's actions do not always indicate their state of mind. Here again, self-report instruments can be designed to measure psychological characteristics through direct communication with the subject.

Self-reports are also versatile with respect to content coverage. People can be asked to report on facts about their personal backgrounds; facts about other people known to them; facts about events or environmental conditions; beliefs about what the facts are; attitudes, feelings, and opinions; reasons for opinions, attitudes, or behaviors; level of knowledge about conditions, situations, or practices; and intentions for future behaviors.

Despite these advantages, verbal report instruments share a number of weaknesses. The most serious issue is the question of the validity and accuracy of self-reports: How can we really be sure that respondents feel or act the way they say they do? How can we trust the information that respondents provide, particularly if the questions could potentially require them to reveal an unpopular position on a controversial issue or to admit to socially unacceptable behavior? Investigators often have no alternative but to assume that most of their respondents have been frank. Yet we all have a tendency to want to present ourselves in the best light, and this may conflict with the truth. Researchers who find it necessary or appropriate to gather self-report data should be cognizant of the limitations of this method and should be prepared to take these shortcomings into consideration when interpreting the results. Likewise, consumers of research reports should be alert to potential biases introduced when subjects are asked to describe themselves, particularly with respect to behaviors or feelings that our society judges to be wrong or unusual.

Observation

For certain types of research problems, an alternative to self-reports is direct *observation* of people's behavior. Various types of information required by nurse researchers as evidence of nursing effectiveness or as clues to improving nursing practices can be obtained through direct observation. Suppose, for instance, that we were interested in studying mental patients' methods of defending their personal territory, or children's reactions to the removal of a leg cast, or a patient's mode of emergence from anesthesia. These phenomena are all amenable to direct observation. Within nursing research, observational methods have broad applicability, particularly for clinical inquiries. Observational methods can be used fruitfully to gather a variety of information, including information on charac-

teristics and conditions of individuals (e.g., the sleep/wake state of patients); verbal communication behaviors (e.g., exchange of information at change-of-shift report); nonverbal communication behaviors (e.g., facial expressions); activities (e.g., geriatric patients' self-grooming activities); and environmental conditions (e.g., architectural barriers in the homes of disabled people).

Observations can be made in laboratory or in natural settings. In addition, observation can be done directly through the human senses or with the aid of technical apparatus, such as video equipment and tape recorders. Thus, observational methods are an extremely versatile approach to data collection.

Like self-report techniques, observational methods can vary in the degree of structure the researcher imposes. That is, a researcher could observe nurses' methods of touching patients in an unstructured manner, taking detailed narrative notes regarding their use of touch. Alternatively, the researcher could tabulate the frequency of the nurses' use of specific types of touching.

The field of nursing is particularly well suited for observational research. Nurses are in an advantageous position to observe, relatively unobtrusively, the behaviors and activities of patients, their families, and hospital staff. Moreover, nurses may by training be especially sensitive observers. Many nursing problems are better suited to an observational approach than to self-report techniques. Whenever people cannot be expected to describe adequately their own behaviors, observational methods may be needed. This may be the case when people are unaware of their own behavior (e.g., manifesting preoperative symptoms of anxiety), when people are embarrassed to report their activities (e.g., displays of aggression or hostility), when behaviors are emotionally laden (e.g., grieving behavior among the bereaved), or when people are not capable of articulating their actions (e.g., young children or the mentally ill). Observational methods have an intrinsic appeal with respect to their ability to capture a record of behaviors and events directly. Furthermore, with an observational approach, humans—the observers—are used as measuring instruments and provide a uniquely sensitive and intelligent (if fallible) tool.

Several of the shortcomings of the observational approach include possible ethical difficulties, distorted behavior on the part of the person being observed when the observer is conspicuous, and a high rate of refusals to being observed. However, one of the most pervasive problems is the vulnerability of observational data to *observer biases*. A number of factors interfere with objective observations, including the following:

- Emotions, prejudices, attitudes, and values of the observer may result in faulty inference.
- Personal interest and commitment may color what is seen in the direction of what the observer wants to see.
- Anticipation of what is to be observed may affect what is observed.
- Hasty decisions before adequate information is collected may result in erroneous classifications or conclusions.

Observational biases probably cannot be eliminated completely, but they can be minimized through the careful training of observers.

Biophysiologic Measures

The trend in nursing research has been toward increased clinical, patient-centered investigations, and this trend is likely to continue in years to come. One result of this trend is an expanded use of measures to assess the physiologic status of subjects. Physiologic and physical variables typically require specialized technical instruments and equipment for their measurement and, generally, specialized training for the interpretation of results. Settings in which nurses operate are usually filled with a wide variety of technical instruments for measuring physiologic functions. In comparison with other types of data collection tools, the equipment for obtaining physiologic measurements is costly.

However, because such equipment is generally available in health care settings, the costs to nurse researchers may be small or nonexistent.

A major strength of biophysiologic measures is their objectivity. Nurse A and nurse B, reading from the same spirometer output, are likely to record the same or highly similar tidal volume measurements for a patient. Furthermore, barring the possibility of equipment malfunctioning, two different spirometers are likely to produce identical tidal volume readouts. Another advantage of physiologic measurements is the relative precision and sensitivity that they normally offer. By relative, we are implicitly comparing physiologic instruments with devices for obtaining various psychological measurements, such as self-report measures of anxiety, pain, attitudes, and so forth. Patients are unlikely to be able to deliberately distort measurements of physiologic functioning. Furthermore, researchers are generally confident that physiologic instrumentation provides measures of those variables in which they are interested: thermometers can be depended on to measure temperature and not blood volume, and so forth. For nonphysiologic measurements, the question of whether a measuring tool is really measuring the target concept is a continuously perplexing problem.

Physiologic measures also have some disadvantages. For example, the highly technical nature of the equipment may constitute a difficulty because the failure of nonengineers to understand the limitations of the instruments may result in greater faith in their accuracy than is warranted. Another problem, which physiologic measures share with other data collection approaches, is the effect that the measuring tool itself has on the variables it is attempting to measure. For instance, a flow transducer located in a blood vessel partially blocks that vessel and, hence, alters the pressure–flow characteristics being measured. Another difficulty is that there are normally interferences that create artifacts in physiologic measurements. For example, the subject may create artifactual signals, particularly when the subject's movements result in movements of sensing devices. Finally, energy must often be applied to the organism when making the physiologic measurements, which means that extreme caution must continually be exercised to avoid the risk of damaging cells by high-energy concentrations. Any researcher utilizing electrical equipment should be thoroughly familiar with safety rules and considerations such as grounding specifications.

❖ DEVELOPING A DATA COLLECTION PLAN

Sometimes the nature of the research question dictates which specific method of data collection to use and where along the four continua described in the first section the methods should lie. Often, however, the researcher has considerable latitude in selecting or designing a data collection plan. In all cases, the plan should strive to yield accurate, trustworthy, and meaningful data that are maximally effective in answering the research questions. These are rigorous requirements, and to be successful, the researcher usually needs to devote considerable time and effort. This section discusses steps that are often undertaken in the development of a data collection plan. Figure 12-1 provides on overview of the procedures often used in developing such a plan for quantitative studies.

Identifying Data Needs

The researcher must generally begin by identifying the types of data that are needed to complete the study successfully. Typically, the researcher needs to gather information about more than just the main study variables. Advance planning may help the researcher avoid "if only" disappointments at the analysis stage.

In a quantitative study, the researcher should give thoughtful consideration to what the data needs are for accomplishing the following:

1. *Testing the hypotheses or addressing all the research questions*. The researcher must

include one or more measures of all the independent and dependent variables. Multiple measures of some variables may be required if a variable is complex and multifaceted or if there are concerns about the accuracy of a single measure.

2. *Describing the main characteristics of the sample*. Information should normally be gathered about major demographic characteristics of the sample and about relevant aspects of the subjects' health status. It is almost always advisable to gather information about the subjects' age, gender, race or ethnicity, educational background, marital status, and income level or type of occupation. This information is critical in interpreting the results and in understanding the population to whom the findings can be generalized. If the sample includes subjects with a health problem, data on the nature of that problem also should be gathered (e.g., length of illness, severity of health problem, types of treatment obtained, length of stay in hospital, and so on).

3. *Controlling for important sources of extraneous variables*. As discussed in Chapter 10, various approaches can be used to control extraneous variables, and many of them require the measurement of those variables. For example, when analysis of covariance is used, each of the variables that is statistically controlled must be measured. Even if a researcher uses a design that does not control all important extraneous variables, it is usually a good idea to measure them because then their relationship with the key research variables can be examined. Thought should be given to gathering data on both external and intrinsic factors that could influence the outcomes.

4. *Analyzing potential biases*. Ideally, data that can help the researcher to identify potential biases should be collected. For example, in a nonequivalent control group design, the researcher should gather infor-

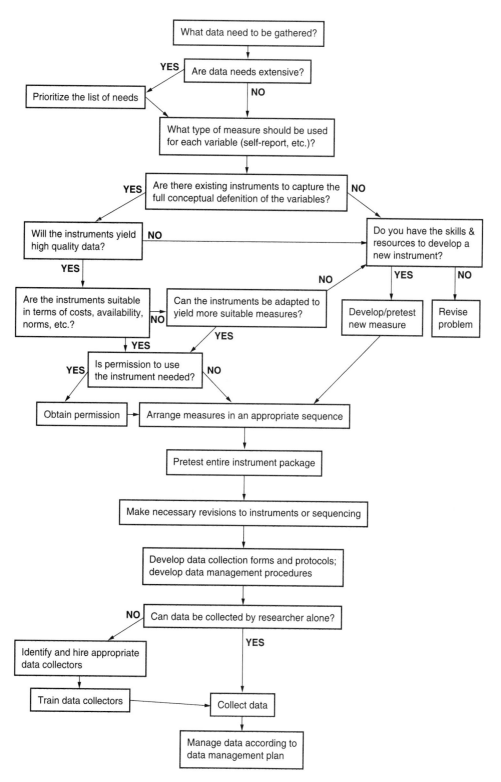

Figure 12-1. *Developing a data collection plan for quantitative studies.*

mation that would help to identify selection biases. As another example, if the researcher is collecting self-report data about a socially unacceptable characteristic or behavior, it might be advisable to administer a special test (e.g., the Marlowe-Crowne Social Desirability Scale) to determine whether respondents have a tendency to give responses that are biased in the direction of "looking good." In general, the researcher should give some thought to what potential sources of biases may arise and then determine whether or not they can be measured.

5. *Understanding subgroup effects.* It is often desirable to answer the research questions not only for the entire sample of subjects but also for certain subgroups of subjects. For example, we may wish to know if a special intervention for indigent pregnant women is equally effective for primiparas and multiparas. In such a situation, we would need to collect information about the subjects' childbearing history so that we could divide the sample and analyze for separate *subgroup effects.*

6. *Interpreting the results.* The researcher should try to anticipate alternative patterns of results and then determine what types of data would best help in interpreting those results. For example, if we hypothesized that the presence of school-based clinics in high schools would lower the incidence of sexually transmitted diseases among students but found that the incidence remained constant after the clinic was established, what type of information would we want to have to help us interpret this result (e.g., information about the students' frequency of intercourse, number of partners, use of condoms, and so on)?

7. *Checking on the manipulation.* When a researcher manipulates the independent variable, it is sometimes advisable to gather information to determine if the manipulation was successful. Such a *manipulation check* provides a mechanism for in-

terpreting negative results. As an example, if a researcher were studying the impact of a new hospital policy on the morale of the nursing staff, it might be important to determine the nurses' level of awareness of the new policy because if the results indicate no change in staff morale, this could reflect lack of awareness of the policy rather than dissatisfaction with it.

8. *Obtaining administrative information.* It is almost always necessary to gather various types of administrative information to help in the management of the project. For example, if there are multiple observers, it is desirable to record separate identification numbers for each one on all observational forms. Other types of administrative information might include subject identification numbers, dates of attempted contact with subjects, dates of actual data collection, where the data collection occurred, when the data collection session began and ended, reasons that a potential subject did not participate in the study, and contact information if the study is longitudinal.

The list of possible data needs may seem daunting, but in actuality, many categories overlap. For example, variables that are useful in describing subject characteristics are often important extraneous variables or are useful in the creation of subgroups. If time or resource constraints make it impossible to collect the full range of variables, then the researcher should prioritize data needs and be aware of how the absence of certain variables will affect the study's integrity. The important point here is that researchers should understand what their data needs are and take steps to ensure the fullest possible coverage.

In qualitative studies, the data collection plan usually is more fluid, with decisions about types of data to collect often evolving in the field. For example, as the researcher begins to gather and digest information, it may become apparent that it would be fruitful to pursue a certain line of questioning that had not originally been anticipated. However, even while allowing and profiting from this flexibility, qualitative researchers should make some up-front decisions about the type of data they will need to obtain initially (e.g., data on sample characteristics, administrative information, and so on).

Selecting Types of Measures

After data needs have been identified, the next step is to select a method to measure each variable and to determine where on the four dimensions mentioned earlier (structure, quantifiability, obtrusiveness, and objectivity) the variables will lie. It is common, and often advantageous, to use a multi-method approach. Researchers have profitably combined self-reports, observations, and physiologic measures in a single study. Researchers have also combined measures that vary in terms of the four basic dimensions. In reviewing the data needs, the researcher should determine how best to capture each of the variables of interest in terms of its conceptual or theoretical definition.

Research considerations, unfortunately, are not the only factors that drive decisions about the specific methods to use in collecting data. The decisions must also be guided by ethical considerations, cost constraints, the availability of appropriate staff to help with data collection, time constraints on the researcher's part, and the anticipated burden to the subjects and to others not associated with the project, such as hospital staff or the subject's family.

Data collection is typically the costliest and most time-consuming portion of a study. Because of this, the researcher is likely to have to make a number of compromises about the type or amount of data collected.

Selecting and Developing Instruments

Once preliminary decisions have been made regarding the basic data collection methods to be used, the researcher should determine if there are instruments already available to measure the constructs of interest for those variables being measured in a structured fashion. For most constructs, existing instruments will be available and should be reviewed. In the next three chapters, we provide sources for locating existing self-report, observational, and other measures.

After potential data collection instruments have been identified and retrieved, they should be carefully reviewed to determine their appropriateness for the study. The primary consideration is whether the instrument is conceptually relevant: Does the instrument capture your conceptual definition of the variable? The next factor to consider is whether the instrument is likely to yield data of a sufficiently high quality. Approaches to evaluating data quality for both qualitative and quantitative data collection methods are discussed in detail in Chapter 16. Six other issues that often affect the researcher's decisions in selecting an instrument are as follows:

1. *Resources.* Resource constraints sometimes make it impossible to use ideal measures. There may be some direct costs associated with the measure (e.g., some psychological tests must be purchased from publishers, or some physiologic equipment may have to be rented). The biggest data collection cost often involves compensation to the people who are collecting data if the researcher cannot do it single-handedly (e.g., hired interviewers or observers). In such a situation, the length of the instrument and time it takes to administer may determine whether it can be used. Also, if the data collection procedures are considered burdensome, it may be necessary to pay a respondent stipend. All the associated costs of data collection should be carefully considered, especially if the use of time-consuming or expensive measures means that the investigator will be forced to cut costs elsewhere (e.g., by using a smaller sample).

2. *Availability and familiarity.* In selecting measures, the researcher may want to consider how readily available or accessible various tools are, especially if they are biophysiologic in nature. Similarly, data collection strategies with which the researcher is familiar or has had experience are generally preferable to new measures because administration is generally smoother and more efficient in such cases.

3. *Norms and comparability.* A researcher may find it desirable to select a measure for which there are relevant norms. *Norms* indicate the "normal" values and distribution of values on the measure with respect to a specified population. For example, most standardized tests (such as the Scholastic Aptitude Test) have national norms. The availability of norms is often useful because norms offer, in essence, a built-in comparison group. For similar reasons, a researcher may decide that it is useful to adopt a specific instrument because it was used in other similar studies and therefore offers a supplementary basis for putting the study findings in context. Indeed, when a study is an intentional replication, it is often essential to use the same instruments as were used in the original study, even if higher-quality measures are available.

4. *Population appropriateness.* The measure should be chosen with the characteristics of the target population in mind. Characteristics of special importance include the age of the subjects, their intellectual abilities or reading skills, and their cultural or ethnic background. If there is concern about the reading skills of the research sample, it may be necessary to calculate the *readability* of a prospective instrument using procedures such as those described in Gunning (1968) or Fry (1968). If the subjects include members of minority groups, the researcher should strive to identify instruments that are not culturally biased, especially if racial or ethnic comparisons will

be made. If non–English-speaking subjects are included in the sample, then the selection of a measure may be based, in part, on the availability of a translated version of the measure.

5. *Administration issues.* An important consideration often relates to the instrument's requirements for obtaining high-quality data. For example, in obtaining information about the developmental status of children, the researcher may want to consider whether the administration of a given measure requires the skills of a professional psychologist or whether an interviewer with adequate training can obtain high-quality data. Another administration issue concerns constraints on where the data must be collected. Certain instruments may require or assume stringent conditions with regard to the time of administration, privacy of the setting, and so on. In such a case, requirements for obtaining valid measures must match the characteristics of the intended research setting.

6. *Reputation.* Instruments designed to measure the same construct often differ in the kinds of reputation they enjoy among specialists working in a field, even if they are comparable with regard to quality. Therefore, a researcher selecting an instrument should seek the advice of knowledgeable individuals, preferably people with personal, direct experience in using the instruments.

Based on such considerations, you may conclude that existing instruments are not suitable for all your research variables. In such a situation, you will be faced with either adapting an existing instrument to make it more appropriate or developing a new one. The development of a new instrument should be considered a last resort, especially for novice researchers, because it is extremely difficult to develop accurate and valid measuring tools. However, there are situations in which there is no acceptable alternative. In the next few chapters, we provide some guidance for those who elect to construct a new instrument, but in some cases, it may make more sense to modify the research question so that existing instruments can be used.

If you are fortunate in identifying an existing instrument that is suitable for your study, it is likely that your next step will be to obtain written permission to use or adapt it from the person who developed it (or from the publisher, if it is a commercially distributed instrument). In general, copyrighted materials always require permission. Instruments that have been developed under a federal grant are usually in the public domain, and so do not require permission, because they have been supported with taxpayers' dollars. When in doubt, however, it is best to obtain permission. By contacting the author of an instrument to obtain permission, it is likely that you will also obtain more detailed information about the instrument and its quality than was available in a published report.

Pretesting the Data Collection Package

Researchers who develop their own instrument typically subject it to rigorous *pretesting* so that it can be evaluated and refined. However, even when the data collection plan involves the use of existing instruments, it is usually wise to conduct a small pretest.*

One purpose of a pretest is to determine the length of time it takes to administer the entire instrument package and whether subjects feel that the time burden is too great. Typically, the researcher uses more than one instrument because there are usually many variables to be measured. It is often difficult to estimate in advance how long it will take to administer a complete package of instruments, and such esti-

---

* Some writers use the terms *pretest* and *pilot study* interchangeably. That is, some researchers say that they undertook a pilot study to test their instruments, while others say that they pretested their instruments. However, a pilot study often involves a small-scale test of the entire study, that is, a testing of not only instruments but also the sampling plan, the intervention, the study procedures, and so on.

mates may be required for informed consent purposes or for developing a more realistic project budget. If the pretest instruments require more time than is considered acceptable, it may be necessary to eliminate certain variables or instruments, guided by the prioritization list established early in the process.

Pretests can serve many other purposes, including the following:

- Identifying any parts of the instrument package that are difficult for the particular population of subjects to read or understand
- Identifying any parts of the data collection package that the subjects find objectionable or offensive
- Determining if the sequencing of instruments within the data collection package is smooth and effective
- Determining needs for the training of the data collection staff
- Determining if the measures yield data with sufficient variability

The last purpose requires a bit of explanation. For most research questions, the instruments should ideally discriminate among subjects with different levels of an attribute. If we are asking, for example, whether women experience greater depression than men when they learn of a cancer diagnosis, we need an instrument capable of distinguishing between people with higher and lower levels of depression. If an instrument yields data with limited variability, then it will be impossible to detect a difference in depression between men and women—even when such a difference actually exists. Thus, a researcher should look at pretest variation in key research variables. If, to pursue the example, the entire pretest sample looks very depressed (or not at all depressed), it may be necessary to modify the instruments.

Developing Data Collection Forms and Procedures

After the instrument package has been finalized, the researcher is faced with a number of tasks that are primarily administrative in nature. First, appropriate forms for the collection of the instrument must be developed for data collected in a structured manner. In some studies, many forms have to be developed, for example, forms for screening potential subjects to determine their eligibility, informed consent forms, forms for explaining the study to prospective subjects, records of attempted contacts with subjects, forms for recording actual research data, contact information forms, and administrative logs for recording the receipt of research forms. The researcher should ensure that forms that will actually be used by subjects are attractively formatted, legible, and inviting to use. Care should also be taken to design forms in such a way that confidentiality can be ensured. For example, identification information such as names and addresses is often recorded on a separate page that can be detached and kept separate from other types of data.

In most quantitative studies, the researcher also develops protocols that spell out the procedures to be used in data collection. These protocols describe such considerations as the following:

- Specification of any conditions that must be met for collecting the data (e.g., Can others be present at the time of data collection? Where must data collection occur?)
- Specific procedures for collecting the data, including requirements for sequencing instruments and recording information
- Standard information to provide subjects who ask routine questions about the study. These questions may include the following: How will the information from this study be used? How did you get my name and why are you asking me? How long will this take? Who will have access to this information? What are the possible benefits and risks?
- Procedures to follow in the event that the subject becomes distraught, disoriented, or for any other reason cannot complete the data collection
- A full listing of all materials that will be required during each data collection session

(forms, notebooks, writing materials, stipends, and so on).

Finally, procedures and forms may need to be developed for managing data as they are gathered, especially if data are being gathered from multiple sites or over an extended period. For example, in an observational study, a data management form might record, for each case, the date the observation was scheduled to take place, the date it actually took place, the date the observation forms were received back in some central location, whether all forms were received, and the date the data were coded and the information entered onto a computer file.

In qualitative studies, there is usually considerably less emphasis on the development of specific forms and protocols because data collection strategies evolve in the field. Nevertheless, the researcher may need to develop a few forms, such as a form for gathering demographic and administrative information or logbook forms for recording narrative information. Also, a preliminary list of questions to be asked or types of observation to be made during the initial data collection is usually useful. Finally, the researcher should make a list of everything that will be needed during data collection, including forms, clipboards, pencils, recording equipment such as tape recorders or cameras, gifts or stipends, and computer equipment.

❖ IMPLEMENTING A DATA COLLECTION PLAN

The quality of data for a research project is affected by the decisions that shape the data collection plan. Data quality is also affected by how the plan is actually implemented.

Selecting Research Personnel

An important decision concerns who will actually collect the research data. In many small research projects, the researchers in charge of the study collect the data themselves. In larger studies, however, this may not be feasible. When data are to be collected by others, great care must be taken to select appropriate research staff. In most studies, the research staff should be neutral agents through whom the data will pass—that is, the characteristics or behavior of the research personnel should not alter or affect the data in any way. Some of the considerations that should be kept in mind when selecting research personnel are as follows:

- *Experience.* Ideally, the research staff should have prior experience with data collection. For example, for a self-report study, it is advantageous to use data collectors who have experience conducting interviews. If it is necessary to use an inexperienced person, it is important to look for someone who can readily acquire the necessary skills (e.g., an interviewer should have good reading and verbal skills).
- *Congruity with sample characteristics.* To the extent possible, it is strongly recommended that staff be hired to match the backgrounds of the subjects with respect to such characteristics as racial or cultural background, gender, and age. In some studies, this is an absolute requirement (e.g., hiring a person who speaks the language of an immigrant sample). The greater the sensitivity of the research questions, the greater the desirability of matching characteristics. For example, in a study of the sexual behavior of pregnant African American teenagers, the data collectors would ideally be African American women in their twenties.
- *Unremarkable appearance.* Extremes of appearance should generally be avoided because subjects may react to extremes and may alter their behavior or responses accordingly. For example, data collectors should generally not be very old or very young. They should not dress extremely casually (e.g., in shorts and tee shirts), nor very formally (e.g., with elaborate jewelry). While on the job, data collectors should never wear any article that would convey their political or social views (e.g., political buttons, jewelry with peace symbols, and so on).
- *Personality.* Data collectors should be pleasant (but not effusive); sociable (but not overly talkative or overbearing); and nonjudgmental (but not apathetic or unfeeling about the subjects' lives). The goal is to have nonthreatening data collectors who can encourage candor and put subjects at ease without interjecting their own values and biases.
- *Availability.* Data collectors should ideally be available for the entire data collection period to avoid having to recruit and train new staff. If the study is longitudinal, it is advantageous to hire data collectors who could potentially be available for subsequent rounds of data collection.

In some situations, the researcher will not be able to select research personnel. For example, the data collectors may be the staff nurses employed at a hospital or graduate students in the school of nursing. Particularly in such situations, training of the data collection staff is important.

Training Data Collectors

Depending on the prior experience of the research personnel, training will need to cover both general procedures (e.g., how to conduct an interview) and procedures specific to the study (e.g., how to administer a particular set of questions or make certain observations). Training can often be accomplished in a single day, but in complex projects, it may require more time. The lead researcher is usually the best person to conduct the training and to develop training materials.

The data collection protocols, as discussed in the previous section, are usually a good foundation for the development of a *training manual*. The manual normally includes background materials, general instructions, specific instructions, and copies of all the data collection and administrative forms. Table 12-1 presents an

Table 12-1. *Example of a Table of Contents: Training Manual for an Interview Study*

example of a table of contents for a training manual for an interview study.

The heart of a training manual is the detailed instructions relating to the administration of the specific data collection instruments (in Table 12-1, these appear in section IV.C). These instructions are usually intended to provide complete information about exactly what the researcher is looking for so that there is no ambiguity about the nature of the data to be obtained. As an example, Table 12-2 provides a *Q-by-Q* (question-by-question instruction) for two structured questions.

The agenda for the training should generally cover the content of the training manual, elaborating on any portion that is especially difficult or complex. The training often includes demonstrations by the research team of fictitious data collection episodes, performed either live or on videotape. Finally, the training usually involves having the trainees do trial runs of data collection in front of the trainers to demonstrate their understanding of the instructions.

❖ TIPS FOR DEVELOPING AND IMPLEMENTING DATA COLLECTION PLANS

Much of this chapter was devoted to guidance on how to develop and implement a data collection plan. We offer here a few additional tips.

- Although the flow chart in Figure 12-1 suggests a fairly linear process, the development of a data collection plan is often an iterative one. Be prepared to backtrack and make adjustments, recognizing that the ultimate goal is not to get to the bottom of the list of steps but rather to ensure that the process yields conceptually relevant data of the highest possible quality.
- If compromises have to be made between data quality and data quantity, it is usually preferable to forego quantity. For example, it is better to have an excellent measure of the dependent variable with no supplementary measures to help in interpreting outcomes than to have mediocre measures of all desired variables. When data quality for key variables is poor, the results cannot be trusted, so additional information cannot possibly help to clarify the findings.
- Try to avoid, to the fullest extent possible, reinventing the wheel. It is inefficient and unnecessary to start from scratch—not only in developing an instrument but also in developing specific forms, protocols, training materials, and so on. Ask seasoned researchers if they have any materials that you

Table 12-2. *Examples of Question-by-Question Specifications*

Question: During the past year, did your child have an injury, poisoning, or other accident that required medical attention?

Q-by-Q: This question asks whether the respondent's child had an injury, poisoning, or other type of accident that required *medical* attention. Included would be examination or treatment by a doctor, nurse, emergency medical technician, or other trained person—not simply application of a bandage at home or something else the respondent might do herself or himself. The response should be "yes" *only* if the injury, poisoning, or accident occurred within the 12 months before the date of the interview.

Question: During your current pregnancy, have you made any visits to a doctor or nurse for prenatal care, that is, to be examined or talk about your pregnancy?

Q-by-Q: This question asks if the respondent obtained prenatal care during this pregnancy. Being tested for pregnancy does *not* by itself constitute prenatal care, nor does obtaining pregnancy or abortion counseling. Prenatal care is concerned with the health and well-being of the mother and fetus and with a successful birth outcome. Prenatal care can be provided by a doctor, nurse, or midwife.

may borrow or adapt for your study. Much of the material relating to data collection plans will *not* be available in published research articles (although it may be available in dissertations or research reports to federal funding agencies).

• Document what you are doing as you develop and implement your data collection plan—and save your documentation. You may need the information later in writing your research report, in requesting funding for a follow-up study, or in helping another researcher.

❖ RESEARCH EXAMPLES

Data collection procedures are often not described in detail in research reports owing to space constraints in journals. However, a few examples of exemplary data collection procedures that were described in research journals are presented in Table 12-3. The examples represent efforts the researchers made to achieve high-quality data. The following is a more detailed example of the data collection plan used in a nursing study.

Mercer, Ferketich, and DeJoseph (1993) examined partner relationships among 371 pregnant women. They tested a conceptual model of the influence of antepartal stress on partner relationships during pregnancy and early parenthood among those in high-risk and low-risk pregnancies. The model was based on earlier research of the study team.

Data were collected longitudinally through interviews and self-administered questionnaires with the pregnant women and, when possible, with their partners. Data were collected at five points in time: before delivery, during postpartal hospitalization, and at 1, 4, and 8 months after delivery.

The authors indicated that six criteria were used to select their battery of instruments: 1) evidence from prior studies that the instrument yielded high-quality data; 2) conceptual congruence with the theoretical underpinnings of the researcher's model; 3) standardization of the instruments for both men and women; 4) previous use in studies of child-bearing families; 5) the clarity of individual questions in the instruments; and 6) instrument brevity. As an example of an instrument they selected, the dependent variable (partner relationship) was operationalized by the Locke-Wallace Marital Adjustment Test, a relatively brief measure of dyadic adjustment that had previously demonstrated adequate data quality. The investigators conducted a pilot study to test the clarity and acceptability of the instrument package to subjects.

The interviewers for this study were primarily graduate nursing students, all of

Table 12-3.   *Examples of Exemplary Data Collection Procedures*

RESEARCH QUESTION	DATA COLLECTION PROCEDURE
What is the efficacy of specialized and traditional AIDS education programs for impoverished women of color? (Nyamathi, Leake, Flaskerud, Lewis, & Bennett, 1993)	Trained African American and Latina nurses and outreach workers (i.e., culturally matched to subjects) collected all data.
Can a reliable and useful measure of impaired cognition among the elderly, using everyday indicators of impairment, be developed? (Algase & Beel-Bates, 1993)	Trained nurses with clinical geriatric experience collected the data by interview. If a subject became restless or uncooperative, data collection was stopped and reattempted after a half-hour interval.
What are the ways in which primary caregivers to older relatives manage the caregiving experience? (Langner, 1993)	In-depth interview guides were developed based on a literature review and the researcher's clinical experience. A pilot study was used to refine the guide for clarity, content, and length. As the qualitative study progressed, new questions evolved and were added to the interview.
What factors influence the behaviors of institutional caregivers when they interact with institutionalized, cognitively impaired elders? (Burgener & Shimer, 1993)	Observations were made as unobtrusively as possible; to decrease sensitivity of subjects to the research team's presence, researchers spent time in the units before data collection. Every week during data collection, observers simultaneously observed the same episode and compared their observations to ensure a continuing level of consistency and objectivity.
What is the level of maternal confidence among Latina mothers with low-birthweight infants? (Zahr, 1993)	Self-report data were collected by a Latina research assistant who spoke fluent Spanish. Observational data were collected by six nurses who were trained in the use of the observational instrument and achieved adequate levels of agreement with the trainer on observational ratings.

whom were trained and supervised by the project director. Team meetings were frequently held during the data collection period to ensure that consistent approaches to interviewing were maintained.

❖ SUMMARY

In developing a *data collection plan*, nurse researchers have available to them a wide variety of data collection approaches. Data collection methods vary along four important dimensions: structure, quantifiability, researcher obtrusive-

ness, and objectivity. Qualitative studies tend to be low on these dimensions, while quantitative studies tend to be high on them, but the researcher often has latitude in customizing a strategy. When research is highly structured, the researcher often uses formal data collection *instruments* or *tools*.

The three principal data collection approaches are self-report, observation, and biophysiologic measures. Most nursing research studies involve the use of *self-reports*, that is, data obtained by directly questioning subjects regarding the phenomena of interest. The self-report method is strong with respect to its di-

rectness and versatility, but the major drawback is the potential for deliberate or unconscious distortions on the part of respondents. *Observational methods* are techniques for obtaining data through the direct observation of phenomena. A wide variety of human activity and traits are amenable to observation, including phenomena that may otherwise be impossible to measure in any other fashion. However, observation is subject to a variety of *observer biases* and may also result in distorted behavior on the part of subjects. *Biophysiologic measures*, which are being used with greater frequency in clinical studies, tend to yield data that are objective and valid, although they are not immune to a variety of technical problems.

Qualitative studies often adopt data collection plans that are flexible and that evolve as the study progresses. Most quantitative studies, however, require considerable advance planning and progress through a series of specific steps—the first of which is a thorough identification and prioritization of all data needs. In addition to data for answering research questions, data may be needed to describe the sample, control extraneous variables, analyze biases, understand *subgroup effects*, interpret results, perform *manipulation checks*, and obtain administrative information.

Once the researcher has made decisions about data needs and data collection methods, existing measures of the variables should be sought for use or adaptation. The construction of new instruments requires considerable time and skill and should be undertaken only as a last resort. The selection of existing instruments should be based on such considerations as conceptual appropriateness, expected data quality, cost, population appropriateness, and reputation. Even when existing instruments are used, the instrument package should usually be pretested to determine its length, clarity, and overall suitability.

Before implementing the data collection plan, the researcher usually must develop data collection protocols, data collection forms, and data management procedures. When the re-searcher cannot collect the data without assistance, he or she should carefully select and train the data collection staff.

❖ STUDY SUGGESTIONS

Chapter 12 of the accompanying *Study Guide for Nursing Research, Principles and Methods, 5th ed.*, offers various exercises and study suggestions for reinforcing the concepts presented in this chapter. Additionally, the following study questions can be addressed:

1. Indicate which method of data collection (self-report, observation, etc.) you would use to operationalize the following variables, and why you have made that choice:
   a. Stress in hospitalized children
   b. Activity level among the noninstitutionalized elderly
   c. Pain in cancer patients
   d. Body image among obese individuals
2. Read a recent research report in a nursing journal, paying especially close attention to the data collection plan. What information about procedures that may affect data quality is missing from the report? How, if at all, does this absence affect your acceptance of the researchers' conclusions?
3. Read the following article and indicate which types of data (according to those listed in the section entitled Identifying Data Needs) were collected: Maloni, J. A., Chance, B., Zhang, C., Cohen, A. W., Betts, D., & Gange, S. J. (1993). Physical and psychosocial side effects of antepartum hospital bed rest. *Nursing Research, 42,* 297–303.

❖ SUGGESTED READINGS

METHODOLOGICAL REFERENCES

Brown, J. S., Tanner, C. A., & Padrick, K. (1984). Nursing's search for scientific knowledge. *Nursing Research, 33,* 26–32.

Collins, C., Given, B., Given, C. W., & King, S. (1988). Interviewer training and supervision. *Nursing Research, 37,* 122–124.

Davis, L. L. (1992). Instrument review: Getting the most from a panel of experts. *Applied Nursing Research, 5,* 194–197.

Fry, E. (1968). A readability formula that saves time. *Journal of Reading, 11,* 513–515.

Gunning, R. (1968). *The technique of clear writing* (rev. ed.). New York: McGraw Hill.

Jacobson, S. F. (1988). Evaluating instruments for use in clinical nursing research. In M. Frank-Stromberg (Ed.), *Instruments for clinical nursing research.* Norwalk, CT: Appleton & Lange.

Marlowe, D. P., & Crowne, D. (1960). A new scale of social desirability independent of psychopathology. *Journal of Consulting Psychology, 24,* 349–354.

Martin, P. A. (1993). Data management for surveys. *Applied Nursing Research, 6,* 142–144.

Reineck, C. (1991). Nursing research instruments: Pathway to resources. *Applied Nursing Research, 4,* 34–45.

Rew, L., Bechtel, D., & Sapp, A. (1993). Self-as-instrument in qualitative research. *Nursing Research, 42,* 300–301.

SUBSTANTIVE REFERENCES

Algase, D. L., & Beel-Bates, C. A. (1993). Everyday indicators of impaired cognition: Development of a new screening scale. *Research in Nursing and Health, 16,* 57–66.

Burgener, S. C., & Shimer, R. (1993). Variables related to caregiver behaviors with cognitively impaired elders in institutional settings. *Research in Nursing and Health, 16,* 193–202.

Langner, S. R. (1993). Ways of managing the experience of caregiving to elderly relatives. *Western Journal of Nursing Research, 15,* 582–594.

Mercer, R. T., Ferketich, S. L., & DeJoseph, J. F. (1993). Predictors of partner relationships during pregnancy and infancy. *Research in Nursing and Health, 16,* 45–56.

Nyamathi, A. M., Leake, B., Flaskerud, J, Lewis, C., & Bennett, C. (1993). Outcomes of specialized and traditional AIDS counseling programs for impoverished women of color. *Research in Nursing and Health, 16,* 11–21.

Zahr, L. K. (1993). The confidence of Latina mothers in the care of their low birth weight infants. *Research in Nursing and Health, 16,* 335–342.

Chapter 13

SELF-REPORTS

Self-report data can be gathered either orally by interview or in writing by questionnaire. Interviews (and, to a lesser extent, questionnaires) can vary considerably with respect to their degree of structure and their question type. We begin by reviewing various alternatives to collecting unstructured self-report data.

❖ UNSTRUCTURED AND SEMI-STRUCTURED SELF-REPORT TECHNIQUES

Unstructured or loosely structured self-report methods offer the researcher flexibility in gathering information from research subjects. When these methods are used, the researcher generally does not have a specific set of questions that must be asked in a specific order and worded in a given way. Instead, the researcher starts with some general questions or topics and allows the respondents (or *informants,* as they are often called in such studies) to tell their stories in a narrative fashion. Unstructured or semi-structured interviews, in other words, tend to be conversational and interactive in nature. Qualitative

self-report studies almost always use such an approach to gathering data.

Types of Unstructured Self-Reports

Researchers use various approaches in collecting unstructured or semi-structured self-report data. The main methods are briefly described next.

1. *Unstructured interview.* When a researcher proceeds with no preconceived view of the content or flow of information to be gathered, he or she may conduct unstructured interviews with respondents. *Unstructured interviews* are conversational and typically are conducted in naturalistic settings. Their aim is to elucidate the respondents' perceptions of the world without imposing any of the researcher's views on them. A researcher using a completely unstructured approach may informally ask a broad question (sometimes called a *grand tour question*) relating to the topic under investigation, such as, "Tell me

about what happened when you first learned you had AIDS?" Subsequent questions are more focused and are guided by responses to the broad question. Ethnographic and phenomenological studies generally rely heavily on unstructured interviews.

2. *Focused interview.* A researcher often wants to be sure that a given set of topics is covered in interviews with research subjects. In a *semi-structured* or *focused interview,* the interviewer is given a list of areas or questions to be covered with each respondent; the list is referred to as a *topic guide.* The interviewer's function is to encourage participants to talk freely about all the topics on the list and to record the responses, usually by tape recorder. Focused interviews are the most widely used method of collecting unstructured self-report data.

3. *Focus group interview.* A variant of the focused interview is the focus group interview, a technique that is becoming increasingly popular in the study of some health problems. In a *focus group interview,* a group of usually 5 to 15 people is assembled for a group discussion. The interviewer (often called a *moderator*) guides the discussion according to a written set of questions or topics to be covered. A major advantage of a group format is that it is efficient—the researcher obtains the viewpoints of many individuals in a short time. One disadvantage is that some people are uncomfortable about expressing their views in front of a group.

4. *Life histories. Life histories* are narrative self-disclosures about a person's life experiences. Anthropologists frequently use the life history approach to learn about cultural patterns. With this approach, the researcher asks the respondents to provide, in chronologic sequence, a narration of their ideas and experiences regarding some theme, either orally or in writing. Leininger (1985) noted that comparative life histories are especially valuable for the study of the patterns and meanings of health and health care among elderly people. Her highly regarded essay provides a protocol for obtaining a life health care history.

5. *Critical incidents.* The *critical incidents technique* is a method of gathering information about people's behaviors by examining specific incidents relating to the behavior under investigation. The technique, as the name suggests, focuses on a factual incident, which may be defined as an observable and integral episode of human behavior. The word critical means that the incident must have a discernible impact on some outcome; it must make either a positive or negative contribution to the accomplishment of some activity of interest. For example, if we were interested in understanding why patients do not always follow their medication regimen, we might ask a sample of patients the following questions: "Think of the last time you failed to take your medications as prescribed. What led up to the situation? Exactly what did you do? Why did you feel it would be all right to miss taking the medicine?" The technique differs from other self-report approaches in that it focuses on something specific about which the respondent can be expected to testify as an expert witness. As an example, Janson-Bjerklie and her colleagues (1993) used the critical incidents technique to examine asthmatic episodes in a sample of asthmatic adults.

6. *Diaries.* Personal diaries have long been used as a source of data in historical research. It is also possible to generate new data for a nonhistorical study by asking subjects to maintain a diary over a specified period. The diaries may be completely unstructured; for example, individuals who have undergone an organ transplantation could be asked simply to spend 10 minutes a day jotting down their thoughts and feelings. Frequently, however, sub-

jects are requested to make entries into a diary regarding some specific aspect of their experience, sometimes in a semi-structured format. For example, studies of the effect of nutrition during pregnancy on fetal outcomes frequently require subjects to maintain a complete diary of everything they ate over a 1- to 2-week period. Nurse researchers have used health diaries to collect information about how people prevent illness, maintain health, experience morbidity, and treat health problems.

Gathering Unstructured Self-Report Data

In most cases, the primary purpose of gathering unstructured self-report data is to enable the researcher to construct reality in ways that are consistent with the construction of the people being studied. This goal requires the researcher to take steps to overcome communication barriers and to enhance the flow of meaning. An important issue is that the researcher and the respondents should have a common vocabulary. If the researcher is studying a different culture or a subgroup that uses distinctive terms or slang, efforts should be made even before data collection to understand those terms and their nuances.

Although unstructured interviews are conversational in nature, this does not mean that they should be entered into casually. The conversations are purposeful ones that require advance thought and preparation. For example, careful thought should be given to the wording of questions. To the extent possible, the wording should make sense to the respondent and reflect his or her world view.

In addition to being a good questioner, the interviewer must be a good listener. Only by attending carefully to what the respondent is saying can the in-depth interviewer develop appropriate follow-up questions. Even when a topic guide is used, the interviewer must not let the flow of dialogue be bound by those questions. In unstructured interviews on a particular theme, many questions that appear on a topic guide are answered spontaneously over the course of the interview, usually out of sequence.

The researcher generally prepares for the interview by developing (mentally or in writing) the broad questions to be asked, and often by practicing the interview with a stand-in respondent. The researcher must also prepare respondents for the interview by putting them at ease insofar as is possible. Part of this process involves sharing pertinent information about the study (e.g., about the study aims and protection of confidentiality). Another part of this process is using the first few minutes for pleasantries and ice-breaking exchanges of conversation before the actual questioning begins.

Unstructured interviews are typically long—sometimes lasting up to several hours. Researchers often find that the respondents' construction of their experience only begins to emerge after lengthy, in-depth dialogues. The issue of how best to record such abundant information is a difficult one. Some researchers take sketchy notes as the interview progresses, filling in the details as soon as is practical after the interview is completed. Others prefer tape recording the interviews for later full transcription. Although some respondents balk or are overly self-conscious when their conversation is recorded, respondents typically forget about the presence of recording equipment after a few minutes. It is often useful to both tape record the interview and to take notes during its progress (or immediately after its completion) to ensure the highest possible reliability of data.

The interviewer should also strive for a positive closure to the interview. In many cases, this involves providing the respondents with a summary of the important features of the interview, giving them ample opportunity to clarify, refine, or correct the interviewer's summary.

Evaluation of Unstructured Approaches

Unstructured interviews are an extremely flexible approach to gathering data and, in many research contexts, offer distinct advantages. In clinical situations, for example, it may be appropriate to let individuals talk freely about their problems and concerns, allowing them to take much of the initiative in directing the flow of information. In general, unstructured interviews are of greatest utility, from a researcher's point of view, when a new area of research is being explored. In such situations, an unstructured approach may allow the investigator to ascertain what the basic issues or problems are, how sensitive or controversial the topic is, how easy it is to secure respondents' cooperation in discussing the issues, how individuals conceptualize and talk about the problems, and what range of opinions or behaviors exist that are relevant to the topic. Unstructured methods may also help elucidate the underlying meaning of a pattern or relationship repeatedly observed in more structured research.

On the other hand, unstructured methods are extremely time-consuming and demanding of the researcher's skill in analyzing and interpreting the resulting qualitative data. Samples tend to be small because of the quantity of information produced, so it may be difficult to know whether findings are reliable and could be generalized. Unstructured methods do not usually lend themselves to the rigorous testing of hypotheses concerning cause-and-effect relationships.

❖ RESEARCH EXAMPLES OF SEMI-STRUCTURED AND UNSTRUCTURED SELF-REPORTS

An increasing number of published nursing studies are based on unstructured or semi-structured self-report methods. Table 13-1 briefly describes the research problem and data collection approach used in five such studies. A more detailed description of a study using semi-structured interviews follows.

Gloersen and her colleagues (1993) undertook a 2-year investigation into the phenomenon of "doing well" in people with AIDS. Their study sought to identify the processes that enhance AIDS patients' states of well-being. An in-depth focused interview approach was used "to generate an understanding of the concept of doing well because of its focus on exploring perceptions of well-being rather than on quantitative measures that would verify and define wellness a priori" (p. 47).

Five investigators conducted the interviews with a sample of 16 AIDS victims, who were selected based on their ability to articulate and discuss their experience of doing well with AIDS. The interviews averaged about 90 minutes in length. Among the questions posed to the respondents were the following: What is your experience of doing well with AIDS? What kinds of things have helped you to do well? What things have you done to help yourself do well? How is the experience of doing well changing over time? What helps you to continue to do well? Respondents were asked to elaborate on any aspect that was considered relevant to the general topic. Follow-up interviews were conducted with 8 of the 16 informants. All interviews were tape recorded and later transcribed. The interviewers supplemented the transcripts with their own field notes.

The researchers found that the AIDS victims used several dynamic processes to develop a sense of well-being. For example, every study participant identified accepting as an important concept. Other important processes included being active; mastering life; relating mind and body; being positive; participating in health care; and experiencing support.

❖ STRUCTURED SELF-REPORT INSTRUMENTS

A researcher using a structured approach always operates with a formal, written instrument,

Table 13-1. *Examples of Nursing Studies Using Unstructured or Semi-Structured Self-Reports*

RESEARCH QUESTION	SAMPLE	SELF-REPORT METHOD
What is the nature of caregiving practice among male and female caregivers of confused older people in relation to gender roles? (Opie, 1994)	28 female and male caregivers from New Zealand	Unstructured personal interviews
What is the effect of maternal activity restriction for preterm labor on the expectant father? (May, 1994)	30 men whose partners had an activity-restricted pregnancy	Focus group interviews (and focused interviews)
What are the health beliefs of Latina women regarding the causes of and treatments for AIDS? (Flaskerud & Calvillo, 1991)	59 low-income Latina women	Focus group interviews
What are the life experiences of women who are substance abusers? (Woodhouse, 1992)	26 women in treatment for substance abuse	Life histories
What is the process by which women progress in a healthy fashion through their experience of living with chronic pain? (Howell, 1994)	19 women living with chronic nonmalignant pain	Critical incident diaries

known as an *interview schedule*, when the questions are asked orally in either a face-to-face or telephone format. The instrument is called a *questionnaire* (or sometimes an *SAQ*, self-administered questionnaire) when the respondents complete the instrument themselves, usually in a paper-and-pencil format but occasionally directly onto a computer. Some studies embed an SAQ into an interview schedule, with interviewers asking some questions orally but relying on respondents to answer others in writing.

Structured instruments consist of a set of questions (also known as *items*) in which the wording of both the question and, in most cases, the response alternatives is predetermined. When structured interviews or questionnaires are used, subjects are asked to respond to the same questions, in the same order, and they have the same set of options for their responses. Most nurse researchers who collect self-report data use instruments with a moderate to high degree of structure. In developing structured instruments, a great deal of effort is usually devoted to the content, form, and wording of the questions.

Question Form

Structured instruments themselves vary in their degree of structure through their combination of open-ended and closed-ended questions. *Open-ended* questions allow subjects to respond in their own words. The question, "What was the biggest problem you faced after your open-heart surgery?" is an example of an open-ended question. In questionnaires, the respondent is asked to give a written reply to open-ended items and, therefore, adequate space must be provided to allow a full response. In interviews, the interviewer is normally expected to quote the response verbatim or as closely as possible.

Closed-ended (or *fixed-alternative*) questions offer respondents a number of alternative replies from which the subjects must choose the one that most closely matches the appropriate answer. The alternatives may range from the simple yes or no variety ("Have you smoked a cigarette within the past 24 hours?") to complex expressions of opinion or behavior.

Both open- and closed-ended questions have certain strengths and weaknesses. Closed-ended items are difficult to construct but easy to administer and, especially, to analyze. With closed-ended questions, the researcher needs only to tabulate the number of responses to each alternative to gain some understanding about what the sample as a whole thinks about an issue. The analysis of open-ended items, on the other hand, is often difficult and time-consuming. The procedure that is normally followed is the development of categories and the assignment of the open-ended responses to those categories. That is, the researcher essentially transforms the open-ended responses to fixed categories in a post hoc fashion so that tabulations can be made. This classification process takes considerable time and skill.

Closed-ended items are generally more efficient than open-ended questions in the sense that a respondent is normally able to complete more closed- than open-ended questions in a given amount of time. In questionnaires, subjects may be less willing to compose a written response than to simply check off or circle the appropriate alternative. With respondents who are unable to express themselves well verbally, closed-ended items have a distinct advantage. Furthermore, there are some types of questions that may seem less objectionable in closed form than in open form. Take the following example:

1. What was the gross annual income of your family last year?
2. In what range was your family's gross annual income last year?
   ( ) under $20,000
   ( ) $20,000 to $39,999
   ( ) $40,000 to $59,999
   ( ) $60,000 or over

The second question is more likely to be answered by respondents because the range of options allows them a greater measure of privacy than the blunter open-ended question.

These various advantages of the fixed-alternative question are offset by some corresponding shortcomings. The major drawback of closed-ended questions lies in the possibility of the researcher neglecting or overlooking some potentially important responses. It is often difficult to see an issue from multiple points of view. The omission of possible alternatives can lead to inadequate understanding of the issues and to outright bias if the respondents choose an alternative that misrepresents their position. When the area of research is relatively new, open-ended questions may be more suitable than closed-ended items for avoiding bias.

Another objection to closed-ended items is that they are sometimes considered superficial. Open-ended questions allow for a richer and fuller perspective on the topic of interest, if the respondents are verbally expressive and cooperative. Some of this richness may be lost when the researcher later tabulates answers by developing a system of classification, but excerpts taken directly from the open-ended responses can be extremely valuable in a research report in imparting the flavor of the replies.

Finally, some respondents may object to being forced into choosing from among responses that do not reflect their opinions precisely. Open-ended questions give a lot of freedom to the respondent and, therefore, offer the possibility of spontaneity, which is unattainable when a set of responses is provided.

The decision to use open- and closed-ended questions is based on a number of important considerations such as the sensitivity of the topic, the verbal ability of the respondents, the amount of time available, and so forth. Combinations of both types are highly recommended to offset the strengths and weaknesses of each. Questionnaires typically use fixed-alternative questions predominantly to minimize the respondent's writing burden. Interview schedules, on the other hand, are more variable in their mixture of these two question types.

Specific Types of Closed-Ended Questions

It is often difficult to create good-quality closed-ended questions because the researcher must pay careful attention to the wording of the question and to the content, wording, and formatting of the response options. Nevertheless, the analytic advantages of closed-ended questions make it compelling to include them on structured instruments. Various types of closed-ended questions, many of which are illustrated in Table 13-2, are discussed below.

1. *Dichotomous items* require the respondent to make a choice between two response alternatives, such as yes/no or male/female. Dichotomous questions are considered most appropriate for gathering factual information.
2. *Multiple-choice questions* offer more than two response alternatives. Dichotomous items often are considered too restrictive by respondents, who may resent being forced to see an issue as either yes or no. Graded alternatives are preferable for opinion or attitude questions because they give the researcher more information (intensity as well as direction of opinion) and because they give the respondent the opportunity to express a range of views. Multiple-choice questions most commonly offer three to five alternatives.
3. *Cafeteria questions* are a special type of multiple-choice question that asks respondents to select a response that most closely corresponds to their view. The response options are generally full expressions of a position on the topic of interest.
4. *Rank-order questions* ask respondents to rank target concepts along some continuum, such as most favorable to least favorable or most to least important. Respondents are asked to assign a 1 to the concept that is most important, a 2 to the concept that is second in importance, and so on. Rank-order questions can be useful but need to be handled carefully because they are often misunderstood by respondents. Rank-order questions should not ask respondents to rank more than about 10 alternatives.
5. *Forced-choice questions* require respondents to choose between two alternative statements that represent polar positions or characteristics. Several personality tests use a forced-choice format.
6. *Rating questions* ask respondents to judge something along an ordered dimension. Rating questions are typically bipolar in nature, with the end points specifying the opposite extremes of a continuum. Rating questions require labeling of the end points, but sometimes intermediary points along the scale are also labeled. The number of gradations or points along the scale can vary but should always be an odd number, such as 7, 9, or 11, to allow for a neutral midpoint. (In the example in Table 13-2, the rating question has 11 points, numbered 0 to 10).
7. *Checklists* are items that encompass several questions on a topic and require the same response format. A checklist is often a two-dimensional arrangement in which a series of questions is listed along one dimension (usually vertically) and response alternatives are listed along the other. This two-dimensional character of checklists has led some people to call these *matrix questions*. Checklists are relatively efficient

Table 13-2.   *Examples of Closed-Ended Question Types*

1. Dichotomous Question
   Have you ever been hospitalized?
   ( ) 1. Yes
   ( ) 2. No
2. Multiple-Choice Question
   How important is it to you to avoid a pregnancy at this time?
   ( ) 1. Extremely important
   ( ) 2. Very important
   ( ) 3. Somewhat important
   ( ) 4. Not at all important
3. Cafeteria Question
   People have different opinions about the use of estrogen-replacement therapy for
   women in menopause. Which of the following statements best represents your
   point of view?
   ( ) 1. Estrogen replacement is dangerous and should be totally banned.
   ( ) 2. Estrogen replacement may have some undesirable side effects that suggest
          the need for caution in its use.
   ( ) 3. I am undecided about my views on estrogen-replacement therapy.
   ( ) 4. Estrogen replacement has many beneficial effects that merit its promotion.
   ( ) 5. Estrogen replacement is a wonder cure that should be administered
          routinely to menopausal women.
4. Rank-Order Question
   People value different things about life. Below is a list of principles or ideas that
   are often cited when people are asked to name things they value most. Please
   indicate the order of importance of these values to you by placing a 1 beside the
   most important, 2 beside the next most important, and so forth.
   ( ) Achievement and success
   ( ) Family relationships
   ( ) Friendships and social interaction
   ( ) Health
   ( ) Money
   ( ) Religion
5. Forced-Choice Question
   Which statement most closely represents your point of view?
   ( ) 1. What happens to me is my own doing.
   ( ) 2. Sometimes I feel I don't have enough control over my life.
6. Rating Question
   On a scale from 0 to 10, where 0 means extremely dissatisfied and 10 means
   extremely satisfied, how satisfied are you with the nursing care you received
   during your hospitalization?
   Extremely dissatisfied   Extremely satisfied
            0   1   2   3   4   5   6   7   8   9   10

and easy for respondents to understand, but because they are difficult for an interviewer to read, they are used more frequently in self-administered questionnaires than in interviews. Figure 13-1 presents an example of a checklist.

8. *Calendar questions* are being used increas-ingly when researchers want to obtain retrospective information about the chronology of different events and activities in people's lives. Questions about start dates and stop dates of events are asked and recorded on a calendar grid, such as the one shown in Figure 13-2. Calendars are

Here are some characteristics of birth-control devices that are of varying importance to different people. How important a consideration has each of these been for you in choosing a birth-control method?

	Of Very Great Importance	Of Great Importance	Of Some Importance	Of No Importance
1. Comfort				
2. Cost				
3. Ease of use				
4. Effectiveness				
5. Noninterference with spontaneity				
6. Safety to you				
7. Safety to partner				

Figure 13-1.   *Example of a checklist.*

useful to respondents because they can often better reconstruct the dates of events when several events are recorded in juxtaposition.

9. *Visual analogue scales (VASs)* have come into increased use to measure subjective experiences, such as pain, fatigue, nausea, and dyspnea. The VAS is a straight line, the end anchors of which are labeled as the extreme limits of the sensation or feeling being measured. Subjects are asked to mark a point on the line corresponding to the amount of sensation experienced. Traditionally, the VAS line is 100 mm in length, which facilitates the derivation of a score from 0 to 100 through simple measurement of the distance from one end of the scale to the subject's mark on the line. An example of a VAS is presented in Figure 13-3.

Composite Scales

A *scale* is a device designed to assign a numerical score to subjects to place them on a continuum with respect to attributes being measured, like a scale for measuring people's weight. Many studies that collect data through self-report use a composite psychosocial scale, the purpose of which is to quantitatively discriminate among people with different attitudes,

fears, motives, perceptions, personality traits, and needs. Scales are generally created by combining several closed-ended items (such as those described in the previous section) into a single composite score. Scales are often incorporated into questionnaires and interview schedules, but they may be used independently. Many sophisticated scaling techniques have been developed, only two of which are discussed here.*

LIKERT SCALES

The most widely used scaling technique is the *Likert scale*, named after the psychologist Rensis Likert. A Likert scale consists of several declarative items that express a viewpoint on a topic. Respondents are asked to indicate the degree to which they agree or disagree with the

---

* Among the earliest types of attitude scale were the *Thurstone scales*, named after the psychologist L. L. Thurstone. The Thurstone approach to scaling is elaborate and time-consuming and has fallen into relative disuse. Another scaling method, developed by Louis Guttman in the 1940s, is known as the *Guttman* or *cumulative scales*. Advanced scaling procedures include ratio scaling, multidimensional scaling, and multiple scalogram analysis. Textbooks on psychological scaling and psychometric procedures should be consulted for more information about these alternative scaling strategies.

Figure 13-2. Example of a calendar question (completed).

	1993												1994												1995											
	J	F	M	A	M	J	J	A	S	O	N	D	J	F	M	A	M	J	J	A	S	O	N	D	J	F	M	A	M	J	J	A	S	O	N	D
Pregnancy (Code no. is Pregnancy no.)	1						1								1														2							2
Employment 1 = Employed (Write in name of each employer)									1 *Central Bank*													1							1 *Acme Insurance*							
Child Care																						6			6 / 7					7						

Employment
1 = Employed
(Write in name of each employer)

Child Care
1 = Kindergarten / elementary school
2 = After/before school program
3 = Summer program/day camp
4 = Head Start
5 = Day care center/nursery school/preschool
6 = Family day care/baby-sitter
7 = Grandparent
8 = Other relative
9 = Boyfriend/husband

(For each period, enter code in beginning month and end month, and connect with solid line)

Case # _____

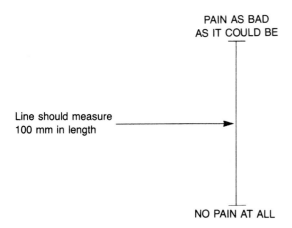

Figure 13-3.   *Example of a visual analogue scale.*

opinion expressed by the statement. Table 13-3 presents an illustrative six-item Likert scale for measuring attitudes toward the mentally ill. Ten to 15 statements are generally recommended for a good Likert scale; the example in Table 13-3 is shown only to illustrate key features. A number of features of the table are discussed in the following paragraphs; first let us briefly discuss the procedure for constructing a Likert scale.

The first step is to develop a large pool of items or statements that clearly state different positions regarding the issue under consideration. Neutral statements or statements so extreme that virtually everyone would agree or disagree with them should be avoided. The aim is to spread out people with various attitudes or traits along a continuum. About equal numbers of positively and negatively worded statements should be chosen to avoid biasing the responses.*

There are differences of opinion concerning the appropriate number of response alternatives to use. Likert used five categories of agreement–disagreement, such as are shown in Table 13-3. Some investigators prefer a seven-point

scale, adding the alternatives "slightly agree" and "slightly disagree." There is also a diversity of opinion about the advisability of including an explicit category labeled "uncertain." Some researchers argue that the inclusion of this option makes the task less objectionable to people who cannot make up their minds or have no strong feelings about an issue. Others, however, feel that the use of this undecided category encourages fence-sitting, or the tendency to not take sides. Investigators who do not give respondents an explicit alternative for indecision or uncertainty proceed in principle as though they were working with a five- or seven-point scale, even though only four or six alternatives are given: nonresponse to a given statement is *scored* as though the neutral response were there and had been chosen.

After the Likert scale is administered to subjects, the responses must be scored. Typically, the responses are scored in such a way that endorsement of positively worded statements and nonendorsement of negatively worded statements are assigned a higher score. Table 13-3 illustrates what this procedure involves. The first statement is positively phrased so that agreement indicates a favorable attitude toward the mentally ill. The researcher, therefore, would assign a higher score to a person agreeing with this statement than to someone disagreeing with it. Because the item has five response alternatives, a score of 5 would be given to someone strongly agreeing, 4 to someone agreeing, and so forth. The responses of two hypothetical respondents are shown by a check or an X, and their score for each item is shown in the right-hand columns of the table. Person 1, who agreed with the first statement, is given a score of 4, while person 2, who strongly disagreed, is given a score of 1. The second statement is negatively worded, and so the scoring is reversed—a 1 is assigned to those who strongly agree, and so forth. This reversal is necessary so that a high score will consistently reflect positive attitudes toward the mentally ill. When each item has been handled in this manner, a person's total score can be determined by adding

*The advanced student who is developing a Likert scale for general use should consult a reference on psychometric procedures, such as *Psychometric Theory* by Nunnally (1978).

Table 13-3.   *Example of a Likert Scale To Measure Attitudes Toward the Mentally Ill*

DIRECTION OF SCORING*	ITEM	RESPONSES†					SCORE	
		SA	A	?	D	SD	Person 1 (√)	Person 2 (X)
+	1. People who have had a mental illness can become normal, productive citizens after treatment.		√			X	4	1
−	2. People who have been patients in mental hospitals should not be allowed to have children.			X		√	5	3
−	3. The best way to handle patients in mental hospitals is to restrict their activity as much as possible.		X		√		4	2
+	4. Many patients in mental hospitals develop normal, healthy relationships with staff members and other patients.			√	X		3	2
+	5. There should be an expanded effort to get the mentally ill out of institutional settings and back into their communities.	√				X	5	1
−	6. Because the mentally ill cannot be trusted, they should be kept under constant guard.		X			√	5	2
	TOTAL SCORE						26	11

*Researchers would not indicate the direction of scoring on a Likert scale administered to subjects. The scoring direction is indicated in this table for illustrative purposes only.

†SA, strongly agree; A, agree; ?, uncertain; D, disagree; SD, strongly disagree.

together individual item scores. Because total scores are computed in this manner, the term *summated rating scale* is sometimes used for such scales. The total scores of the two hypothetical respondents to the items in Table 13-3 are shown at the bottom of that table. These scores reflect a considerably more positive attitude toward the mentally ill on the part of person 1 than person 2.

The summation feature of Likert scales makes it possible to make fine discriminations among people with different points of view. A single Likert question allows people to be put into only five categories. A six-item scale, such as the one in Table 13-3, permits much finer gradation—from a minimum possible score of 6 (6 × 1) to a maximum possible score of 30 (6 × 5).

Likert scales are popular among nurse researchers. Kidd and Huddleston (1994), for example, developed a 10-item Driving Practices Scale to measure risky driving. The items in the scale were developed on the basis of unstructured interviews with hospitalized trauma patients who had sustained injuries while driving.

SEMANTIC DIFFERENTIAL SCALES

Another technique that one encounters in the research literature is known as the *semantic differential* (SD). With the SD, the respondent is asked to rate a given concept (e.g., primary nursing, team nursing) on a series of bipolar adjectives, such as effective/ineffective, good/bad, important/unimportant, or strong/weak. Respondents are asked to place a check at the appropriate point on 7-point rating scales that extend from one extreme of the dimension to the other. An example of the format for an SD is shown in Figure 13-4.

The semantic differential has the advantage of being highly flexible and easy to construct. The concept being rated can be virtually anything—a person, place, situation, abstract idea, controversial issue, and so forth. Typically, several concepts are included on the same schedule so that comparisons can be made across concepts (e.g., male nurse, female nurse, male physician, and female physician).

The researcher also has considerable freedom in constructing the bipolar scales. However, two considerations should guide the selection of the adjectives. First, the adjectives should be appropriate for the concepts being used and for the information being sought. The addition of the adjective pair tall/short in Figure 13-4 would add little understanding of how people react to the role of nurse practitioners.

The second consideration in the selection of adjective pairs is the extent to which the adjectives are measuring the same dimension or aspect of the concept. Osgood and his colleagues (1957), through extensive research with semantic differential scales, found that adjective pairs tend to cluster along three principal and independent dimensions that they labeled evaluation, potency, and activity. The most important group of adjectives are those that are evaluative, such as valuable/worthless, good/bad, fair/unfair, and so forth. Potency adjectives include strong/weak and large/small, and examples of activity adjectives are active/passive and fast/slow. The reason these three dimensions need to be considered separately is that a person's evaluative rating of a concept is independent of the activity or potency ratings of that

NURSE PRACTITIONERS

competent	7*	6	5	4	3	2	1	incompetent
worthless	1	2	3	4	5	6	7	valuable
important								unimportant
pleasant								unpleasant
bad								good
cold								warm
responsible								irresponsible
successful								unsuccessful

*The score values would not be printed on the form administered to actual subjects. The numbers are presented here solely for the purpose of illustrating how semantic differentials are scored.

Figure 13-4. *Example of a semantic differential.*

concept. For example, two people who associate high levels of activity with the concept of nurse practitioner might have divergent views with regard to how valuable they perceive the concept of nurse practitioner. The researcher must decide whether to represent all three of these dimensions or whether only one or two are needed. Each dimension or aspect must be scored separately.

The scoring procedure for SD responses is essentially the same as for Likert scales. Scores from 1 to 7 are assigned to each bipolar scale response, with higher scores generally associated with the positively worded adjective. Responses are then summed across the bipolar scales to yield a total score.

Semantic differentials have been used in a number of nursing studies. For example, Ganong (1993) developed a 40-item SD instrument called the First Impression Questionnaire, designed to measure attitudes toward an individual. He used the instrument to study whether nurses stereotype pregnant patients on the basis of their marital status.

EXISTING SELF-REPORT SCALES AND PSYCHOLOGICAL MEASURES

Many social–psychological states and traits are of interest to those engaged in clinical nursing research, and many self-report scales have been developed to measure them, often using a Likert-type format. Table 13-4 illustrates a number of important constructs that have been measured with an existing composite scale by nurse researchers.

A special suggested readings section at the end of this chapter provides references for locating existing self-report scales. Additionally, both the nursing and nonnursing indexes and abstracting services should be consulted for references to studies that have developed scales. Information on standardized tests and psychological measures can be retrieved through a computerized literature search of the data base called *Mental Measurement Yearbook*, produced by the Buros Institute of Mental Measure-

ments, or through *Health and Psychological Instruments Online*.

Developing Structured Instruments

A careful, well-developed interview schedule or questionnaire cannot be prepared in minutes or even in hours. A researcher interested in designing a useful and accurate instrument must devote considerable time to analyzing the research requirements and attending to minute details. The steps in developing a structured instrument follow closely the steps outlined in Chapter 12. However, a few additional considerations should be mentioned.

Once data needs have been identified, it is often useful to cluster related constructs together as a basis for separate *modules* or areas of questioning in the instrument. For example, an interview schedule may consist of a module on demographic information, another on health symptoms, a third on stressful life events, and a fourth on health-promoting activities.

Before actually developing questions or selecting existing scales, it is necessary to decide whether to collect the data by means of interview or questionnaire because questions must often be worded somewhat differently depending on the mode of administration. The advantages and disadvantages of each are described in a later section.

Some thought needs to be given to the sequencing of modules and questions within modules to arrive at an order that is psychologically meaningful to respondents and encourages candor and cooperation. For example, the schedule should begin with questions that are interesting and motivating. The instrument also needs to be arranged in such a way that distortions and biases are minimized. The possibility that earlier questions might influence replies to the subsequent questions should be kept in mind. Whenever both general and specific questions about a topic are to be included, the general question should be placed first to avoid putting ideas into people's heads.

Table 13-4. *Examples of Concepts Frequently Measured With Composite Scales*

CONCEPT	RESEARCH EXAMPLE REFERENCE	INSTRUMENT USED
Anxiety	Erler & Rudman, 1993 Littlefield, Chang, & Adams, 1990	State-Trait Anxiety Inventory (STAI) Multiple Affect Adjective Checklist
Body image	Nicholas & Leuner, 1992 Mock, 1993	Body Cathexis Scale (BCS) Body Image Scale
Coping	Hahn, Brooks, & Hartsough, 1993 Herth, 1990	Lazarus Ways of Coping Scale Jalowiec Coping Scale
Depression	Fogel, 1993 Buchanan, Cowan, Burr, Waldron, & Kogan, 1993	{ Center for Epidemiological Studies Depression Scale (CES-D) Beck Depression Inventory (BDI)
Family functioning	Stuifbergen, 1990 Woods, Haberman, & Packard, 1993	Family Environment Scale (FES) Family Adaptibility & Cohesion Evaluation Scales (FACES)
Hope	Farran, Salloway, & Clark, 1990 Christman, 1990	Stoner Hope Scale Beck Hopelessness Scale
Life satisfaction	Topp & Stevenson, 1994 Foster, 1992	Life Satisfaction Scale (LSS) Life Satisfaction Index (LSI)
Mood states	Crumlish, 1994 King, Porter, Norsen, & Reis, 1992	Profile of Mood States (POMS) Bipolar Profile of Mood States (POMS-BI)
Pain	Neill, 1993	McGill Pain Questionnaire
Psychosomatic symptoms	Cossette & Levesque, 1993	Symptom Checklist-90 (SCL-90)
Self-care agency	Jirovec & Kasno, 1993 Behm & Frank, 1992	Appraisal of Self Care Agency Exercise of Self-Care Agency (ESCA)
Self-esteem	Weaver & Narsavage, 1992 Walsh, 1993	Rosenberg Self-Esteem Scale Coopersmith Self-Esteem Inventory
Social support	White, Richter, & Fry, 1992 Dodd, Dibble, & Thomas, 1993	Personal Resource Questionnaire (PRQ85) Norbeck Social Support Questionnaire
Stress	Gardner, 1991 Gennaro, Brooten, Roncoli, & Kumar, 1993	Hospital Stress Rating Scale Life Experiences Survey

Every schedule should be prefaced by introductory comments about the nature and purpose of the study. In interviews, the introductory comments would normally be read to the respondents by the interviewer and often incorporated into an informed consent form. In questionnaires, the introduction usually takes the form of a *cover letter* that accompanies the instrument. The introduction should be given considerable care and attention because it represents the first point of contact between the researcher and potential respondents. An example of a cover letter accompanying a mailed questionnaire is presented in Figure 13-5.

When a first draft of the instrument is in reasonably good order, critically discuss it with individuals who are knowledgeable about the construction of questionnaires and with people who are familiar with the substantive content of your schedule. The instrument should also be

reviewed by someone who is capable of detecting technical difficulties such as spelling mistakes, grammatical errors, and so forth. When these various people have provided feedback, a revised version of the instrument can be pretested. The pretest should be administered to individuals who are similar to those who will ultimately participate in the study. Ordinarily, 10 to 20 pretested schedules is sufficient.*

❖ ADMINISTRATION OF SELF-REPORT INSTRUMENTS

Interview schedules and questionnaires require different skills and different considerations in their administration. Both the quantity and the

---

* If a new composite scale is being developed, a much larger pretest sample is advisable.

Dear _____ :

   We are conducting a study to examine how women who are approaching retirement age (age 55 to 65) feel about various issues relating to health and health care. This study, which is sponsored by the State Department of Health, will enable health-care providers to better meet the needs of women in your age group. Would you please assist us in this study by completing the enclosed questionnaire? Your opinions and experiences are very important to us and are needed to give an accurate picture of the health-related needs of women in the greater Middletown area.

   Your name was selected at random from a list of residents in your community. The questionnaire is completely anonymous, so you are not asked to put your name on it or to identify yourself in any way. We therefore hope that you will feel comfortable about giving your honest opinions. If you prefer not to answer any particular question, please feel perfectly free to leave it blank. Please do answer the questions if you can, though, and if you have any comments or concerns about any question, just write your comments in the margin.

   A postage-paid return envelope has been provided for your convenience. We hope that you will take a few minutes to complete and return the questionnaire to us—it should take only about 15 minutes of your time. To analyze the information in a timely fashion, we ask that you return the questionnaire to us by May 12.

   Thank you very much for your cooperation and assistance in this endeavor. If you would like a copy of the summary of the results of this study, please check the box at the bottom of page 10.

Figure 13-5. *Fictitious example of a cover letter for a mailed questionnaire.*

quality of the data gathered are influenced by the data collection procedures and the competencies of the research personnel. In this section, we examine the problems involved in instrument administration and ways of handling those difficulties.

Collecting Interview Data

The quality of interview data depends to a great extent on the proficiency of the interviewers. Interviewers for large survey organizations receive extensive general training in addition to specific training for individual studies. Although this introductory book cannot adequately cover all the principles of good interviewing, it can identify some of the major issues.

A primary task of the interviewer is to put respondents at ease so that they will feel comfortable in expressing their honest opinions. The respondents' personal reaction to the interviewer can seriously affect their willingness to participate. Interviewers, therefore, should always be punctual (if an appointment has been made), courteous, and friendly. The interviewer should strive to appear unbiased and to create a permissive atmosphere that encourages candor. All opinions of the respondents should be accepted as natural—the interviewer generally should not express surprise, disapproval, or even approval.

When a structured interview schedule is being used, interviewers should follow the wording of the questions in the schedule precisely. Similarly, interviewers should not offer spontaneous explanations of what the questions mean. Repetitions of the questions are usually adequate to dispel any misunderstanding, particularly if the instrument has been properly pretested. The interviewer should not read the questions from the schedule mechanically. A naturalistic, conversational tone is essential in building rapport with respondents, and this tone is impossible to achieve if the interviewer is not thoroughly familiar with the questions.

When closed-ended questions with lengthy or complicated response alternatives

are posed, the interviewer should hand the subjects a *show card* that lists all the options. Individuals cannot be expected to remember detailed unfamiliar material and are sometimes inclined to choose the last alternative if they cannot recall earlier ones. Closed-ended items can be recorded by checking or circling the appropriate alternative, but responses to open-ended questions need to be recorded in full or tape recorded for later transcription. The interviewer should not paraphrase or summarize the respondent's reply.

Interviewers typically find that obtaining complete and relevant responses to open-ended questions is not always an easy matter. Respondents often reply to seemingly straightforward questions with irrelevant discussions or partial answers, or they may say, "I don't know" to avoid giving their opinions on sensitive topics or to stall while they think over the question. In such cases, the job of the interviewer is to probe. The purpose of a *probe* is to elicit more useful information from a respondent than was volunteered during the first reply. A probe can take many forms: sometimes it involves a repetition of the original question and sometimes it is a long pause intended to communicate to respondents that they should continue. Frequently, it is necessary to encourage a more complete response by a nondirective supplementary question such as, "How is that?" The interviewer must be careful to use only *neutral* probes that do not influence the content of the subject's response. Box 13-1 gives some examples of neutral, nondirective probes that are used by professional interviewers in getting more complete responses to questions. The ability to probe well is perhaps the greatest test of an interviewer's skill. To know when to probe and how to select the best probes, the interviewer must comprehend fully the purpose of each question and the type of information being sought, as spelled out in the question-by-question instructions (Q-by-Qs).

The guidelines for handling telephone interviews are essentially the same as those for face-to-face interviews, although additional ef-

---

BOX 13-1.   EXAMPLES OF NEUTRAL, NONDIRECTIVE PROBES

Is there anything else?
Go on.
Are there any other reasons?
How do you mean?
Could you tell me more about that?
Why do you feel that way?
Would you tell me what you have in mind?
There are no right or wrong answers; I'd just
   like to get your thinking.
Could you please explain that?
Could you give me an example?

---

fort usually is required to build rapport over the telephone. In both cases, the interviewer should strive to make the interview a pleasant and satisfying experience in which respondents are made to feel as though the information they are providing is important.

Collecting Questionnaire Data

Self-administered questionnaires can be distributed in a number of ways. The most convenient procedure is to distribute the questionnaires to a group of respondents who complete the instrument together at the same time. This approach has the obvious advantages of maximizing the number of completed questionnaires and allowing the researcher to clarify any possible misunderstandings about the instrument. Group administrations are often possible in educational settings and might also be feasible in some hospital or community situations.

Personal presentation of questionnaires to individual respondents is another alternative. Personal contact with respondents has been found to have a positive effect on the rate of questionnaires returned. Furthermore, the availability of the researcher or an assistant can be an advantage in terms of explaining and clarifying the purposes of the study or particular items. This method may be relatively time-consuming and expensive if the questionnaires have to be delivered and picked up at respondents' homes. The distribution of questionnaires in a clinical setting, on the other hand, is often inexpensive and efficient and likely to yield a high rate of completed questionnaires.

Questionnaires are often mailed to respondents. A problematic feature of this approach is that the *response rates* tend to be low. When only a small subsample of respondents return their questionnaires, it may be unreasonable to assume that those who did respond were somehow typical of the sample as a whole. In other words, the researcher is faced with the possibility that those individuals who did not complete a questionnaire would, as a group, have answered the questions differently from those who did return the schedule.

If the response rate is high, the risk of serious response bias may be negligible. A response rate greater than 60% is probably sufficient for most purposes, but lower response rates are common. The researcher generally should attempt to discover how representative the respondents are, relative to the target population, in terms of basic demographic characteristics such as age, gender, marital status, and the like. This comparison may lead the researcher to conclude that respondents and nonrespondents are similar enough to assume the absence of serious biases. If demographic differences are found, the investigator will at least be in a position to make some inferences about the direction of the biases.

The response rate can be affected by the manner in which the questionnaires are designed and mailed. The physical appearance of the questionnaire can influence its appeal, so some thought should be given to the layout, quality and color of paper, method of reproduction, and typographic quality of the instrument. The standard procedure for distributing the questionnaire is to include with the instrument a cover letter and a stamped, addressed return envelope. Failure to enclose a return envelope could have a serious effect on the response rate.

The use of *follow-up reminders* has been found to be effective in achieving higher response rates for mailed questionnaires. This procedure involves the mailing of additional letters urging nonrespondents to complete and return their forms. Follow-up letters or notices are typically sent 2 to 3 weeks after the initial mailing. Sometimes the reminder simply involves a letter of encouragement to nonrespondents. It is preferable, however, to enclose a second copy of the questionnaire with the reminder letter because most nonrespondents will have misplaced the original copy. Telephone follow-ups can be successful, but they are costly and involve a considerable amount of time. With anonymous questionnaires, the investigator may be unable to distinguish respondents and nonrespondents for the purpose of sending follow-up letters. In such a situation, the simplest procedure is to send out a follow-up letter to the entire sample, thanking those individuals who have already answered and asking others to cooperate.

As questionnaires are returned, the investigator should keep a log of the incoming receipts on a daily basis. Each questionnaire should be opened, checked for usability, and assigned an identification number. Such record-keeping will assist the researcher in assembling the results, monitoring the response rate, and making decisions about the timing of follow-up mailings and cutoff dates.

The problems associated with mailed questionnaires are not ones that can be handled using interpersonal skills. Building rapport in a questionnaire situation to enhance the response rate is difficult and often depends on attention to details. Even though these procedural matters may seem trivial, the success of the project may depend on their careful execution.

❖ QUESTIONNAIRES VERSUS INTERVIEWS: AN ASSESSMENT

Self-administered questionnaires offer a number of advantages over personal interviews, but they have some drawbacks as well. Let us consider some of the following strong points of questionnaires:

1. *Cost.* Questionnaires, relative to interviews, are generally much less costly and require less time and energy to administer. Group-administered questionnaires are clearly the least expensive and time-consuming of any procedure. With a fixed amount of funds or time, a larger and more geographically diverse sample can usually be obtained with mailed questionnaires than with interviews.

2. *Anonymity.* Questionnaires, unlike interview schedules, offer the possibility of complete anonymity. Sometimes a guarantee of anonymity is crucial in obtaining candid responses, particularly if the questions are of a highly personal or sensitive nature. Anonymous questionnaires often result in a higher proportion of socially unacceptable responses (i.e., responses that place the respondent in an unfavorable light) than face-to-face interviews.

3. *Interviewer bias.* The absence of an interviewer ensures that there will be no *interviewer bias.* Ideally, an interviewer is a neutral agent through whom questions and answers are passed. Studies have shown, however, that this ideal is difficult to achieve. Respondents and interviewers interact as humans, and this interaction can affect the subject's responses. This problem clearly is not present for questionnaires.

Despite these advantages, the strengths of interviews far outweigh those of questionnaires. It is true that interviews are costly, prevent respondent anonymity, and are subject to interviewer biases. Nevertheless, the numerous advantages described as follows have led many researchers to conclude that interviews are superior to questionnaires for most research purposes:

1. *Response rates.* The response rate tends to be high in face-to-face interviews. Respondents are apparently more reluctant to refuse to talk to an interviewer who is directly in front of them than to discard or ig-

nore a questionnaire. A well-designed and properly conducted interview study normally achieves a response rate in the vicinity of 80% to 90%. Because nonresponse is not a random process, low response rates may introduce serious biases.

2. *Audience.* Many individuals simply cannot fill out a questionnaire. Examples include young children and blind, elderly, illiterate, or uneducated individuals. Interviews, on the other hand, are normally feasible with most people.

3. *Clarity.* Interviews offer some protection against ambiguous or confusing questions. The interviewer can determine whether questions have been misunderstood and can clarify matters. In questionnaires, items that are misinterpreted may go undetected by the researchers, and thus the responses may lead to erroneous conclusions.

4. *Depth of questioning.* The information obtained from questionnaires tends to be somewhat more superficial than interview data, partly because questionnaires ordinarily contain a preponderance of closed-ended items. Open-ended questions often engender resentment among questionnaire respondents, who dislike having to compose and write out a reply. Much of the richness and complexity of the human experience can be lost if closed-ended items are used exclusively. Furthermore, interviewers can enhance the quality of the self-report data through probing.

5. *Missing information.* Respondents are less likely to give "I don't know" responses or to leave a question unanswered in an interview situation than on questionnaires.

6. *Order of questions.* In an interview, the researcher has strict control over the order of presentation of the questions. Questionnaire respondents are at liberty to skip around from one section of the instrument to another. It is possible that a different ordering of questions from the one originally intended could bias the responses.

7. *Sample control.* Interviews permit greater control over the sample in the sense that the interviewer knows whether the person being interviewed is the intended respondent. It is not unusual to have individuals who receive questionnaires pass the instrument on to a friend, relative, secretary, and so forth. This kind of activity can change the characteristics of the sample.

8. *Supplementary data.* Finally, face-to-face interviews have an advantage in their ability to produce additional data through observation. The interviewer is in a position to observe or judge the respondents' level of understanding, degree of cooperativeness, social class, lifestyle, and so forth. These kinds of information can be useful in interpreting the responses.

Many of the advantages of face-to-face interviews also apply to telephone interviews. Complicated or detailed schedules or ones with sensitive questions are not well suited for telephone interviewing, but for relatively brief instruments, the telephone interview is more economical than personal interviews and tends to yield a higher response rate than mailed questionnaires.

❖ RESPONSE BIASES

Although self-reports represent a powerful mechanism for obtaining data, researchers who use this approach should always be aware of the risk of *response biases*—that is, the tendency of some respondents to distort their responses. Perhaps the most pervasive problem is a person's tendency to present a favorable image of himself or herself. The *social desirability* response bias refers to the tendency of some individuals to misrepresent their responses consistently by giving answers that are congruent with prevailing social mores. This problem is often difficult to combat. Subtle, indirect, and delicately worded questioning sometimes can help to alleviate this response bias. The creation of a permissive atmosphere and provisions for respondent anonymity also encourage frankness.

Some response biases are most commonly observed in connection with composite scales. These biases are sometimes referred to as *response sets*. Scale scores are seldom entirely accurate and pure measures of the critical variable. A number of irrelevant factors are also being measured at the same time. Because these response-set factors can sometimes influence or bias responses to a considerable degree, investigators who construct scales must attempt to eliminate them or reduce their impact.

Extreme responses are an example of such a response set. This biasing factor results from the fact that some individuals consistently express their attitudes in terms of extreme response alternatives (e.g., "strongly agree"), and others characteristically endorse middle-range alternatives. This response style is a distorting influence in that extreme responses may not necessarily signify the most intense attitude toward the phenomenon under investigation. There appears to be little that a researcher can do to counteract this bias, although there are procedures for detecting its existence.

Some people have been found to agree with statements regardless of the content. In the research literature, these people are sometimes referred to as *yea-sayers*, and the bias is known as the *acquiescence response set*. A less common problem is the opposite tendency for other individuals, called *nay-sayers*, to disagree with statements independently of the question content. Although there apparently are some people for whom such tendencies are stable and enduring personality characteristics, acquiescence and its opposite counterpart can often be avoided or minimized by the simple strategy of *counterbalancing* positively and negatively worded statements.

The effects of response biases should not be exaggerated, but it is important that researchers who are using self-reports give these issues some thought. If an instrument or scale is being developed for general use by other researchers, it is recommended that evidence be gathered demonstrating that the scale is sufficiently free from the influence of response biases to measure the critical variable.

❖ TIPS FOR DEVELOPING SELF-REPORT INSTRUMENTS

Although we all are accustomed to asking questions, the proper phrasing of questions in a research study is a delicate task. In this section, we provide some tips on the wording of questions and response options for self-report instruments. Although some of the advice is specific to structured self-reports, many of the suggestions are equally appropriate for unstructured interviews.

Tips for Wording the Questions

In wording questions for research purposes, the researcher must keep four important considerations in mind.

1. *Clarity.* Questions should be worded clearly and unambiguously—often a difficult task because respondents do not necessarily understand what information is needed and do not always have the same mind-set as the researcher.
2. *Ability of respondents to give information.* The researcher needs to consider whether the respondents can be expected to understand the question or are qualified to provide meaningful information.
3. *Bias.* Questions should be worded in a manner that will minimize the risk of response biases.
4. *Sensitive information.* In developing questions, the researcher should strive to be courteous, considerate, and sensitive to the needs and rights of respondents, especially when asking questions of a highly private nature.

Here are some specific suggestions to keep in mind with regard to these four considerations:

- Clarify in your own mind the information that you are trying to obtain. The question, "When do you usually eat your evening meal?" might elicit such responses as "around 6 PM" or "when my son gets home from soccer practice" or "when I feel like cooking." The question itself contains no words that are difficult, but the question is unclear because the intent of the researcher is not apparent.
- Try to state your questions in the affirmative rather than the negative, and particularly avoid sentences with double negatives.
- Avoid long sentences or phrases, and avoid technical terms if more common terms are equally appropriate. Try to use words that are simple enough for the *least* educated respondents in your sample. Do not assume that even members of your own profession will have extensive knowledge on all aspects of nursing and medical terminology.
- Avoid "double-barreled" questions that contain two distinct ideas or concepts. The statement, "The mentally ill are essentially incapable of caring for themselves and should, therefore, be denied of any responsibilities or rights," might lead to conflicts of opinion in a single person, who might only agree with one part of the statement.
- Do not assume that respondents will be aware of, or informed about, issues or questions in which you are interested. Furthermore, avoid giving the impression that respondents *ought* to have the information. Questions on complex or specialized issues can be worded in such a way that a respondent will be comfortable admitting ignorance (e.g., "Many people have not had an opportunity to learn much about the physiologic side-effects of oral contraceptives, but some people have picked up information on this subject. Do you happen to know of any such side effects?"). Another approach is to preface a question by a short statement of explanation about terminology or issues.
- Avoid leading questions that suggest a particular kind of answer. A question such as, "Do you agree that nurse–midwives play an indispensable role in the health team?" is not neutral.
- State a range of alternatives within the question itself when possible. For instance, the question, "Do you normally prefer to get up early in the morning on weekends?" is more suggestive of the "right" answer than "Do you normally prefer to get up early in the morning or to sleep late on weekends?"
- For questions that deal with socially unacceptable behavior or attitudes (e.g., excessive drinking habits, noncompliance with physician's instructions, and the like), closed-ended questions are often useful because it is easier to check off having engaged in socially disapproved actions than to verbalize those actions in response to an open-ended question. Furthermore, when the unacceptable behavior is actually presented to respondents as an option, they are more likely to realize that they are not alone in their behaviors or attitudes, and admissions of nonstandard behavior becomes less difficult.
- Impersonal wording of a question is sometimes useful in minimizing embarrassment and encouraging honesty. To illustrate this point, compare these two statements with which respondents would be asked to agree or disagree: 1) "I am personally dissatisfied with the nursing care I received during my hospitalization." 2) "The quality of nursing care in this hospital is unsatisfactory." A respondent might feel more comfortable about admitting dissatisfaction with nursing care in the less personally worded second question.

Tips for Preparing Response Alternatives

If closed-ended questions are used, the researcher also needs to make decisions about the form that the response alternatives will take. Below are some suggestions for preparing alternatives to closed-ended items.

- The responses options should adequately cover all the significant alternatives. If respondents are forced to choose a response from among options provided by the researcher, they should feel reasonably comfortable with the available options. As a safety measure, the researcher can have as one response option a phrase such as "other—please specify."

- The alternatives should be mutually exclusive (e.g., the following categories for a question on a person's age are *not* mutually exclusive: 30 or younger, 30–40, 40–50, 50 or older).

- There should be some underlying rationale for the order in which the alternatives are presented to the respondent. Often the options can be placed in order of decreasing or increasing favorability, agreement, or intensity. When the respondent is asked to choose from options that have no natural sequence or order, alphabetic ordering of the alternatives is less likely to lead the respondent to a particular response (e.g., see question 4 in Table 13-2).

- The response alternatives should not be too lengthy. One sentence or phrase for each alternative should almost always be sufficient to express a concept. In general, the response alternatives should be approximately equal in length.

Tips for Formatting an Instrument

The appearance and layout of the schedule may seem a matter of minor administrative importance. However, a poorly designed format can have substantive consequences if respondents (or interviewers) become confused, miss questions, or answer questions that they should have omitted. The format is especially important in the case of questionnaires because respondents who are unfamiliar with the researcher's intent will not usually have an opportunity to ask questions. The following suggestions may be helpful in laying out a schedule:

- Try not to compress too many questions into too small a space. An extra page of questions is better than a schedule that appears cluttered and confusing and that provides inadequate space for responses to open-ended questions.

- Set off the response options from the question or stem itself in formatting alternative responses. These options are usually aligned vertically (Box 13-2). In a questionnaire, respondents can be asked either to circle the appropriate answer or to place a check in the appropriate box.

- Give special care to formatting *filter questions,* which are designed to route respondents through different sets of questions depending on their response to earlier items. In interview schedules, the most typical procedure is to use *skip patterns* that instruct the interviewers to skip to a specific place in the schedule (e.g., SKIP TO Q10). In self-administered questionnaires, such skip patterns may be confusing, and it may be better to set off questions appropriate to only a subset of respondents apart from the main series of questions, as illustrated in Box 13-2.

- Avoid forcing all readers to go through inapplicable questions in a questionnaire. That is, question 2 in Box 13-2 could have been worded as follows: "If you are a member of the American Nurses' Association, for how long have you been a member?" The person who is not a member may not be sure how to handle this question and may be annoyed at having to read through material that is irrelevant.

❖ *RESEARCH EXAMPLE: STRUCTURED SELF-REPORT*

Structured self-report instruments are the most commonly used method of collecting data for nursing research studies. Table 13-5 presents some examples of studies that have used structured interviews or questionnaires, together

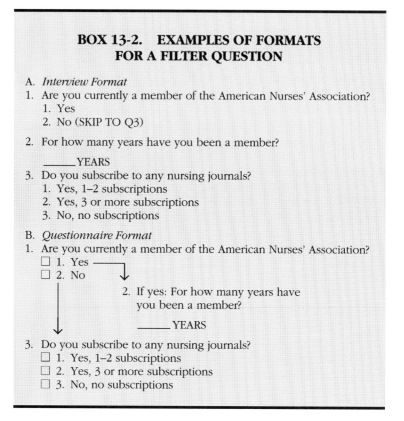

with information on response rates. A more detailed description of a questionnaire study follows.

Vortherms, Ryan, and Ward (1992) conducted a survey of nurses to determine their knowledge of, attitudes toward, and perceived barriers to pharmacologic management of pain in cancer patients. Using a number of questions from other instruments, the researchers developed an 82-item questionnaire. The questionnaire consisted of four modules, including a module on background and demographic questions; knowledge of the pharmacologic management of cancer pain; liberalness in pain management; and perceived barriers to pain management in the nurses' practice settings.

The researchers developed a 32-item knowledge test, comprising three subtests: knowledge of opioids, of pain, and of medication scheduling regimens. Test scores were computed in terms of percentage of correct responses. Five items (with response options ranging from 1 to 5) were used to measure liberalness of nurses' attitudes in pain management. This summated rating scale (scores ranged from 0 to 24) was adapted from a scale previously used to measure physicians' liberalness in pain management. The questions on perceived barriers were all rating questions, in which respondents were asked to rate nine factors as to whether each was a barrier to pain management in their setting, and also to rate other nurses and physicians in their settings on adequacy of pain management. Five pain management experts reviewed a draft of the questionnaire for clarity and appropriateness of the content, and survey experts reviewed it with respect to format and style. The questionnaire was pretested with a sample of nurses with oncology experience.

Table 13-5.   *Examples of Nursing Studies Using Structured Self-Reports*

RESEARCH QUESTION	SAMPLE	SELF-REPORT METHOD	RESPONSE RATE
What is the relationship between physical health and psychological well-being in elderly women? (Heidrich, 1993)	243 elderly women	Questionnaires	92%
What is the relationship between background variables and coping effectiveness in postmyocardial infarction patients? (Bennett, 1993)	81 patients	Mailed questionnaires	43%
What are the primary barriers to recruiting RNs in rural areas? (Stratton, Dunkin, Juhl, & Geller, 1993)	556 directors of nursing	Telephone interviews	90%
What are the levels of satisfaction with and perceived barriers to health care among women in a Medicaid prepaid plan versus regular fee-for-service Medicaid program? (Reis, 1990)	98 Medicaid clients	Personal interviews	89%

The questionnaire, a cover letter, a stamped self-addressed return envelope, and a stamped self-addressed postcard were mailed to a systematic sample of 1173 nurses holding active licensure in Wisconsin. To encourage cooperation, the cover letter was printed on Pain Research Group/World Health Organization Collaborating Center letterhead. Anonymity was maintained by the use of a separate return postcard by which respondents indicated that they had sent in their questionnaires. Second and third mailings (with duplicate questionnaires and postcards) were sent at 6-week intervals to those who had not yet returned the postcards. A total of 790 nurses (68%) returned a completed questionnaire.

The researchers found that 59% of the nurses had worked with cancer patients in the prior 6 months, although only 7% worked in oncology settings. The scores on the knowledge test ranged from 11% to 93% correct. In general, nurses believed that a substantial minority of patients overreported pain, although they had fairly liberal attitudes toward pain management.

❖ SUMMARY

Self-report data are collected by means of an oral interview or written questionnaire. Self-reports vary widely in terms of their degree of structure or standardization. Unstructured methods provide both respondent and interviewer latitude in the formulation of questions and answers. Methods of collecting unstructured or loosely structured self-report data include: 1) *unstructured interviews,* which are conversational discussions on the topic of interest; 2) *semi-structured* or *focused interviews,* in which the interviewer is guided by a broad *topic guide* of questions to be asked; 3) *focus group interviews,* which involve discussions with small groups about topics covered in a topic guide; 4) *life histories,* which encourage respondents to narrate, in chronologic sequence, their life experiences regarding some theme; 5) the *critical incidents method,* which involves probes about the circumstances surrounding a behavior or incident that is critical to some outcome of interest; and 6) *diaries,* in which respondents are asked to maintain daily records about some aspects of their lives. Unstructured methods tend to yield data of considerable depth and are useful in gaining an understanding about little-researched phenomena, but they are time-consuming and yield data that are challenging to analyze.

Most self-report data in nursing studies are collected through structured interview schedules or questionnaires. Questions in the instrument also vary in their degree of structure. *Open-ended questions* permit respondents to reply to questions in their own words. *Closed-ended* (or *fixed-alternative*) *questions* offer a number of alternative responses from which respondents are instructed to choose.

Closed-ended questions can take a number of different forms. The simplest type of fixed alternative (*dichotomous items*) requires a choice between two options, such as yes or no. *Multiple-choice questions* provide respondents with a range of alternatives. *Cafeteria questions* are a special type of multiple-choice item in which respondents are asked to select a statement that best represents their view. Respondents are sometimes requested to *rank-order* a list of alternatives along a continuum, usually from most favorable to least favorable. *Forced-choice questions* require respondents to choose between two competing positions. *Rating questions* ask respondents to judge something along an ordered, bipolar dimension. A *checklist* groups together several questions that require the same response format and that can be answered by placing a check in the appropriate space on a *matrix. Calendar questions* ask for information about the stop and start dates of various events, recorded on a calendar grid. *Visual analogue scales* are often used for the measurement of subjective experiences such as pain and nausea.

Composite psychosocial *scales* are multi-item self-report tools for quantitatively measuring the degree to which individuals possess or are characterized by target traits or attributes. The most common type of composite scale is the *Likert scale,* or *summated rating scale.* Likert scales present the respondent with a series of items that are worded either favorably or unfavorably toward some phenomenon. Respondents are asked to indicate their degree of agreement or disagreement with each statement. A total score is derived by the summation of scores assigned to all items, which in turn are scored according to the direction of favorability expressed. The *semantic differential* is a second scaling procedure used for measuring the meaning of concepts to individuals. The technique consists of a series of bipolar rating scales on which respondents are asked to indicate their reaction toward some phenomenon. The scales may be measuring an evaluation (e.g., good/bad); activity (e.g., active/passive); or potency (e.g., strong/weak) dimension. Scoring of the SD proceeds in a fashion similar to that of Likert scales.

The quality of interview data depends heavily on the interpersonal skills of the interviewer. The interviewer must endeavor to put respondents at ease and build rapport with them. When respondents give incomplete or irrelevant replies to a question, the interviewer must use a technique known as *probing* to solicit additional information.

Self-administered questionnaires can be distributed in various ways. Group administration to an intact group is the most convenient and economical procedure. Another approach is to mail questionnaires to individuals. The main problem with mailed questionnaires is that many people fail to respond to them, leading to the risk of a biased sample. A number of techniques, such as the use of *follow-up reminders* and good *cover letters*, are designed to increase the *response rate.*

On the whole, interviews suffer from fewer weaknesses than questionnaires. Questionnaires are less costly and time-consuming than interviews, offer the possibility of anonymity, and do not run a risk of interviewer bias. However, interviews yield a higher response rate, are suitable for a wider variety of individuals, are less likely to lead to misinterpretations of questions, and provide richer data than questionnaires.

The researcher interested in using self-reports must contend with the possibility of reporting biases, which are often called *response-set* biases in the context of scales. This problem concerns the tendency of certain individuals to respond to items in characteristic ways, independently of the item's content. The *social desirability* response bias stems from a person's desire to appear in a favorable light. The *extreme response set* results when a person characteristically endorses extreme response alternatives. Another type of response bias is known as *acquiescence,* which designates an individual's tendency to agree with statements regardless of their content. A converse problem arises less frequently when a person disagrees with most statements.

❖ STUDY SUGGESTIONS

Chapter 13 of the accompanying *Study Guide for Nursing Research: Principles and Methods, 5th ed.,* offers various exercises for reinforcing the concepts presented in this chapter. Additionally, the following study questions can be addressed:

1. Identify which unstructured methods of self-report might be appropriate for the following research problems:
   a. What are the coping strategies of parents who have lost a child through sudden infant death syndrome?
   b. How do nurses in emergency rooms make decisions about their activities?
   c. What are the health beliefs and practices of Haitian immigrants in the United States?
2. The underutilization of nursing skills because of voluntary nonemployment is sometimes the cause of some concern. Suppose that you were planning to conduct a state-wide study concerning the plans and intentions of nonemployed registered nurses in your state. Would you

adopt an interview or questionnaire approach? How structured would your schedule be? Why?
3. Suppose that the investigation of nonemployed nurses were to be accomplished by means of a mailed questionnaire. Draft a cover letter to accompany the schedule.
4. Suppose that you were interested in studying the attitudes of men toward witnessing the birth of their children in a hospital delivery room. Develop five positively worded and five negatively worded statements that could be used in constructing a Likert scale for such a study.
5. List 10 pairs of bipolar adjectives that would be appropriate for rating *all* the following concepts for an SD scale: cigarettes, alcohol, marijuana, heroin, cocaine.
6. Suggest ways of improving the following questions:
   a. When do you usually administer your injection of insulin?
   b. Would you disagree with the statement that nurses should not unionize?
   c. Do you agree or disagree with the following statement?: Alcoholics deserve more pity than scorn and should be encouraged to seek medical rather than spiritual assistance.
   d. What is your opinion about the new health reform bill?
   e. Don't you think that the role of nurses ought to be expanded?

❖ SUGGESTED READINGS

METHODOLOGICAL REFERENCES

General References on Self-Reports

Bradburn, N. M., & Sudman, S. (1979). *Improving interview method and questionnaire design.* San Francisco: Jossey-Bass.

Collins, C., Given, B., Given, C. W., & King, S. (1988). Interviewer training and supervision. *Nursing Research, 37,* 122–124.

Denzin, N. K. (1989). *The research act* (3rd ed.). New York: McGraw-Hill.

Dillman, D. (1978). *Mail and telephone surveys: The total design method*. New York: John Wiley.

Flanagan, J. C. (1954). The critical-incident technique. *Psychological Bulletin, 51,* 327–358.

Gift, A. G. (1989). Visual analogue scales: Measurement of subjective phenomena. *Nursing Research, 38,* 286–288.

Goldman, A. E., & McDonald, S. S. (1987). *The group depth interview: Principles and practice*. Englewood Cliffs, NJ: Prentice-Hall.

Gordon, R. L. (1980). *Interviewing: Strategy, techniques and tactics* (3rd ed.). Homewood, IL: Dorsey Press.

Institute for Social Research. (1976). *Interviewer's manual, Survey Research Center* (rev. ed.). Ann Arbor: University of Michigan.

Kingry, M. J., Fiedje, L. B., & Friedman, L. L. (1990). Focus groups: A research technique for nursing. *Nursing Research, 39,* 124–125.

Krueger, R. A. (1988). *Focus groups: A practical guide for applied research*. San Mateo: Sage.

Lee, K. A., & Kieckhefer, G. M. (1989). Measuring human responses using visual analogue scales. *Western Journal of Nursing Research, 11,* 128–132.

Leininger, M. M. (1985). Life-health-care history: Purposes, methods and techniques. In M. M. Leininger (Ed.), *Qualitative research methods in nursing*. New York: Grune & Stratton.

McCracken, G. (1988). *The long interview*. Newbury Park, CA: Sage.

Morgan, D. L. (1988). *Focus groups as qualitative research*. Newbury Park, CA: Sage.

Nunnally, J. C. (1978). *Psychometric theory*. New York: McGraw-Hill.

Osgood, C. E., Suci, G. J., & Tannenbaum, P. H. (1957). *The measurements of meaning*. Urbana, IL: University of Illinois Press.

Paterson, B., & Bramadat, I. J. (1992). Use of the preinterview in oral history. *Qualitative Health Research, 2,* 99–115.

Payne, S. (1951). *The art of asking questions*. Princeton, NJ: Princeton University Press.

Reiskin, H. (1992). Focus groups: A useful technique for research and practice in nursing. *Applied Nursing Research, 5,* 197–201.

Schuman, H., & Presser, S. (1981). *Questions and answers in attitude surveys: Experiments in questions form, wording and context*. New York: Academic Press.

Spradley, J. (1979). *The ethnographic interview*. New York: Holt Rinehart & Winston.

Waltz, C. F., Strickland, O. L., & Lenz, E. R. (1991). *Measurement in nursing research*. (2nd ed.). Philadelphia: F. A. Davis.

Woods, N. F. (1981). The health diary as an instrument for nursing research. *Western Journal of Nursing Research, 3,* 76–92.

Wykle, M. L., & Morris, D. L. (1988). The health diary. *Applied Nursing Research, 1,* 47–48.

References for Locating Scales and Psychological Measures

Anastasi, A. (1988). *Psychological testing* (6th ed.). New York: Macmillan.

Beere, C. A. (1979). *Women and women's issues: A handbook of tests and measures*. San Francisco: Jossey-Bass.

Buros, O. K. (1974). *Tests in print II*. Highland Park, NJ: Gryphon Press.

Cattell, J. B., & Warburton, F. W. (1967). *Objective personality and motivation tests*. Chicago: University of Illinois Press.

Chun, K. T., Cobb, S., & French, J. R. P., Jr. (1975). *Measures for psychological assessment*. Ann Arbor: Survey Research Center.

Corcoran, K., & Fischer, J. (1987). *Measures for clinical practice: A sourcebook*. New York, NY: Macmillan.

Frank-Stromberg, M. (Ed.). (1988). *Instruments for clinical nursing research*. Norwalk, CT: Appleton and Lange.

Keyser, D. J., & Sweetland, R. C. (Eds.) (1988). *Test critiques*. (Vol. 7). Kansas City, MO: Test Corporation of America.

McDowell, I., & Newell, C. (1987). *Measuring health: A guide to rating scales and questionnaires*. New York, NY: Oxford University Press.

Mitchell, J. V., Jr. (Ed.) (1985). *The ninth mental measurements yearbook*. Lincoln, NE: University of Nebraska Press.

Reineck, C. (1991). Nursing research instruments: Pathway to resources. *Applied Nursing Research, 4,* 34–38.

Robinson, J. P., & Shaver, P. R. (1973). *Measures of social psychological attitudes* (rev. ed.). Ann Arbor: University of Michigan.

Shaw, M. E., & Wright, J. M. (1967). *Scales for the measurement of attitudes*. New York: McGraw-Hill.

Strickland, O. L., & Waltz, C. (1988). *Measurement of nursing outcomes: Vol. II. Measuring nursing performance*. New York: Springer.

Touliatos, J., Perlmutter, B. F., & Straus, M. A. (Eds.) (1990). *Handbook of family measurement techniques*. Newbury Park, CA: Sage.

Waltz, C. F., & Strickland, O. L. (1988). *Measurement of nursing outcomes: Vol. I. Measuring client outcomes*. New York: Springer.

Ward, M. J., & Felter, M. E. (1979). *Instruments for use in nursing education research*. Boulder, CO: Western Interstate Commission for Higher Education.

Ward, M. J., & Lindeman, C. A. (Eds.). (1978). *Instruments for measuring nursing practice and other health variables*. Washington, DC: U.S. Government Printing Office.

SUBSTANTIVE REFERENCES

Behm, L. K., & Frank. D. I. (1992). The relationship between self-care agency and job satisfaction in public health nurses. *Applied Nursing Research, 5,* 28–29.

Bennett, S. J. (1993). Relationships among selected antecedent variables and coping effectiveness in postmyocardial infarction patients. *Research in Nursing and Health, 16,* 131–139.

Buchanan, L. M., Cowan, M., Burr, R., Waldron, C., & Kogan, H. (1993). Measurement of recovery from myocardial infarction using heart rate variability and psychological outcomes. *Nursing Research, 42,* 74–78.

Christman, N. J. (1990). Uncertainty and adjustment during radiotherapy. *Nursing Research, 39,* 17–20.

Cossette, S., & Levesque, L. (1993). Caregiving tasks as predictors of mental health of wife caregivers of men with chronic obstructive pulmonary disease. *Research in Nursing and Health, 16,* 251–263.

Crumlish, C. M. (1994). Coping and emotional response in cardiac surgery patients. *Western Journal of Nursing Research, 16,* 57–68.

Dodd, M. J., Dibble, S. L., & Thomas, M. L. (1993). Predictors of concerns and coping strategies of cancer chemotherapy outpatients. *Applied Nursing Research, 6,* 2–7.

Erler, C. J., & Rudman, S. D. (1993). Effect of intensive care simulation on anxiety of nursing students in the clinical ICU. *Heart and Lung, 22,* 259–265.

Farran, C. J., Salloway, J. C., & Clark, D. C. (1990). Measurement of hope in a community-based older population. *Western Journal of Nursing Research, 12,* 42–59.

Flaskerud, J.H., & Cavillo, E. R. (1991). Beliefs about AIDS, health, and illness among low income Latina women. *Research in Nursing and Health, 16,* 431–438.

Fogel, C. I. (1993). Pregnant inmates: Risk factors and pregnancy outcomes. *Journal of Obstetric, Gynecologic, and Neonatal Nursing, 22,* 33–39.

Foster, M. F. (1992). Health promotion and life satisfaction in elderly black adults. *Western Journal of Nursing Research, 14,* 444–465.

Ganong, L. (1993). Nurses' perceptions of married and unmarried pregnant patients. *Western Journal of Nursing Research, 15,* 352–362.

Gardner, K. (1991). A summary of findings of a five-year comparison study of primary and team nursing. *Nursing Research, 40,* 113–116.

Gennaro, S., Brooten, D., Roncoli, M., & Kumar, S. P. (1993). Stress and health outcomes among mothers of low-birth-weight infants. *Western Journal of Nursing, 15,* 97–113.

Gloersen, B., Kendall, J., Gray, P., McConnell, S., Turner, J., & Lewkowicz, J. W. (1993). The phenomena of doing well in people with AIDS. *Western Journal of Nursing Research, 15,* 44–54.

Hahn, W. K., Brooks, J. A., & Hartsough, D. M. (1993). Self-disclosure and coping styles in men with cardiovascular reactivity. *Research in Nursing and Health, 16,* 275–282.

Heidrich, S. M. (1993). The relationship between physical health and psychological well-being in elderly women. *Research in Nursing and Health, 16,* 123–130.

Herth, K. (1990). Relationship of hope, coping styles, concurrent losses, and setting to grief resolution in the elderly widower. *Research in Nursing and Health, 13,* 109–117.

Howell, S. L. (1994). A theoretical model for caring for women with chronic nonmalignant pain. *Qualitative Health Research, 4,* 94–122.

Janson-Bjerklie, S., Ferketich, S., & Benner, P. (1993). Predicting the outcomes of living with asthma. *Research in Nursing and Health, 16,* 241–250.

Jirovec, M. M., & Kasno, J. (1993). Predictors of self-care abilities among the institutionalized elderly. *Western Journal of Nursing Research, 15*, 314–324.

Kidd, P., & Huddleston, S. (1994). Psychometric properties of the Driving Practices Questionnaire: Assessment of risky driving. *Research in Nursing and Health, 17*, 51–58.

King, K. B., Porter, L. A., Norsen, L. H., & Reis, H. T. (1992). Patient perceptions of quality of life after coronary artery surgery: Was it worth it? *Research in Nursing and Health, 15*, 327–334.

Littlefield, V. M., Chang, A., & Adams, B. N. (1990). Participation in alternative care: Relationship to anxiety, depression, and hostility. *Research in Nursing and Health, 13*, 17–25.

May, K. A. (1994) Impact of maternal activity restriction for preterm labor on the expectant father. *Journal of Obstetric, Gynecologic, and Neonatal Nursing, 23*, 246–251.

Mock, V. (1993). Body image in women treated for breast cancer. *Nursing Research, 42*, 153–157.

Neill, K. M. (1993). Ethnic pain styles in acute myocardial infarction. *Western Journal of Nursing Research, 15*, 531–543.

Nicholas, P. K., & Leuner, J. D. (1992). Relationship between body image and chronic obstructive pulmonary disease. *Applied Nursing Research, 5*, 83–88.

Opie, A. (1994). The instability of the caring body: Gender and caregivers of confused older people. *Qualitative Health Research, 4*, 31–50.

Price, M. J. (1993). An experiential model of learning diabetes self-management. *Qualitative Health Research, 3*, 29–54.

Reis, J. (1990). Medicaid maternal and child health care: Prepaid plans vs. private fee-for-service.

Research in Nursing and Health, 13, 163–171.

Stratton, T. D., Dunkin, J. W., Juhl, N., & Geller, J. M. (1993). Recruiting registered nurses to rural practice settings. *Applied Nursing Research, 6*, 64–70.

Stuifbergen, A. K. (1990). Patterns of functioning in families with a chronically ill parent. *Research in Nursing and Health, 13*, 35–44.

Topp, R., & Stevenson, J. S. (1994). The effects of attendance and effort on outcomes among older adults in a long-term exercise program. *Research in Nursing and Health, 17*, 15–24.

Vortherms, R., Ryan, P., & Ward, S. (1992). Knowledge of, attitudes toward, and barriers to pharmacologic management of cancer pain in a statewide random sample of nurses. *Research in Nursing and Health, 15*, 459–466.

Walsh, S. M. (1993). Future images: An art intervention with suicidal adolescents. *Applied Nursing Research, 6*, 111–118.

Weaver, T. E., & Narsavage, G. L. (1992). Physiological and psychological variables related to functional status in chronic obstructive pulmonary disease. *Nursing Research, 41*, 286–291.

White, N. E., Richter, J. M., & Fry, C. (1992). Coping, social support, and adaptation to chronic illness. *Western Journal of Nursing Research, 14*, 211–224.

Woodhouse, L. D. (1992). Women with jagged edges: Voices from a culture of substance abuse. *Qualitative Health Research, 2*, 262–281.

Woods, N. F., Haberman, M. R., & Packard, N. J. (1993). Demands of illness and individual, dyadic, and family adaptation in chronic illness. *Western Journal of Nursing Research, 15*, 10–25.

Chapter 14

OBSERVATIONAL METHODS

Scientific observation involves the systematic se-lection, observation, and recording of behav-iors, events, and settings relevant to a problem under investigation. Like self-report methods, observational methods can vary in terms of structure, from highly unstructured to highly structured approaches. Both structured and un-structured methods are discussed in this chap-ter. First, however, we present an overview of some general issues.

❖ OBSERVATIONAL ISSUES

When a nurse researcher observes an event—such as a nurse administering an injection to a patient—he or she typically has a clear idea about what is to be observed and under what circumstances it will be done. The researcher cannot absorb and record an infinite number of details and must, therefore, have some guide-lines specifying the manner in which the obser-vations are to be focused and recorded. In this section, we indicate the versatility of observa-tional methods and point out some considera-tions for observing phenomena in a research context.

Phenomena Amenable to Observations

Nurse researchers usually make observa-tional records of either human behaviors or the characteristics of individuals, events, environ-ments, or objects. The following list of observ-able phenomena is meant to be suggestive rather than exhaustive:

1. *Characteristics and conditions of individu-als.* A broad variety of information about people's attributes and states can be gath-ered by direct observation. We refer not only to relatively enduring traits of individ-uals, such as their physical appearance, but also to more temporary conditions, such as physiologic symptoms that are amenable to observation. We include here physiologic conditions that can be ob-served either directly through the senses, or with the aid of observational apparatus, such as a radiograph. To illustrate this class of observable phenomena, the following could be used as dependent or indepen-dent variables in a nursing research inves-tigation: the sleep or wake state of pa-

tients, the presence of edema in congestive heart failure, turgor of the skin in dehydration, the manifestation of decubitus ulcers, alopecia during cancer chemotherapy, or symptoms of infusion phlebitis in hospitalized patients. For example, Ziemer and Pigeon (1993) observed and documented skin changes in mothers' nipples during the first week of lactation in relation to changes in pain.

2. *Verbal communication behaviors.* The content and structure of people's conversations are readily observable, easy to record, and, thus, an obvious source of data. Among the kinds of verbal communications that a nurse researcher may be interested in observing are information-giving of nurses to patients, nurses' conversations with grieving relatives, exchange of information among nurses at change of shift report, the dialogue of residents in a nursing home, and conversations in a rural public health clinic. For example, Morse and McHutchion (1991), in their study of the effects of releasing restraints among the elderly, observed the verbal behavior of patients in a psychogeriatric ward.

3. *Nonverbal communication behaviors.* People communicate their fears, wants, and emotions in many ways other than just with words. For nurse researchers, nonverbal communication represents an extremely fruitful area for research because nurses are often called on to be sensitive to nonverbal cues. The kinds of nonverbal behavior amenable to observational methods include facial expressions, touch, posture, gestures and other body movements, and extralinguistic behavior (i.e., the manner in which people speak, aside from the content, such as the intonation, loudness, and continuity of the speech). As an example, Sawada and her colleagues (1992) studied patterns of nonverbal communication between nurses and preoperative patients.

4. *Activities.* Many actions are amenable to observation and constitute valuable data for nurse researchers. Activities that serve as an index of health status or physical and emotional functioning are particularly important. As illustrations, the following kinds of activities lend themselves to an observational study: patients' eating habits and trends, bowel movements in postsurgical patients, length and number of visits by friends and relatives to hospitalized patients, and aggressive actions among children in the hospital playroom. Lucero and her co-researchers (1993), for example, studied the motor and self-care activities among institutionalized Alzheimer's disease patients.

5. *Skill attainment and performance.* Nurses and nurse educators are routinely called on to develop skills among clients and students. The attainment of these skills is often manifested behaviorally, and in such cases, an observational assessment is appropriate. For example, a nurse researcher might want to observe the following kinds of behaviors: the ability of nursing students to properly insert a urinary catheter, the ability of stroke patients to scan a food tray if homonymous hemianopia is present, the ability of diabetics to test their urine for sugar and acetone, or the ability of a newborn to exhibit sucking behavior when positioned for breastfeeding. Glass and colleagues (1993), for example, used observations to study nurses' ability to achieve hyperventilation and hyperoxygenation with a manual resuscitation bag during endotracheal suctioning.

6. *Environmental characteristics.* An individual's surroundings may have a profound effect on his or her behavior, and a number of studies have explored the relationship between certain observable attributes of the environment on the one hand and human beliefs, actions, and needs on the other. Examples of observable environmental attributes include the following: the

noise levels in different areas of a hospital, the decor in a nursing home, the safety hazards in an elementary school classroom, or the cleanliness of the homes in a community. For example, Kinzel (1991), in her in-depth field study, observed the environmental characteristics of the shelters and streets where the homeless live.

Units of Observation

In selecting behaviors, attributes, or situations to be observed, the investigator must decide what constitutes a unit. There are two basic approaches, which are best considered as the end points of a continuum. The *molar approach* entails observing large units of behavior and treating them as a whole. For example, psychiatric nurse researchers might engage in a study of patient mood swings. An entire constellation of verbal and nonverbal behaviors might be construed as signaling aggressive behaviors, and another set might constitute passive behaviors. At the other extreme, the *molecular approach* uses small and highly specific behaviors as the unit of observation. Each movement, action, gesture, or phrase is treated as a separate entity, or perhaps broken down into even smaller units. The choice of approaches depends to a large degree on the nature of the problem and the preferences of the investigator. The molar approach is more susceptible to observer errors and distortions because of the greater ambiguity in the definition of the units. On the other hand, in reducing the observations to more concrete and specific elements, the investigator may lose sight of the activities that are at the heart of the inquiry.

The Observer–Observed Relationship

The observer–researcher can interact with individuals in the observational setting to varying degrees. The issue of the relationship between the observer and those observed is an important one, and one that has stirred much

controversy. Two important aspects of this issue concern intervention and concealment. The decisions a researcher makes in establishing a strategy for handling these considerations should be based on an understanding of the ethical and methodological implications.

In observational studies, intervention may involve an experimental intervention of the type described in Chapter 8 on experimental designs. For example, a nurse researcher may observe patients' postoperative behaviors after an intervention designed to improve the patients' ability to cough and breathe after surgery. In observational studies, however, the researcher sometimes intervenes to structure the research setting without necessarily introducing an experimental treatment, that is, without manipulating the independent variable. This approach is sometimes referred to as the use of *directed settings*. For instance, researchers sometimes stage a situation to provoke specific behavioral patterns. Certain events or activities are rare in naturalistic settings, and therefore, it becomes inexpedient to await their manifestation. For example, a number of social psychologic investigations have studied the behavior of bystanders in crisis situations. Because crises are unpredictable and infrequent, investigators have staged emergencies to observe helping behavior (or lack of it) among onlookers. Such studies are considered high on the intervention dimension. Studies in which the researcher intervenes to elicit behaviors of interest may be practical when there is little opportunity to observe activities or events as they unfold naturalistically. However, such studies are sometimes criticized on the grounds of artificiality and may suffer from serious problems of external validity.

The second dimension that concerns the relationship between the observer and the observed is the degree to which subjects are aware of the observation and their subject status. In naturalistic settings, researchers are often concerned that their presence, if known, would alter the behaviors under observation. In some situations, therefore, observers may adopt a completely passive role, attempting insofar as possible to become unobtrusive bystanders. The problem of behavioral distortions owing to the known presence of an observer has been called a reactive measurement effect or, more simply, *reactivity*. One approach to minimizing the problem of reactivity is to make the observations without the subjects' knowledge, through some type of concealment. For example, a nurse could monitor patients' conversations surreptitiously by means of the call system located at the nurses' station. In laboratory environments or in some directed settings, concealed observations can be accomplished through the use of one-way mirrors.

Concealment offers the researcher a number of distinct advantages, even beyond the reduction of reactivity. Some individuals might deny a researcher the privilege of observing them altogether so that the alternative to concealed observation might be no observation at all. Total concealment, however, may be difficult to attain except in highly structured or active observational settings. Furthermore, concealed observation, without the knowledge and consent of those observed, is ethically problematic (see Chapter 6).

A second situation is one in which the subjects are aware of the researcher's presence but may not be aware of the investigator's underlying motives. This approach offers the researcher the opportunity of getting more in-depth information than is usually possible with total concealment. Also, because the researcher is not totally concealed, there may be fewer ethical problems. Nevertheless, the issues of subject deception and failure to obtain informed voluntary consent remain thorny ones. Furthermore, a serious drawback of this second approach is the possibility that the interaction between the observer and the observed will alter the subjects' behavior. Even when the observed individuals are unaware of being participants in a research study, there is always a risk that the researcher's presence will alter their normal activities, mannerisms, or conversations.

The researcher will be confronted with methodological, substantive, or ethical issues at every point along the concealment and intervention dimensions. Some of these problems will be irrelevant in particular projects, but the careful investigator should assess the relative weaknesses of an approach against the possible advantages it might offer.

❖ OBSERVATIONAL METHODS: UNSTRUCTURED OBSERVATIONS

Qualitative studies sometimes involve the collection of unstructured or loosely structured observational data, often as an important supplement to self-report data. The aim of qualitative research is typically to understand the behaviors and experiences of people as they actually occur in naturalistic settings. Therefore, the qualitative researcher's aim is to observe and record information about people and their environments with a minimum of structure and researcher-imposed interference.

Unstructured observational data are often gathered in field settings through a process referred to as *participant observation*. In participant observation research, the investigator participates in the functioning of the social group under investigation and strives to observe and record information within the contexts, structures, and symbols that are relevant to the group members. Although it is beyond the scope of this book to describe in detail the methods used in participant observation research, we describe some of the salient issues.

The Observer–Participant Role

The role that an observer plays in the social group under investigation is important because the social position of the observer determines what he or she is likely to see. That is, the behaviors that are likely to be available for observation will depend on the observer's position in a network of relations.

Leininger (1985) noted that the observer's role typically evolves through a sequence of four phases:

1. Primarily observation
2. Primarily observation with some participation
3. Primarily participation with some observation
4. Reflective observation

In the initial phase, the researcher observes and listens to those under study to obtain a broad view of the situation. This phase allows both observers and subjects to "size up" each other, to become acquainted, and to become more comfortable in interacting. In phase 2, observation is enhanced by a modest degree of participation. As the researcher participates more actively in the activities of the social group, the reactions of people to specific researcher behaviors can be more systematically studied. In phase 3, the researcher strives to become a more active participant, learning by the actual experience of doing rather than just by watching and listening. In phase 4, the researcher reflects on the total process of what transpired and how people interacted with and reacted to the researcher.

The observer must overcome at least two major hurdles in assuming a satisfactory role regarding subject-informants. The first is to gain entrée into the social group under investigation; the second is to establish rapport and develop trust within the social group. Without gaining entrée, the study cannot proceed; but without the trust of the group, the researcher will typically be restricted to what Leininger (1985) refers to as "front stage" knowledge, that is, information that is distorted by the group's protective facades. The goal of the participant observer is to "get back stage"—to learn about the true realities of the group's experiences and behaviors. On the other hand, being a fully participating member does not *necessarily* offer the best perspective for studying a phenomenon—just as being an actor in a play does not offer the most advantageous view of the performance.

Interpersonal skills play an important part in developing the appropriate role in participant observation research. Wilson (1985) noted that successful participant observation research may require researchers to "go through channels, cultivate relationships, contour [their] appearances, withhold evaluative judgments, and be as unobtrusive and charming as possible" (p. 376).

Gathering and Recording Unstructured Observational Data

During the initial phase of a naturalistic inquiry, it is often useful to gather some written or pictorial descriptive information that provides an overview of the environment. In an institutional setting, for example, it may be helpful to obtain a floor plan, an organizational chart, an annual report, and so on. Then, a preliminary personal tour of the site should be undertaken to gain familiarity with the ambience of the site and to note major activities, social groupings, transactions, and events.

The next step is to identify a meaningful way to sample observations and to select observational locations. Sampling by time and by event are common strategies for observational sampling (these strategies are discussed later in this chapter). It is generally useful to use a combination of positioning approaches in selecting observational locations. *Single positioning* means staying in a single location for a period to observe behaviors and transactions in that location. *Multiple positioning* involves moving around the site to observe behaviors from different locations. *Mobile positioning* involves following a person throughout a given activity or period.

Because participant observers cannot spend a lifetime in one site and because they cannot be in more than one place at a time, observation is almost always supplemented with information obtained in unstructured interviews or conversations. For example, an informant may be asked to describe what went on in a meeting that the observer was unable to attend, or informants may be asked to describe an event that occurred before the observer entered the field. In such a case, the informant functions as the observer's observer.

The participant observer typically places few restrictions on the nature of the data collected, in keeping with the goal of minimizing observer-imposed meanings and structure. Nevertheless, participant observers often have a broad plan for the types of information to be gathered. Among the aspects likely to be considered relevant are the following:

1. *The physical setting.* What are the main features of the physical setting? What is the context within which human behavior unfolds? What types of behaviors and characteristics are promoted (or constrained) by the physical environment?
2. *The participants.* What are the characteristics of the people being observed? How many people are there? What are their roles? Who is given free access to the setting—who "belongs"? What brings these people together?
3. *Activities and interactions.* What is going on—what are the participants doing? Is there a discernible progression of activities? How do the participants interact with one another? What methods do they use to communicate, and how frequently do they do so? What type of affect is manifested during their interactions? How are the participants interconnected to one another or to the activities underway?
4. *Frequency and duration.* When did the activity or event begin, and when is it scheduled to end? How much time has elapsed? Is the activity a recurring one, and if so, how regularly does it recur? How typical of such activities is the one that is under observation?
5. *Intangible factors.* What did *not* happen (especially if it ought to have happened)? Are the participants saying one thing verbally but communicating other messages nonverbally? What types of things were disruptive to the activity or situation?

The most common forms of record-keeping in participant observation studies are logs and field notes. A *log* is a daily record of events

and conversations. *Field notes* may include the daily log but tend to be much broader, more analytic, and more interpretive than a simple listing of occurrences. Field notes represent the participant observer's efforts to record information and also to synthesize and understand the data.

Field notes are sometimes categorized according to the purpose they will serve during the analysis and integration of information. *Observational notes* are objective descriptions of events and conversations; information such as time, place, activity, and dialogue are recorded as completely and objectively as possible. *Theoretical notes* are interpretive attempts to attach meaning to observations. *Methodological notes* are instructions or reminders about how subsequent observations will be made. *Personal notes* are comments about the researcher's own feelings during the research process. Table 14-1 presents some examples of all four types of field notes from a fictitious study of an in vitro fertilization treatment facility.

The success of any participant observation study depends heavily on the quality of the logs and field notes. It is essential to record observations while the researcher is still in the process of collecting information because the memory is bound to fail if there is too long a delay. On the other hand, the participant observer cannot usually perform the recording function by openly carrying a clipboard, pens, and paper because this action would undermine the observer's role as an ordinary participant of the group. The researcher, therefore, must develop the skill of making detailed mental notes that can later be committed to paper or recorded on tape. Alternatively, the observer can try to jot down unobtrusively a phrase or sentence that will later serve as a reminder of an event, conversation, or impression. At a later point—preferably as soon as possible—the observer can use the brief notes and mental recordings to develop the more extensive field notes. The use of portable computers with word processing capabilities can greatly facilitate the recording and organization of notes in the field.

Table 14-1. *Example of Field Notes: Study of an In Vitro Fertilization (IVF) Facility*

Observational Notes	Couple A entered the center for the first time at around 7 PM on a Tuesday evening. Mrs. A sat very stiffly on the chair next to the receptionist's desk, and Mr. A sat beside her. Both parties looked uncomfortable and tense. There was little interaction between them until they were called in for the initial consultation. While in the waiting area, Mrs. A picked up several magazines, thumbed through them absently, and then put them down again. Mr. A spent most of the time smoking cigarettes, staring at the ceiling or at the entrance to the office. Couple A spent about 15 minutes in the waiting area. When their name was called, Mrs. A jumped as though startled and then moved quickly toward the door. She turned back once to make sure Mr. A was following, and when she saw that he was just rising, motioned for him to follow her.
Theoretical notes	Tension is a common feature among couples waiting for their initial consultation. However, the tension seems to stem from different sources and manifests itself in different ways. Some couples seem not to be persuaded that IVF is right for them; these couples seem embarrassed and tend not to communicate with one another. The source of tension seems to stem less from conflict about whether to try IVF but rather from the fear of disappointment. These couples tend to engage in continuous *sotto voce* discussions about what they've heard about IVF while waiting for their intake.
Methodological notes	I decided yesterday to make more systematic observations of couples immediately after they complete their initial interview. This decision was spurred by an incident yesterday in which both partners left the office in tears.
Personal notes	My progress in understanding what these couples seeking IVF treatment are going through is very uneven. Two days ago, I was confident that patterns were falling into place. But this afternoon, a little girl in the waiting room (an adopted daughter of a couple undergoing treatment) made me painfully aware of how much more complex the phenomenon of infertility and its social and psychological meanings really are.

Evaluation of Unstructured Observation

Unstructured observation is a method of collecting research data that has both opponents and proponents. Researchers who support the use of unstructured methods point out that these techniques usually provide a deeper and richer understanding of human behaviors and social situations than is possible with more standardized procedures. Participant observation is particularly valuable, according to this view, for its ability to "get inside" a particular situation and lead to a more complete understanding of its complexities. Furthermore, unstructured observational approaches are inherently flexible and, therefore, permit the observer greater freedom to reconceptualize the problem after becoming more familiar with the situation. Advocates of qualitative observational research also claim that structured, quantitatively oriented methods are too mechanistic and superficial to render a meaningful account of the intricate nature of human behavior.

Critics of the unstructured approach point out a number of methodological shortcomings. Observer bias and observer influence are prominent difficulties. Not only is there a concern that the observer may lose objectivity in recording actual observations, there is also the possibility that the observer will inappropriately sample events and situations to be observed. Once the researcher begins to participate in a group's activities, the risk of emotional involvement becomes a salient issue. The researcher in the new member role may fail to attend to many scientifically relevant aspects of the situation or may develop a myopic view on issues of importance to the group. Participant observation techniques, thus, may be an unsuitable approach to study problems when one suspects that the risk of identification is strong. Finally, unstructured observational methods depend more on the observational and interpersonal skills of the observer than do highly structured techniques—skills that may be difficult to cultivate.

On the whole, it appears that unstructured observational methods are extremely profitable for exploratory research in which the investigator wishes to establish an adequate conceptualization of the important variables in a social setting or wants to develop a set of hypotheses. The more structured observational methods discussed in the next section are probably better suited in most cases to the testing of research hypotheses.

❖ OBSERVATIONAL METHODS: STRUCTURED OBSERVATIONS

Structured observational methods differ from unstructured techniques in the specificity of behaviors or events selected for observation, in the advance preparation of record-keeping forms, and in the kinds of activities in which the observer engages. The observer using a structured observational procedure may still have room for making inferences and exercising judgment but is restrained with regard to the kinds of phenomena that will be watched and recorded. The creativity of structured observation lies not in the observation itself but rather in the formulation of a system for accurately categorizing, recording, and encoding the observations and sampling the phenomena of interest. Because structured techniques depend on plans developed before observation, they are not considered appropriate when the investigator has limited knowledge about the phenomena under investigation.

Categories and Checklists

The most common approach to making structured observations of ongoing events and behaviors consists of the construction of a category system to which the observed phenomena can be assigned. A *category system* represents an attempt to designate in a systematic or quantitative fashion the qualitative behaviors and events transpiring within the observational setting.

CONSIDERATIONS IN USING CATEGORY SYSTEMS

One of the most important requirements of a category system is the careful and explicit definition of the behaviors and characteristics to be observed. Each category should be explained in detail with an operational definition so that observers will have relatively clearcut criteria for assessing the occurrence of the phenomenon in question. For example, Hurley and her colleagues (1992) developed an observational scale for measuring discomfort in noncommunicative patients with advanced Alzheimer's disease. An example of a behavioral indicator for the Discomfort Scale is "noisy breathing," which is defined as follows:

> Noisy breathing: negative sounding noise on inspiration or expiration; breathing looks strenuous, labored, or wearing; respirations sound loud, harsh, or gasping; difficulty breathing or trying hard at attempting to achieve good gas exchange; episodic bursts of rapid breaths or hyperventilation. (Hurley, Volicer, Hanrahan, Houde, & Volicer, 1992, p. 373)

In developing or selecting a categorization scheme, the researcher must make a number of important decisions. One decision concerns the exhaustiveness of the phenomena to be observed and the number of categories to be included. Some category systems are constructed such that *all* observed interactive behaviors can be classified into one (and only one) category.

A contrasting technique is to develop a nonexhaustive system in which only particular types of behavior are categorized. For example, if we were observing the aggressive behavior of autistic children, we might develop such categories as "strikes another child," "kicks or hits walls or floors," "calls other children names," "throws objects around the room," and so forth. In this restricted category system, many behaviors (all those that are nonaggressive) would not be classified. Such nonexhaustive systems are adequate for many research purposes. However, they run the risk of providing data that are difficult to interpret. When a large number of observed behaviors are unclassified, the investigator may have difficulty in placing the categorized behaviors into a proper perspective.

Virtually all category systems require that some inferences be made on the part of the observer, but there is considerable variability on this dimension. Weiss' (1992) Tactile Interaction Index (TII) for observing patterns of interpersonal touch is an example of a system that requires a modest amount of inference. For example, one dimension of the TII concerns the location or part of an individual's body that is touched, classified in one of 19 relatively straightforward categories (e.g., abdomen, arm, back, and so on). On the other hand, a category system such as the Abnormal Involuntary Movement Scale (AIMS) requires considerably more inference. The AIMS system, which was developed by the National Institute for Mental Health and used by Whall and associates (1989) for studying tardive dyskinetic movements over time during the day, contains such broad categories as "incapacitation due to abnormal movements." Even when such categories are accompanied by detailed definitions and descriptions, there is a heavy inferential burden placed on the observer. The decision concerning how much observer inference is appropriate depends on a number of factors, including the research purposes and the skills of the observers. Beginning researchers are advised to construct or use category systems that require only a moderate degree of inference. In general, category systems that use molecular units of behavior tend to require less inference than those that use molar units.

Once a category system has been developed or selected, the researcher can proceed to construct a *checklist,* which is the instrument used by the observer to record observed phenomena. Whether one constructs a new category system or uses an existing one, the system should be subjected to pilot runs to assess its suitability for the intended study.

CHECKLISTS FOR EXHAUSTIVE SYSTEMS

When an observer uses an exhaustive system (i.e., when all behaviors of a certain type—such as verbal interaction—are observed and recorded), the researcher must be especially careful to define the categories in such a way that the observers know when one behavior ends and a new one begins. Another essential feature of exhaustive systems is that the referent behaviors should be mutually exclusive. If overlapping categories are not eliminated, then the observer may have difficulty in deciding how to classify a particular observation. The underlying assumption in the use of such a category system is that behaviors, events, or attributes that are allocated to a particular category are equivalent to every other behavior, event, or attribute in that same category.

The checklist is generally formatted with the list of behaviors or events from the category system on the left and space for tallying the frequency or duration of occurrence of behaviors on the right. In complex social situations with multiple actors, the right-hand portion may be divided into panels according to characteristics of the actors (e.g., nurse/physician; male patients/female patients) or by individual subjects' names or identification numbers.

The task of the observer using this approach is to place all behaviors in only one category for each element. By *element,* we refer to either a unit of behavior, such as a sentence in a conversation, or to a time interval. To illustrate, suppose that we were interested in studying the problem-solving behavior of a group of public health workers developing a maternal–child health program in a rural area. We might construct a category system such as the following: 1) information seeking; 2) information giving; 3) problem describing; 4) suggestion proposing;

5) suggestion opposing; 6) suggestion supporting; 7) summarizing; and 8) miscellaneous. The observer would be required to classify every group member's contribution—using, for example, each sentence as the element—to the problem-solving process in terms of one of these eight categories. By employing such a system, it would be possible to analyze, for example, the relationship between a group member's role, status, or characteristics on the one hand and the types of problem-solving behaviors engaged in on the other.

The second manner in which this approach can be used is to categorize the relevant behaviors at regular time intervals. For example, in an observational system for analyzing the motor activity of infants, the researcher might want to use 15-second time intervals as the basic recording unit. That is, the observer would be expected to record infant movements occurring within a 15-second period. Checklists based on exhaustive category systems are demanding of the observer because the recording task is continuous.

CHECKLISTS FOR NONEXHAUSTIVE SYSTEMS

The second approach, which is sometimes referred to as a *sign system,* begins with a listing of categories of behaviors that may or may not be manifested by the subjects. The observer's task is to watch for instances of the behaviors on the list. When a behavior occurs, the observer either places a check mark beside the appropriate behavior to designate its occurrence or makes a cumulative tally of the number of times the behavior was witnessed. The product of this type of endeavor is a kind of demography of events transpiring within the observational period. With this type of checklist, the observer does not classify *all* the behaviors or characteristics of the individuals being observed but rather identifies the occurrence and frequency of particular behaviors. A hypothetical example of a checklist using the sign system for describing patients' ability to perform selected activities of daily living is presented in Table 14-2.

Rating Scales

Structured observations can be recorded in a number of ways other than through the use of category systems and checklists. The major alternative is to use *rating scales* that require the observer to rate some phenomenon in terms of points along a descriptive continuum. The ratings usually are quantified during the subsequent analysis of the observational data.

Rating scales normally are used in one of two ways. The observer may be required to make ratings of behavior or events at frequent intervals throughout the observational period in much the same way that a checklist would be used. Alternatively, the observer may use the rating scales to summarize an entire event or transaction after the observation is completed. Postobservation ratings require the observer to integrate a number of activities and to judge which point on a scale most closely resembles

Table 14-2. *Example of Categories for a Sign System*

ACTIVITY	FREQUENCY
EATING BEHAVIORS	
Eats with hand	
Eats with spoon or fork	
Cuts soft food	
Cuts meat	
Drinks from a straw	
Drinks from a cup or glass	
HYGIENE	
Washes hands or extremities	
Brushes teeth	
Cleans fingernails	
Brushes or combs hair	
Shaves	
DRESSING SKILLS	
Fastens or unfastens buttons	
Fastens or unfastens snaps	
Pulls zipper up or down	
Ties or unties shoelace	
Puts on or takes off eyeglasses	
Fastens or unfastens buckle	
Puts in or takes out dentures	

the interpretation given to the overall situation. For example, suppose that we were interested in comparing the behaviors of nurses working in intensive care units with those of nurses in other units. After 15-minute observation sessions, the observer might be asked to rate the perceived anxiety level of the nursing staff in each unit as a whole, or that of individual members. The rating scale item might take the following form:

According to your perceptions, how tense were the nurses in the observed unit?

1. Extremely relaxed
2. Rather relaxed
3. Somewhat relaxed
4. Neither relaxed nor tense
5. Somewhat tense
6. Rather tense
7. Extremely tense

The same information could be solicited using a graphic rating scale format:

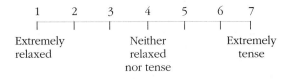

Rating scales can also be used as an extension of checklists wherein the observer records not only the occurrence of some behavior but also some qualitative aspect of it, such as its magnitude or intensity. Weiss' (1992) TII once again provides a good example. Her category scheme comprises four dimensions: location (part of body touched); action (the specific gesture or movement used, such as grabbing, hitting, patting, and so on); duration (temporal length of the touch); and intensity. Observers using the index must both classify the nature and duration of the touch *and* rate the intensity on a four-point scale: light, moderate, strong, and deep. When rating scales are coupled with a category scheme in this fashion, considerably more information about the phenomena under investigation can be obtained. The disadvantage of this approach is that it places an immense burden on the observer, particularly if there is an extensive amount of activity.

Constructing Versus Borrowing Structured Observational Instruments

The development, testing, refining, and retesting of a new category scheme or rating scale may require weeks or even months of effort, particularly if the system is intended to be used in a variety of settings and with a variety of subjects. In some cases, a researcher may have no alternative but to design new observational instruments. For example, the researcher may be investigating a relatively new area or may be expanding an area of inquiry with a new population of subjects for whom existing tools may be inappropriate. As in the case of self-report instruments, however, we encourage researchers to explore the literature fully for potentially usable observational instruments.

Many observational systems have been constructed with the intent of being applied to a variety of research situations. Generalized systems, such as the AIMS system described earlier, should be scrutinized before proceeding to design a new system. The use of an existing system not only saves a considerable amount of work but also facilitates comparisons among investigations.

A few source books describe available observational checklists for certain research applications. For example, the reference books by Frank-Stromberg (1988) and Strickland and Waltz (1988), which describe instruments for measuring variables of relevance to nursing, include some observational instruments. Perhaps the best source for such tools, however, is the current research literature on the topic of interest. For example, if you wanted to conduct an observational study of maternal–infant bonding behavior, a good place to begin would be to review recently completed research on this or similar topics to get clues about how maternal bonding was operationalized. Table 14-3 provides examples of some concepts of interest to nurse researchers for which observational instruments have been developed and lists a recent study that used these instruments.

Table 14-3.   *Examples of Observational Instruments Used by Nurse Researchers*

CONCEPT	RESEARCH EXAMPLE REFERENCE	NAME OF INSTRUMENT
Caregiver behaviors	Burgener & Shimer, 1993	Interaction Behavior Measure (IBM)
Children's development	Youngblut, Loveland-Cherry, & Horan, 1993	Bayley Scales of Infant Development
Confusion	Foreman, Theis, & Anderson, 1993	Clinical Assessment of Confusion
Elderly's functional ability	Burgener & Shimer, 1993	Barthel Self-Care Index (BSCI)
Infant behavioral organization	Becker, Grunwald, Moorman, & Stuhr, 1991	Brazelton Neonatal Behavioral Assessment Scales (NBAS)
Infant's medical complications	Harrison, Leeper, & Yoon, 1991	Neonatal Morbidity Scale (NBS)
Infant–mother attachment	Quinn, 1991	Attachment-Separation-Individuation Scale (ASI)
Infant stress, crying	Treloar, 1994	Anderson Behavioral State Scale (ABSS)
Pain	Maikler, 1991	Maximally Discriminative Facial Movement Coding System (MAX)
Pressure ulceration	Foreman, Theis, & Anderson, 1993	Braden Scale
Quality of nursing care	Gardner, 1991	Quality of Patient Care Scale (QualPacs)

Observational Sampling

Structured observational methods rarely involve the recording of all behaviors or activities that occur in a given situation. The investigator must often decide how and when the system will be applied. Observational sampling methods represent a mechanism for obtaining representative examples of the behavior being observed without having to observe for prolonged periods.

The most frequently used system is the *time-sampling method*. This procedure involves the selection of periods during which the observations will occur. The timeframes may be systematically selected (e.g., every 30 seconds at 2-minute intervals) or may be selected at random. As a hypothetical example, suppose we were studying the interaction patterns of mothers and their handicapped children. Some of the mothers have received specific preparation from a community health nurse for dealing with their conflict over the child's dependence–independence needs, and a control group of mothers has not received this intervention. To examine the effects of this special program, the behavior of the mothers and children are observed in a playground setting. During a 1-hour observation period, we decide to sample behaviors rather than to observe the entire session. For the sake of simplicity, let us say that 3-minute observations will be made. If we use a systematic sampling approach, we would observe for 3-minutes, then cease observing for a prespecified period, say 3 minutes. Using this scheme, a total of 10 3-minute observations would be made. A second approach is to sample randomly 3-minute periods from the total of 20 such periods in an hour. The decision with regard to the length and number of periods for creating a suitable sample must be influenced by the aims of the research. In establishing time units, one of the most important considerations is determining a psychologically meaningful timeframe. A good deal of pretesting and experimentation with different sampling plans is essential in developing or adapting observational strategies.

Event sampling is a second system for obtaining a set of observations. This approach selects integral behaviors or events of a prespecified type for observation. Event sampling requires that the investigator either have some knowledge concerning the occurrence of events or be in a position to await their occurrence. Examples of integral events that may be suitable for event sampling include shift changes of nurses in a hospital, cast removals of pediatric patients, epileptic seizures, and cardiac arrests in the emergency room. This sampling approach is preferable to time sampling when the events of principal interest are infrequent throughout the day and are at risk of being missed if specific time-sampling frames are established. In addition, event sampling has the advantage that the observation treats situations in their entirety rather than fragmenting them into discontinuous segments. Still, when behaviors and events are relatively frequent, time sampling does have the virtue of enhancing the representativeness of the observed behaviors. Time sampling and event sampling can sometimes be profitably combined.

Structured Observations by Nonresearch Personnel

The research we have discussed thus far involves situations in which the researcher (or an observer assistant) observes ongoing events or behaviors of relevance to the research problem and then codes information relating to what has been seen in some specified period. Other forms of observational data-gathering methods provide more global information about the characteristics and behaviors of individuals. Often such methods involve asking nonresearch personnel to summarize on structured scales their knowledge of a person or group, based on their own observations. This method has much in common (in terms of format and scoring procedures) with the self-report scales described in Chapter 13; the primary difference is that the person completing the scale describes the attributes and behaviors of people other than himself or herself, based on observation. For example, a mother might be asked to describe the temperament of her infant, staff nurses might be asked to evaluate the functional capacity of nursing home residents, or a nursing supervisor might be asked to assess the nursing competency of nurses on the unit. As with self-report instruments, researchers might decide to construct their own behavior-rating scale for a specific research purpose, or they might choose to use or adapt an existing scale. Some of the references cited in Chapter 13 and at the end of this chapter identify such observational instruments.

The use of nonresearch personnel to provide observational data has a number of practical advantages. It is an economical method compared with using trained observers. For example, an observer might have to watch children for hours or days to describe fully the nature and intensity of certain behavior problems when a parent or teacher could readily do this. In some situations, the behaviors of interest might never be capable of observation by an outsider because of reactivity problems, because they occur in private situations, or because they constitute rare events (e.g., sleep-walking). Also, self-report data cannot be obtained for some populations, such as infants, the mentally retarded, or the very old.

On the other hand, such methods may have all the same problems as self-report scales (such as response-set biases) in addition to the problem of observer bias. Nonresearch observers are typically not trained, and interobserver agreement usually cannot be determined. Thus, this approach has a number of problems but will inevitably continue to find many research applications because, in many cases, there are no alternatives.

Several nurse researchers have used third-party observers to collect research data. For example, Swanson and her colleagues (1994) asked Alzheimer's disease patients' primary nurses to rate the patients' functional abilities using the Geriatric Rating Scale and the Functional Abilities Checklist. Hall and her colleagues (1991) asked mothers to record their observations of their children's behavior using the Preschool Behavior Questionnaire. Meininger, Stashinko, and Hayman (1991) used teacher ratings of children's competence in their study of children with Type A behavior.

❖ MECHANICAL AIDS IN OBSERVATIONS

Our discussion has focused on those types of observations that are made by observers directly through the use of their sensory organs. In this section, we look at mechanical devices or other equipment that can be used either as an extension of the human senses or as a means of securing permanent records of observational data.

The health care field has a rich store of devices and equipment designed to make available to observers conditions or attributes that are ordinarily imperceptible. Nasal specula, stethoscopes, bronchoscopes, radiographic and imaging equipment, ultrasound technology, and a myriad of other medical instruments make it possible for health care personnel to gather ob-

servational information concerning the health status and bodily functioning of patients.

In addition to equipment for enhancing physiologic observations, several mechanical devices are available for recording behaviors and events. These techniques make possible categorization at a later time. When the behavior of interest is primarily auditory, tape recordings can be obtained and used as a permanent observational record. Transcripts from such recordings can then be prepared to facilitate the coding or classification process. Other technological instruments to aid auditory observation have been developed, such as laser devices that are capable of recording sounds by being directed on a window to a room, and voice tremor detectors that are sensitive to stress.

When a visual record is desired, videotapes are likely to be the most suitable media. In addition to being permanent, videotapes offer the possibility of capturing complex behaviors that would elude categorization by an on-the-spot observer. Visual records are also capable of capturing finer units of behavior, such as micromomentary facial expressions, than the naked eye. Videotapes offer the possibility of checking the accuracy of the coders and, thus, are useful as an aid to training. Finally, it is often easier to conceal a camera than a human observer, and in some situations, this feature would constitute a major advantage. Video records also have a number of drawbacks, some of which are fairly technical, such as lighting requirements, lens limitations, and so forth. Other serious problems result from the fact that the camera angle adopted could present a lopsided view of an event or situation. Still, for many applications, permanent visual records offer unparalleled opportunities to expand the range and scope of observational studies.

Also of interest is the growing technology for assisting with the encoding and recording of observations made directly by on-the-spot observers. For example, there is equipment that permits the observer to enter observational data directly into a computer as the observation occurs, and in some cases, the equipment can be used to record physiologic data concurrently. Such a system was used in an interesting nursing study by White and her colleagues (1990), who tested whether a taped bedtime story read to hospitalized children by their parents would help to ease separation anxiety.

❖ OBSERVER BIASES

Although observation is an extremely important method of data collection, it must be acknowledged that observational data are vulnerable to many distortions and biases. Human perceptual errors and inadequacies are a continuous threat to the quality of obtained information. Observation and interpretation are demanding tasks, requiring attention, sensation, perception, and conception. To accomplish these activities in a completely objective fashion is probably impossible, although structured category systems are designed to reduce observer subjectivity.

Several types of observational biases are especially common. One bias is referred to as the *enhancement of contrast effect*. The observer may tend to distort the observation in the direction of dividing the content into clearcut entities. The converse effect—a bias toward *central tendency*—occurs when extreme events are distorted toward a middle ground. A series of biases are in a category described as *assimilatory*. The observer may tend to distort observations in the direction of identity with previous inputs. This bias would have the effect of miscategorizing information in the direction of regularity and orderliness. Assimilation to the expectations and attitudes of the observer also occurs.

Rating scales are susceptible to several distinct types of bias. The *halo effect* refers to the tendency of the rater to be influenced by one characteristic in rating other unrelated characteristics. For example, if we formed a positive general impression of a person, we would probably be likely to rate that person as intelligent, loyal, and dependable simply because these traits are positively valued. Rating scales may reflect the

personality traits of the observer. The *error of leniency* is the tendency for the observer to rate everything positively, and the *error of severity* is the contrasting tendency to rate too harshly.

Needless to say, these biases are much more likely to operate when a high degree of observer inference is required by the observational tasks. The careful construction and pretesting of checklists and rating scales, the development of an adequate sampling plan, and the proper training of observers are techniques that can play an important role in minimizing or estimating these problematic biases. Although the degree of observer bias is not necessarily a function of the degree of structure imposed on the observation, it is generally more difficult to assess the extent of bias when using unstructured methods.

❖ TIPS FOR GATHERING OBSERVATIONAL DATA

By the time we reach adulthood, many of us have lost some of our native ability to learn through careful observation. We may even have to "unlearn" habits of filtering out details of the world around us. Below are some suggestions for how to proceed in an observational study.

- As in the case of interviewers, observers should accept the behaviors and events under observation in a neutral and nonjudgmental fashion. The people being observed are more likely to mask their emotions or behave in an atypical fashion if they think they are being evaluated or critically appraised. Even positive cues (such as nodding approval) should be withheld because approval may induce repetition of a behavior that might not otherwise have occurred.
- The adequate training and preparation of observers is essential to the collection of high-quality observational data. If people are to become good instruments for collecting observational data, then they must be trained to observe in such a way that accuracy is maxi-

mized and biases are minimized. Even when the investigator who designed the study does most or all of the observations, self-training and dry runs are essential. The setting during the trial period should resemble as closely as possible the settings that will be the focus of the actual observations.

- Ideally, training should include practice sessions during which the comparability of the observers' recordings is assessed. That is, two or more observers should watch a trial event or situation, and observations should then be compared. Procedures for establishing the *interrater reliability* of structured observational instruments are described in Chapter 16.
- With both structured and unstructured methods of observation, it is usually useful to spend a period of time with subjects before the actual observations and recording of

data. Having a warm-up period helps to relax subjects (especially if audio or video equipment is being used) and can be extremely helpful to observers (e.g., if the subjects have a linguistic style to which the observer must adjust, such as a strong regional accent).

❖ *RESEARCH EXAMPLES*

Table 14-4 presents several examples of observational studies conducted by nurse researchers. Two other examples that illustrate observational research in greater detail follow.

Unstructured Observation

Aroian (1992) conducted an in-depth, qualitative study regarding the process of adaptation among Polish immigrants to the United

Table 14-4.   *Examples of Observational Studies*

RESEARCH QUESTION	TYPE OF OBSERVATION	PHENOMENA OBSERVED
What are the behaviors that occur between hospitalized premature infants and their nurse caregivers? (Pickler, 1993)	Unstructured	Nurse–infant interactions
What is the nature of the interactions between migrant farmworkers and health care providers? (Jezewski, 1990)	Participant observation	Interactions during clinic sessions
Do high-risk infants who receive developmental care in the neonatal intensive care unit show improvements in their motor behavior and behavioral state organization? (Becker, Grunwald, Moorman, & Stuhr, 1993)	Structured categorization	Infant motor activity, infant behavioral state, nurse caregiving behaviors
What is the effectiveness of a special program to teach children with disabilities about handwashing? (Day, Arnaud, & Monsma, 1993)	Structured checklist	Handwashing behaviors
Does nurturant performance of the maternal role during acts of caregiving predict children's later social competence and behavioral problems? (Walker & Montgomery, 1994)	Structured ratings	Mother–infant interactions

States. Although much of Aroian's data were gathered through interviews with the immigrants, observations were also an important part of her data collection plan.

Participant observation of a Polish community in Seattle occurred over a 13-month period. According to the researcher, "participant observation . . . provided macrolevel community assessment and contextual validation of interview data" (p. 185). The researcher participated in a wide variety of quasi-public functions in the community and observed patterns of social interaction. These functions included Sunday masses, a Solidarity picnic, cabarets, bazaars, and political celebrations. The researcher also participated in less public family activities, including dinners and weddings. The investigator's observations and her interpretations were recorded as field notes. The observations helped Aroian to understand sources of social support among the immigrants and how social relationships facilitated psychosocial adaptation.

Structured Observation

Miller and Holditch-Davis (1992) compared the interactions of preterm infants and their parents with the infants' interactions with nurses. A sample of 29 high-risk preterm infants were observed weekly from 7:00 PM to 11:00 PM. All infants received at least 2 minutes of parental care and 2 minutes of nursing care during the observational session. During the observations, occurrences of infant and caregiver behaviors were recorded every 10 seconds, according to a behavioral scoring system that had been developed by other researchers. There was an audible signal at the end of each 10-second epoch, at which time the observer recorded the behaviors on a computer used as an event recorder. Each observation was conducted by one of two observers.

The researchers measured various dimensions of behaviors. One dimension was caregiver involvement. For this variable, infant time spent with parents and nurses was divided into four mutually exclusive levels of involvement: contact (touching, holding); routine care (feeding, changing diaper); low-level nursing care (e.g., taking vital signs); and high-level nursing care (e.g., respiratory care). Contact was scored only if no other type of involvement occurred in the 10-second epoch; if one of the other three levels occurred in the same epoch, the one that occupied the greatest amount of time was scored. Other dimensions scored included the infant's behavior, the infant's sleep–wake state, and caregiver stimulation.

The researchers found that nurses and parents provided different types of stimulation to the infants. Nurses were more likely to engage in procedural care, and parents were more likely to hold, talk to, move, and touch the infants affectionately. The infants demonstrated more large body movements and jitters when they were with the nurses and more active sleep and smiles when they were with the parents.

❖ SUMMARY

Observational methods are techniques for acquiring information for research purposes through the direct observation and recording of phenomena. In any observational setting— whether it be in a natural field situation or laboratory setup—the observer must have a plan regarding the nature of the phenomena to be observed. The researcher usually selects an appropriate *unit of observation*. The *molar approach* entails the observation of large segments of behaviors and events as integral units. The *molecular approach,* on the other hand, treats small, specific actions as separate entities.

The investigator must make decisions concerning the relationship between the observer and the subjects. The decisions relate primarily to the dimensions of concealment and intervention. *Concealment* refers to the degree to which the observed people are aware that they are being observed or that they are the subjects of a research study. The problem of behavioral distortions stemming from the presence of an observer (known as *reactivity*) is a major reason for making concealed observations. *Intervention* refers to the degree to which the investigator structures the observational setting in line with research demands as opposed to being a passive observer.

Like self-reports, observational methods vary in terms of structure. Qualitative studies generally collect unstructured observational data, often using a procedure known as participant observation. *Participant observation* is a method that has been used by anthropologists and sociologists as a means of understanding cultures, institutions, and social groups. The participant observer endeavors to obtain information about the dynamics of the social group within the subject's own frame of reference, without imposing a preconceived structure based on the researcher's world view.

In the initial phase of a participant observation study, the researcher is primarily an observer and gathers a preliminary understanding of the site. As time passes, the researcher typically becomes a more active participant and also develops a plan for sampling events and selecting observational positions. The observer usually combines *single positioning, multiple positioning,* and *mobile positioning.* The final phase of the research involves reflective observation about the activities that transpired.

Participant observers typically collect information about the setting, participants, activities and interactions, frequency and duration of events, and intangible factors. *Logs* of daily events and *field notes* are the major methods of recording data. Field notes have multiple purposes and may be categorized as *observational notes, theoretical notes, methodological notes,* and *personal notes.*

Proponents of the participant observation approach claim it represents both a source of data *and* a basis for understanding what the data mean. Although participant observation and other unstructured methods can yield extremely rich and useful information, particularly when used by insightful observers, they are nevertheless subject to a number of methodological difficulties. The most prominent difficulties are

observer bias in sampling, recording, and interpreting phenomena; observer influence (reactivity); and observer identification with the observed group.

Structured observational methods impose a number of constraints on the observer for the purpose of maximizing observer accuracy and objectivity and for obtaining an adequate representation of the phenomena of interest. Two types of data collection forms are used most commonly by observers in structured situations. *Checklists* are tools for recording the appearance or frequency of prespecified behaviors, events, or characteristics. Checklists are based on the development of *category systems* for encoding the observed phenomena. The researcher constructing a category system must make a number of decisions concerning its exhaustiveness, generality, inference requirements, and training demands. One type of checklist is based on the *sign system* and is used as a demographic record of the types of behavior that occurred during the observational session. A second format is used to exhaustively analyze ongoing events and activities.

Rating scales are the second most common record-keeping tool for structured observations. The observer using a rating scale is required to rate some phenomenon according to points along a dimension that is typically bipolar (e.g., passive/aggressive or excellent health/poor health). Ratings are generally made either during the observational setting at specific intervals (e.g., every 5 minutes) or after the observation is completed.

Most structured observations make use of some form of sampling plan for selecting the behaviors, events, and conditions to be observed. The most frequently used approach is *time sampling,* which involves the specification of the duration and frequency of both the observational periods and the intersession intervals. *Event sampling* selects integral behaviors or events of a special type for observation.

Technological advances have greatly augmented the researcher's capacity to collect, record, and preserve observational data. Such devices as tape recorders, movie cameras, videotape cameras, laser devices, and so forth permit behaviors and events to be categorized after their occurrence.

Observational methods, while extremely valuable to nurse researchers, are subject to a variety of biasing effects. The greater the degree of observer inference and judgment, the more likely it is that perceptual errors and distortions will occur. Among the most prevalent observer biases are the *enhancement of contrast effect, central tendency bias,* the *halo effect, assimilatory biases, errors of leniency,* and *errors of severity.*

❖ STUDY SUGGESTIONS

Chapter 14 of the accompanying *Study Guide for Nursing Research: Principles and Methods, 5th ed.,* offers various exercises and study suggestions for reinforcing the concepts presented in this chapter. Additionally, the following study questions can be addressed:

1. Suppose you were interested in observing the behavior of fathers in the delivery room during the birth of their first child. Identify the observer–observed relationship or the concealment and intervention dimensions that you would recommend adopting for such a study, and defend your recommendation. What are the possible drawbacks of your approach, and how might you deal with them?

2. Would a psychiatric nurse researcher be well suited to conduct a participant observation study of the behavior of psychiatric nurses and their interactions with clients? Why or why not?

3. A nurse researcher is planning to study temper tantrums displayed by hospitalized children. Would you recommend using a time-sampling approach? Why or why not?

4. Below is a list of problem statements. Indicate which of these problems could be studied by using some form of observational method. For each problem that is amenable to observation, specify whether you think a structured or unstructured approach would be preferable.

   a. Does team nursing versus primary nursing affect the type of communication patterns between nurses and patients?

   b. Is there a relationship between prenatal instruction and delivery room behaviors of primiparas?

   c. Is the number of hours of direct clinical practice for student nurses related to their performance on the licensure examination?

   d. Do the attitudes of nurses toward abortion affect the quality of care given to abortion patients?

   e. Do industrial alcohol programs have a positive impact on on-the-job accident rates?

   f. Is the touching behavior of nurses related to their ethnic or cultural background?

❖ SUGGESTED READINGS

METHODOLOGICAL REFERENCES

Dowrick, P., & Biggs, S. J. (Eds.). (1983). *Using video: Psychological and social applications.* New York: John Wiley and Sons.

Frank-Stromberg, M. (Ed.). (1988). *Instruments for clinical nursing research.* Norwalk, CT: Appleton & Lange.

Kerlinger, F. (1986). *Foundations of behavioral research* (3rd ed.). New York: Holt, Rinehart & Winston.

Leininger, M. (1985). Ethnography and ethnonursing: Models and modes of qualitative data analysis. In M. Leininger (Ed.), *Qualitative research methods in nursing.* New York: Grune & Stratton.

Lobo, M. L. (1992). Observation: A valuable data collection strategy for research with children. *Journal of Pediatric Nursing, 7,* 320–328.

Lofland, J., & Lofland, L. (1984). *Analyzing social settings: A guide to qualitative observation and analysis.* Belmont, CA: Wadsworth.

McCall, G. J., & Simmons H. L. (Eds.). (1969). *Issues in participant observation: A text and reader.* Reading, MA: Addison-Wesley.

Morrison, E. F., Phillips, L. R., & Chal, Y. M. (1990). The development and use of observational measurement scales. *Applied Nursing Research, 3,* 73–86.

Schatzman, L., & Strauss, A. (1982). *Field research: Strategies for a natural sociology* (2nd ed.). Englewood Cliffs, NJ: Prentice-Hall.

Strickland, O. L., & Waltz, C. (Eds.). (1988). *Measurement of nursing outcomes.* New York: Springer.

Ward, M. J., & Lindemann, C. (Eds.). (1979). *Instruments for measuring nursing practice and other health care variables.* Hyattsville, MD: Department of Health, Education and Welfare.

Wilson, H. S. (1985). *Research in nursing.* Menlo Park, CA: Addison-Wesley.

SUBSTANTIVE REFERENCES

Aroian, K. J. (1992). Sources of social support and conflict for Polish immigrants. *Qualitative Health Research, 2,* 178–207.

Becker, P. T., Grunwald, P. C., Moorman, J., & Stuhr, S. (1991). Outcomes of developmentally supportive nursing care for very-low-birth-weight infants. *Nursing Research, 40,* 150–156.

Becker, P. T., Grunwald, P. C., Moorman, J., & Stuhr, S. (1993). Effects of developmental care on behavioral organization in very-low-birth-weight infants. *Nursing Research, 42,* 214–220.

Burgener, S. C., & Shimer, R. (1993). Variables related to caregiver behaviors with cognitively impaired elders in institutional settings. *Research in Nursing and Health, 16,* 193–202.

Day, R. A., Arnaud, S. S., & Monsma, M. (1993). Effectiveness of a handwashing program. *Clinical Nursing Research, 2,* 24–40.

Foreman, M. D., Theis, S. L., & Anderson, M. A. (1993). Adverse events in the hospitalized elderly. *Clinical Nursing Research, 2,* 360–370.

Gardner, L. (1991). A summary of findings of a five-year comparison study of primary and team nursing. *Nursing Research, 40,* 113–116.

Glass, C., Grap, M. J., Corley, M. C., & Wallace, D. (1993). Nurses' ability to achieve hyperinflation and hyperoxygenation with a manual resuscitation bag during endotracheal suctioning. *Heart and Lung, 22,* 158–165.

Hall, L. A., Gurley, D. N., Sachs, B., & Kryscio, R. J. (1991). Psychosocial predictors of maternal depressive symptoms, parenting attitudes, and child behavior in single-parent families. *Nursing Research, 40,* 214–219.

Harrison, L. L., Leeper, J., & Yoon, M. (1991). Preterm infants' physiologic responses to early parent touch. *Western Journal of Nursing Research, 13,* 698–713.

Hurley, A. C., Volicer, B. J., Hanrahan, P. A., Houde, S., & Volicer, L. (1992). Assessment of discomfort in advanced Alzheimer patients. *Research in Nursing and Health, 15,* 369–377.

Jezewski, M. A. (1990). Culture brokering in migrant farmworker health care. *Western Journal of Nursing Research, 12,* 497–513.

Kinzel, D. (1991). Self-identified concerns of two homeless groups. *Western Journal of Nursing Research, 13,* 181–190.

Lucero, M., Hutchinson, S., Leger-Krall, S., & Wilson, H. S. (1993). Wandering in Alzheimer's dementia patients. *Clinical Nursing Research, 2,* 160–175.

Maikler, V. E. (1991). Effects of a skin refrigerant/anesthetic and age on the pain responses of infants receiving immunizations. *Research in Nursing and Health, 14,* 397–402.

Meininger, J. C., Stashinko, E. E., & Hayman, L. L. (1991). Type A behavior in children. *Nursing Research, 40,* 221–227.

Miller, D. B., & Holditch-Davis, D. (1992). Interactions of parents and nurses with high-risk preterm infants. *Research in Nursing and Health, 15,* 187–197.

Morse, J. M., & McHutchion, E. (1991). Releasing restraints: Providing safe care for the elderly. *Research in Nursing and Health, 14,* 187–196.

Pickler, R. H. (1993). Premature infant-nurse caregiver interaction. *Western Journal of Nursing Research, 15,* 548–559.

Quinn, M. M. (1991). Attachment between mothers and their Down syndrome infants. *Western Journal of Nursing Research, 13,* 382–396.

Sawada, N. O., Mendes, I. A., Galvao, C. M., & Treizan, M. A. (1992). The importance of nonverbal communication during the preanesthesia period. *Clinical Nursing Research, 1,* 207–213.

Swanson, E. A., Maas, M. L., & Buckwalter, K. C. (1994). Alzheimer's residents' cognitive and functional measures. *Clinical Nursing Research, 3,* 27–41.

Treloar, D. M. (1994). The effect of nonnutritive sucking on oxygenation in healthy, crying full-term infants. *Applied Nursing Research, 7*, 52–58.

Walker, L. O., & Montgomery, E. (1994). Maternal identity and role attainment: Long-term relations to children's development. *Nursing Research, 43*, 105–110.

Weiss, S. J. (1992). Measurement of the sensory qualities in tactile interaction. *Nursing Research, 41*, 82–86.

Whall, A., Booth, D., Kosinski, J. Donbroski, D., Zakul-Krupa, I., & Weissfeld, L. (1989). Tardive dyskinetic movements over time. *Applied Nursing Research, 2*, 128–134.

White, M. A., Williams, P. D., Alexander, D. J., Powell-Cope, G. M., & Conlon, M. (1990). Sleep onset latency and distress in hospitalized children. *Nursing Research, 39*, 134–139.

Youngblut, J. M., Loveland-Cherry, C. J., & Horan, M. (1993). Maternal employment, family functioning, and preterm infant development at 9 and 12 months. *Research in Nursing and Health, 16*, 33–43.

Ziemer, M. M., & Pigeon, J. G. (1993). Skin changes and pain in the nipple during the first week of lactation. *Journal of Obstetric, Gynecologic, and Neonatal Nursing, 22*, 247–256.

Chapter 15

Biophysiologic and Other Data Collection Methods

Most nursing research studies involve the collection of data by means of self-report and observational methods. However, other methods of collecting data are available, and several of these are reviewed in this chapter. The most important alternative method is the use of biophysiologic measures.

❖ BIOPHYSIOLOGIC MEASURES

The trend in nursing research has been toward increased clinical, patient-centered investigations, and this trend is likely to continue in years to come. One result of this trend is an expanded use of measures to assess the physiologic status of subjects. In this section, we discuss a particular class of measures, namely those physiologic and physical variables that require specialized technical instruments and equipment for their measurement and, generally, specialized training for the interpretation of results.

Settings in which nurses operate are typically filled with a wide variety of technical instruments for measuring physiologic functions. It is beyond the scope of this book to describe in any detail the many kinds of biophysiologic measures available to nurse researchers. Our objectives are to present an overview of potential measures for clinical nursing studies, to illustrate their usage in a research context, and to direct the interested reader to supplementary sources for further information.

Many variables that are of interest in clinical research do not require biophysiologic instrumentation for their measurement. Data on physiologic activity or dysfunction can often be gathered through direct observation. For example, phenomena such as vomiting, cyanosis, postcardiotomy delirium, edema, and wound status can be observed for presence or absence and intensity. Other biophysiologic data can be gathered by asking people directly. Examples of possible self-report measures include assessment of pain, ratings of fatigue, and reports of nausea. This section focuses on biophysiologic phenomena that require the use of specialized technical apparatus that yield quantitative measures.

Polit DF, Hungler BP: NURSING RESEARCH: PRINCIPLES
AND METHODS, 5th ed. © 1995 J. B. Lippincott Company.

Purposes of Biophysiologic Measures

Clinical nursing studies often involve specialized equipment and instruments both for creating independent variables (e.g., an intervention using biofeedback equipment) and for measuring dependent variables. For the most part, our discussion focuses on the use of biophysiologic measures as outcome or dependent variables.

Most nursing studies in which biophysiologic measures have been used fall into one of five classes.

1. Studies of basic physiologic processes that have relevance for nursing care. Such studies often involve subjects who are healthy and normal or some subhuman animal species. For example, Kasper and co-researchers (1993) studied impaired physical mobility and the resulting skeletal muscle atrophy in a rat model. Brown and her colleagues (1993) studied the incidence and pattern of jaundice, using a transcutaneous bilirubinometer, in healthy breastfed infants during the first month of life.

2. Explorations of the ways in which nursing actions or medical interventions affect the health outcomes of patients. For example, Potempa and co-researchers (1993) evaluated the relationship of blood pressure reactivity during exercise to treatment responsiveness to two commonly used β-blockers (propranolol and pindolol). Kirchhoff and her colleagues (1990) examined the necessity of restricting ice water for patients with acute myocardial infarction by examining the effects of small and moderate amounts of ingested ice water on the electrocardiograms (ECGs) of myocardial infarction patients.

3. Evaluations of a specific nursing procedure or intervention. These studies differ from the studies in the second class in that they generally involve a hypothesis stating that an innovative nursing procedure will result in improved biophysiologic outcomes among patients. For example, Rogers and Aldrich (1993) used electroencephalogram (EEG), electrooculogram (EOG), and electromyogram (EMG) recordings in their evaluation of the effectiveness of nap therapy for narcoleptic patients. Nelson, Thomas, and Stein (1992) evaluated the effect of hooding infant incubators on the infants' body temperature.

4. Studies to improve the measurement and recording of biophysiologic information regularly gathered by nurses. For example, Klein and her colleagues (1993) compared tympanic membrane temperature with pulmonary artery and rectal temperature to determine consistency among the measures. Cole (1993) studied the effect of ingesting iced water on the length of time required for oral temperature measurements to return to baseline.

5. Studies of the correlates of physiological functioning in patients with health problems. For example, Griego (1993) studied the physiologic factors (oxygen saturation, functional status) that were correlated with depression among patients who had had a myocardial infarction a year earlier. Medoff-Cooper, Verklan, & Carlson (1993) examined the physiologic correlates (heart rate, oxygen saturation, blood pressure) of nutritive sucking patterns in very-low-birthweight babies.

The physiologic phenomena that interest nurse researchers run the full gamut of available measures. Some of these measures are discussed in the next section.

Types of Biophysiologic Measures

Physiologic measurements can be classified in one of two major categories. *In vivo measurements* are those that are performed directly within or on living organisms themselves. One example of an in vivo measure is oxygen saturation measurement through a pulse oximeter.

An *in vitro measurement,* by contrast, is performed outside the organism's body, as in the case of measuring serum potassium concentration in the blood drawn from a patient.

IN VIVO MEASURES

In vivo measures often involve the use of highly complex instrumentation systems. An *instrumentation system* is the apparatus and equipment used to measure one or more attributes of a subject and the presentation of that measurement data in a manner that humans can interpret. Organism–instrument systems involve up to six major components: 1) stimulus, 2) subject, 3) sensing equipment, 4) signal-conditioning equipment, 5) display equipment, and 6) recording, data processing, and transmission equipment. These components and their interrelationships are presented in Figure 15-1. The role of each component is briefly described as follows:

1. *Stimulus.* Many physiologic measurements require some type of external stimulus. The stimulation may be engendered by another human, as in the case of requests for deep and rapid breathing by the patient when recording electrical activity from the brain. The stimulus may also be produced by electrical or mechanical equipment, such as an external pacemaker and cardiac defibrillator.

2. *Subject.* Human bodies consist of chemical, electrical, mechanical, thermal, hydraulic, pneumatic, and other systems interacting with each other and with the outside world. Communication of the human organism with the external environment consists of various inputs (e.g., sensory inputs, inspired air, or liquid and food intake) and outputs (e.g., speech, body movements, expired air, or wastes). Most of these inputs and outputs are easily amenable to measurements. The major bodily systems—circulatory, respiratory, and so forth—also communicate with each other internally, as do smaller subsystems, such as organs and cells. Biomedical instrumentation constitutes the tools for measuring the information communicated by these diverse elements.

3. *Sensing equipment.* Sensing equipment normally consists of one or more transducers. Generally defined, a *transducer* is a device that converts one form of energy

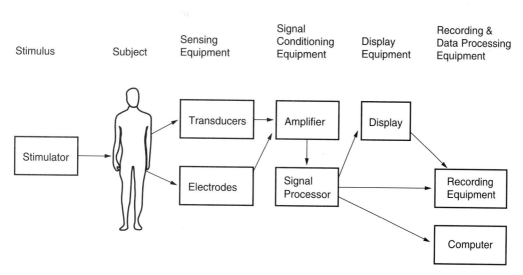

Figure 15-1. *Schema of the organism–instrument system*

into another. Transducers are used in organism–instrument systems to measure physical phenomena by producing an electrical signal proportional to these phenomena. Electrical signals permit presentations of the desired physiologic information in a highly useful form. With an electrical analogue of the critical physiologic event, the scientist can store the event on a computer file for later inspection and analysis.

4. *Signal-conditioning equipment.* In virtually all physiologic measurements, two signals are produced by the subject: the key physiologic signal—such as the ECG signal—and an interference signal. An important function of signal-conditioning equipment is to reject the interference signal and to amplify the desired physiologic signal from the transducer.

5. *Display equipment.* Display devices convert the modified electrical signals into visual or auditory output. For example, an *oscilloscope* is a device that allows for the visual observation of the wave form of a signal. It is used to display and measure the time, phase, voltage, or frequency of a physiologic signal. With sophisticated equipment, a television monitor that shows interpretation of the various physiologic functions under scrutiny is often available.

6. *Recording, data processing, and transmission equipment.* For research purposes, it is usually necessary to obtain a permanent record of the physiologic measurements for subsequent scrutiny and analysis. The recording equipment can be either a unit separate from the display device or integrated with it. The use of computer-linked equipment has the advantage of permitting information to be transmitted and replayed for convenient and detailed analysis.

Not all instrumentation systems involve all six components. Some systems, such as an electronic thermometer, are simple; other systems are extremely complex. For example, there are some electronic monitors that, although they are miniaturized and can be put into place during ambulation, yield simultaneous measures of such physiologic variables as cardiac responsivity, respiratory rate and rhythm, core temperature, and muscular activity.

In vivo instruments have been developed to measure all bodily functions, and technological improvements continue to advance our ability to measure biophysiologic phenomena more accurately, more conveniently, and more rapidly than ever before. The uses to which such instruments have been put by nurse researchers is richly diverse and impressive. Table 15-1 presents examples of research questions that have been posed by nurse researchers relating to the various physiologic systems, together with a list of the physiologic variables measured. Of course, most nurse researchers who have gathered physiologic data have used data from two or more physiologic systems. For example, it is common for nurses to use data on vital signs (e.g., temperature, heart rate, or blood pressure) in their investigations. It is also common for nurses to combine information from in vivo measures with that from in vitro measures.

IN VITRO MEASURES

With in vitro measures, data are gathered from subjects by extracting some physiologic material from subjects and submitting it for laboratory analysis. Nurse researchers may or may not be involved in the extraction of the material; however, the analysis is normally done by highly specialized laboratory technicians. Generally, each laboratory establishes a range of normal values for each measurement, and this information is critical for interpreting the results of laboratory tests.

Several classes of laboratory analysis have been used in studies by nurse researchers. These include:

- *Chemical measurements,* such as the measure of hormone levels, sugar levels, or potassium levels

Table 15-1.　　*Examples of Nursing Studies Using In Vivo Measures*

RESEARCH QUESTIONS	MEASUREMENTS
What are the effects of iced and room temperature injectate on the cardiac output measurements in critically ill patients? (Wallace & Winslow, 1993)	Circulatory function: cardiac output and cardiac index measures, using a cardiac output computer; heart rate; pulmonary artery diastolic and systolic blood pressure
Do patients who receive a preoperative bolus of epidural morphine have better pulmonary function over the first 2 days after a colectomy than patients who do not? (Simpson, Wahl, DeTraglia, Speck, & Taylor, 1993)	Respiratory function: forced vital capacity; respiratory rate; forced expiratory volume in 1 second; and inspiratory capacity, using a portable spirometer
Can the relationship between axillary and tympanic core temperature readings be used to detect and categorize thermal state in full-term infants? (Bliss-Holtz, 1993)	Neurological function: core body temperature, using First Temp infrared tympanic thermometer; axillary temperature, using mercury-in-glass thermometer
What are the physical and psychosocial side effects of antepartum hospital bedrest on pregnant women? (Maloni, Chance, Zhang, Cohen, Betts, & Gange, 1993)	Musculoskeletal function: range of motion/muscle flexibility, using a Jamar goniometer; gastrocnemius muscle function, using a hemoglobin/myoglobin spectrophotometer
What is the level of agreement between two methods of measuring gastric pH in critically ill patients? (Neill & Rice, 1993)	Gastrointestinal function: gastric pH, using an intragastric probe with pH sensor, attached to a pH meter
What is the relationship between the frequeny of urinary incontinence in older women and various functional, urologic, and environmental characteristics? (Wyman, Elswick, Ory, Wilson, & Fantl, 1993)	Genitourinary function: maximal cystometric bladder capacity, using saline infusion cystometry

- *Microbiologic measures,* such as bacterial counts and identification
- *Cytologic or histologic measures,* such as tissue biopsies

Because nurse researchers as a rule are not responsible for the analysis of in vitro extractions, it is unnecessary to explain relevant instrumentation or procedures, and it is impossible to catalog the thousands of laboratory tests available. To give students a flavor of how in vitro measures have been used by nurse researchers, we present some examples in Table 15-2. Laboratory analyses of blood and urine samples are the most frequently used in vitro measures in nursing investigations.

Selecting a Biophysiologic Measure

For nurses unfamiliar with the hundreds of biophysiologic measures available in institutional settings, the selection of one or more appropriate measures of important research variables may pose a real challenge. There are, unfortunately, no comprehensive handbooks to guide interested researchers to the measures, in-

Table 15-2.   *Examples of Nursing Studies Using In Vitro Measures*

TYPE OF TEST	RESEARCH QUESTION	MEASUREMENT
Blood tests	Do diabetics who implement behavioral strategies for self-management of their diabetes have better outcomes than those who do not? (Boehm, Schlenk, Raleigh, & Ronis, 1993)	Changes in levels of glycocylated hemoglobin (GHb)
	Are there differences in the effectiveness of low-dose heparin therapy when administered in three different subcutaneous sites? (Fahs & Kinney, 1991)	Coagulation test: activated partial thromboplastin time
Urine tests	Is there a difference in the duration and amount of menses in women runners who run at different levels of intensity? (Estok, Rudy, Kerr, & Menzel, 1993)	Serum progesterone levels
	What are the effects of menstrual cycle phase on gastrointestinal symptoms in dysmenorrheic women? (Heitkemper, Jarrett, Bond, & Turner, 1991)	Urine catecholamine levels
Saliva tests	What are the factors that contribute to nicotine dependence among African American women smokers? (Ahijevych & Wewers, 1993)	Salivary cotinine levels
Bacterial cultures	What is the extent to which two types of infusion devices allow the persistence of inoculated microorganisms? (Larson, Cheng, Choo, & Merz, 1993)	Count of coagulase-negative staphylococci and *Enterobacter aerotgenes*
	Does the type of wrapper on gauze sponges affect the incidence of strikethrough contamination? (Alexander, Gammage, Nichols, & Gaskins, 1992)	Count of *Staphylococcus epidermidis* and *Escherichia coli*
Cell histology	What is the effect of noise stress on leukocyte function in rats? (McCarthy, Ouimet, Daun, 1992)	Cell culture for lymphocyte proliferation, interleukin-1 secretion, and superoxide release

struments, and interpretations that may be required in collecting physiologic data. Probably the best approach is to consult a knowledgeable colleague or an expert at a local institution. It also may be possible to obtain useful information on biophysiologic measures from original research articles on a problem similar to your own, a review article on the central phenomenon under investigation, manufacturers' catalogs, and exhibits of manufacturers at professional conferences.

Obviously, the most basic issue to address in selecting a physiologic measure is whether the measure will yield good information about the research variable under investigation. In some cases, the researcher will need to consider whether the variable should be measured by observation or self-report instead of (or in addition to) using biophysiologic equipment or apparatus. For example, stress could be measured by asking people questions (e.g., using the State–Trait Anxiety Inventory); by observing their behavior during exposure to stressful stimuli; or by measuring heart rate, blood pressure, or levels of adrenocorticotropic hormone in urine samples.

Several other considerations should be kept in mind in selecting a biophysiologic measure, several of which have been noted by Lindsey and Stotts (1989). These include the following:

- Is the equipment or laboratory analysis you will need readily available to you? If not, can it be borrowed, rented, or purchased?
- If equipment must be purchased, is it affordable? Can funding be acquired to cover the purchase (or rental) price?
- Can you operate the required equipment and interpret its results, or will you need training? Are there resources available to help you with operation and interpretation?
- Will you encounter any difficulties in obtaining permission to use the necessary equipment from an Institutional Review Board or other institutional authority?
- Does the measure need to be direct (e.g., a direct measure of blood pressure by way of an arterial line), or is an indirect measure (e.g., blood pressure measurement by way of a sphygmomanometer) sufficient?
- Will continuous monitoring be necessary (e.g., ECG readings), or is a point-in-time measure adequate?
- Will your activities during data collection permit you to record data simultaneously, or will you need an instrument system with recording equipment (or a research assistant)?
- Will a mechanical stimulus be needed to get appropriate or meaningful measurements? Does available equipment include the required stimulus?

- Will a single measure of your dependent variable be sufficient, or is it preferable to operationalize your research variable using multiple measures? If multiple measures are better, what burden does this place on you as a researcher and on patients as research subjects?
- Are your measures likely to be influenced by *reactivity* (i.e., the subjects' awareness of their subject status)? If so, can alternative or supplementary nonreactive measures be identified, or can the extent of reactivity bias be assessed?
- Can your research variable be measured using a noninvasive procedure, or is an invasive procedure required?
- Is the measure you plan to use sufficiently accurate and sensitive to variation?
- Are you thoroughly familiar with rules and safety precautions, such as grounding procedures, especially when using electrical equipment?

The difficulty in choosing biophysiologic measures for nursing research investigations lies not in their shortage, nor in their questionable utility, nor in their inferiority to other methods. Indeed, they are plentiful, often highly reliable and valid, and extremely useful in clinical nursing studies. However, great care must be exercised in selecting appropriate instruments or laboratory analyses with regard to practical, ethical, medical, and technical considerations.

Research Example

Topf (1992) used an experimental design to test whether sleep was affected by a person's ability to control hospital noises. Subjects were randomly assigned to three groups: 1) those who received instruction in control over critical care unit (CCU) sounds and were subjected to a noisy condition; 2) those who received no instruction and were subjected to a noisy condition; or 3) those who were subjected to a quiet condition. Data were collected in a sleep laboratory that simulated a CCU environment so that actual noise levels could be controlled.

Twenty different measures of sleep were used in this study, one of which was a self-reported rating of sleep quality and 19 of which were physiologic. The physiologic measures included sleep efficiency; minutes in bed, asleep and awake in various sleep stages; and number of stage shifts, intrasleep awakenings, and rapid-eye-movement periods. The physiologic data were obtained through polysomnograph equipment, which included EEG, EMG, and EOG recordings. The recordings yielded 1000-page sleep records. The unit of analysis for coding the sleep records was each page of the record. The stage of sleep of each page was recorded on a sleep summary sheet using well-established sleep stage criteria.

Subjects in all three groups changed into sleep wear around 9:30 PM, and then the polysomnograph technician taped EEG, EOG, and EMG electrodes in place. At 10:25 PM, subjects were instructed to retire for the night, and the polysomnograph wires were connected to wall outlets in the subjects' rooms. The polysomnograph equipment was calibrated by the technician, who then recorded sleep according to standardized procedures. The technician also turned on an amplifier and audiotape recorder with CCU nighttime sounds for subjects in the two noise conditions.

The actual measures were derived through scoring by a doctorally prepared polysomnograph specialist. A second doctorally prepared polysomnographer scored some records (one sleep record randomly selected out of every five) to establish inter-scorer agreement. Agreement between the two scorers ranged between 78% and 94%.

The findings indicated that subjects' sleep patterns were strongly related to whether or not there was noise in the laboratory, but not as a function of the instruction.

❖ *RECORDS AND AVAILABLE DATA*

Thus far we have examined a number of data collection strategies for which it was assumed that the researcher would be responsible for actually collecting the data and, in some cases, de-veloping the data collection instruments. However, it is not always necessary for a researcher to collect new data. A wealth of data is gathered for nonresearch purposes and can be fruitfully exploited to answer research questions. Nurse researchers are particularly fortunate in the amount and quality of existing data available to them for exploration. Hospital records, patient charts, physicians' order sheets, care plan statements, and so forth all constitute rich data sources to which nurse researchers may have access.

Data Sources

The places where a nurse researcher is likely to find useful records are too numerous to list here, but a few suggestions may be helpful. Within a hospital or other health care setting, excellent records are kept routinely and systematically. In addition to medical and nursing records, hospitals maintain financial records, personnel records, nutritional records, and so forth. Educational institutions maintain various records. For example, most schools of nursing have permanent files on their students. Public school systems also keep records, including both academic and health-related information. Industries and businesses normally maintain a variety of records that may interest industrial nurse researchers, such as information on employees' absenteeism, health status, on-the-job accidents, job performance ratings, alcoholism or drug problems, and so forth. In addition to institutional records, personal documents such as diaries and letters should be considered as possible data sources. Table 15-3 illustrates some of the data sources and types of variables measured in nursing studies that have used existing records.

Advantages and Disadvantages of Using Records

The use of information from records is advantageous to the researcher for several reasons. The most salient advantage of existing records is that they are an economical source of

Table 15-3.   *Examples of Nursing Studies Using Existing Institutional Records*

RESEARCH QUESTION	DATA SOURCE	TYPE OF DATA USED
How effective is the Creighton model ovulation method of natural family planning in avoiding and achieving a pregnancy? (Fehring, Lawrence, & Philpot, 1994)	Clinic logbooks	Number of clinic sessions attended; reason for program withdrawal; pregnancies; pregnancy outcomes; referral codes
Do falls among older nursing home residents predict subsequent disease onset? (Miceli, Waxman, Cavalieri, & Lage, 1994)	Physician progress notes; medical records; physician order sheets; nursing assessment records	Onset of new medical conditions; incidence of falling; circumstance of any fall; cognitive and functional status; medication use; activity; restraint use; fatality
What is the effect of a preterm infant's physical condition on nipple-feeding practices? (Pridham, Sondel, Chang, & Green, 1993)	Physicians' notes; nurses' flow sheets	Infant's attributes at birth (weight, gestational age, Apgar scores, medical condition); nipple-feeding practices
What are the organizational and personal demographic factors that are correlated with nurses' turnover, absenteeism, and reduced work schedules? (Wise, 1993)	Hospital personnel records	Nurses' background information (age, tenure, gender); organizational factors (type of unit, shift); and withdrawal behavior (absenteeism, turnover, reduced schedules)

information; the collection of original data is often time-consuming and costly. The use of preexisting records also permits an examination of trends over time, if the information is of the type that is collected repeatedly. Problems of reactivity and response biases may be completely absent when the researcher obtains information from records. Furthermore, the investigator does not have to be concerned with obtaining cooperation from participants.

On the other hand, because the researcher has not been responsible for the collection and recording of information, he or she may be unaware of the limitations, biases, or incompleteness of the records. Two of the major sources of bias in records are *selective deposit* and *selective survival*. If the records available for use do not constitute the entire set of all possible such records, the investigator must somehow deal with the question of how representative the existing records are. Many record keepers intend to maintain an entire universe or set of records rather than a sample but may fail to adhere to this ideal. The lapses from the ideal may be the result of some systematic biases, and the careful researcher should attempt to learn just what those biases may be.

An additional problem with which researchers must contend is the increasing reluctance of institutions to make their records available for scientific studies. The Privacy Act, a federal regulation enacted to protect individuals against possible misuse of records, has made hospitals, agencies, schools, and industrial organizations sensitive to the possibility of legal action from individuals who think that their right to privacy has been violated. The major issue here is the divulgence of an individual's identity.

If records are maintained with an identifying number rather than a name, permission to use the records may be readily granted. However, most institutions *do* maintain records by their clients' names. In such a situation, the researcher may need the assistance of personnel at the institution to maintain client anonymity, and some organizations may be unwilling to use their personnel for such purposes.

A number of other difficulties in the use of records for research purposes may be relevant. Sometimes the records have to be verified in terms of their authenticity, authorship, or accuracy, a task that may be difficult to execute if the records are old. The researcher using records must be prepared to deal with forms and file systems that he or she does not understand. Codes and symbols that had meaning to the record keeper may have to be translated to be usable. In using records to study trends, the researcher should always be alert to the possibility of changes in record-keeping procedures. For example, does a dramatic increase or decrease in the incidence of sudden infant death syndrome reflect changes in the causes or cures of this problem, or does it reflect a change in diagnosis or record-keeping?

These considerations suggest that, although existing records may be plentiful, inexpensive, and accessible, they should not be used without paying attention to potential problems and weaknesses.

Research Example

Davis and Nomura (1990) were concerned about the appropriate frequency for assessing patients' vital signs after surgery. They noted that hospitals typically have protocols governing the frequency of this monitoring but that the frequencies specified vary considerably from hospital to hospital, and such variations appear to be based on tradition rather than on scientific data. The purpose of their investigation was to determine whether the protocol in effect in one specific hospital (a 450-bed acute care hospital in a large urban area) was appropriate for class I surgical patients. The protocol in effect was q 15 minutes × 4, q ½ hour × 2, q 1 hour × 1, and q 4 hours × 4.

Various hospital records were obtained for 250 surgical patients who were determined to be class I by an anesthesiologist. Charts of patients over a 1-year period for those undergoing five different types of surgical procedures were randomly selected. Data were gathered from the admit/discharge sheet; surgical permit; anesthesia record; recovery room record; unit record of temperature, pulse, respiration, and blood pressure; intake/output sheet; medication record; doctor's progress notes; and nurses' notes.

The investigators' analysis focused primarily on the timing of vital signs outside abnormal parameters and the occurrence of abnormal signs and symptoms such as nausea and vomiting and urinary retention. The pattern of findings revealed a dramatic reduction in vital signs outside normal parameters between the first and second hour after surgery, with few signs occurring at hour 4 or beyond. Newly occurring abnormal vital signs appeared in only 2% of the sample in hour 3 on the unit, and none of these patients had recurrences in the following hour. Based on this analysis, the protocol in the hospital in which the study was conducted was changed. Unless otherwise ordered by the physician, the new frequency is q 15 minutes × 1, q 30 minutes × 2, q 1 hour × 1, q 4 hours × 4.

❖ Q METHODOLOGY

Q methodology is the term used by William Stephenson (1975) to refer to a constellation of substantive, statistical, and psychometric concepts relating to research on individuals. Q methodology utilizes a procedure known as the *Q sort,* which involves the sorting of a deck of cards according to specified criteria.

Q-Sort Procedures

In a Q sort, the subject is presented with a set of cards on which words, phrases, statements, or other messages are written. The subject is then asked to sort the cards according to a particular dimension, such as approval/disapproval, most like me/least like me, or highest priority/lowest priority. The number of cards to be sorted is typically between 60 and 100. Usually, the subject sorts the cards into 9 or 11 piles, with the number of cards placed in each pile determined by the researcher. A common practice is to have the subjects distribute the cards such that fewer cards are placed at either of the two extremes and more cards are placed toward the middle. Table 15-4 shows a hypothetical distribution of 60 cards, with the specification of the number of cards to be placed in each of the nine piles.

The sorting instructions and the objects to be sorted in a Q-sort investigation vary according to the requirements of the research. Attitudes can be studied by asking subjects to sort statements in terms of agreement/disagreement or approval/disapproval. The researcher can study personality by developing cards on which personality characteristics are described. The subject can then be requested to sort items on a very much like me to not at all like me continuum. Self-concept can be explored by comparing responses to this "like me" dimension to responses elicited when the instructions are to sort cards according to what subjects consider ideal personality traits. Q sorts can be used to great advantage in studying individuals in depth. For example, subjects could be asked to sort traits as they apply to themselves in different roles such as employee, parent, spouse, friend, and so forth. The technique can also be used to gain information concerning how individuals see themselves, how they perceive others seeing them, how they believe others would

like them to be, and so forth. Other applications include asking patients to rate nursing behaviors on a continuum of most helpful to least helpful; asking nursing students to rate aspects of their educational preparation along a most useful to least useful continuum; and asking cancer patients to rate various aspects of their treatment in terms of a most distressing to least distressing dimension.

The number of cards in a Q sort varies according to the research problem. However, it is unwise to use fewer than 50 or 60 items because it is difficult to achieve stable and reliable results with a smaller number. On the other hand, 100 to 150 cards are normally considered the upper limit because the task becomes tedious and difficult with larger numbers.

The analysis of data obtained through Q sorts is a somewhat controversial matter. The options range from the most elementary, descriptive statistical procedures, such as rank ordering, averages, and percentages, to highly complex procedures, such as factor analysis. Factor analysis, a procedure designed to reveal the underlying dimensions or common elements in a set of items, is described in Chapter 19. Some researchers insist that factor analysis is essential in the analysis of Q-sort data.

Evaluation of Q Methodology

Q methodology can be a powerful methodological tool, but like other data collection techniques, it has a number of drawbacks as well. On the plus side, we have seen that Q sorts are extremely versatile and can be applied to a wide variety of problems. Unlike many other clinical approaches, we find in Q methodology an objective and (usually) reliable pro-

Table 15-4.   *Example of a Distribution of Q-Sort Cards*

	APPROVE OF LEAST								APPROVE OF MOST
Category	1	2	3	4	5	6	7	8	9
Number of Cards	2	4	7	10	14	10	7	4	2

cedure for the intensive study of an individual. Q sorts have been used effectively to study the progress of people during different phases of therapy, particularly psychotherapy. The requirement that individuals place a predetermined number of cards in each pile virtually eliminates response-set biases that often characterize responses to written scale items. Furthermore, the task of sorting cards may be more agreeable to some subjects than completing a paper-and-pencil instrument.

On the other hand, it is difficult and time-consuming to administer Q sorts to a large sample of individuals. Without a sizable sample, it may be problematic to generalize the results of the study. The sampling problem is further compounded by the fact that Q sorts cannot normally be administered through the mail, thereby resulting in difficulties in obtaining a geographically diverse sample of subjects. Some critics have argued that the forced procedure of distributing cards according to the researcher's specifications is artificial and actually excludes information concerning how the subjects would ordinarily distribute their opinions.

Another criticism of Q-sort data relates to permissible statistical operations. Most statistical tests and procedures assume that responses to items are independent of one another. Likert-type scales exemplify items that are totally independent: a person's response of agree/disagree to one item does not in any way restrict responses to other items. Techniques of this type are known as *normative measures*. Normative measures can be interpreted by comparing individual scores with the average score for a group. The Q-sort technique is a forced-choice procedure, wherein a person's response to one item depends on, and is restricted by, responses to other items. Referring to Table 15-4, a respondent who has already placed two cards in category 1 ("approve of least") is not free to place another item in this same category.* Such an approach produces what is known as *ipsative*

measures. With ipsative measures, the average of a group is an irrelevant point of comparison because the average is identical for all individuals. With a nine-category Q sort such as is shown in Table 15-4, the average value of the sorted cards will always be five. (The average value of a *particular item* can be meaningfully computed and compared among individuals or groups, however.) Strictly speaking, ordinary statistical tests of significance are inappropriate for use with nonindependent ipsative measures. In practice, many researchers feel that the violation of assumptions in applying standard statistical procedures to Q-sort data is not a serious transgression, particularly if the number of items is large.

Research Example

Von Essen and Sjödén (1993) compared the perceptions of psychiatric inpatients and nursing staff regarding the importance of various nurse caring behaviors. A total of 61 patients and 63 nurses in four psychiatric short-term hospital wards in Sweden were the subjects in this study.

Data were collected by means of a Q-sort instrument called the Caring Assessment Instrument (CARE-Q), modified for this study and translated into Swedish. The CARE-Q consists of 50 caring behaviors that subjects were asked to place on a seven-point continuum from most important to least important. The cards had to be placed to conform to a symmetric distribution with 1, 4, 10, 20, 10, 4, and 1 cards in the respective piles. The patients were asked: "In order to make you feel cared for, how important is it that the staff . . . ?"

The CARE-Q items designated nursing behaviors conceptualized as comprising six subscales: Accessible; Explains and Facilitates; Comforts; Anticipates; Monitors; and Trusting relationship. For example, the Comfort subscale consists of nine items, such as "touches the patient when he/she needs comfort" and "sits down with the patient." In the version used by the in-patients, the word *patient* was replaced by the word *you*. Each behavior was given a value from 1 to 7,

---

* Subjects are usually told, however, that they can move cards around from one pile to another until the desired distribution is obtained.

corresponding to the subject's placement of it in the distribution.

The findings indicated that patients assigned a higher average value to the Explains and Facilitates subscale than nurses did. Nursing behaviors in this category were ranked as number 1 by patients and as number 6 by staff. By contrast, staff gave a higher average value to the Comforts subscale than did the patients.

❖ PROJECTIVE TECHNIQUES

Questionnaires, interview schedules, and psychological tests and scales normally depend on the respondents' capacity for self-insight or willingness to share personal information with the researcher. *Projective techniques* include a variety of methods for obtaining psychological measures with only a minimum of cooperation required of the person. Projective methods give free play to the subjects' imagination and fantasies by providing them with a task that permits an almost unlimited number and variety of responses. The rationale underlying the use of projective techniques is that the manner in which a person organizes and reacts to unstructured stimuli is a reflection of the person's needs, motives, attitudes, values, or personality characteristics. A stimulus of low structure is sufficiently ambiguous that respondents can read in their own interpretations and in this way provide the researcher with information about their perception of the world. In other words, people project part of themselves into their interaction with phenomena, and projective techniques represent a means of taking advantage of this fact.

Types of Projective Techniques

Projective techniques are highly flexible because virtually any unstructured stimuli or situation can be used to induce projective behaviors. One class of projective methods uses pictorial materials. One particularly useful *pictorial device* is the Thematic Apperception Test (TAT). The TAT materials consist of 20 cards that con-

tain pictures. The subject is requested to make up a story for each picture, inventing an explanation of what led up to the event shown, what is happening at the moment, what the characters are feeling and thinking, and what kind of outcome will result. The responses are then scored according to some scheme for the variables of interest to the researchers. Variables that have been measured by TAT-type pictures are achievement motivation, need for affiliation, parent–child relationships, attitude toward minority groups, creativity, attitude toward authority, and fear of success.

Verbal projective techniques present subjects with an ambiguous verbal stimulus rather than a pictorial one. There are two classes of verbal methods: association techniques and completion techniques. An example of an association technique is the *word-association method*, which presents subjects with a series of words, to which subjects respond with the first thing that comes to mind. The word list often combines both neutral and emotionally tinged words, which are included for the purpose of detecting impaired thought processes or internal conflicts. The word-association technique has also been used to study creativity, interests, and attitudes.

The most common completion technique is *sentence completion*. The person is supplied with a set of incomplete sentences and is asked to complete them in any desired manner. This approach is frequently used as a method of measuring attitudes or some aspect of personality. Some examples of incomplete sentences include the following:

> When I think of a nurse, I feel. . . .
> The thing I most admire about nurses is. . . .
> A good nurse should always. . . .

The sentence stems are designed to elicit responses toward some attitudinal object or event in which the investigator is interested. Responses are typically categorized or rated according to a prespecified plan.

A third class of projective measures falls into a category known as *expressive methods*.

These techniques encourage self-expression, in most cases, through the construction of some product out of raw materials. The major expressive methods are play techniques, drawing and painting, and role playing. The assumption is that people express their feelings, needs, motives, and emotions by working with or manipulating various materials.

Evaluation of Projective Measures

Projective measures are among the most controversial in the behavioral sciences. Critics point out that it is difficult to score projective techniques objectively. A high degree of inference is required in gleaning information from projective tests, and the quality of the data depends heavily on the sensitivity and interpretive skill of the investigator or analyst. It has been pointed out that the interpretation of the responses by the researcher is almost as projective as the subjects' reactions to original stimuli.

Another problem with projective techniques is that there have been difficulties in demonstrating that they are, in fact, measuring the variables that they purport to measure. If a pictorial device is used to score aggressive expressions, can the researcher be confident that individual differences in aggressive responses really reflect underlying differences in aggressiveness?

Projective techniques have supporters as well as critics in the research community. People have advocated using projective devices, arguing that they probe the unconscious mind, encompass the whole personality, and provide data of a breadth and depth unattainable by more traditional methods. One useful feature of projective instruments is that they are less susceptible to faking than self-report measures. Another strength is that it is often easier to build rapport and gain the subject's interest with a projective measure than with a questionnaire or scale. Finally, some projective techniques are particularly useful with special groups, especially with children.

Research Example

Janelli (1993) undertook a study to determine whether there is a difference between how older men and older women perceive their body image. The sample consisted of 89 older men and women from several long-term care facilities.

One of the measures that Janelli used to measure body image perception was the Draw-A-Person (DAP) Technique, a paper-and-pencil projective test. Each older person was instructed to "draw a person: You may make it any way you wish, but draw a whole person, not just the face" (p. 332). Based on the drawings, three variables were created: (1) area, considered to reflect self-assessment in relation to the environment; (2) height, interpreted as an indication of feelings of self-significance; and (3) centeredness, considered to reflect the person's general security level and orientation to reality. The area measure was obtained by placing a transparency of graphic paper measured in quarter-inch squares over the drawing. Height was measured from top to bottom of the figure with a ruler, to the nearest quarter of an inch. Centeredness was measured by how far the center of the drawing was from the center of the page. Janelli, who acknowledged that "no consensus exists among researchers that the DAP Technique represents a projection of a person's own body image" (p. 332) also administered the self-report Body Cathexis Scale (BCS) as a supplementary measure of body image.

The findings indicated that men and women had comparable scores on the BCS. However, on the DAP measures, the men drew figures that were larger in area, taller, and more centered than the drawings of the women. Janelli concluded that the women had a poorer body image perception than the men, as measured by the DAP Technique.

❖ *VIGNETTES*

The final data collection alternative we examine is called vignettes.

Uses of Vignettes

Vignettes are brief descriptions of an event or situation to which respondents are asked to react. The descriptions can either be fictitious or based on fact, but are always structured to elicit information about respondents' perceptions, opinions, or knowledge about some phenomenon under study. The vignettes are often written, narrative descriptions, but researchers have also begun to use videotaped vignettes that portray a specific situation. The questions posed to respondents after the presentation of the vignettes are usually closed-ended (e.g., "On the nine-point scale below, rate how well you believe the nurse in this story handled the situation"). Normally, the number of vignettes included in a study ranges from 4 to 10.

The purpose of the study in which vignettes are used is sometimes not revealed to subjects. This technique has sometimes been used as an indirect measure of attitudes, prejudices, and stereotypes through the use of embedded or hidden descriptors. For example, a researcher interested in exploring attitudes toward, or stereotypes of, male nurses could present subjects with a series of vignettes describing fictitious nurses in terms of, say, their education, family background, nursing experience, and so forth. For each vignette, the nurse would be described as a male half the time (at random) and as a female the other half. The subjects could then be asked to describe the fictitious nurses in terms of likableness, friendliness, cheerfulness, effectiveness, and so forth. Any differences in the subjects' descriptions presumably result from attitudes toward appropriate sex-role behavior.

Evaluation of Vignettes

Vignettes are often an economical means of eliciting information about how people might behave in situations that would be difficult to observe in daily life. For example, we might want to assess how patients would react to or feel about nurses with different types of personalities and personal styles of interaction. In clinical settings, it would be difficult to expose patients to many different nurses, all of whom have been evaluated as having different personalities. Another advantage of vignettes is that it is possible to manipulate the stimuli (the vignettes) experimentally by randomly assigning vignettes to groups, as in the example about male nurses. Furthermore, vignettes often represent an interesting task for subjects. Finally, vignettes can be incorporated into mailed questionnaires and are therefore an inexpensive data collection strategy.

Vignettes are handicapped by some of the same problems as other self-report techniques. The principal problem is that of response biases. If a respondent describes how he or she would react in a situation portrayed in the vignette, how accurate is that description of the respondent's actual behavior? Thus, although the use of vignettes can be profitable, researchers should consider how to minimize or at least assess potential response biases.

Research Example

McDonald and Bridge (1991) were interested in examining the effect of gender stereotyping on nursing care. Using a factorial design, they created an experimental manipulation that involved the use of a written vignette.

The vignette, which described a 3-day postoperative colostomy patient, simulated a typical shift report for a medical-surgical patient. Eight separate packets, corresponding to eight different experimental conditions, were created. The vignettes in the packet appeared to be identical but differed in three ways: gender of the patient (male versus female); patient health status (described as stable or unstable); and memory load (high versus low). With respect to the latter, subjects in the low memory load condition read only the colostomy vignette, while those in the high memory load condition read several other vignettes. Box 15-1 presents a sample vignette from this study, for the unstable female condition.

BOX 15-1   EXAMPLE OF A VIGNETTE

Mary B. is a 48-year-old with colon cancer. She had surgery 3 days ago creating a permanent colostomy. Today she says her pain is "8" (on a 1–10 scale with 1, *no pain*, and 10, *unbearable pain*). She has received Demerol, 75 mg IM every 6 hours for the past 24 hours. Yesterday she was up to the chair three times for 30 minutes each, and walked the hallway three times for 10 minutes each. Thirty minutes ago Mary's temperature spiked unexpectedly to 102°F.

McDonald, D.D., & Bridge, R.G. (1991). Gender stereotyping and nursing care. *Research in Nursing and Health, 124,* 375.

The sample of 160 female medical-surgical nurses was randomly assigned to one of the eight conditions (2 × 2 × 2). After reading their vignette package, nurses were instructed to estimate to the nearest minute the time they would plan for each of 16 nursing actions (e.g, patient ambulation, patient chair time, emotional support). The results indicated that nurses planned significantly more ambulation, analgesic administration, and emotional support for the patient described as male than for the same patient described as female.

❖ TIPS FOR COLLECTING DATA WITH ALTERNATIVE METHODS

The methods described in this chapter represent important data collection alternatives to self-report and observations. Below are a few suggestions regarding the use of these alternative methods.

• Sometimes the methods used in this chapter are attractive because they are unusual and may therefore seem like a more creative approach to collecting data than self-report and observational methods. However, the prime considerations in selecting a data collection method should always be conceptual congruence between the constructs of interest and the method, and the quality of data that the method yields.

• If you decide to use an alternative method such as a projective technique or a Q sort, a good strategy might be to supplement it with a more traditional measure of the construct, as a means of assessing the validity of the alternative approach.

• Most of the techniques described in this chapter yield quantitative data. However, several can also yield qualitative data. Records, for example, may be narrative accounts, such as nurses' notes. Projective techniques are often scored quantitatively but almost always yield narrative data that can be analyzed qualitatively. The questions asked of subjects after they read a vignette could also be open-ended questions amenable to qualitative analysis (e.g., "How would you recommend handling the situation described here?").

• As in other methods of data collection, the importance of adequate training of the data collectors cannot be overemphasized. Even when using existing records, the data collectors need to be trained with respect to the extraction of relevant information and the recording of that information on appropriate forms.

❖ SUMMARY

This chapter reviewed several data collection strategies that are used less frequently than those described in Chapters 13 and 14. For certain research problems, these alternative techniques—and especially biophysiologic measures—may be strong candidates as methods of collecting data.

The trend in nursing research is toward increasing numbers of clinical, patient-centered investigations in which biophysiologic indicators of patients' health status are used as dependent variables. Many examples of instruments and laboratory tests used in nursing studies were described. Particular attention was paid to the *instrumentation systems* used for *in vivo measurements* (those performed within or on living organisms). The components of an organism–instrument system are the stimulus, subject, sensing equipment, signal-conditioning equipment, display equipment, and recording equipment. Blood tests and urine tests are the most frequently used *in vitro measurements* (those performed outside the organism's body). Despite the clearcut utility of biophysiologic measures for nursing science, great care must be taken in selecting such measures with regard to practical, technical, and ethical considerations.

Existing *records* are often used by researchers in the conduct of scientific investigations. Such records provide an economical source of information. In using records, the researcher should try to determine how representative and accurate they are. Two major sources of bias in records are *selective deposit* and *selective survival*.

Q sorts involve having the subject sort a set of statements into piles according to specified criteria. Attitudes, personality, and self-concept are some of the traits that may be measured by Q methodology. One limitation in the use of Q sorts is that it produces *ipsative measures*, wherein the average across cards is an irrelevant basis of comparison inasmuch as the forced-choice approach produces the same average for all subjects. This differs from other techniques that produce *normative measures* because each choice is independent of other choices.

Projective techniques encompass a variety of data collection methods that rely on the subject's projection of psychological traits or states in response to vaguely structured stimuli. *Pictorial methods* present a picture or cartoon and ask the subject to describe what is happening, what led up to the event, or what kind of action is needed. *Verbal methods* present the subject with an ambiguous verbal stimulus rather than a picture. Two types of verbal methods are *word association* and *sentence completion*. *Expressive*

methods take the form of play, drawing, or role playing.

Vignettes are brief descriptions of some event, person, or situation to which respondents are asked to react. Vignettes are often incorporated into questionnaires or interview schedules. They may be used to assess respondents' hypothetical behaviors, opinions, and perceptions.

❖ STUDY SUGGESTIONS

Chapter 15 of the accompanying *Study Guide for Nursing Research: Principles and Methods, 5th ed.*, offers various exercises and study suggestions for reinforcing the concepts presented in this chapter. Additionally, the following study questions can be addressed:

1. Formulate a research problem in which each of the following could be used as the measurements for the dependent variable:
   a. Blood pressure
   b. EMGs
   c. Thermograms
   d. Blood sugar levels

2. Identify some of the in vivo or in vitro measures you might use to address the following research questions:
   a. Does clapping the lungs before suctioning result in better patient outcomes than suctioning without clapping?
   b. What is the effect of various bed positions on the development of respiratory acidosis or alkalosis?
   c. What are the cardiovascular effects of administering liquid potassium chloride in three different solutions (orange juice, fruit punch, cranberry juice)?
   d. What is the rate of respiratory increase for designated decreases in the pH level of cerebrospinal fluid?

3. Suppose that you were interested in studying the following variables: professionalism

in nurses, fear of death in patients, achievement motivation in nursing students, job satisfaction among industrial nurses, fathers' reactions to their newborn infants, and patients' needs for affiliation. Describe at least two ways of collecting data relating to these concepts, using the following approaches:

    a. Vignettes
    b. Verbal projective techniques
    c. Pictorial projective techniques
    d. Records
    e. Q sorts

❖ SUGGESTED READINGS

METHODOLOGICAL REFERENCES

Biophysiologic References

Abbey, J. (Guest Ed.). (1978). Symposium on bio-instrumentation for nurses. *Nursing Clinics of North America, 13,* 561–640.

Bauer, J. D., Ackermann, P. G., & Toro, G. (1982). *Clinical laboratory methods* (9th ed.). St. Louis: C. V. Mosby.

Cromwell, L., Weibell, F. J., & Pfeiffer, E. A. (1980). *Biomedical instrumentation and measurements* (2nd ed.). Englewood Cliffs, NJ: Prentice-Hall.

Ferris, C. D. (1980). *Guide to medical laboratory instruments.* Boston: Little, Brown.

Fischbach, F. (1992). *A manual of laboratory diagnostic tests* (4th ed.). Philadelphia: J. B. Lippincott.

Kraemer, H. C. (1992). *Evaluating medical tests.* Newbury Park, CA: Sage.

Lindsey, A. M. (1984). Research for clinical practice: Physiological phenomena. *Heart and Lung, 13,* 496–507.

Lindsey, A. M., & Stotts, N. A. (1989). Collecting data on biophysiologic variables. In H. S. Wilson, *Research in nursing* (2nd ed.). Menlo Park, CA: Addison-Wesley.

Pagana, K. D., & Pagana, T. J. (1993). *Diagnostic testing and nursing implications: A case study approach* (4th ed.). St. Louis: C. V. Mosby.

Weiss, M. D. (1973). *Biomedical instrumentation.* Philadelphia: Chilton Book Company.

Widmann, F. K. (1983). *Clinical interpretation of laboratory tests* (9th ed.). Philadelphia: F. A. Davis.

Other Data Collection Methods

Aaronson, L. S., & Burman, M. E. (1994). Use of health records in research: Reliability and validity issues. *Research in Nursing and Health, 17,* 67–74.

Anastasi, A. (1988). *Psychological testing.* (6th ed.). New York: Macmillan.

Angell, R. C., & Freedman, R. (1953). The use of documents, records, census materials, and indices. In L. Festinger & D. Katz (Eds.), *Research methods in the behavioral sciences* (pp. 300–326). New York: Holt, Rinehart & Winston.

Block, J. (1978). *The Q-Sort method in personality assessment and psychiatric research.* (2nd ed.). Springfield, IL: Charles C. Thomas.

Flaskerud, J. H. (1979). Use of vignettes to elicit responses toward broad concepts. *Nursing Research, 28,* 210–212.

Kerlinger, F. N. (1986). *Foundations of behavioral research* (3rd ed.). New York: Holt, Rinehart & Winston.

Lanza, M. L. (1988). Development of a vignette. *Western Journal of Nursing Research, 10,* 346–351.

Semeomoff, B. (1976). *Projective techniques.* New York: John Wiley and Sons.

Simpson, S. H. (1989). Use of Q-sort methodology in cross-cultural nutrition and health research. *Nursing Research, 38,* 289–290.

Stephenson, W. (1975). *The study of behavior: Q technique and its methodology.* Chicago: University of Chicago Press.

Tetting, D. W. (1988). Q-sort update. *Western Journal of Nursing Research, 10,* 757–765.

Waltz, C. F., Strickland, O. L., & Lenz, E. R. (1991). *Measurement in nursing research* (2nd ed.). Philadelphia: F. A. Davis.

SUBSTANTIVE REFERENCES

Biophysiologic Studies

Ahijevych, K., & Wewers, M. E. (1993). Factors associated with nicotine dependence among African American women cigarette smokers. *Research in Nursing and Health, 16,* 283–292.

Alexander, D., Gammage, D., Nichols, A., & Gaskins, D. (1992). Analysis of strike-through contamination in saturated sterile dressings. *Clinical Nursing Research, 1,* 28–34.

Bliss-Hotz, J. (1993). Determination of thermoregulatory state in full-term infants. *Nursing Research, 42*, 204–207.

Boehm, S., Schlenk, E. A., Raleigh, E., & Ronis, D. (1993). Behavioral analysis and behavioral strategies to improve self-management of type II diabetes. *Clinical Nursing Research, 2*, 327–344.

Brown, L. P., Arnold, L., Allison, D., Klein, M. E., & Jacobsen, B. (1993). Incidence and pattern of jaundice in healthy breast-fed infants during the first month of life. *Nursing Research, 42*, 106–110.

Cole, F. L. (1993). Temporal variation in the effects of iced water on oral temperature. *Research in Nursing and Health, 16*, 107–111.

Estok, P. J., Rudy, E. B., Kerr, M. E., & Menzel, L. (1993). Menstrual response to running: Nursing implications. *Nursing Research, 42*, 158–165.

Fahs, P. S., & Kinney, M. R. (1991). The abdomen, thigh and arm as sites for subcutaneous sodium heparin injections. *Nursing Research, 40*, 204–207.

Griego, L. C. (1993). Physiologic and psychologic factors related to depression in patients after myocardial infarction. *Heart and Lung, 22*, 392–400.

Heitkemper, M., Jarrett, M., Bond, E. F., & Turner, P. (1991). GI symptoms, function, and psychophysiological arousal in dysmenorrheic women. *Nursing Research, 40*, 20–26.

Kasper, C. E., McNulty, A. L., Otto, A. J., & Thomas, D. P. (1993). Alterations in skeletal muscle related to impaired mobility: An empirical model. *Research in Nursing and Health, 16*, 265–273.

Kirchhoff, K., Holm, K., Foreman, M., & Rebenson-Piano, M. (1990). Electrocardiographic response to ice water ingestion. *Heart and Lung, 19*, 41–48.

Klein, D. G., Mitchell, C., Petrinec, A., Monroe, M. K., Oblak, M., Ross, B., & Youngblut, J. M. (1993). A comparison of pulmonary artery, rectal, and tympanic membrane measurement in the ICU. *Heart and Lung, 22*, 435–441.

Larson, E. L., Cheng, G., Choo, J. T. E., & Merz, W. (1993). In vitro survival of skin flora in heparin locks and needleless valve infusion devices. *Heart and Lung, 22*, 459–462.

Maloni, J. A., Chance, B., Zhang, C., Cohen, A. W., Betts, D., & Gange, S. J. (1993). Physical and psychosocial side effects of antepartum hospital bed rest. *Nursing Research, 42*, 197–203.

McCarthy, D. O., Ouimet, M. E., & Daun, J. M. (1992). The effects of noise stress on leukocyte function in rats. *Research in Nursing and Health, 15*, 131–137.

Medoff-Cooper, B., Verklan, T., & Carlson, S. (1993). The development of sucking patterns and physiologic correlates in very-low-birth-weight infants. *Nursing Research, 42*, 100–105.

Neill, K. M., & Rice, K. T. (1993). Comparison of two methods of measuring gastric pH. *Heart and Lung, 22*, 349–355.

Nelson, H., Thomas, K., & Stein, M. (1992). Thermal effects of hooding incubators. *Journal of Obstetric, Gynecologic, and Neonatal Nursing, 5*, 377–381.

Potempa, K. M., Fogg, L. F., Fish, A. F., & Kravitz, H. M. (1993). Blood pressure reactivity in the evaluation of resting blood pressure and mood response to pindolol and propranolol in hypertensive patients. *Heart and Lung, 22*, 383–391.

Rogers, A. E., & Aldrich, M. S. (1993). The effect of regularly scheduled naps on sleep attacks and excessive daytime sleepiness associated with narcolepsy. *Nursing Research, 42*, 111–117.

Simpson, T., Wahl, G., DeTraglia, M., Speck, E., & Taylor, D. (1993). A pilot study of pain, analgesia use, and pulmonary function after colectomy with or without a preoperative bolus of epidural morphine. *Heart and Lung, 22*, 316–327.

Topf, M. (1992). Effects of personal control over hospital noise on sleep. *Research in Nursing and Health, 15*, 19–28.

Wallace, D. C., & Winslow, E. H. (1993). Effects of iced and room temperature injectate on cardiac output measurements in critically ill patients with low and high cardiac outputs. *Heart and Lung, 22*, 55–63.

Wyman, J. F., Elswick, R. K., Ory, M. G., Wilson, M. S., & Fantl, J. A. (1993). Influence of functional, urological, and environmental characteristics on urinary incontinence in community dwelling older women. *Nursing Research, 42*, 270–275.

Studies Using Other Data Collection Methods

Davis, M. J., & Nomura, L. A. (1990). Vital signs of class I surgical patients. *Western Journal of Nursing Research, 12*, 28–41.

Fehring, R. J., Lawrence, D., & Philpot, C. (1994). Use effectiveness of the Creighton model ovulation method of family planning. *Journal of Obstetric, Gynecologic, and Neonatal Nursing, 23,* 303–309.

Janelli, L. M. (1993). Are there body image differences between older men and women? *Western Journal of Nursing Research, 15,* 327–339.

McDonald, D. D., & Bridge, R. G. (1991). Gender stereotyping and nursing care. *Research in Nursing and Health, 14,* 373–378.

Miceli, D. L., Waxman, H., Cavalieri, T., & Lage, S. (1994). Prodromal falls among older nursing home residents. *Applied Nursing Research, 7,* 18–27.

Pridham, K. F., Sondel, S., Chang, A., & Green, C. (1993). Nipple feeding for preterm infants with bronchopulmonary dysplasia. *Journal of Obstetric, Gynecologic, and Neonatal Nursing, 22,* 147–155.

von Essen, L., & Sjödén, P. (1993). Perceived importance of caring behaviors to Swedish psychiatric inpatients and staff, with comparisons to somatically-ill samples. *Research in Nursing and Health, 16,* 293–303.

Wise, L. C. (1993). The erosion of nursing resources: Employee withdrawal behaviors. *Research in Nursing and Health, 16,* 67–75.

Chapter 16

ASSESSING DATA QUALITY

Data collection methods vary considerably in their ability to capture adequately the constructs in which nurse researchers are interested. An ideal data collection procedure is one that results in measures of the constructs that are relevant, credible, accurate, unbiased, and sensitive. For most concepts of interest to nurse researchers, there are few, if any, data collection procedures that match this ideal. Biophysiologic methods have a much higher chance of success in attaining these goals than self-report or observational methods, but no method is perfect. In this chapter, we discuss criteria for evaluating the quality of data obtained in a research project. Because most data collected by nurse researchers are quantitative, we begin with a discussion of the principles of measurement.

❖ MEASUREMENT

Measurement may be defined as follows: "Measurement consists of rules for assigning numbers to objects to represent quantities of attributes" (Nunnally, 1978, p. 2). As this definition implies, quantification is intimately associated with measurement. An often-quoted statement by early American psychologist L. L. Thurstone

advances a position assumed by many researchers: "Whatever exists, exists in some amount and can be measured." The notion underlying this statement is that attributes of objects are not constant: they vary from day to day, from situation to situation, or from one object to another. This variability is capable of a numerical expression that signifies *how much* of an attribute is present in the object. Quantification is used to communicate that amount. The purpose of assigning numbers, then, is to differentiate between people or objects that possess varying degrees of the critical attribute.

Rules and Measurement

The definition of measurement indicates that numbers must be assigned to objects according to specified rules rather than haphazardly. Quantification in the absence of rules would be meaningless. The rules for measuring temperature, weight, blood pressure, and other physical attributes are familiar to us. Rules for measuring many variables for nursing research studies, however, have to be invented. Whether the data are collected by way of observation, self-report, or some other method, the researcher must specify under what conditions

Polit DF, Hungler BP: NURSING RESEARCH: PRINCIPLES AND METHODS, 5th ed. © 1995 J. B. Lippincott Company.

and according to what criteria the numerical values are to be assigned to the characteristic of interest.

As an example, suppose we were studying attitudes toward the distribution of condoms in school-based clinics and asked parents to express their extent of agreement with the following statement:

> Teenagers should be taught to "say no" rather than having contraceptives available to them in schools.
> {   } Strongly agree
> {   } Agree
> {   } Slightly agree
> {   } Undecided
> {   } Slightly disagree
> {   } Disagree
> {   } Strongly disagree

The responses to this question can be quantified by developing a system for assigning numbers to them. Note that *any* rule would satisfy the definition of measurement. We could assign the value of 30 to "strongly agree," 27 to "agree," 24 to "slightly agree," and so on, but there is no apparent justification for doing so. Therefore, in measuring attributes, we must strive not only to develop rules but also to develop good, meaningful rules. A simplified scheme of assigning a 1 to "strongly agree" and a 7 to "strongly disagree" is probably the most defensible procedure for the question at hand. This rule would quantitatively differentiate, in increments of one point, among people who have seven different reactions to the statement. In developing a new set of rules for measuring attributes, the researcher seldom knows in advance if his or her rules really are the best possible. In essence, a new set of measurement rules constitutes a researcher's hypothesis concerning how an attribute functions and varies. The adequacy of the hypothesis—that is, the worth of the measuring tool—needs to be assessed empirically.

In developing rules, the researcher must strive to link the numerical values to reality. To state this requirement somewhat more technically, the measurement procedures must be isomorphic to reality. The term *isomorphism* signifies equivalence or similarity between two phenomena. A measurement tool cannot be of scientific utility unless the measures resulting from it have some correspondence with the real world.

To illustrate the concept of isomorphism, suppose the Scholastic Aptitude Test (SAT) were administered to 10 people, who obtained the following scores: 345, 395, 430, 435, 490, 505, 550, 570, 620, and 640. These values are shown at the top of Figure 16-1. Let us further suppose that in reality the true scores of these same 10 people on a hypothetically perfect test of scholastic aptitude were as follows: 360, 375, 430, 465, 470, 500, 550, 610, 590, and 670. These values are shown at the bottom of Figure 16-1.

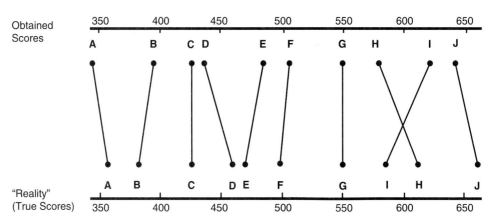

Figure 16-1.   *Relationship between obtained and true scores for a hypothetical set of test scores*

This figure shows that, while not perfect, the test came fairly close to representing the true scores of the 10 subjects. Only two individuals (H and I) were improperly ordered as a result of the actual test. This example illustrates a measure whose isomorphism with reality is fairly high, but improvable.

The researcher almost always works with fallible measures. Measuring instruments that measure psychological phenomena are less likely to correspond to reality than physical measures, but few instruments are totally immune from error. Techniques for evaluating how much error is present in a measuring instrument are discussed later in this chapter.

Advantages of Measurement

What exactly does measurement accomplish? Consider how handicapped nurses and doctors—and, of course, researchers—would be in the absence of measurement. What would happen, for example, if there were no measures of weight, temperature, or blood pressure? Only intuition, guesses, personal judgments, and subjective evaluations would remain.

One of the principle strengths of measurement is that it removes much of the guesswork in gathering information. Because measurement is based on explicit rules, the information tends to be objective. An objective measure is one that can be independently verified by others. Two people measuring the weight of a subject using the same scale would be likely to get identical results. Two people scoring a standardized self-report stress scale would be likely to arrive at identical scores. Not all scientific measures are completely objective, but most are likely to incorporate rules for minimizing subjectivity.

An additional advantage is that quantitative measurement makes it possible to obtain reasonably precise information. Instead of describing Nathan as rather tall, we can depict him as a man who is 6 feet 2 inches tall. If we chose, or if the research requirements demanded it, we could obtain even more precise height measurements. Because of the possibility for preci-

sion, the researcher's task of differentiating among objects that possess different degrees of an attribute becomes considerably easier.

Finally, measurement constitutes a language of communication. Numbers are much less vague than words and therefore are capable of communicating information to a broad audience. If a researcher reported that the average oral temperature of a sample of postoperative patients was somewhat high, different readers might develop different conceptions about the physiologic state of the sample. However, if the researcher reported an average temperature of 99.6°F, there is no possibility of ambiguity and subjective interpretations.

Errors of Measurement

The measurement of attributes does not occur in a vacuum. Both the procedures involved in applying the measurement and the object being measured are susceptible to numerous influences that could alter the resulting information. Some of the factors that impinge on the measurement process can be controlled to a certain degree, and attempts should always be made to do so, but such efforts are rarely completely successful.

If an instrument is not perfectly accurate, then the measures it yields can be said to contain a certain degree of error. Conceptually, an *observed* or *obtained score* can be decomposed into two parts—an error component and a true component. This can be written symbolically as follows:

$$\text{Obtained score} = \text{True score} \pm \text{Error}$$
$$\text{or}$$
$$X_O = X_T \pm X_E$$

The first term in this equation represents the actual, observed score for some measurement. For example, it could represent a patient's systolic blood pressure or a score on a scale of subjective pain. The X_T stands for the true value that would be obtained if it were possible to arrive at an infallible measure. The *true score* is a hypothetical entity—it can never be known because measures are *not* infallible. The final term in the equation is the *error of measurement*. The difference between true and obtained scores is the result of factors that affect the measurement and result in distortions.

Decomposing obtained scores in this fashion brings to light an important point. When a researcher measures an attribute of interest, he or she is also *measuring* attributes that are not of interest. The true score component is what one hopes to isolate; the error component is a composite of other factors that are also being measured, contrary to the desires of the researcher. This concept can be illustrated with an exaggerated example. Suppose a researcher were measuring the weight of 10 people on a spring scale. As each subject steps on the scale, our fictitious researcher places a hand on the subject's shoulder and applies some pressure. The resulting measures (the X_Os), will all be biased in an upward direction because the scores reflect the influence of both the subject's actual weight (X_T) and the researcher's pressure (X_E). Errors of measurement are problematic because they represent an unknown quantity and also because they are variable. In this example, the amount of pressure applied would undoubtedly vary from one subject to the next. In other words, the proportion of true score component in an obtained score varies from one person to the next.

Many factors contribute to errors of measurement. Among the most common are the following seven factors:

1. *Situational contaminants*. Scores can be affected by the conditions under which they are produced. The subject's awareness of an observer's presence (the reactivity problem) is one source of bias. The anonymity of the response situation, the friendliness of the researchers, or the location of the data gathering can all affect a subject's responses. Other environmental factors, such as the temperature, humidity, lighting, time of day, and so forth, can represent sources of measurement error.

2. *Response-set biases*. A number of relatively enduring characteristics of the respondents can interfere with accurate measures of the target attribute. Response sets such as social desirability, extreme responses, and acquiescence are potential problems in self-report measures, particularly in psychological scales (see Chapter 13).

3. *Transitory personal factors*. The scores of an individual may be influenced by a variety of temporary personal states such as fatigue, hunger, anxiety, mood, and so forth. In some cases, these factors can affect a measurement directly, as in the case of anxiety affecting a measurement of pulse rate. In other cases, temporary personal factors can alter individuals' scores by influencing their motivation to cooperate, act naturally, or do their best.

4. *Administration variations*. Alterations in the methods of collecting data from one subject to the next could result in variations in obtained scores that have little to do with variations in the target attribute. If observers alter their coding categories or definitions, if interviewers improvise the wording of a question, if test administrators change the test instructions, or if some physiologic measures are taken before a feeding and others are taken after a feeding, then measurement errors can potentially occur.

5. *Instrument clarity*. If the directions for obtaining measures are vague or poorly understood, then scores may reflect this ambiguity and misunderstanding. For example, questions in a self-report instrument may sometimes be interpreted differently by different respondents, leading to a distorted measure of the critical variable. Observers may miscategorize observations if the classification scheme is unclear.

6. *Item sampling*. Sometimes errors are introduced as a result of the sampling of items used to measure an attribute. For example, a nursing student's score on a 100-item test of general nursing knowledge will be influenced to a certain extent by *which* 100

questions are included on the examination. A person might get 95 questions correct on one test but only get 90 right on another similar test.

7. *Instrument format.* Several technical characteristics of an instrument can influence the obtained measurements. Open-ended questions may yield information different from closed-ended questions. Oral responses to a specific question may be at odds with responses to a written form of the same question. The ordering of questions within an instrument may also influence responses.

This list represents a sampling of the sources of measurement error with which a researcher must deal. Other common problems will come to light in other sections of this chapter.

❖ RELIABILITY OF MEASURING INSTRUMENTS

The reliability* of an instrument that yields quantitative data is a major criterion for assessing its quality and adequacy. Essentially, the *reliability* of an instrument is the degree of consistency with which it measures the attribute it is supposed to be measuring. If a scale gave a reading of 120 pounds for a person's weight one minute, and a reading of 150 pounds in the next minute (barring any tampering with the instrument or subject), we would naturally be wary of using that scale because the information would be unreliable. The less variation an instrument produces in repeated measurements of an attribute, the higher its reliability. Thus, reliability can be equated with the stability, consistency, or dependability of a measuring tool.

Another way of defining reliability is in terms of accuracy. An instrument can be said to

be reliable if its measures accurately reflect the true scores of the attribute under investigation. This definition links reliability to the issues raised in the discussion of measurement error. We can make this relationship clearer by stating that an instrument is reliable to the extent that errors of measurement are absent from obtained scores. A reliable measure is one that maximizes the true score component and minimizes the error component. The greater the error, the greater the unreliability.

These two ways of approaching the concept of reliability (consistency and accuracy) are not so different as they might at first appear. The errors of measurement that impinge on an instrument's accuracy also affect its consistency. The example of the scale that produced variable weight readings should clarify this point. Suppose that the true weight of a subject is 125 pounds, but that two independent measurements yielded 120 and 150 pounds. In terms of the equation presented in the previous section, we could express the measurements as follows:

$$120 = 125 - 5$$
$$150 = 125 + 25$$

The values of the errors of measurement for the two trials are -5 and $+25$, respectively. These errors produced scores that are both inconsistent and inaccurate. We must conclude that our fictitious spring scale is highly unreliable.

The reliability of a measuring tool can be assessed in several different ways. The method chosen depends to a certain extent on the nature of the instrument but also on the aspect of the reliability concept that is of greatest interest. The aspects that have received major quantitative attention are stability, internal consistency, and equivalence.

Stability

The *stability* of a measure refers to the extent to which the same results are obtained on repeated administrations of the instrument. The

---

* The discussion of reliability presented here is based entirely on classic measurement theory. Readers concerned with assessing the reliability of instructional measures that can be classified as mastery-type or criterion-referenced should consult Thorndike and Hagen (1990).

estimation of reliability here focuses on the instrument's susceptibility to extraneous factors from one administration to the next.

Assessments of the stability of a measuring tool are derived through procedures that evaluate *test–retest reliability.* The researcher administers the same test to a sample of individuals on two occasions and then compares the scores obtained. The comparison procedure is performed objectively by computing a *reliability coefficient,* which is a numerical index of the magnitude of the test's reliability.

We must pause at this point to briefly explain the concepts underlying the statistic known as the *correlation coefficient.** We have pointed out repeatedly in this text that a scientist often strives to detect and explain the relationships among phenomena: Is there a relationship between patients' gastric acidity levels and incidents of emotional upset? Is there a relationship between body temperature and perceptions of the passage of time? The correlation coefficient is an important tool for quantitatively describing the magnitude and direction of a relationship. The computation of this index does not concern us here. It is more important to understand how to read a correlation coefficient.

Two variables that are obviously related to one another are the height and weight of individuals. Tall people tend, on the average, to be heavier than short people. We would say that there was a *perfect relationship* if the tallest person in the world were the heaviest, the second tallest person were the second heaviest, and so forth. The correlation coefficient summarizes how perfect a relationship is. The possible values for a correlation coefficient range from a −1.00 through 0.0 to +1.00. If height and weight were perfectly correlated, then the correlation coefficient expressing this relationship would be 1.00. Because the relationship does exist but is not perfect, the correlation coefficient is probably in the vicinity of .50 or .60. The relationship between height and weight would

be described as a *positive relationship* because increases in height tend to be associated with increases in weight.

When two variables are totally unrelated, the correlation coefficient is equal to zero. One might anticipate that a woman's dress size is unrelated to her intelligence. Large women are as likely to perform well on tests of ability as small women. The correlation coefficient summarizing such a relationship would presumably be in the vicinity of 0.0.

Correlation coefficients running from 0.0 to −1.00 express what is known as *inverse* or *negative relationships.* When two variables are inversely related, increases in one variable are associated with decreases in the second variable. Suppose that there is an inverse relationship between a nurse's age and attitude toward abortion. This means that, on the average, the greater the age of the nurse, the *less* favorable the attitude. If the relationship were perfect (i.e., if the oldest nurse had the least favorable attitude and so on), then the correlation coefficient would be equal to −1.00. In actuality, the relationship between age and abortion attitudes is probably modest—in the vicinity of −.20 or −.30. A correlation coefficient of this magnitude describes a weak relationship wherein older nurses tend to be unfavorable and younger nurses tend to be favorable toward abortion, but a "crossing of lines" is not unusual. That is, a number of younger nurses oppose abortion, and a number of older nurses support it.

Now we are prepared to discuss the use of correlation coefficients to compute reliability estimates. In the case of test–retest reliability, a sample of subjects is exposed to the administration of the instrument on two occasions. Let us say we are interested in the stability of a scale to measure self-esteem in adolescents. Because self-esteem is presumably a fairly stable attribute that does not change markedly from one day to the next, we would expect a measure of it to yield consistent scores on two separate tests. As a check on the instrument's stability, we might arrange to administer the scale 3 weeks apart to a sample of teenagers. Fictitious data for this

---

* Computational procedures and additional information concerning correlation coefficients (Pearson's *r*) are presented in Chapter 17.

example are presented in Table 16-1. It can be seen that, generally, the differences in the scores on the two testings are not large. The reliability coefficient for test–retest estimates is the correlation coefficient between the two sets of scores. In this example, the computed reliability coefficient is .95, which is high.

The value of the reliability coefficient theoretically can range between −1.00 and +1.00, just as in the case of other correlation coefficients. A negative coefficient would have been obtained in the self-esteem example if teenagers who had the highest self-esteem scores at time 1 had the lowest scores at time 2. In practice, reliability coefficients normally range between 0.0 and 1.00. The higher the coefficient, the more stable the measure. For most purposes, reliability coefficients above .70 are considered satisfactory. In some situations, a higher coefficient may be required, or a lower one may be considered acceptable.

The test–retest method is a relatively easy and straightforward approach to estimating reliability. It is a method that can be used with self-report, observational, and physiologic measures. However, the test–retest approach has certain disadvantages. One problem is that many traits of interest *do* change over time, independently of the stability of the measure. Attitudes, behaviors, moods, knowledge, physical

Table 16-1. *Fictitious Data for Test–Retest Reliability of Self-Esteem Scale*

SUBJECT NUMBER	TIME 1	TIME 2	
1	55	57	
2	49	46	
3	78	74	
4	37	35	
5	44	46	
6	50	56	
7	58	55	
8	62	66	
9	48	50	
10	67	63	$r = .95$

condition, and so forth can be modified by intervening experiences between the two testings. The procedures used to estimate stability confound changes resulting from random fluctuations and those resulting from true modifications in the attribute being measured. Still, there are many attributes (such as self-esteem) that are relatively enduring characteristics for which a test–retest approach is suitable.

Stability estimates suffer from other problems, however. One possibility is that the subjects' responses or observer's coding on the second administration will be influenced by the memory of their responses or coding on the first administration, regardless of the actual values on the second day. This memory interference will result in a spuriously high reliability coefficient. Another difficulty is that subjects may actually change as a result of the first administration. Finally, people may not be as careful using the same instrument a second time. If they find the procedure boring on the second occasion, then the responses could be haphazard, resulting in a spuriously low estimate of stability.

In summary, the test–retest approach is a procedure for estimating the stability of a measure over time. On the whole, reliability coefficients tend to be higher for short-term retests than for long-term retests (i.e., those greater than 1 or 2 months) because of actual changes in the attribute being measured. Stability indexes are most appropriate for relatively enduring characteristics such as personality, abilities, or certain physical attributes such as height.

Internal Consistency

Composite scales and tests are often evaluated in terms of their internal consistency. Ideally, scales designed to measure an attribute are composed of a set of items, all of which are measuring the critical attribute and nothing else. On a scale to measure empathy in nurses, it would be inappropriate to include an item that is a better measure of diagnostic competence than empathy. An instrument may be said to be *internally consistent* or *homogeneous* to the extent that all of its subparts are measuring the same characteristic.

The internal consistency approach to estimating an instrument's reliability is probably the most widely used method among researchers today. The reason for the popularity of the procedures is not only that they are economical (they require only one test administration) but also that they are the best means of assessing one of the most important sources of measurement error in psychosocial instruments, the sampling of items.

One of the oldest methods for assessing internal consistency is the *split-half technique.* In this approach, the items composing a test are split into two groups and scored independently, and the scores on the two half-tests are used to compute a correlation coefficient. To illustrate this procedure, the fictitious scores from the first administration of the self-esteem scale are reproduced in the second column of Table 16-2. For the sake of simplicity, we will say that the total instrument consists of 20 questions. To compute a split-half reliability coefficient, the items must be divided into two groups of 10. Although a large number of possible splits is possible, the usual procedure is to use odd items versus even items. One half-test, therefore, con-

sists of items 1, 3, 5, 7, 9, 11, 13, 15, 17, and 19, and the even-numbered items compose the second half-test. The scores on the two halves for our example are shown in the third and fourth columns of Table 16-2. The correlation coefficient describing the relationship between the two half-tests is an estimate of the internal consistency of the self-esteem scale. If the odd items are measuring the same attribute as the even items, then the reliability coefficient should be high. The correlation coefficient computed on the fictitious data is .67.

The correlation coefficient computed on split-halves of a measure tends to underestimate systematically the reliability of the entire scale. Other things being equal, longer scales are more reliable than shorter ones. The correlation coefficient computed on the data in Table 16-2 is an estimate of reliability for a 10-item instrument, not a 20-item instrument. To overcome this difficulty, a formula has been developed for adjusting the correlation coefficient to give an estimate of reliability for the entire test. The correction equation, which is known as the *Spearman-Brown prophecy formula,* is as follows:

$$r^1 = \frac{2r}{1 + r}$$

Table 16-2.   *Fictitious Data for Split-Half Reliability of the Self-Esteem Scale*

SUBJECT NUMBER	TOTAL SCORE	ODD-NUMBERS SCORE	EVEN-NUMBERS SCORE	
1	55	28	27	
2	49	26	23	
3	78	36	42	
4	37	18	19	
5	44	23	21	
6	50	30	20	
7	58	30	28	
8	62	33	29	
9	48	23	25	
10	67	28	39	$r = .80$

where r = the correlation coefficient computed on the split halves

r^1 = the estimated reliability of the entire test

Using the formula, the reliability for our hypothetical 20-item measure of self-esteem would be

$$r^1 = \frac{(2)(.67)}{1 + .67} = .80$$

The split-half technique is easy to use and eliminates most of the problems associated with the test–retest approach. However, the split-half technique is handicapped by the fact that different reliability estimates can be obtained by using different splits; that is, it makes a difference whether one uses an odd–even split, a first-half–second-half split, or some other method of dividing the items into two groups. For this reason, the split-half approach is increasingly being replaced by formulas that compensate for this deficiency.

The two most widely used methods are *coefficient alpha* (or *Cronbach's alpha*) and the *Kuder-Richardson formula 20* (abbreviated KR-20). It is beyond the scope of this text to explain in detail the application of these formulas. However, because coefficient alpha is a widely used index of reliability, the reader may wish to consult an advanced text on psychometrics, such as Cronbach (1990) or Nunnally (1978).*

Both the coefficient alpha and KR-20 produce a reliability coefficient that can be interpreted in the same fashion as other reliability

* The coefficient alpha equation, for the advanced student, is as follows:

$$r = \frac{k}{k-1}\left[1 - \frac{\Sigma\sigma_1^2}{\sigma y^2}\right]$$

where r = the estimated reliability

k = the total number of items in the test

σ_1^2 = the variance of each individual item

σy^2 = the variance of the total test scores

Σ = the sum of

coefficients described here. That is, the normal range of values is between 0.0 and +1.00, and higher values reflect a higher degree of internal consistency. Coefficient alpha (and KR-20, which is actually a special case of the more general coefficient alpha used with dichotomous items) is preferable to the split-half procedure because it gives an estimate of the split-half correlation for *all possible* ways of dividing the measure into two halves.

In summary, indices of homogeneity or internal consistency estimate the extent to which different subparts of an instrument are equivalent in terms of measuring the critical attribute. The split-half technique frequently has been used to estimate homogeneity, but the coefficient alpha is a preferable method. None of these approaches considers fluctuations over time as a source of unreliability.

Equivalence

A researcher may be interested in estimating the reliability of a measure by way of the *equivalence* approach under one of two circumstances: 1) when different observers or researchers are using an instrument to measure the same phenomena at the same time or 2) when two presumably parallel instruments are administered to individuals at about the same time. In both situations, the aim is to determine the consistency or equivalence of the instruments in yielding measurements of the same traits in the same subjects.

In Chapter 14, which covers observational methods, it was pointed out that a potential weakness of this data collection approach is the fallibility of the observer. The greater the interpretive burden on the observer, the higher is the risk of observer error or bias. The accuracy of observer ratings and classifications can be enhanced by careful training, the development of clearly defined and nonoverlapping categories, the use of a small number of categories, and the use of behaviors that tend to be molecular rather than molar. Even when care is taken to design an observational system that minimizes the possibility of error, the researcher should assess the reliability of the instrument. In this case, the instrument includes both the category system developed by the researcher and the observer making the measurements.

Interrater (or *interobserver*) *reliability* is estimated by having two or more trained observers watching some event simultaneously and independently recording the relevant variables according to a predetermined plan or coding system. The resulting records can then be used to compute an index of equivalence or agreement. Several procedures for arriving at such an index are possible. For certain types of observational data (e.g., ratings and frequency counts within a category system), correlation techniques are often suitable. That is, a correlation coefficient may be computed to demonstrate the strength of the relationship between one observer's ratings or frequencies and another's.

Another procedure is to compute reliability as a function of agreements, using the following equation:

$$\frac{\text{Number of agreements}}{\text{Number of agreements} + \text{disagreements}}$$

This simple formula unfortunately tends to overestimate observer agreements. If the behavior under investigation is one that observers code for absence or presence every, say, 10 seconds, then by chance alone, the observers will agree 50% of the time. Other approaches for estimating interrater reliability may be of interest to advanced students. Techniques such as analysis of variance, intraclass correlations, and rank-order correlations have been used to assess the reliability of observational measures.

The second situation in which the equivalence of measures is evaluated is when two alternative, parallel forms of a single instrument are available. This type of research problem is unlikely to present itself frequently in nursing research, except in methodological studies or in an educational context. For example, alternate forms of a test of nursing knowledge might be needed. In such a case, the two forms should be administered to a sample of individuals in immediate succession, randomly alternating the order of presentation of the forms. The correlation coefficient between the two sets of scores would be an index of reliability of equivalence. This procedure is adopted to determine whether the two instruments are, in fact, measuring the same attribute. The researcher uses this technique to assess the errors of measurement resulting from errors in item sampling.

Interpretation of Reliability Coefficients

The reliability coefficients computed according to the procedures just described can be used as an important indicator of the quality of an instrument. A measure that is unreliable interferes with an adequate testing of a researcher's hypotheses. If data fail to confirm a research prediction, one possibility is that the measuring tools were unreliable—not necessarily that the expected relationships do not exist. There is no standard for what an acceptable reliability coefficient should be. If a researcher is only interested in making group-level comparisons, then coefficients in the vicinity of .70 or even .60 would probably be sufficient. By group-level comparisons, we mean that the investigator is interested in comparing the scores of such groups as male versus female, smoker versus nonsmoker, experimental versus control, and so forth. However, if measures were to be used as a basis for making decisions about individuals, then the reliability coefficient should be .90 or better. For instance, if a score on a test were to be used as a criterion for admission to a graduate nursing program, then the accuracy of the test is of critical importance to both individual applicants and the school of nursing.

The reliability coefficient has a special interpretation that should be briefly explained without elaborating on technical details. This interpretation relates to the earlier discussion of decomposing an observed score into an error component and a true component. Suppose that we have just administered to 50 nurses a scale that measures empathy. It would be expected that the scores would vary from one nurse to another because some nurses are more empathic than others. Some of the variability in scores is true variability, reflecting real individual differences in the attribute being measured; some of the variability, however, is error. Thus,

$$V_O = V_T + V_E$$

where V_O = observed total variability in scores
V_T = true variability
V_E = variability owing to random errors

A reliability coefficient is directly associated with this equation. *Reliability is the proportion of true variability to the total obtained variability,* or

$$r = \frac{V_T}{V_O}$$

If, for example, the reliability coefficient were .85, then 85% of the variability in obtained scores could be said to represent true individual differences, and 15% of the variability would reflect random, extraneous fluctuations. Looked at in this way, it should be a bit clearer why in-

struments with reliability of .60 or lower are risky to use.

Table 16-3 illustrates different forms of reliability evaluations that nurse researchers have used to assess instruments that they or others developed.

❖ *VALIDITY*

The second important criterion by which a quantitative instrument's adequacy is evaluated is its validity. *Validity* refers to the degree to which an instrument measures what it is supposed to be measuring. When a researcher develops an instrument to measure patients' hopelessness, how can its developer really know that the resulting scores validly reflect this construct and not something else, such as depression? Problems of validity relate to the question, Are we really measuring the attribute we think we are measuring?

Like reliability, validity has a number of different aspects and assessment approaches. Unlike reliability, however, the validity of an instrument is extremely difficult to establish. Solid evidence supporting the validity of most psychologically oriented measures is rarely available. There are no formulas or equations that can easily be applied to the scores of the hypo-

Table 16-3.   *Examples of Reliability Assessments by Nurse Researchers*

INSTRUMENT	TYPE OF RELIABILITY	RELIABILITY COEFFECIENT	REFERENCE
Perceived Conflict Scale— a 16-item self-report scale	Test–retest (2 weeks) Cronbach's alpha	.77 .81	Gardner, 1992
Discomfort Scale for Alzheimer patients (DS-DAT)— a 9-item observational scale	Test–retest (1 hour) Cronbach's alpha Interrater reliability	.60 .87 .90	Hurley, Volicer, Hanrahan, Houde, & Volicer, 1992
Breast-Self Examination/ Health Belief Model Scale— a 45-item self-report scale	Test–retest (2–8 weeks) Cronbach's alpha	.45–.70* .80–.93	Champion, 1993

*This is the range of coefficients for different subscales of the instrument.

thetical hopefulness scale to estimate how good a job the scale is doing in measuring the critical variable.

The reliability and validity of an instrument are not totally independent qualities of an instrument. *A measuring device that is unreliable cannot possibly be valid.* An instrument cannot validly be measuring the attribute of interest if it is erratic, inconsistent, and inaccurate. An unreliable tool would be measuring too many other factors associated with random error to be considered a valid indicator of the target variable. However, an instrument can be reliable without being valid. Suppose we had the idea to measure anxiety in patients by measuring the circumference of their wrists. We could obtain highly accurate, consistent, and precise measurements of the wrist circumferences, but such measures would not be valid indicators of anxiety. Thus, the high reliability of an instrument provides no evidence of its validity for an intended purpose; the low reliability of a measure *is* evidence of low validity.

The methodological literature abounds with terms relating to different facets of the validity question. One aspect is known as face validity. *Face validity* refers to whether the instrument looks as though it is measuring the appropriate construct. Although face validity should not be considered as acceptable evidence for the quality of an instrument, it may be helpful for a measure to have face validity if other types of validity have also been demonstrated. For example, it might be easier to persuade administrators to undertake an evaluation if the evaluation instruments have face validity. Three other aspects of validity are of greater importance in assessments of an instrument: content validity, criterion-related validity, and construct validity.

Content Validity

Content validity is concerned with the sampling adequacy of the content area being measured. Content validity is of special relevance to individuals designing a test to measure knowledge in a specific content area. In such a context, the validity question being asked is, How representative are the questions on this test of the universe of all questions that might be asked on this topic? Suppose we were interested in testing the knowledge of a group of lay people concerning the seven danger signals of cancer identified by the American Cancer Society. To be representative, or content valid, the questions on the test would have to include items from each of the seven danger signals, or "CAUTION":

*C*hange in bowel or bladder habits
A sore that does not heal
*U*nusual bleeding or discharge
*T*hickening or lump in breast or elsewhere
*I*ndigestion or difficulty in swallowing
*O*bvious change in wart or mole
*N*agging cough or hoarseness

The issue of content validity also arises in conjunction with measures of attributes other than knowledge, such as in attitudinal measures. For example, Frank-Stromberg (1989) made efforts to enhance the content validity of her Reaction to the Diagnosis of Cancer Questionnaire. She began by asking 340 cancer patients the following open-ended question: "What do you remember of your feelings when first told you had cancer?" Prevalent themes that emerged in the responses to this question were then incorporated into items in the scale, thus reflecting the major content areas experienced by cancer patients.

The content validity of an instrument is necessarily based on judgment. There are no completely objective methods of assuring the adequate content coverage of an instrument. Experts in the content area may be called on to analyze the items to see if they represent adequately the hypothetical content universe in the correct proportions. The researcher developing a test or scale, in writing or selecting items for inclusion in an instrument, should aim to build in content validity by careful planning and the careful execution of a prespecified plan.

Criterion-Related Validity

The *criterion-related* approach to validity assessment is a pragmatic one. The researcher attempting to establish the criterion-related validity of an instrument is not seeking to ascertain how well the tool is measuring a particular theoretical trait. The emphasis is on establishing the relationship between the instrument and some other criterion. The instrument, whatever abstract attribute it is measuring, is said to be valid if its scores correlate highly with some criterion. For example, if a measure of birth control use among sexually active teenaged girls correlates highly with subsequent premarital pregnancies, then the birth control measure could be described as having good validity. In terms of the criterion-related validation approach, the key issue is whether the instrument is a useful predictor of subsequent behaviors, experiences, or conditions.

One requirement of the criterion-related approach to validation is the availability of a reasonably reliable and valid criterion with which the measures on the target instrument can be compared. This is, unfortunately, seldom easy. If we were developing an instrument to predict the nursing effectiveness of nursing students, we might use subsequent supervisory ratings as our criterion. However, how can we be sure that these ratings are themselves valid and reliable? In fact, the supervisory ratings might themselves be in need of validation. Usually the researcher must be content with less than perfect criteria.

Once the criterion is selected, the validity can be assessed easily and straightforwardly. The scores on the predictor instrument are correlated with scores on the criterion variable. The magnitude of the correlation coefficient is a direct estimate of how valid the instrument is, according to this method of validation. To illustrate, suppose a team of nurse researchers developed a scale to measure professionalism among nurses. They administer the instrument to a sample of nurses and at the same time ask the nurses to indicate how many articles they have published. The publications variable was chosen as one of many potential objective criteria of professionalism. Fictitious data are presented in Table 16-4. The correlation coefficient of .83 indicates that the professionalism scale correlates reasonably well with the number of articles a nurse has published. Whether the scale is really measuring professionalism is a somewhat different issue—an issue that is the concern of construct validation discussed in the next section.

Sometimes a distinction is made between two types of criterion-related validity. The dis-

Table 16-4. *Fictitious Data for Criterion-Related Validity Example*

SUBJECT	SCORE ON PROFESSIONALISM SCALE	NUMBER OF PUBLICATIONS
1	25	2
2	30	4
3	17	0
4	20	1
5	22	0
6	27	2
7	29	5
8	19	1
9	28	3
10	15	1 $r = .83$

tinction is not usually an important one, but the terms are used frequently enough to warrant their mention. *Predictive validity* refers to the adequacy of an instrument in differentiating between the performance or behaviors of individuals on some future criterion. When a school of nursing correlates the incoming SAT scores of students with subsequent grade point averages, the predictive validity of the SATs for nursing school performance is being evaluated. *Concurrent validity* refers to the ability of an instrument to distinguish individuals who differ in their present status on some criterion. For example, a psychological test to differentiate between those patients in a mental institution who can and cannot be released could be correlated with current behavioral ratings of health care personnel. The difference between predictive and concurrent validity, then, is the difference in the timing of obtaining measurements on a criterion.

Validation by means of the criterion-related approach is most often used in applied or practically oriented research. Criterion-related validity is helpful in assisting decision makers by giving them some assurance that their decisions will be effective, fair, and, in short, valid.

Construct Validity

Validating an instrument in terms of *construct validity* is a difficult and challenging task. The instrument designer adopting this approach is concerned with the questions: What is this measuring device really measuring? Is the abstract concept under investigation being adequately measured with this instrument? Unlike criterion-related validity, construct validity is more concerned with the underlying attribute than with the scores that the instrument produces. The scores are of interest only insofar as they constitute a valid basis for inferring the degree to which a subject possesses some characteristic. Unfortunately, the more abstract the concept, the more difficult it is to establish the construct validity of the measure; at the same time, the more abstract the concept, the less suitable it is to validate a measure by the crite-

rion-related approach. Actually, it is really not just a question of suitability but also of feasibility. What objective criterion is there for such concepts as empathy, grief, role conflict, or separation anxiety?

Despite the obstacles and difficulties encountered in assessing the construct validity of instruments, this activity is a vital component of scientific progress. The constructs in which scientists are interested must be reliably and validly measured. The significance of construct validity is in its linkage with theory and theoretical conceptualization. In validating a measure of death anxiety, we would probably be less concerned with the adequate sampling of items or with relating the resultant scores to a criterion than with the extent to which the measure corresponds to a theory of death anxiety that is acceptable to us.

Construct validation can be approached in several ways, but there is always an emphasis on logical analysis and the testing of relationships predicated on the basis of theoretical considerations. Constructs are usually explicated in terms of other concepts; therefore, the researcher should be in a position to make predictions about the manner in which the construct will function in relation to other constructs. One common approach to construct validation is the *known-groups technique*. In this procedure, groups that are expected to differ on the critical attribute because of some known characteristic are administered the instrument. For instance, in validating a measure of fear of the labor experience, one might contrast the scores of primiparas and multiparas. Because one would expect that women who had never given birth would experience more fears and anxiety than women who had already had children, one might question the validity of the instrument if such differences did not emerge. There is not necessarily an expectation that the differences would be great. It would be expected that some primiparas would feel no anxiety at all, and some multiparas would express some fears. On the whole, however, it would be anticipated that some group differences would be reflected in the average scores. As another example of the known-groups technique, consider the example of validating a measure concerning limitations in functional ability. One might choose people with emphysema and people without emphysema to validate the instrument. The validity of the instrument might be questioned if differences in scores between the two groups did not occur because one would expect that people with emphysema would have experienced limitations in functional ability.

Another method of construct validation consists of an examination of relationships based on theoretical predictions, which is really a variant of the known-groups approach. A researcher might reason as follows:

- According to theory, construct X is positively related to construct Y;
- instrument A is a measure of construct X, and instrument B is a measure of construct Y;
- scores on A and B are correlated positively, as predicted by the theory;
- therefore, it is inferred that A and B are valid measures of X and Y.

This logical analysis is fallible and does not constitute proof of construct validity but is important as a type of evidence, nevertheless.

A significant advance in the area of construct validation is the procedure developed by Campbell and Fiske (1959) known as the *multitrait–multimethod matrix method*. This procedure makes use of the concepts of convergence and discriminability. *Convergence* refers to evidence that different methods of measuring a construct yield similar results. Different approaches to measurement should converge on the construct. *Discriminability* refers to the ability to differentiate the construct being measured from other similar constructs. Campbell and Fiske argued that evidence of both convergence and discriminability should be brought to bear in the construct validity question.

To help explain the multitrait–multimethod approach, fictitious data from a study to validate a "need for autonomy" measure are presented in Table 16-5. In using this approach, the researcher must measure the critical concept by two or more methods. Suppose we measured need for autonomy in a sample of nursing home residents by having the residents respond to a self-report summated rating scale (the measure we are attempting to validate); having nurses rate each person after observing him or her in a task designed to elicit different degrees of autonomy; and having the residents respond to a pictorial (projective) stimulus depicting an autonomy-relevant situation. A second requirement of the multitrait–multimethod approach is that we must also measure constructs from which we wish to differentiate the key con-

Table 16-5. *Multitrait–Multimethod Matrix*

METHOD*	TRAITS†	METHOD 1		METHOD 2		METHOD 3	
		A_1	B_1	A_2	B_2	A_3	B_3
Method 1	A_1	(.88)					
	B_1	−.38	(.86)				
Method 2	A_2	.60	−.19	(.79)			
	B_2	−.21	.58	−.39	(.80)		
Method 3	A_3	.51	−.18	.55	−.12	(.74)	
	B_3	−.14	.49	−.17	.54	−.32	(.72)

* Methods: 1, self-report summated scale; 2, observational rating; 3, projective test.
† Traits: A, need for autonomy trait; B, need for affiliation trait.

struct, using the same measuring methods. In the current example, suppose that we decided to differentiate need for autonomy from need for affiliation. The two concepts are related: one would expect, on the average, that people who exhibited a high degree of need for autonomy would be relatively low in terms of need for affiliation. The point of including both concepts in a single validation study is to gather evidence that the two concepts are, in fact, distinct rather than two different labels for the same underlying attribute.

The numbers in Table 16-5 represent the correlation coefficients between the scores on the six different measures (two traits × three methods). For instance, the coefficient of $-.38$ at the intersection of A1–B1 expresses the relationship between the self-report scores on the need for autonomy and need for affiliation measures. Recall that a minus sign before the correlation coefficient signifies an inverse relationship. In this case, the $-.38$ tells us that there was a slight tendency for people scoring high on the need for autonomy scale to score low on the need for affiliation scale. The numbers in parentheses along the diagonal of this matrix are the reliability coefficients.

Various aspects of the multitrait–multimethod matrix have a bearing on the construct validity question. The most direct evidence (convergence) comes from the correlations between two different methods for measuring the same trait. In the case of A1–A2, the coefficient is .60, which is reasonably substantial. Convergent validity should be sufficiently large to encourage further scrutiny of the matrix. Second, the convergent validity entries should be higher (in terms of absolute magnitude*) than those correlations between measures that have neither method nor trait in common. That is, A1–A2 should be greater than A2–B1 or A1–B2. Inspection of the table reveals that, indeed, .60 surpasses the "heterotrait–heteromethod" values

of $-.21$ and $-.19$. This requirement is a minimum one, which, if failed, should cause the researcher to have serious doubts about the validity of the measures. Third, the convergent validity coefficients should be greater than the coefficients between measures of different traits by a single method. Once again, the matrix in Table 16-5 fulfills this criterion: A1–A2 (.60) and A2–A3 (.55) are higher than A1–B1 ($-.38$), A2–B2 ($-.39$) and A3–B3 ($-.32$). The last two requirements provide some evidence for discriminant validity.

The multitrait–multimethod approach can be extended to include more traits and more methods. The difficulty is in administering a large number of measures to a sample of subjects. Also, the evidence is seldom as clearcut as in this contrived example, and therefore, additional measures may create undesirable confusion. The full matrix as exemplified in Table 16-5 represents a valuable and perhaps unparalleled tool for exploring the validity of instruments. The researcher should not abandon attempts to utilize the concepts underlying the procedure even when the full model is not feasible. Perhaps in some cases only an A1–B1 type of combination is possible, whereas in others, A1–A2–A3 would be manageable. Without any doubt, the execution of any portion of the model is better than no effort to estimate construct validity and generally is preferable to a content validity approach for most concepts of interest to nurse researchers.

Another approach to construct validation employs a statistical procedure known as factor analysis. Although factor analysis, which will be discussed in Chapter 19, is computationally complex, it is conceptually rather simple. *Factor analysis* is essentially a method for identifying clusters of related variables. Each cluster, called a *factor*, represents a relatively unitary attribute. The procedure is used to identify and group together different measures of some underlying attribute. In effect, factor analysis constitutes another means of looking at the convergent and discriminant validity of a large set of measures.

---

* The *absolute magnitude* refers to the value without a plus or minus sign. A value of $-.50$ is of a higher absolute magnitude than $+.40$.

In summary, construct validation uses both logical and empirical procedures. Like content validity, construct validity requires a judgment pertaining to what the instrument is measuring. Unlike content validity, however, the logical operations required by construct validation are typically linked to a theory or conceptual framework. Construct and criterion-related validity share an empirical component, but in criterion-related validity, there is usually a pragmatic, objective criterion with which to compare a measure rather than a second measure of an abstract theoretical construct.

Interpretation of Validity

Like reliability, validity is not an all-or-nothing characteristic of an instrument. An instrument cannot really be said to possess or lack validity; it is a question of degree. Furthermore, although we have referred to the process of testing the validity of an instrument as validation, it is inappropriate to speak of the process as yielding proof of validity. Like all tests of hypotheses, the testing of an instrument's validity is not proved, established, or verified but rather supported to a greater or lesser degree by evidence.

Strictly speaking, a researcher does not validate the instrument per se but rather some application of the instrument. A measure of anxiety may be valid for presurgical patients on the day before an operation but may not be valid for nursing students on the morning of a final examination. Of course, some instruments may be valid for a wide range of uses with different types of samples, but each use requires new supporting evidence. In a sense, validation is a never-ending process. The more evidence that can be gathered that an instrument is measuring what it is supposed to be measuring, the more confidence researchers will have in its validity.

Nurse researchers have become increasingly sophisticated in assessing the validity of measures. Table 16-6 presents some examples of measures that have been subjected to a validation process by nurse researchers.

❖ OTHER CRITERIA FOR ASSESSING QUANTITATIVE MEASURES

Reliability and validity are the two most important aspects to consider in evaluating a measuring instrument. If a measure can be shown to be

Table 16-6. *Examples of Validity Assessments by Nurse Researchers*

INSTRUMENT	TYPE OF VALIDITY	PROCEDURE
The Pain-O-Meter, a device for recording sensory and affective components of pain (Gaston-Johansson, Franco, & Zimmerman, 1992)	Construct	Known groups (scores before and after pain-relieving analgesics)
	Criterion	Relation to scores on other pain measures
Mastery of Stress Instrument— a 60-item self-report scale for adults (Younger, 1993)	Content	Review by panel of 18 experts
	Concurrent	Correlation with Mastery Scale
	Construct	Relation to other personal characteristics; factor analysis
Work Assessment Scale— a 53-item self-report scale for multiple sclerosis (MS) patients (Gulick, 1991)	Content	Content analysis of MS patients' open-ended responses
	Criterion	Relation to scores on functional ability scales
	Construct	Factor analysis

reasonably reliable and valid for a specific purpose, then the researcher can have some assurance that the results of a study will be meaningful. High reliability and validity are a necessary, though insufficient, condition for good scientific research.

Sometimes a researcher needs to consider other qualities of an instrument in addition to its validity and reliability. These additional criteria are by no means a substitute for reliability and validity but may in some cases be equally important. Indeed, several of these qualities are directly related to the issues raised in the preceding two sections.

Efficiency

Instruments of comparable reliability and validity may still differ in their efficiency. An instrument that requires 10 minutes of a subject's time to measure his or her coping capacity is efficient in comparison with an instrument to measure the same attribute that requires 30 minutes to complete. One aspect of efficiency is the number of items incorporated in an instrument. Long instruments tend to be more reliable than shorter ones. There is, however, a point of diminishing returns. As an example, consider a 40-item scale to measure feelings of guilt among parents of handicapped children. Let us say that we find a reliability of .94 for the scale, using coefficient alpha as our index of internal consistency. Using the Spearman-Brown formula, we can estimate how reliable the scale would be with only 30 items:

$$r^1 = \frac{kr}{1 + [(1 - k)r]} = \frac{.75\,(.94)}{1 - [.25\,(.94)]} = .92$$

where k = the factor by which the instrument is being incremented or decreased; in this case, $k = 30 \div 40 = .75$

As this calculation shows, a 25% reduction in the length of the instrument resulted in this case in a negligible decrease in reliability, from .94 to .92. Most researchers probably would be willing to sacrifice a modest amount of reliability in exchange for the opportunity to substantially reduce the subjects' response burden and data collection costs.

Efficiency is more characteristic of certain types of data collection procedures than others. In a questionnaire or interview, closed-ended questions are more efficient than open-ended items. Self-report scales tend to be less time-consuming than projective instruments for a comparable amount of information. Of course, a researcher may decide that other advantages (such as depth of information) offset a certain degree of inefficiency. Other things being equal, however, it is desirable to select as efficient an instrument as possible.

Sensitivity

The sensitivity of an instrument affects how small a variation in an attribute can be reliably detected and measured. A yardstick marked off with only three divisions for feet would result in a highly insensitive measure of a person's height. The yardstick could be made more sensitive to variations in height by subdividing each foot into 12 equal sections for inches, and the process could be continued until a sufficiently sensitive measuring tool were obtained for the purposes needed. Unfortunately, it is not this easy to increase the sensitivity of most instruments.

The sensitivity of an instrument determines how discriminating its measurements will be between individuals with differing amounts of an attribute. Using the yardstick marked off in feet only, it would be impossible to discriminate between a person who is 5 feet 8 inches tall and one who is 6 feet 3 inches tall: both would be measured as 6 feet, measuring to the nearest foot. There are statistical procedures that permit a researcher to enhance the sensitivity of paper-and-pencil measures by assessing the degree to which each item is contributing to the instrument's power to make discriminations. These *item analysis techniques* are described in detail in texts on measurement and psychometric theory. Several references are noted at the end of this chapter.

The sensitivity of an instrument is most likely to become an issue in certain kinds of situations. When changes in the level of an attribute are being closely monitored, as in the case of many physiologic measurements, then it is important to use a sensitive device. If important decisions are to be based on the measures resulting from an instrument, then the sensitivity of the instrument could have serious consequences. Experimenters must also be concerned with the sensitivity of measuring tools whenever the treatments they are introducing are not markedly different from their control conditions. In the nursing research literature, there are many examples of studies in which differences between conditions were not detected. Part of the difficulty in many nursing intervention studies is that new interventions are compared with older interventions rather than with no intervention at all. When experimental and control conditions are not maximally different—as must often be the case in nursing research—then highly sensitive instruments may be required to detect differences in the effects of the treatments.

Other Criteria

There is no need to elaborate in detail on the few remaining qualities that should be considered in assessing a quantitative instrument. Most of the following 10 criteria are actually aspects of the reliability and validity issues:

1. *Objectivity.* There should be as little room as possible for disagreements between two or more independent researchers applying the instrument to measure the same phenomenon.
2. *Comprehensibility.* The subject or the researcher should be able to comprehend the behaviors required to secure accurate and valid measures.
3. *Balance.* The instrument designer should strive for a balanced measure to minimize response-set biases and to facilitate content validity.
4. *Speededness.* For most types of instruments, the researcher should be sure that adequate time is allowed to obtain complete measurements without rushing the measuring process.
5. *Unidimensionality.* A measuring tool should be designed to produce separate scores for unitary concepts that can be isolated.
6. *Range.* The instrument should be capable of achieving a meaningful measure from the smallest expected value of the variable to the largest.
7. *Linearity.* A researcher normally strives to construct measures that are equally accurate and sensitive over the entire range of values.
8. *Signal-to-noise ratio.* In physiologic measures, it is important to use instruments and procedures that maximize the signal reading and minimize the interference noise.
9. *Reactivity.* The instrument should, insofar as possible, avoid affecting the attribute that is being measured.
10. *Simplicity.* Other things being equal, a simple instrument is more desirable than a complex instrument inasmuch as complicated measures run a greater risk of having errors.

❖ ASSESSMENT OF QUALITATIVE DATA

The methods of assessment described in this chapter apply primarily to structured data collection instruments that yield quantitative scores. For the most part, these procedures cannot be meaningfully applied to such qualitative materials as unstructured interview responses or narrative descriptions from a participant observer's field notes. However, this does not imply that qualitative researchers are unconcerned with the quality of their data collection techniques. The central question underlying the concepts of reliability and validity is: Do the data collected by the researcher reflect the truth? Certainly, qualitative researchers are as eager as quantitative researchers to have their findings reflect the true state of human experience.

Many qualitative nurse researchers seek to evaluate the quality of their data and their findings through procedures that have been outlined by Lincoln and Guba (1985), two proponents of the naturalistic paradigm of inquiry. These researchers have suggested four criteria for establishing the *trustworthiness* of qualitative data: credibility, transferability, dependability, and confirmability.

Credibility

Careful qualitative researchers take steps to improve and evaluate the *credibility* of their data and conclusions, which refers to confidence in the truth of the data. Lincoln and Guba point out that the credibility of an inquiry involves two aspects: first, carrying out the investigation in such a way that the believability of the findings is enhanced, and second, taking steps to demonstrate credibility.

Lincoln and Guba suggest a variety of techniques for improving and documenting the credibility of qualitative research. First, they recommend activities that make it more likely that credible data and interpretations will be produced. This includes *prolonged engagement*—the investment of sufficient time in the data collection activities to learn the culture of the group under study, to test for misinformation and distortions, and to build trust with informants.

The technique known as triangulation is also used to improve the likelihood that qualitative findings will be found credible. *Triangulation* refers to the use of multiple referents to draw conclusions about what constitutes the truth. Denzin (1989) identified four types of triangulation:

1. *Data triangulation*: the use of multiple data sources in a study (e.g., interviewing multiple key informants about the same topic)
2. *Investigator triangulation*: the use of multiple individuals to collect, analyze, and interpret a single set of data

3. *Theory triangulation*: the use of multiple perspectives to interpret a single set of data
4. *Method triangulation*: the use of multiple methods to address a research problem (e.g., observations plus interviews)

The purpose of using triangulation is to provide a basis for convergence on the truth. In other words, by using multiple methods and perspectives, it is hoped that true information can be sorted out from error information.

Two other techniques that Lincoln and Guba recommend for establishing credibility include debriefing with peers to provide an external check on the inquiry process, and debriefing with informants (or *member checks*). Member checking can be carried out both informally in an ongoing way as data are being collected and more formally after data have been collected and analyzed. Member checking is a particularly important technique for establishing the credibility of qualitative data.

Transferability

In Lincoln and Guba's framework, *transferability* refers essentially to the generalizability of the data, that is, the extent to which the findings from the data can be transferred to other settings or groups. This is, to some extent, a sampling and design issue rather than an issue relating to the soundness of the data per se. However, as Lincoln and Guba note, the responsibility of the investigator is to provide sufficient descriptive data in the research report so that consumers can evaluate the applicability of the data to other contexts: "Thus the naturalist cannot specify the external validity of an inquiry; he or she can provide only the thick description necessary to enable someone interested in making a transfer to reach a conclusion about whether transfer can be contemplated as a possibility" (p. 316).

Dependability

The *dependability* of qualitative data refers to the stability of data over time and over conditions. One approach to assessing the dependability of data is to undertake a procedure referred to as *stepwise replication*. This approach, which is conceptually similar to the conventional split-half technique, involves having a research group of two or more people who can be divided into two teams. These teams deal with data sources separately and conduct, essentially, independent inquiries through which data can be compared. Ongoing, regular communication between the teams is essential for the success of this procedure. Another technique relating to dependability is the *inquiry audit*, which consists of a scrutiny of the data and relevant supporting documents by an external reviewer, an approach that also has a bearing on the confirmability of the data.

Confirmability

Confirmability is a concept that refers to the objectivity or neutrality of the data, such that there would be agreement between two or more independent people about the data's relevance or meaning. Inquiry audits can be used to establish both the dependability and confirmability of the data. In an inquiry audit, the investigator must develop an *audit trail*, that is, a systematic collection of materials and documentation that will allow an independent auditor to come to conclusions about the data. The inquiry auditor then proceeds to audit, in a fashion analogous to a financial audit, the trustworthiness of the data and the meanings attached to them. Although the auditing task is complex, it can serve as an invaluable tool for persuading others that qualitative data are worthy of confidence.

❖ TIPS FOR ASSESSING DATA QUALITY

Researchers can place little confidence in their findings if their data collection instruments and procedures yield data that are of poor quality. With quantitative instruments, it has become a customary procedure for the developers to estimate the validity and reliability of their tools before making them available for general use. Such an evaluation is often referred to as a *psychometric assessment* of an instrument. However, it is the responsibility of all researchers—not just the researchers who develop instruments—to ensure high-quality data. In this section, we provide some additional guidance relating to data quality.

- If you are using an existing quantitative instrument, you should always choose a measure with demonstrated high reliability and validity. This information is usually available in reports of methodological studies. If you are considering an instrument for which you can find no published psychometric information, it is wise to contact the developer of the instrument and ask about evidence of validity and reliability.

- As Table 16-3 illustrates, reliability estimates vary according to the procedures used to obtain them. In selecting an instrument, the researcher needs to determine which aspect of reliability (stability, internal consistency, or equivalence) is most relevant to the attribute and instrument under consideration.

- Even if you choose an instrument that previously was demonstrated to be reliable, this is no guarantee of its high quality for your study. An instrument's reliability is not a fixed entity. *The reliability of an instrument is a property not of the instrument but rather of the instrument when administered to a certain sample under certain conditions.* A scale developed to measure dependence in hospitalized adults may be unreliable for use with hospitalized adolescents, or for the elderly in nursing homes, and so forth. This means that you should always learn about the characteristics of the group with whom or for whom the instrument was developed. If the original group was similar to the researcher's target group, then the reliability estimate provided by the scale developer is probably a reasonably good index of the instrument's accuracy and consistency for your study.

- The prudent researcher should not be satisfied with an instrument that will *probably* be reliable in his or her study. The recommended procedure is to compute estimates of reliability whenever data are collected for a scientific investigation. For physiologic measures that are relatively impervious to random fluctuations stemming from personal or situational factors, this procedure may be unnecessary. However, observational tools, self-report measures, tests of knowledge or ability, and projective tests—all of which are highly susceptible to errors of measurement—should be subjected to a reliability check as a routine step in the research process.

- If you are developing a new composite self-report or observational scale (or modifying an existing one), you should be aware that the reliability of such scales is partly a function of their length or number of items. To improve the reliability, more items tapping the same concept should be added.

- The reliability of an instrument is related in part to the heterogeneity of the sample with which it is used. The more homogeneous the sample (i.e., the more similar their scores), the lower the reliability coefficient will be. This is because instruments are designed to measure differences among those being measured. If the sample is homogeneous, then it is more difficult for the instrument to reliably discriminate among those who possess varying degrees of the attribute being measured.

- The development of adequate measuring tools is probably the single most pressing problem in the field of nursing research, as it is in other disciplines concerned with human behavior. Given the improbability of ever finding *the* perfect criterion measure, researchers should often use *multiple criterion measures,* each of whose measurement strengths complement one another. This strategy is basically triangulation—an approach that qualitative researchers have long advocated and used.

- Many qualitative researchers fail to include information on data quality in their research reports—although this situation is changing. When information on data quality is totally absent in qualitative reports, readers have no way of knowing how trustworthy the data are, and this makes the utilization of the knowledge more problematic.

❖ RESEARCH EXAMPLES

In this section, we describe the efforts of a team of researchers to develop and evaluate a structured observational instrument, and of another researcher to evaluate her qualitative data.

Assessment of a Structured Scale

Prescott and her colleagues (1991) undertook several activities to develop and refine the Patient Intensity for Nursing Index (PINI). The PINI is a 10-item scale for nurses to use in evaluating the intensity of nursing care and the nursing skill level needed by individual patients. The PINI includes items relating to severity of illness, dependency, complexity of care, and time.

After an initial development study, the research team performed an extensive psychometric evaluation. Interrater reliability was assessed by having day and evening RNs from one unit in each of five hospitals use the PINI on the same 150 patients as closely in time as possible (i.e., late in the shift for day nurses, early in the shift for night nurses). The overall interrater reliability was .62. Internal consistency of the PINI was also assessed. The reliability coefficient, based on the Cronbach alpha method, was .85.

Four substudies were undertaken for the validity testing, using data on 6445 patients collected by 487 RNs. The nurses worked in various clinical units of five hospitals in several states. The first study involved a factor analysis, which revealed that the PINI measures three underlying constructs: severity of illness, dependency, and complexity. The second substudy involved the testing of six hypotheses that predicted the relationship of PINI scores to other existing measures, such as length of hospital stay and scores on the hospital patient classification. All the hypotheses were supported. The third substudy involved comparing PINI scores for two groups of patients with different requirements, based on diagnostic-related group ratings. The low and high nursing intensity groups had substantially different PINI scores, as expected. Finally, the fourth substudy involved comparing nurses' ratings of one item on the PINI—hours of care—with observer-recorded time data. Although nurses completing the PINI tended to overestimate time requirements, agreement between the nurses and the observers was reasonably high. The researchers concluded that "the psychometric evaluation of the PINI as a measure of nursing intensity has been very positive" (p. 219).

Assessment of Qualitative Data

Gagliardi (1991) conducted an in-depth inquiry to better understand the experience of families living with a child with Duchenne muscular dystrophy. Three families that had a young boy (aged 7 to 9 years) with Duchenne were included in the study. The researcher visited each family weekly over a 10-week period and engaged in participant observation, including involvement in play activities, trips to summer camps, watching television with family members, and participation in family conversations. Logs of the observations were maintained the same day. Periodically, the researcher wrote analytic memoranda that were used to examine the researcher's emotions, biases, and conflicts.

In-depth unstructured interviews with family members were also conducted; the interviews were taped and later transcribed. Interviews were conducted twice over the 10-week period, and then a third time 1 year later.

Gagliardi used several procedures to evaluate and document data quality. First, triangulation was used: data triangulation was achieved by interviewing multiple members of the family, and method triangulation

was achieved by collecting both observational and self-report data. Member checks were undertaken by having family members verify themes emerging in the data during the second and third interviews. The grouping of narrative materials into themes was also verified by having two external auditors and several colleagues independently categorize a sample of the data, resulting in a 90% rate of agreement. The researcher met with her colleagues every 3 weeks to explore areas of disagreement and to help further reduce bias.

❖ SUMMARY

Measurement involves a set of rules according to which numerical values are assigned to objects to represent varying degrees of some attribute. Measurement is advantageous to researchers because it offers objectivity, precision, and a tool for communication. However, researchers must strive to develop or use measurements whose rules are *isomorphic* with reality.

Few, if any, measuring instruments used by researchers are pure or infallible. *Obtained scores*—that is, the actual measurements obtained through the administration of the instruments—can be decomposed into a true score and an error component. The *true score* is a hypothetical entity that represents the value that would be obtained if it were possible to arrive at a perfect measure. The error component, or *error of measurement,* represents the inaccuracies present in the measurement process. Sources of measurement error include situational contaminants, response-set biases, transitory personal factors, and several others.

One important characteristic of a measuring tool is its *reliability,* which refers to the degree of consistency or accuracy with which an instrument measures an attribute. The higher the reliability of an instrument, the lower the amount of error present in the obtained scores. Several empirical methods assess various aspects of an instrument's reliability. The *stability* aspect, which concerns the extent to which the instrument yields the same results on repeated administrations, is evaluated by *test–retest* procedures. The *internal consistency* or *homogeneity* aspect of reliability refers to the extent to which all the instrument's subparts or items are measuring the same attribute. Internal consistency may be evaluated using either the *split-half reliability* technique or *Cronbach's alpha* method. When the focus of a reliability assessment is on establishing *equivalence* between observers in rating behaviors, estimates of *interrater* or *interobserver reliability* may be obtained. Most of the methods of estimating reliability rely on the calculation of a *reliability coefficient,* an index that reflects the proportion of true variability in a set of scores to the total obtained variability. Reliability coefficients generally range in value from a low of .00 to 1.00, with higher values reflecting increased reliability.

Validity refers to the degree to which an instrument measures what it is supposed to be measuring. *Face validity* refers to whether the instrument appears, on the face of it, to be measuring the appropriate construct. *Content validity* is concerned with the sampling adequacy of the content being measured. *Criterion-related validity* focuses on the relationship or correlation between the instrument and some outside criterion. *Construct validity* refers to the adequacy of an instrument in measuring the abstract construct of interest. One approach to assessing the construct validity of a measuring tool is the *known-groups technique,* which contrasts the scores of groups that are presumed to differ on the attribute. Another construct validity approach is the *multitrait–multimethod matrix* technique, which is based on the concepts of convergence and discriminability. *Convergence* refers to evidence that different methods of measuring the same attribute yield similar results. *Discriminability* refers to the ability to differentiate the construct being measured from other similar concepts. Another approach is to use a statistical procedure known as *factor analysis.*

Although high reliability and validity are essential criteria for assessing the quality of an instrument, other characteristics of the tool may also be important. Other criteria for evaluating a measuring tool include its efficiency, sensitivity, objectivity, comprehensibility, balance, speededness, unidimensionality, range, linearity, signal-to-noise ratio, frequency response, reactivity, and simplicity.

Data quality is equally important to qualitative and quantitative research. In both, the fundamental issue is whether one can have confidence that the data represent the true state of the phenomena under study. The criteria often used to assess the trustworthiness of qualitative data are *credibility, transferability, dependability*, and *confirmability.* Various procedures have been devised to establish data quality in qualitative studies, including independent *inquiry audits* by external auditors; *member checks,* wherein informants are asked to comment on the data and their interpretation; and procedures referred to as triangulation. *Triangulation* is the process of using multiple referents to draw conclusions about what constitutes the truth. The four major forms are *investigator triangulation, data triangulation, theoretical triangulation,* and *method triangulation.*

❖ *STUDY SUGGESTIONS*

Chapter 16 of the accompanying *Study Guide for Nursing Research: Principles and Methods, 5th ed.,* offers various exercises and study suggestions for reinforcing the concepts presented in this chapter. Additionally, the following study questions can be addressed:

1. Explain in your own words the meaning of the following correlation coefficients:
   a. The relationship between intelligence and grade point average was found to be .72.
   b. The correlation coefficient between age and gregariousness was − .20.
   c. It was revealed that patients' compliance with nursing instructions was re-

lated to their length of stay in the hospital ($r = -.50$).

2. Suppose the split-half reliability of an instrument to measure attitudes toward contraception was .70. Calculate the reliability of the full scale by using the Spearman-Brown formula.

3. If a researcher had a 20-item scale whose reliability was .60, about how many items would have to be added to achieve a reliability of .80?

4. An instructor has developed an instrument to measure knowledge of research terminology. Would you say that more reliable measurements would be yielded before or after a year of instruction on research methodology, using the exact same test, or would there be no difference? Why?

5. What types of groups do you feel might be useful for a known-groups approach to validating a measure of emotional maturity; attitudes toward alcoholics; territorial aggressiveness; job motivation; and subjective pain?

❖ SUGGESTED READINGS

METHODOLOGICAL REFERENCES

Armstrong, G. D. (1981). The intraclass correlation as a measure of interrater reliability of subjective judgments. *Nursing Research, 30,* 314–315.

Banik, B. J. (1993). Applying triangulation in nursing research. *Applied Nursing Research, 6,* 47–52.

Berk, R. A. (1990). Importance of expert judgment in content-related validity evidence. *Western Journal of Nursing Research, 12,* 659–670.

Brink, P. J. (1991). Issues of reliability and validity. In J. M. Morse (Ed.), *Qualitative nursing research: A contemporary dialogue.* Newbury Park, CA: Sage.

Campbell, D. T., & Fiske, D. W. (1959). Convergent and discriminant validation by the multitrait–multimethod matrix. *Psychological Bulletin, 56,* 81–105.

Cronbach, L. J. (1990). *Essentials of psychological testing* (5th ed.). New York: Harper & Row.

Davis, L.L., & Grant, J. S. (1993). Guidelines for using psychometric consultants in nursing studies. *Research in Nursing and Health, 16,* 151–155.

DeKeyser, F. G., & Pugh, L. C. (1990). Assessment of the reliability and validity of biochemical measures. *Nursing Research, 39,* 314–317.

Denzin, N. K. (1989). *The research act* (3rd ed.). New York: McGraw-Hill.

Ferketich, S. L., Figueredo, A., & Knapp, T. R. (1991). The multitrait-multimethod approach to construct validity. *Research in Nursing and Health, 14,* 315–319.

Garvin, B. J., Kennedy, C. W., & Cissna, K. N. (1988). Reliability in category coding systems. *Nursing Research, 37,* 52–55.

Goodwin, L. D., & Goodwin, W. L. (1991). Estimating construct validity. *Research in Nursing and Health, 14,* 235–243.

Guilford, J. P. (1964). *Psychometric methods* (2nd ed.). New York: McGraw-Hill.

Hoffart, N. (1991). A member check procedure to enhance rigor in naturalistic research. *Western Journal of Nursing Research, 13,* 522–534.

Hutchinson, S., & Wilson, H. S. (1992). Validity threats in scheduled semistructured research interviews. *Nursing Research, 41,* 117–119.

Kerlinger, F. N. (1986). *Foundations of behavioral research* (3rd ed.). New York: Holt, Rinehart & Winston.

Kirk, J., & Miller, M. L. (1985). *Reliability and validity in qualitative research.* Beverly Hills, CA: Sage.

Laschinger, H. K. S. (1992). Intraclass correlations as estimates of interrater reliability in nursing research. *Western Journal of Nursing Research, 14,* 246–251.

Lincoln, Y. S., & Guba, E. G. (1985). *Naturalistic inquiry.* Newbury Park, CA: Sage.

Lowe, N. K., & Ryan-Wenger, N. M. (1992). Beyond Campbell and Fiske: Assessment of convergent and discriminant validity. *Research in Nursing and Health, 15,* 67–75.

Lynn, M. R. (1986). Determination and quantification of content validity. *Nursing Research, 35,* 382–385.

Nunnally, J. (1978). *Psychometric theory.* New York: McGraw-Hill.

Rodgers, B. L., & Cowles, K. V. (1993). The qualitative research audit trail: A complex collection of documentation. *Research in Nursing and Health, 16,* 219–226.

Ryan, J. W., Phillips, C. Y., & Prescott, P. A. (1988). Interrater reliability: The underdeveloped role of rater training. *Applied Nursing Research, 1,* 148–150.

Slocumb, E. M., & Cole, F. L. (1991). A practical approach to content validation. *Applied Nursing Research, 4,* 192–195.

Thomas, S. D., Hathaway, D. K., & Arheart, K. L. (1992). Face validity. *Western Journal of Nursing Research, 14,* 109–112.

Thorndike, R. L., & Hagen, E. (1990). *Measurement and evaluation in psychology and education* (5th ed.). New York: John Wiley and Sons.

Tilden, V. P., Nelson, C. A., & May, B. A. (1990). Use of qualitative methods to enhance content validity. *Nursing Research, 39,* 172–175.

Waltz, C. F., Strickland, O. L., & Lenz, E. R. (1991). *Measurement in nursing research* (2nd ed.). Philadelphia: F. A. Davis.

Washington, C. C., & Moss, M. (1988). Pragmatic aspects of establishing interrater reliability in research. *Nursing Research, 37,* 190–191.

SUBSTANTIVE REFERENCES

Champion, V. L. (1993). Instrument refinement for breast cancer screening behaviors. *Nursing Research, 42,* 139–143.

Frank-Stromberg, M. (1989). Reaction to the diagnosis of cancer questionnaire: Development and psychometric evaluation. *Nursing Research, 38,* 364–369.

Gagliardi, B. A. (1991). The family's experience of living with a child with Duchenne muscular dystrophy. *Applied Nursing Research, 4,* 159–164.

Gardner, D. L. (1992). Conflict and retention of new graduate nurses. *Western Journal of Nursing Research, 14,* 76–85.

Gaston-Johansson, F., Franco, T., & Zimmerman, L. (1992). Pain and psychological distress in patients undergoing autologous bone marrow transplantation. *Oncology Nursing Forum, 19,* 41–48.

Gulick, E. E. (1991). Reliability and validity of the Work Assessment Scale for persons with multiple sclerosis. *Nursing Research, 40,* 107–112.

Hurley, A. C., Volicer, B. J., Hanrahan, P. A., Houde, S., & Volicer, L. (1992). Assessment of discomfort in advanced Alzheimer patients. *Research in Nursing and Health, 15,* 369–377.

Prescott, P. A., Ryan, J. W., Soeken, K. L., Castorr, A. H., Thompson, K. O., & Phillips, C. Y. (1991). The Patient Intensity for Nursing Index: A validity assessment. *Research in Nursing and Health, 14,* 213–221.

Younger, J. B. (1993). Development and testing of the Mastery of Stress instrument. *Nursing Research, 42,* 68–73.

Part V

THE ANALYSIS OF RESEARCH DATA

Chapter 17

QUANTITATIVE ANALYSIS: DESCRIPTIVE STATISTICS

Statistical analysis is a method for rendering quantitative information meaningful and intelligible. Without the aid of statistics, the quantitative data collected in a research project would be little more than a chaotic mass of numbers. Statistical procedures enable the researcher to reduce, summarize, organize, evaluate, interpret, and communicate numerical information.

Some students are intimidated by statistics, but it may be of some comfort to know that mathematic talent is not required to use or understand statistical analysis. To apply and interpret most statistics, only basic arithmetic skills and logical thinking ability are needed. This textbook does not emphasize the theoretical rationale or mathematic derivation of statistical operations. In fact, even computation is underplayed because this is not a statistics textbook and because statistics are seldom calculated by hand in this era of computers and calculators. Our emphasis is on how to use statistics appropriately in different research situations and how to understand what they mean once they have been applied.

Statistics usually are classified as either descriptive or inferential. *Descriptive statistics* are used to describe and synthesize data. Averages and percentages are examples of descriptive statistics. Actually, when such indexes are calculated on data from a population, they are referred to as *parameters*. A descriptive index from a sample is called a *statistic*. Most scientific questions are about parameters, but researchers usually calculate statistics to estimate those parameters. When researchers use statistics to make inferences or draw conclusions about a population, *inferential statistics* are required. This chapter discusses descriptive statistics, and Chapter 18 focuses on inferential statistics. First, however, we must discuss the concept of levels of measurement.

❖ LEVELS OF MEASUREMENT

Scientists have developed a system for categorizing different types of measures. This classification system is important because the analytic operations that can be performed on data depend on the measurement level used. Four major classes, or levels, of measurement have been identified: nominal, ordinal, interval, and ratio.

Nominal Measurement

The lowest level of measurement is referred to as *nominal measurement.* This level involves the assignment of numbers simply to classify characteristics into categories. Examples of variables amenable to nominal measurement include gender, blood type, religion, and nursing specialty.

The numerical codes assigned in nominal measurement are not intended to convey any quantitative information. If we establish a rule to classify males as 1 and females as 2, the numbers in and of themselves have no meaning. The number 2 here clearly does not mean "more than" 1. It would be perfectly acceptable to reverse the code and use 1 for females and 2 for males. The numbers are merely symbols that represent two different values of the gender attribute. Indeed, instead of numerical codes, we could as easily have chosen alphabetical symbols such as *M* and *F.* We recommend, however, thinking in terms of numerical codes if the subsequent analysis of data involves the use of a computer.

Nominal measurement provides no information about an attribute except that of equivalence and nonequivalence. If we were to measure the gender of Harvey, Cassie, Brigitte, and Brian, we would—according to our rule—assign them the codes, 1, 2, 2, and 1, respectively. Harvey and Brian are considered equivalent with respect to the target attribute but are not equivalent to the other two subjects.

The basic requirements for measuring attributes on the nominal scale are that the classifications must be mutually exclusive and collectively exhaustive. For example, if we were measuring ethnicity, we might establish the following scheme: 1 = whites, 2 = African Americans, 3 = Hispanics. Each subject must be classifiable into one and only one of these categories. The requirement for collective exhaustiveness would not be met if, for example, there were several individuals of Asian descent in the sample.

The numbers used in nominal measurement cannot be treated mathematically. Although it might make perfectly good sense to determine the average weight of a sample of subjects, it is nonsensical to calculate the average gender of a sample. However, the elements assigned to each category can be enumerated, and statements can be made concerning the frequency of occurrence in each class. In a sample of 50 patients, we might find 30 males and 20 females. We could also say that 60% of the subjects are male and 40% are female. However, no further mathematic operations would be meaningful with data from nominal measures.

It may strike some readers as odd to think of the categorization procedure we have been describing as measurement. If the definition of measurement is recalled, however, it can be seen that nominal measurement does, in fact, involve the assignment of numbers to attributes according to rules. The rules are not sophisticated, to be sure, but they are rules nonetheless.

Ordinal Measurement

The next level in the measurement hierarchy is ordinal measurement. *Ordinal measurement* permits the sorting of objects on the basis of their standing relative to each other on a specified attribute. This level of measurement goes beyond a mere categorization: the attributes are *ordered* according to some criterion. If a researcher were to rank-order subjects from the heaviest to the lightest, then we would say that an ordinal level of measurement had been used.

The fundamental difference between nominal and ordinal measurement is that, with ordinal measurement, information concerning not only equivalence but also relative standing or ordering among objects is indicated. When we assign numbers to a person's religious affiliation, the numbers have no inherent meaning or significance. Now, consider this scheme for measuring a client's ability to perform activities of daily living: (1) completely dependent, (2) needs another person's assistance, (3) needs mechanical assistance, (4) completely independent. In this case, the measurement is ordinal. The numbers are not arbitrary—they signify incremental ability to perform the activities of daily living. The individuals assigned a value of four are equivalent to each other with regard to their ability to function *and,* relative to those in all the other categories, have more of that attribute.

Ordinal measurement does not, however, tell us anything about how much greater one level of an attribute is than another level. We do not know if being completely independent is twice as good as needing mechanical assistance, nor do we know if the difference between needing another person's assistance and needing mechanical assistance is the same as that between needing mechanical assistance and being completely independent. Ordinal measurement only tells us the relative ranking of the levels of an attribute.

As in the case of nominal scales, the types of mathematical operations permissible with ordinal-level data are rather restricted. Averages are generally meaningless with rank-order measures. Frequency counts, percentages, and several other statistical procedures to be discussed in Chapter 18 are appropriate for analyzing ordinal-level data.

Interval Measurement

Interval measurement occurs when the researcher can specify both the rank-ordering of objects on an attribute and the distance between those objects. The distances between the numerical values on an interval scale represent equal distances in the attribute being measured. Most psychological and educational tests are based on interval scales. The Scholastic Aptitude Test (SAT) is an example of this level of measurement. A score of 550 on the SAT is higher than a score of 500, which in turn is higher than 450. Additionally, a difference between 550 and 500 on the test is presumably equivalent to the difference between 500 and 450.

Interval measures, then, are more informative than ordinal measures, but one piece of information that interval measures fail to provide is the absolute magnitude of the attribute. The Fahrenheit scale for measuring temperature illustrates this point. A temperature of 60°F is 10°F warmer than 50°F. A 10°F difference similarly separates 40°F and 30°F, and the two differences in temperature are equivalent. However, it cannot be said that 60°F is twice as hot as 30°F, or three times as hot as 20°F. The assignment of numbers to temperature on the Fahrenheit scale involves an arbitrary zero point. Zero on the thermometer does not signify a total absence of heat. In interval scales, there is no real or rational zero point.

The use of interval scales greatly expands the researcher's analytic possibilities. The intervals between numbers can be meaningfully added and subtracted: the interval between 10°F and 5°F is 5°F, or $10 - 5 = 5$. This same operation could not be performed with ordinal measures. Because of this capability, interval-level data can be averaged. It is perfectly reasonable, for example, to compute an average daily temperature for hospitalized patients from whom temperature readings are taken four times a day. Many widely used statistical procedures require that measurements be made on at least an interval scale.

Ratio Measurement

The highest level of measurement is the ratio scale. *Ratio scales* are distinguished from interval scales by virtue of having a rational, meaningful zero. Measures on a ratio scale provide information concerning the rank-ordering of objects on the critical attribute, the intervals between objects, and the absolute magnitude of the attribute for the object. Many physical measures provide ratio-level data. A person's weight, for example, is measured on a ratio scale because zero weight is an actual possibility. It is perfectly acceptable to say that someone who weighs 200 pounds is twice as heavy as someone who weighs 100 pounds.

Because ratio scales have an absolute zero, all arithmetic operations are permissible. One can meaningfully add, subtract, multiply, and divide numbers on a ratio scale. Consequently, all the statistical procedures suitable for interval-level data are also appropriate for ratio-level data. Ratio measurement constitutes the measurement ideal for scientists but is unattainable for most attributes of a psychological nature.

Comparison of the Levels

The four levels of measurement constitute a hierarchy, with ratio scales at the pinnacle and nominal measurement at the base. When one moves from a higher to a lower level of measurement, there is always an information loss. Let us demonstrate this using an example relating to data on the weight of a sample of individuals. Table 17-1 presents fictitious data for 10 subjects. The second column shows the ratio-level data, that is, their actual weight in pounds. The ratio measure gives us complete information concerning the absolute weight of each subject and the differences in weights between all pairs of subjects.

In the third column, the original data have been converted to interval measures by assigning a score of 0 to the lightest individual (Katy), the score of 5 to the person 5 pounds heavier than the lightest person (Lindsay), and so forth. Note that the resulting scores are still amenable to addition and subtraction; the differences in pounds are equally far apart, even though they are at different parts of the scale. The data no longer tell us, however, anything about the absolute weights of the people in this sample. Katy, the lightest individual, might be a 10-pound infant or a 200-pound Weight Watcher.

In the fourth column of Table 17-1, ordinal measurements were assigned by rank-ordering the sample from the lightest, who was assigned the score of 1, to the heaviest, who was assigned the score of 10. Now even more information is missing. The data provide no indication of how much heavier Nathan is than Katy. The difference separating them might be as little as 5 pounds or as much as 150 pounds.

Finally, the fifth column presents nominal measurements in which all subjects were classified as either heavy or light. The criterion applied in categorizing individuals was arbitrarily set as a weight either greater than 150 pounds (2), or less than or equal to 150 pounds (1). The available information is very limited. Within any one category, there are no clues as to who is heavier than whom. With this level of measurement Nathan, Alex, and Kevin are considered equivalent. They are equivalent with regard to

Table 17-1.   *Fictitious Data for Four Levels of Measurement*

SUBJECTS	RATIO-LEVEL	INTERVAL-LEVEL	ORDINAL-LEVEL	NOMINAL
Nathan	180	70	10	2
Katy	110	0	1	1
Alex	165	55	8	2
Lauren	130	20	5	1
Kevin	175	65	9	2
Lindsay	115	5	2	1
Rosanna	125	15	4	1
Chad	150	40	7	1
Tom	145	35	6	1
Megan	120	10	3	1

the attribute heavy/light as defined by the classification criterion.

This example illustrates that at every successive level in the measurement hierarchy, there is a loss of information. It also illustrates another point: When one has information at one level, one can always manipulate the data to arrive at a lower level, but the converse is not true. If we were only given the nominal measurements, it would be impossible to reconstruct the actual weights.

It is not always a straightforward task to identify the level of measurement for a particular instrument. Usually, nominal measures and ratio scales are discernible with little difficulty, but the distinction between ordinal and interval measures is more problematic. Some methodologists argue that most psychological measures that are treated as interval measures are really only ordinal measures. Most writers seem to believe that, although such instruments as Likert scales produce data that are, strictly speaking, ordinal level, the distortion introduced by treating them as interval measures is too small to warrant an abandonment of powerful statistical analyses. Table 17-2 presents examples of con-

Table 17-2.   *Examples of Variables Measured at Different Levels of Measurement*

RESEARCH QUESTION	CONCEPT/MEASURE	LEVEL OF MEASUREMENT	INDEPENDENT (IV) OR DEPENDENT (DV) VARIABLE
What is the effect of a slow stroke effleurage back rub on older adult's anxiety salivary secretory immunoglobulin A (s-IgA) and anxiety? (Groër, Mozingo, Droppleman, Davis, Jolly, Boynton, Davis & Kay, 1994)	Treatment group (experimental vs. control)	Nominal	IV
	Scores on STAI anxiety scale	Interval	DV
	S-IgA concentrations	Ratio	DV
What are the cognitive abilities of Alzheimer's disease patients according to Piaget's stages of child development? (Thornbury, 1992)	Alzheimer status (has the disease or not)	Nominal	IV
	Piagetian stage (sensorimotor, preoperational, concrete operational, formal operational)	Ordinal	DV
	Scores on the Mini-Mental Status Exam	Interval	DV
What factors are related to body satisfaction in edentulous complete-denture-wearing clients? (Rudy, Guckes, Li, McCarthy, & Brahim, 1993)	Chronic illness status (present vs. absent)	Nominal	IV
	Education (high school, college graduate school)	Ordinal	IV
	Body image (Body Cathexis Scale scores)	Interval	DV
What is the effect of crystalloid vs. colloid replacement therapy on cardiac patients? (Ley, Miller, Skov, & Preisig, 1990)	Type of solution for intravenous replacement fluid (crystalloid vs. colloid)	Nominal	IV
	Pulmonary edema (5-point rating scale)	Ordinal	DV
	Blood pressure	Ratio	DV

cepts that nurse researchers have operational-ized at different levels of measurement.

❖ *FREQUENCY DISTRIBUTIONS*

Raw quantitative data that are neither analyzed nor organized are overwhelming. It is not even possible to discern general trends until some order or structure is imposed on the data. Consider the 60 numbers presented in Table 17-3. Let us assume that these numbers represent the scores of 60 nursing students on a 30-item test to measure knowledge about AIDS. Visual inspection of the numbers in this table is not too helpful in understanding how the nurses performed. The data are too numerous to make much sense of them in this form.

A set of data can be completely described in terms of three characteristics: the shape of the distribution of values, central tendency, and variability. Central tendency and variability are dealt with in subsequent sections.

Constructing Frequency Distributions

Frequency distributions represent a method of imposing some order on a mass of numerical data. A *frequency distribution* is a systematic arrangement of numerical values from the lowest to the highest, together with a count of the number of times each value was obtained. The fictitious test scores of the 60 nurses are presented as a frequency distribution in Table 17-4. This organized arrangement makes it convenient to see at a glance how the

students performed. We can see what the highest and lowest scores were, where the bulk of scores tended to cluster, and what the most common score was. None of this was easily discernible before the data were organized.

The construction of a frequency distribution is simple. It consists basically of two parts: the observed values or measurements (the Xs) and the frequency or count of the observations falling in each class (the *f*s). The values are listed in numerical order in one column, and the corresponding frequencies are listed in another. Table 17-4 shows the intermediary step in which the observations were actually tallied by the familiar method of four vertical bars and then a slash for the fifth observation. The only requirement for a frequency distribution is that the classes of observation must be mutually exclusive and collectively exhaustive. The sum of the numbers appearing in the frequency column must be equal to the size of the sample. In less verbal terms, $\Sigma f = n$, which translates as the sum of (signified by the Greek letter sigma, Σ) the frequencies (f) equals the sample size (n).

It is often useful to display not only the frequency counts for different values but also the percentages of the total, as shown in the fourth column of Table 17-4. The percentages are calculated by the simple formula: $\% = (f \div n) \times 100$. Just as the sum of all frequencies should equal n, the sum of all percentages should equal 100.

Rather than listing frequencies in tabular form, some researchers display their data graphically. Graphs have the advantage of being able to communicate a lot of information almost instantaneously. The most widely used types of

Table 17-3.   *AIDS Knowledge Test Scores*

22	27	25	19	24	25	23	29	24	20
26	16	20	26	17	22	24	18	26	28
15	24	23	22	21	24	20	25	18	27
24	23	16	25	30	29	27	21	23	24
26	18	30	21	17	25	22	24	29	28
20	25	26	24	23	19	27	28	25	26

Table 17-4. *Frequency Distribution of Test Scores*

Score (X)	TALLIES	FREQUENCY (f)	PERCENTAGE (%)
15	|	1	1.7
16	| |	2	3.3
17	| |	2	3.3
18	| | |	3	5.0
19	| |	2	3.3
20	| | | |	4	6.7
21	| | |	3	5.0
22	| | | |	4	6.7
23	⊬⊦⊦	5	8.3
24	⊬⊦⊦ | | | |	9	15.0
25	⊬⊦⊦ | |	7	11.7
26	⊬⊦⊦ |	6	10.0
27	| | | |	4	6.7
28	| | |	3	5.0
29	| | |	3	5.0
30	| |	2	3.3
		$n = 60 = \Sigma f$	$\Sigma\% = 100\%$

graphs for displaying interval- and ratio-level data are *histograms* and *frequency polygons*. These two types are actually similar forms of presenting the same data.

Both histograms and frequency polygons are constructed in much the same fashion. First, score classes are placed on a horizontal dimension, with the lowest value on the left, ascending to the highest value on the right. Next, the vertical dimension is used to designate the frequency count or, alternatively, percentages. The numbering of the vertical axis usually begins with zero. Using these dimensions as a base, a histogram is constructed by drawing bars above the score classes to the height corresponding to the frequency for that score class. An example is presented in Figure 17-1, using the same fictitious data on nursing students' AIDS knowledge test scores.

Instead of vertical bars, the frequency polygon uses dots connected by straight lines to show frequencies for score classes. A dot corresponding to the frequency is placed above each score, as shown in Figure 17-2. It is conventional to connect the figure to the base (zero line) at the score below the minimum value ob-

tained and above the maximum value obtained. In this particular example, however, the graph is terminated at 30 and brought down to the base at that point with a dotted line because a score of 31 was not possible.

Shapes of Distributions

A distribution of numerical values such as those displayed in a frequency polygon can assume an almost infinite number of shapes or forms. However, there are general aspects of the shape that can be described verbally. A distribution is said to be *symmetric* in shape if, when folded over, the two halves of the distribution would be superimposed on one another. In other words, symmetric distributions consist of two halves that are mirror images of one another. All the distributions shown in Figure 17-3 are symmetric. With real data sets, the distributions are rarely as perfectly symmetric as shown in this figure. However, minor discrepancies are often ignored in trying to characterize the shape of a distribution.

Asymmetric distributions usually are described as being *skewed*. In skewed distribu-

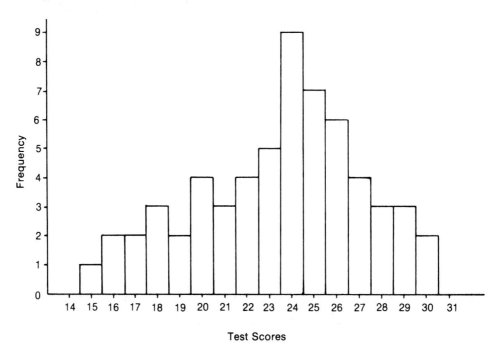

Figure 17-1.   *Histogram of test scores*

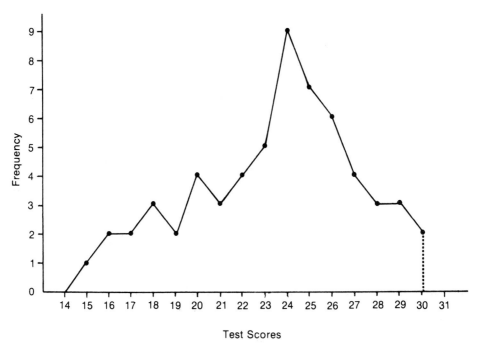

Figure 17-2.   *Frequency polygon of test scores*

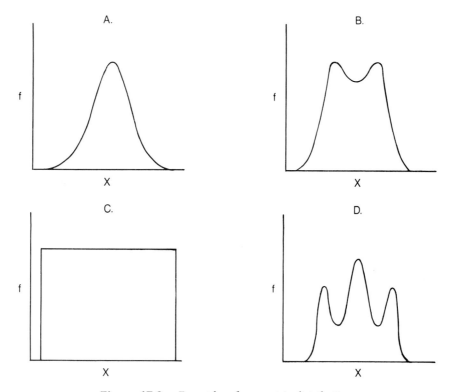

Figure 17-3. *Examples of symmetric distributions*

tions, the peak is off center, and one tail is longer than the other. Distributions that are skewed are usually described in terms of the direction of the skew. When the longer tail is pointing toward the right, the distribution is said to be *positively skewed*. Figure 17-4(*A*) depicts a positively skewed distribution. If, on the other hand, the tail points to the left, the skew is described as negative. A *negatively skewed* distribution is illustrated in Figure 17-4(*B*). An example of an actual attribute that is positively skewed is personal income. The bulk of people have low to moderate incomes, with relatively few people in high-income brackets in the right-hand tail of the distribution. An example of a negatively skewed attribute is age at death. Here, the bulk of people are at the upper end of the distribution, with relatively few people dying at an early age.

A second aspect of a distribution's shape is its modality. A *unimodal* distribution is one that has only one peak or high point (i.e., a value with high frequency), whereas a *multimodal* distribution has two or more peaks (i.e., two or more values of high frequency). The most common type of multimodal distribution is one with two peaks, which is called *bimodal*. Figure 17-3(*A*) is unimodal, as are both graphs in Figure 17-4. Multimodal distributions are illustrated in Figure 17-3(*B*) and (*D*). Symmetry and modality are completely independent aspects of a distribution. Knowledge of skewness does not tell you anything about how many peaks the distribution has.

Some distributions are encountered so frequently that special labels are used to designate them. Of particular interest in statistical analysis is the distribution known as the *normal distri-*

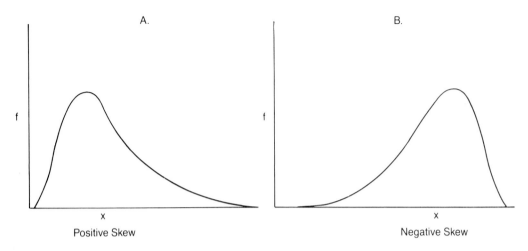

Figure 17-4. *Examples of skewed distributions*

bution (sometimes called a *bell-shaped curve*). A normal distribution is one that is symmetric, unimodal, and not too peaked, as illustrated by the distribution in Figure 17-3(*A*). Many physical and psychological attributes of humans have been found to approximate a normal distribution. Examples include height, intelligence, age at menarche, and grip strength. As we will see in Chapter 18, the normal distribution plays a central role in inferential statistics.

❖ CENTRAL TENDENCY

Frequency distributions are an important means of imposing order on a set of raw data and of clarifying group patterns. For many purposes, however, a group pattern is of less interest to a researcher than an overall summary of a group's characteristics. The researcher usually asks such questions as, "What is the average oxygen consumption of myocardial infarction patients during bathing?" "What is the average blood pressure reading of hypertensive patients during relaxation therapy?" "How much information does the average pregnant teenager have about nutrition?" Such questions seek a single number that best represents a whole distribution of data values. Because an index of typicalness is more

likely to be representative if it comes from the center of a distribution than if it comes from either extreme, such indexes are referred to as measures of *central tendency*. To lay people, the term average is normally used to designate central tendency. Researchers seldom use this term because it is ambiguous, inasmuch as there are three commonly used kinds of averages, or indexes of central tendency: the mode, the median, and the mean. Each can be used as an index to represent a whole set of measurements.

The Mode

The *mode* is that numerical value in a distribution that occurs most frequently. The mode is the simplest to determine of the three measures of central tendency. Actually, the mode is not computed but rather is determined through inspection of a frequency distribution. In the following distribution of numbers, one can readily determine that the mode is 53:

50 51 51 52 53 53 53 53 54 55 56

The score of 53 was obtained four times, a higher frequency than for any other number. In the example presented earlier, the mode of the AIDS knowledge test scores is 24 (see Table 17-4). In multimodal distributions, of course, there is more than one score value that has high frequencies. The mode is seldom used in research reports as the only index of central tendency. Modes are a quick and easy method of determining the most popular score at a glance but are unsuitable for further computation and also are rather unstable. By unstable, we mean that modes tend to fluctuate widely from one sample drawn from a population to another sample drawn from the same population. The mode is infrequently used, except for describing typical values on nominal-level measures. For instance, researchers often characterize their samples by providing modal information on nominal-level demographic variables, as in the following example: "The typical (modal) subject was an unmarried white female, living in an urban area, with no prior history of sexually transmitted diseases."

The Median

The *median* is that point on a numerical scale above which and below which 50% of the cases fall. As an example, consider the following set of values:

2 2 3 3 4 5 6 7 8 9

The value that divides the cases exactly in half is 4.5, which is the median for this set of numbers. The point that has 50% of the cases above and below it is halfway between 4 and 5. An important characteristic of the median is that it does not take into account the quantitative values of individual scores. The median is an index of average *position* in a distribution of numbers. The median is insensitive to extreme values. Let us take the previous example to illustrate this point, making only one small change:

2 2 3 3 4 5 6 7 8 99

Despite the fact that the last value has been increased from 9 to 99, the median remains unchanged at 4.5. Because of this property, the median is often the preferred index of central tendency when the distribution is skewed and when one is interested in finding a typical value for variables measured on an ordinal scale or higher.

The Mean

The *mean* is the point on the score scale that is equal to the sum of the scores divided by the total number of scores. The mean is the index of central tendency that is usually referred to as an average. The computational formula for a mean—which everyone knows, but whose symbols need to be learned—is

$$\overline{X} = \frac{\Sigma X}{n}$$

where $\overline{X}$ = the mean
Σ = the sum of
X = each individual raw score
n = the number of cases

The researcher should become familiar with these symbols because they are used in the research literature.

Let us apply the above formula to calculate the mean weight of eight subjects whose individual weights are as follows:

85 109 120 135 158 177 181 195

$$\overline{X} = \frac{85 + 109 + 120 + 135 + 158 + 177 + 181 + 195}{8} = 145$$

Unlike the median, the mean is affected by the value of each and every score. If we were to exchange the 195-pound subject in this example for a subject weighing 275 pounds, the mean would increase from 145 to 155. A substitution of this kind would leave the median unchanged.

The mean is unquestionably the most widely used measure of central tendency. Many of the important tests of statistical significance, described in Chapter 18, are based on the mean. When researchers work with interval-level or ratio-level measurements, the mean, rather than the median or mode, is almost always the statistic reported.

Comparison of the Mode, Median, and Mean

Of the three indexes of central tendency, the mean is the most stable. If repeated samples were drawn from a given population, the means would vary or fluctuate less than the modes or medians. Because of its stability, the mean is the most reliable estimate of the central tendency of the population.

The arithmetic mean is the most appropriate index in situations in which the concern is for totals or combined performance of a group. If a school of nursing were comparing two graduating classes in terms of scores on a National League for Nursing Achievement Test, then the calculation of two means would be in order. Sometimes, however, the primary concern is learning what a typical value is, in which case a median might be preferred. In efforts to understand the economic well-being of United States citizens, for example, we would get a distorted impression of the financial status of the typical individual by considering the mean. The mean in this case would be inflated by the wealth of a small minority. The median, on the other hand, would reflect more realistically how the average person fared financially.

When a distribution of scores is symmetric and unimodal, the three indexes of central tendency coincide. In skewed distributions, the values of the mode, median, and mean differ. The mean is always pulled in the direction of the long tail, as shown in Figure 17-5.

The level of measurement plays a role in determining the appropriate index of central tendency that can be used to describe a variable. In general, the mode is appropriate for nominal measures, the median is appropriate for ordinal measures, and the mean is appropriate for interval and ratio measures. However, the higher the level of measurement, the greater the flexibility one has in choosing a descriptive statistic. Variables measured on an interval or ratio scale can use any of the three indexes of central tendency, although it is usually preferable to use the mean.

❖ VARIABILITY

Measures of central tendency do not give a total picture of a distribution. Two sets of data with identical means could be different from one another in several respects. For one thing, two distributions with the same mean could be very

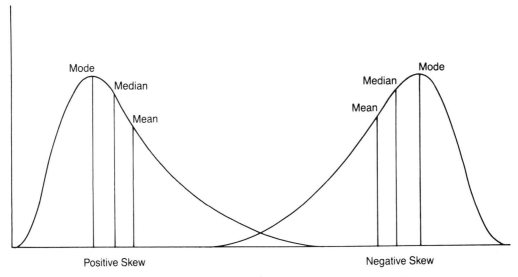

Figure 17-5. *Relationships of central tendency indexes in skewed distributions*

different in shape: they could be skewed in opposite directions, for example. The characteristic of concern in this section is how spread out or dispersed the data are. The *variability* of two distributions can be different, even when the means are identical.

Consider the two distributions in Figure 17-6, which represent the hypothetical scores of freshman students from two schools of nursing on the SAT. Both distributions have an average of 500, but the patterns of scores are clearly different. In school A, there is a wide range of scores: from scores below 300 to some above 700. This school has many students who performed among the best, but also has many students who were well below average. In school B, on the other hand, there are few students at either extreme. School A is said to be more *heterogeneous* than school B, and school B is said to be more *homogeneous* than school A.

To describe a distribution adequately, there is a need for a measure of variability that expresses the extent to which scores deviate from one another. Several such indexes have been developed, the most common of which are the range, semiquartile range, and standard deviation.

The Range

The *range* is simply the highest score minus the lowest score in a given distribution. In the examples shown in Figure 17-6, the range for school A is about 500 (750 − 250), and the range for school B is about 300 (650 − 350). The range indicates the distance on the score scale between the lowest and highest values.

The chief virtue of the range is the ease with which it can be computed. As an index of variability, the shortcomings of the range outweigh this modest advantage. The range, being based on only two scores, is a highly unstable index. From sample to sample drawn from the same population, the range tends to fluctuate considerably. Another difficulty with the range is that it ignores completely variations in scores between the two extremes. In school B of Figure 17-6, suppose that only one student obtained a score of 250 and one other student obtained a score of 750. The range of both schools would then be 500, despite obvious differences in the heterogeneity of scores. For these reasons, the range is used largely as a gross descriptive index and is typically reported in conjunction with, not instead of, other measures of variability.

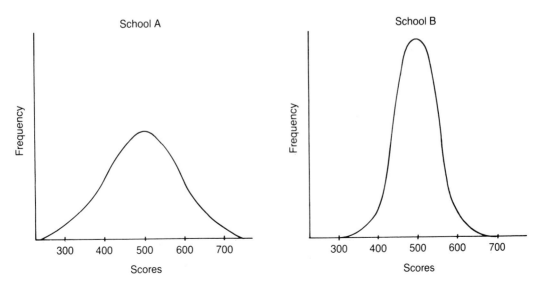

Figure 17-6. *Two distributions of different variability*

Semiquartile Range*

A previous section described the median as the point below which 50% of the cases fall. It is computationally possible to determine the point below which any percentage of the scores fall. For example, an admissions committee for a school of nursing might establish a minimum standard at the 40th percentile on the SAT for its entrants. The *semiquartile range* is calculated on the basis of quartiles within a distribution. The upper quartile (Q3) is the point below which 75% of the cases fall, and the lower quartile (Q1) is the point below which 25% of the scores lie.† The semiquartile range (SQR) is half the distance between Q1 and Q3, or

$$SQR = \frac{Q_3 - Q_1}{2}$$

The semiquartile range indicates half the range of scores within which the middle 50% of scores lie. Because this index is a measure based on middle cases rather than extreme scores, it is considerably more stable than the range. In the case of the two nursing schools in Figure 17-6, school A would have an semiquartile range in the vicinity of 125, and the semiquartile range of school B would be about 75. The addition of one deviant case at either extreme for school B would leave the semiquartile range virtually untouched.

Standard Deviation

With interval or ratio-level data, the most widely used measure of variability is the standard deviation. Like the mean, the standard deviation considers every score in a distribution. The standard deviation summarizes the average amount of deviation of values from the mean.

What is needed in a variability index is some way of capturing the degree to which scores deviate from one another. This concept of deviation is represented in both the range and the semiquartile range by the presence of a minus sign, which produces an index of deviation, or difference, between two score points. The standard deviation is similarly based on score differences. In fact, the first step in calculating a standard deviation is to compute deviation scores for each subject. A *deviation score* (usually symbolized with a small *x*) is the difference between an individual score and the mean. If a person weighed 150 pounds and the sample mean were 140, then the person's deviation score would be +10. Symbolically, the formula for a deviation score is

$$x = X - \overline{X}$$

Because what one is essentially looking for is an average deviation, one might think that a good variability index could be arrived at by summing the deviation scores and then dividing by the number of cases. This gets us close to a good solution, but the difficulty is that the sum of a set of deviation scores is always zero. Table 17-5 presents an example of deviation scores computed for nine numbers. As shown in the second column, the sum of the *x*s is equal to zero. The deviations above the mean always balance exactly those deviations below the mean.

The standard deviation overcomes this problem by squaring each deviation score before summing. After dividing by the number of cases, one takes the square root to bring the index back to the original unit of measurement. The formula for the standard deviation (SD)‡ is

‡ Some statistical texts indicate that the formula for an unbiased estimate of the population SD is

$$SD = \sqrt{\frac{\Sigma x^2}{n - 1}}$$

Knapp (1970) clarifies when n or $n - 1$ should be used in the denominator. He indicates that n is appropriate when the researcher is interested in *describing* variation in sample data.

* Some statistical texts use the term *semiquartile range*, while others refer to this statistic as the *semi-interquartile range* or the *quartile deviation*.

† The computational formulas for percentiles are not presented here. Most standard statistics texts contain this information.

$$SD = \sqrt{\frac{\Sigma x^2}{n}}$$

A standard deviation has been completely worked out in the example in Table 17-5. First, a deviation score is calculated for each of the nine raw scores by subtracting the mean ($\overline{X} = 7$) from them. The third column shows that each deviation score is squared, thereby converting all values to positive numbers. The squared deviation scores are summed ($\Sigma x^2 = 28$), divided by 9 (n), and a square root taken to yield an SD of 1.76.

Most researchers routinely report the standard deviation of a variable along with the mean. Sometimes, however, one will find a reference to an index of variability known as the variance. The *variance* is simply the value of the standard deviation before a square root has been taken. In other words,

$$Variance = \frac{\Sigma x^2}{n} = SD^2$$

In the above example, the variance is $(1.76)^2$, or 3.11. The variance is less widely reported because it is an index that is not in the same unit of measurement as the original data.

Table 17-5. *Computation of a Standard Deviation*

X	$x = X - \overline{X}$	$x^2 = (X - \overline{X})^2$
4	−3	9
5	−2	4
6	−1	1
7	0	0
7	0	0
7	0	0
8	1	1
9	2	4
10	3	9
$\Sigma X = 63$	$\Sigma x = 0$	$\Sigma x^2 = 28$

$\Sigma X / n = \overline{X}$
$= 63/9 = 7$

$$SD = \sqrt{\frac{28}{9}} = \sqrt{3.11} = 1.76$$

The variance, however, is an important component in many inferential statistical tests that will be encountered later.

A standard deviation is typically more difficult for students to interpret than other statistics such as the mean or range. In our previous example, we calculated an SD of 1.76. One might well ask, 1.76 *what?* What does the number mean? We will try to answer these questions from several vantage points. First, as we already know, the standard deviation is an index of the variability of scores in a data set. If two distributions had a mean of 25.0, but one had an SD of 7.0 and the other had an SD of 3.0, then we would immediately know that the second sample was more homogeneous.

A convenient way to conceptualize the standard deviation is to think of it as an average of the deviations from the mean. The mean tells us the single best point for summarizing an entire distribution, whereas a standard deviation tells us how much, on the average, the scores deviate from that mean. A standard deviation might thus be interpreted as an indication of our degree of error when we use a mean to characterize the entire sample.

The standard deviation can also be used in interpreting individual scores from within a distribution. Suppose we had a set of weight measures from a sample whose mean weight was 125 and whose SD was 10. We can think of the standard deviation as actually providing a standard of variability. Weights greater than 1 SD away from the mean (i.e., greater than 135 or less than 115) are greater than the average variability for that distribution. Weights less than 1 SD from the mean, by consequence, are less than the average variability for that sample.

When the distribution of scores is normal, it is possible to say even more about the standard deviation. A normal curve, it will be recalled, is a symmetric, unimodal distribution. There are about 3 SDs above and 3 SDs below the mean with normally distributed data. To illustrate some further characteristics, suppose that we had a normal distribution of scores whose mean was 50 and whose SD was 10, as shown in Figure 17-7. In a normal distribution such as this, a fixed percentage of cases falls within certain distances from the mean. Sixty-eight percent of all cases fall within 1 SD of the mean (34% above and 34% below the mean). In this example, nearly 7 of every 10 scores fall between 40 and 60. Ninety-five percent of the scores in a normal distribution fall within 2 SDs from the mean. Only a handful of cases—about 2% at each extreme—lie more than 2 SDs from the mean. Using this figure, we can see that a person who obtained a score of 70 got a higher score than about 98% of the sample.

In summary, the standard deviation is a useful index of variability that can be used to describe an important characteristic of a distribution and that also can be used to interpret the score or performance of an individual in relation to others in the sample. Like the mean, the standard deviation is a stable estimate of a population parameter and also is used extensively in more advanced statistical procedures. The standard deviation is the preferred measure of a distribution's variability but is appropriate only for variables measured on the interval or ratio scale.

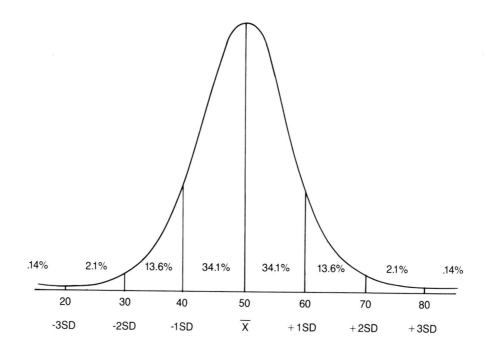

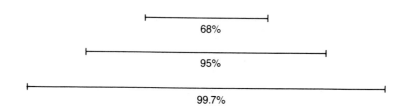

Figure 17-7.   *Standard deviations in a normal distribution*

❖ BIVARIATE DESCRIPTIVE STATISTICS: CONTINGENCY TABLES AND CORRELATION

The discussion has so far focused on a description of single variables. The mean, mode, standard deviation, and so forth are all used in describing data for one variable at a time. We have been examining what is referred to as *univariate* (one-variable) *statistics*. As indicated throughout this text, research usually is concerned with relationships between variables. What is needed then is some method of describing such relationships. In this section, we look at *bivariate* (two-variable) *descriptive statistics*.

Contingency Tables

A *contingency table* is essentially a two-dimensional frequency distribution in which the frequencies of two variables are cross-tabulated. Suppose we had data on subjects' gender and responses to a question on whether they were nonsmokers, light smokers (less than one pack per day), or heavy smokers (one pack per day or more). We might be interested in learning if there is a tendency for members of one gender to smoke more heavily than members of the other gender. Some fictitious data on these two variables are presented in Table 17-6. It is difficult to make sense of these data in their present form. To describe the data, we need a method of organizing this mass of numbers. The best way to do so in a manner that highlights the research question is to construct a contingency table.

A contingency table for the data in Table 17-6 is presented in Table 17-7. Six cells are created by placing one variable (gender) along the horizontal dimension and the other variable (smoking status) along the vertical dimension at the left-hand side. The system of bars and cross-hatches can then be used to tabulate the number of subjects belonging in each cell. The first subject, who has a code of 1 for gender and 1 for smoking status, would be marked in the upper left-hand cell, and so on. After all subjects have

Table 17-6. *Fictitious Data for Gender–Smoking Relationship*

SUBJECT NUMBER	SUBJECT GENDER[*]	SMOKING STATUS[†]
01	1	1
02	2	3
03	2	1
04	1	2
05	1	1
06	2	2
07	2	1
08	2	3
09	1	1
10	2	3
11	1	2
12	1	3
13	1	1
14	2	3
15	2	1
16	2	2
17	2	3
18	1	1
19	2	2
20	1	2
21	1	1
22	1	3
23	1	2
24	2	2
25	2	1
26	1	3
27	2	3
28	1	1
29	1	3
30	1	2
31	2	1
32	1	1
33	2	2
34	1	2
35	1	1
36	2	2
37	2	3
38	2	3
39	2	2
40	1	2
41	1	1
42	2	1
43	1	2
44	2	2

[*]Gender: 1, female; 2, male.

[†]Smoking status: 1, nonsmoker; 2, light smoker; 3, heavy smoker.

Table 17-7.   *Contingency Table for Gender–Smoking Relationship Data*

SMOKING STATUS	GENDER					
	Female		Male		Total	
	N	%	N	%	N	%
Nonsmoker	⊔⊤⊤ ⊔⊤⊤ 10	45%	⊔⊤⊤ ∣ 6	27%	16	36%
Light smoker	⊔⊤⊤ ∣∣∣ 8	36%	⊔⊤⊤ ∣∣∣ 8	35%	16	36%
Heavy smoker	∣∣∣∣ 4	18%	⊔⊤⊤ ∣∣∣ 8	36%	12	27%
Total	22	50%	22	50%	44	100%

been assigned to the appropriate cells, the frequencies can be tabulated and percentages computed. This simple procedure allows us to see at a glance that, in this particular sample, women were more likely to be nonsmokers and less likely to be heavy smokers than men. Contingency tables, or *cross-tabulations* as they are sometimes called, are easy to construct and have the ability to communicate a lot of information. The use of contingency tables usually is restricted to nominal data or to ordinal data that have few values or ranks. In the gender–smoker relationship example, gender is a nominal measure, and smoking status is an ordinal measure. We will encounter contingency tables again in the discussion on inferential statistics in Chapter 18.

Correlation

The most common method of describing the relationship between two measures is through correlation procedures. The computation of a correlation coefficient is normally performed when two variables are measured on either the ordinal, interval, or ratio scale. Correlation coefficients were briefly described in Chapter 16, and this section extends that discussion.

The correlation question asks, To what extent are two variables related to each other? For example: "To what extent are height and weight related?" "To what degree are anxiety test scores and blood pressure measures related?" These

questions can be answered graphically or, more commonly, by the calculation of an index that describes the magnitude of the relationship.

The graphic representation of a correlation between two variables is called a *scatter plot* or *scatter diagram*. To construct a scatter plot, one first sets up a scale for the two variables constructed at right angles, making a rectangular coordinate graph. The range of values for one variable (X) is scaled off along the horizontal axis, while the same is done for the second variable (Y) along the vertical axis. One example is presented in Figure 17-8. To locate the position for subject A, one goes two units to the right along the X axis, and one unit up on the Y axis. The same procedure is followed for all subjects, resulting in the scatter plot shown. The letters shown on the plot in this figure have been included to help identify each point. Normally only the dots appear on the diagram.

From a scatter plot, it is possible to determine both the direction and approximate magnitude of a correlation. The direction of the slope of points indicates the direction of the correlation. It may be recalled from Chapter 16 that correlations can be either positive or negative in direction. A positive correlation is obtained when high values on one variable are associated with high values on the second variable. If the slope of points begins at the lower-left corner and extends to the upper-right corner, then the relationship is positive. In the current example, we would say that X and Y are positively re-

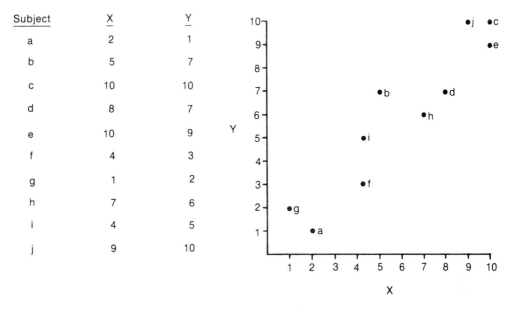

Subject	X	Y
a	2	1
b	5	7
c	10	10
d	8	7
e	10	9
f	4	3
g	1	2
h	7	6
i	4	5
j	9	10

Figure 17-8.   *Construction of a scatter plot*

lated. Inspection of the values shows that, indeed, people who have a high score on variable *X* also tend to have a high score on variable *Y*, and low scorers on *X* tend to score low on *Y*.

A negative (or inverse) relationship is one in which high values on one variable are related to low values on the other. On a scatter plot, negative relationships are depicted by points that slope from the upper-left corner to the lower-right corner. A negative correlation is shown in Figure 17-9(*A*) and (*D*).

Relationships are described as perfect when it is possible to perfectly predict the value of one variable by knowing the value of the second. For instance, if all people who were 6 feet 2 inches tall weighed 180 pounds, and all people who were 6 feet 1 inch tall weighed 175 pounds, and so on, then we could say that weight and height were perfectly, positively related. In such a situation, one would only need to be informed of a person's height to know his or her weight, or vice versa. On a scatter plot, a perfect relationship is represented by a sloped straight line, as shown in Figure 17-9(*C*). When a relationship is not perfect, as is usually the case, one can interpret the degree of correlation from a scatter plot by seeing how closely the

points cluster around a straight line. The more closely packed the points are around a diagonal slope, the higher the correlation. When the points are scattered all over the graph, the relationship is very low or nonexistent. Various degrees and directions of relationships are presented in Figure 17-9.

Usually it is more convenient and more succinct to express the direction and magnitude of a linear relationship by computing a correlation coefficient. As noted in Chapter 16, the correlation coefficient is an index whose values range from −1.0 for a perfect negative correlation, through zero for no relationship, to +1.0 for a perfect positive correlation. All correlations that fall between 0.0 and −1.0 are negative, and all correlations that fall between 0.0 and +1.0 are positive. The higher the absolute value of the coefficient (i.e., the value disregarding the sign), the stronger is the relationship. A correlation of −.80, for instance, is stronger than a correlation of +.20.

The most commonly used correlation index is the *product–moment correlation coefficient*, also referred to as *Pearson's r.* This coefficient is computed when the variables being correlated have been measured on either an

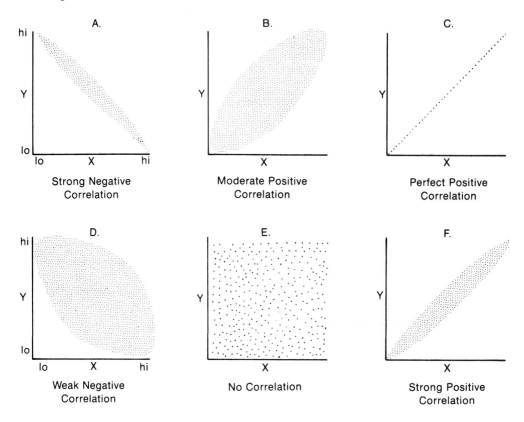

Figure 17-9. *Various relationships graphed on scatter plots*

interval or ratio scale. (The correlation index generally used for ordinal-level measures is *Spearman's rho*, discussed in Chapter 18). The calculation of the *r* statistic is rather laborious and seldom performed by hand.*

Perfect correlations (+1.00 and −1.00) are extremely rare in research with humans. It is dif-

*For those who may wish to understand how a correlation coefficient is computed, we offer the following formula:

$$r_{xy} = \frac{\Sigma (X - \overline{X})(Y - \overline{Y})}{\sqrt{[\Sigma(X - \overline{X})^2][\Sigma(Y - \overline{Y})^2]}}$$

where r_{xy} = the correlation coefficient for variables X and Y

    X = an individual score for variable X
    $\overline{X}$ = the mean score for variable X
    Y = an individual score for variable Y
    $\overline{Y}$ = the mean score for variable Y
    Σ = the sum of

ficult to offer guidelines on what should be interpreted as strong or weak relationships. This determination depends, to a great extent, on the nature of the variables. If we were to measure patients' body temperatures both orally and rectally, a correlation of .70 between the two measurements would be considered low. For most variables of a social or psychological nature, however, an *r* of .70 is high; correlations between variables of a psychosocial nature are typically in the .10 to .40 range.

❖ THE COMPUTER AND DESCRIPTIVE STATISTICS

In the previous sections, we introduced the basic concepts of statistics that are used to organize, summarize, and describe data. In this section, we work through a fictitious example of a study and illustrate these concepts through the use of computer printouts. This section aims to make the concepts less abstract by illustrating them with some data and to familiarize the reader with printouts from a standard computer program called Statistical Package for the Social Sciences (SPSS). Information regarding the use of such programs is described in greater detail in Chapter 20.

Suppose that a nurse researcher were interested in improving the childbirth outcomes among a group of young, low-income pregnant women. A program of intensive health care, nutritional counseling, and contraceptive counseling is implemented, and an experiment is designed to test the effect of the program: half of a sample of pregnant women, assigned randomly, will receive the special treatment, and the other half will be assigned to a group receiving routine care. The two outcomes that the researcher is primarily interested in are the birthweight of the infant and whether or not the young woman becomes pregnant again within 18 months of delivery. Some fictitious data for this example, including data on various maternal characteristics, are presented in Table 17-8.

Figure 17-10 presents a frequency distribution printout for the birthweight variable. Under the term VALUE, each birthweight in the sample is listed in ascending order. In the next column, FREQUENCY, the number of occurrences of each birthweight is indicated. Thus, there was one 76-ounce baby, two 89-ounce babies, and so on. The next column, PERCENT, indicates the percentage of birthweights in each class: 3.3% of the babies weighed 76 ounces at birth, 6.7% weighed 89 ounces, and so on. The next column, VALID PERCENT, shows the percentage in each category after removing any missing data. In this example, birthweights were obtained for all 30 cases, but if one piece of data had been missing, the adjusted frequency for the 76-ounce baby would have been 3.4% (1 ÷ 29 rather than 30). The last column, CUM PERCENT, adds the percentage for a given birthweight value to the percentage for all preceding

values. Thus, we can tell by looking at the row for 99 ounces that, cumulatively, 33.3% of the babies weighed *under* 100 ounces.

The bottom of this printout lists several of the descriptive statistics discussed in this chapter. The MEAN is equal to 104.7, whereas the MEDIAN is 102.5, and the MODE is 99. This suggests that the distribution is somewhat skewed. The RANGE is 52, which is equal to the MAXIMUM of 128 minus the MINIMUM of 76. The SD (STD DEV) is 10.955, and the VARIANCE is 120.010 (10.955^2).

In addition to tabular information, such as that shown in Figure 17-10, many computer programs can produce graphic materials. Figure 17-11 presents a histogram for the variable of a mother's age. In this case, all the values for age are shown on the vertical axis, and the frequency on the horizontal axis. The histogram shows at a glance that the modal age is 19 ($f = 7$) and that this variable is negatively skewed (i.e., there are fewer younger than older girls). Descriptive statistics shown at the bottom of the printout indicate that the mean age for this group is 18.167, with an SD of 2.086.

If we were interested in comparing the repeat-pregnancy experience of the two groups of young women (experimental versus control), we would instruct the computer to cross-tabulate the two variables, as shown in the contingency table in Figure 17-12. This cross-tabulation resulted in four cells: 1) experimental subjects with no repeat pregnancy (upper-left cell); 2) control subjects with no repeat pregnancy (upper-right cell); 3) experimental subjects with a repeat pregnancy (lower-left cell); and 4) control subjects with a repeat pregnancy (lower-right cell). Each cell contains four pieces of information, which we will explain for the first cell. The first number is the number of subjects in that cell. Ten experimental subjects did not have a repeat pregnancy within 18 months of their delivery. The next number is the *row* percentage: 47.6% of the women who did not become pregnant again were in the experimental group (10 ÷ 21). The next number represents the *column* percentage: 66.7% of those in

Table 17-8.   *Fictitious Data on Low-Income Pregnant Women*

GROUP*	INFANT BIRTHWEIGHT	REPEAT PREGNANCY†	MOTHER'S AGE (YEARS)	NO. OF PRIOR PREGNANCIES	SMOKING STATUS‡
1	107	1	17	1	1
1	101	0	14	0	0
1	119	0	21	3	0
1	128	1	20	2	0
1	89	0	15	1	1
1	99	0	19	0	1
1	111	0	19	1	0
1	117	1	18	1	1
1	102	1	17	0	0
1	120	0	20	0	0
1	76	0	13	0	1
1	116	0	18	0	1
1	100	1	16	0	0
1	115	0	18	0	0
1	113	0	21	2	1
2	111	1	19	0	0
2	108	0	21	1	0
2	95	0	19	2	1
2	99	0	17	0	1
2	103	1	19	0	0
2	94	0	15	0	1
2	101	1	17	1	0
2	114	0	21	2	0
2	97	0	20	1	0
2	99	1	18	0	1
2	113	0	18	0	1
2	89	0	19	1	0
2	98	0	20	0	0
2	102	0	17	0	0
2	105	0	19	1	1

*Group: 1, experimental; 2, control.

† Repeat pregnancy: 1, yes; 0, no.

‡ Smoking status: 1, smokes; 0, does not smoke.

the experimental group did not become pregnant (10 ÷ 15). The last number is the *overall* percentage of women in that cell (10 ÷ 30 = 33.3%). This order need not be memorized. It is shown in the upper-left corner of the table:

COUNT
ROW PCT
COL PCT
TOT PCT

Thus, Figure 17-12 indicates that a somewhat higher percentage of experimental subjects (33.3%) than controls (26.7%) experienced a repeat pregnancy. The row totals on the far right indicate that, overall, 30.0% of the sample (N = 9) had a subsequent pregnancy. The column total at the bottom indicates that, overall, 50.0% of the subjects were in the experimental group, and 50.0% were in the control group.

```
------------------------------------------------------------------------
Page    2                        SPSS/PC+
                                                                 3/20/94
WEIGHT      INFANT BIRTH WEIGHT


                                                        Valid      Cum
Value Label                                             Percent    Percent
                       Value  Frequency  Percent
                         76      1         3.3             3.3        3.3
                         89      2         6.7             6.7       10.0
                         94      1         3.3             3.3       13.3
                         95      1         3.3             3.3       16.7
                         97      1         3.3             3.3       20.0
                         98      1         3.3             3.3       23.3
                         99      3        10.0            10.0       33.3
                        100      1         3.3             3.3       36.7
                        101      2         6.7             6.7       43.3
                        102      2         6.7             6.7       50.0
                        103      1         3.3             3.3       53.3
                        105      1         3.3             3.3       56.7
                        107      1         3.3             3.3       60.0
                        108      1         3.3             3.3       63.3
                        111      2         6.7             6.7       70.0
                        113      2         6.7             6.7       76.7
                        114      1         3.3             3.3       80.0
                        115      1         3.3             3.3       83.3
                        116      1         3.3             3.3       86.7
                        117      1         3.3             3.3       90.0
                        119      1         3.3             3.3       93.3
                        120      1         3.3             3.3       96.7
                        128      1         3.3             3.3      100.0
                               -------   -------         -------
                        Total    30       100.0          100.0
------------------------------------------------------------------------
Page    3                        SPSS/PC+
                                                                 3/20/94
WEIGHT      INFANT BIRTH WEIGHT


Mean        104.700      Std err     2.000      Median      102.500
Mode         99.000      Std dev    10.955      Variance    120.010
Kurtosis       .473      S E Kurt     .833      Skewness      -.254
S E Skew       .427      Range      52.000      Minimum      76.000
Maximum     128.000      Sum      3141.000


Valid cases     30      Missing cases       0
------------------------------------------------------------------------
```

Figure 17-10.   *SPSS Computer Printout: Frequency Distribution of Infant Birthweight*

❖ TIPS FOR APPLYING LEVELS OF MEASUREMENT AND DESCRIPTIVE STATISTICS

A knowledge of basic statistical methods is indispensable for those who want to keep abreast of research developments in their field—and for those undertaking a research project. Even researchers who conduct a basically qualitative study typically use some descriptive statistics for characterizing their sample. In this section, we provide some suggestions on the application of descriptive statistics.

• In operationalizing research variables, it is usually best to select or construct measures on as high a level of measurement as possible, especially for measures that will be used as dependent variables. This guideline is based on the fact that higher levels of measurement generally yield more information

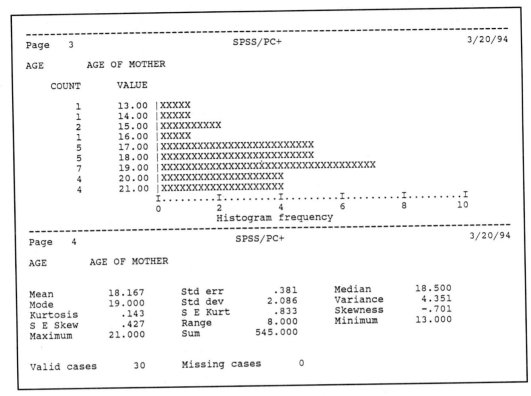

```
------------------------------------------------------------------------
Page    3                      SPSS/PC+                          3/20/94

AGE          AGE OF MOTHER

     COUNT        VALUE

       1        13.00 |XXXXX
       1        14.00 |XXXXX
       2        15.00 |XXXXXXXXXX
       1        16.00 |XXXXX
       5        17.00 |XXXXXXXXXXXXXXXXXXXXXXXXX
       5        18.00 |XXXXXXXXXXXXXXXXXXXXXXXXX
       7        19.00 |XXXXXXXXXXXXXXXXXXXXXXXXXXXXXXXXXXXXX
       4        20.00 |XXXXXXXXXXXXXXXXXXXX
       4        21.00 |XXXXXXXXXXXXXXXXXXXX
                      I........I........I........I........I........I
                      0        2        4        6        8       10
                            Histogram frequency
------------------------------------------------------------------------
Page    4                      SPSS/PC+                          3/20/94

AGE          AGE OF MOTHER


Mean            18.167   Std err        .381   Median        18.500
Mode            19.000   Std dev       2.086   Variance       4.351
Kurtosis          .143   S E Kurt       .833   Skewness       -.701
S E Skew          .427   Range        8.000   Minimum       13.000
Maximum         21.000   Sum        545.000


Valid cases       30     Missing cases       0
```

Figure 17-11.   *SPSS Computer Printout: Histogram of Maternal Age*

and are amenable to more powerful and sensitive analytic procedures than lower levels.

- Although it is generally preferable to use the highest possible level of measurement, there are exceptions to this guideline. For example, researchers sometimes use people's scores on interval- or ratio-level measures to create groups, and sometimes group membership is more meaningful or interpretable than continuous scores. For example, for some research and clinical purposes, it may be more relevant to designate infants as being of low birthweight or normal birthweight (nominal level) than to use actual birthweight values (ratio level).

- Descriptive statistics (percentages, means, standard deviations, and so on) are used for a variety of purposes in research reports. Sometimes—in purely descriptive studies—they are used directly to answer research questions, but inferential statistics (discussed in Chapter 18) are more likely to be used for this purpose. Descriptive statistics are most likely to be used to describe sample characteristics; to provide descriptive information about the distribution of key research variables in the study; and to document certain features of the research methods (e.g., the response rate or the attrition rate).

- When variables are measured on a nominal or ordinal scale, the nature of the measures limits the type of descriptive statistics that is appropriate. However, for variables measured on an interval or ratio scale, the researcher may wish to report multiple measures of central tendency or variability—particularly when the distribution is skewed. With asymmetric distributions, all three indexes of central tendency contain new information.

- In reading (or constructing) tables with descriptive statistics, it is useful to recognize

```
┌─────────────────────────────────────────────────────┐
│ REPEAT   HAD A REPEAT PREGNANCY?  by  GROUP          │
│                                                       │
│                        GROUP        Page 1 of 1       │
│                Count  |                                │
│                Row Pct|EXPERIME CONTROL               │
│                Col Pct|NTAL                Row        │
│                Tot Pct|    1   |    2    | Total       │
│         REPEAT        --------+--------+                │
│                    0  |   10   |   11   |    21        │
│           NO          |  47.6  |  52.4  |  70.0        │
│                       |  66.7  |  73.3  |              │
│                       |  33.3  |  36.7  |              │
│                       +--------+--------+              │
│                    1  |    5   |    4   |     9        │
│           YES         |  55.6  |  44.4  |  30.0        │
│                       |  33.3  |  26.7  |              │
│                       |  16.7  |  13.3  |              │
│                       +--------+--------+              │
│               Column      15       15        30        │
│                Total    50.0     50.0     100.0        │
│                                                       │
│ Number of Missing Observations:  0                    │
└─────────────────────────────────────────────────────┘
```

Figure 17-12. *SPSS Computer Printout: Cross-Tabulation of Repeat Pregnancy, by Group*

that a number of different abbreviations and symbols are used. The most widely used ones are as follows:

Mean: M, $\overline{X}$
Median: Md, Mdn
Standard deviation: SD, s, σ
Variance: σ^2, s^2

❖ RESEARCH EXAMPLES

Bernhard and Sheppard (1993) conducted a study to examine the relationships among perceived health, menopausal symptoms, and self-care activities in perimenopausal and postmenopausal women. A total of 101 women in a large midwestern city responded to a newspaper advertisement for "menopausal women" and completed a self-administered questionnaire. The questionnaire included demographic information and four composite scales: the Health Perceptions Questionnaire (HPQ); the Menopause Symptom Checklist (MSC); the Self-Care Responses Questionnaire (SCR) and the Dyadic Adjustment Scale (DAS).

The research report for this study contained a variety of descriptive statistics, displayed in a number of tables. Table 17-9 shows a portion of their first table, which presented frequency information on sample characteristics. This table indicates that the typical woman who participated in the study was a married white woman with at least some college education.

The researchers then computed measures of central tendency and variability for their primary study variables, as shown in Table 17-10. For each of the four scales included in the questionnaire, the table shows the mean, standard deviation, range, and number of sample members. Note that this last piece of information had to be included as a separate column in this table because varying numbers of respondents completed all four scales.

Information on the extent to which the various scales were intercorrelated is presented in Table 17-11. As is often the case in research reports, correlation coefficients were reported in a two-dimensional *correlation matrix*, in which all correlated variables are displayed in both a row and a column. To read a correlation matrix, one finds the row for one of the variables and reads across until the row intersects with the column for a second variable. Table 17-11 lists, on the left, six variables: responses to a question on self-rated health and scores on the various scales (including total and subscale scores on the MSC). The numbers in the top row, from 1 to 6, correspond to the six variables: 1 is self-rated health, 2 is HPQ scores, and so forth. The correlation matrix shows, in the first col-

Table 17-9. *Demographic Characteristics of Study Participants*

CHARACTERISTIC		% PERCENTAGE (N = 101)
Race	White	96
	Other	4
Marital status	Married	64
	Divorced/Separated	25
	Living together	4
	Widowed	4
	Single	3
Education	Some high school	1
	High school graduate	12
	Some college	49
	College graduate	26
	Graduate degree	12
Religion	Protestant	74
	Catholic	17
	Other	5
	None	4

Adapted from Bernhard, L.A., & Sheppard, L. (1993). Health, symptoms, self-care, and dyadic adjustment in menopausal women. *Journal of Obstetric, Gynecologic, and Neonatal Nursing, 22,* Table 1, with permission.

umn, the value of the correlation coefficient between self-rated health on the one hand and all six variables on the other. At the intersection of row 1 and column 1, we find the value 1.00, which simply indicates that self-rated health scores are perfectly correlated with themselves. The next entry in the first column represents the correlation between self-rated health and HPQ scores; the value of .44 (which can be read as +.44) indicates a moderate and positive relationship between these two variables: Women who rated their health as excellent tended to have higher scores on the HPQ than women who said their health was fair or poor. By contrast, self-rated health was virtually unrelated

Table 17-10. *Descriptive Statistics for Key Study Variables*

VARIABLE	M	SD	RANGE	N
Health perceptions	124.84	10.01	91–144	59*
Menopause symptoms				
Total symptoms	12.99	5.49	0–26	90
Worrisome symptoms	2.49	3.15	0–20	90
Self-care responses	116.19	13.82	72–143	95
Dyadic adjustment	107.25	15.75	57–128	75

*Variations in numbers are due to missing data and to an administrative error with regard to an incorrect form of the Health Perceptions Questionnaire given to 39 women.

Adapted from Bernhard, L.A., & Sheppard, L. (1993). Health, symptoms, self-care, and dyadic adjustment in menopausal women. *Journal of Obstetric, Gynecologic, and Neonatal Nursing, 22,* Table 2, with permission.

Table 17-11.   *Intercorrelations Among Key Study Variables*

VARIABLE	1	2	3	4	5	6
1. Self-rated health	1.00					
2. Health Perceptions Questionnaire	.44	1.00				
3. Menopause Symptom Checklist (total symptoms)	−.30	−.19	1.00			
4. Menopause Symptom Checklist (worrisome symptoms)	−.26	.30	.38	1.00		
5. Self-Care Responses Questionnaire	.12	.43	.03	−.16	1.00	
6. Dyadic Adjustment Scale	−.02	.19	.03	.15	−.14	1.00

Adapted from Bernhard, L.A., & sheppard, L. (1993), Health, symptoms, self-care, and dyadic adjustment in meno-pausal women. *Journal of Obstretic, Gynecologic, and Neonatal Nursing, 22,* Table 3, with permission.

to dyadic adjustment with a partner: Women who had strong dyadic relationships were as likely to rate their health positively as women whose relationships were more troubled ($r = -.02$).

❖ SUMMARY

There are four major *levels of measurement.* *Nominal measurement* classifies characteristics of attributes into mutually exclusive categories. *Ordinal measurement* involves the sorting of objects on the basis of their relative standing to each other on a specified attribute. *Interval measurement* indicates not only the rank-order-ing of objects on an attribute but also the amount of distance between each object. Dis-tances between numerical values on the interval scale represent equivalent distances in the at-tribute being measured. *Ratio-level measure-ments*, which constitute the highest form of measurement, are distinguished from interval measurements by virtue of having a rational zero point.

Descriptive statistics enable the researcher to reduce, summarize, and describe quantitative data obtained from empirical observations and measurements. A *frequency distribution* is one of the easiest methods of imposing some order on a mass of numbers. In a frequency distribu-tion, numerical values are ordered from the low-est to the highest with a count of the number of times each value was obtained. *Histograms* and *frequency polygons* are two common methods of displaying frequency information graphically.

A set of data may be completely described in terms of the shape of the distribution, central tendency, and variability. The most important attributes of the distribution's shape are its sym-metry and modality. A distribution is *symmetric* if its two halves are mirror images of each other. A *skewed distribution,* by contrast, is asymmet-ric, with one tail longer than the other. The modality of a distribution refers to the number of peaks present: a *unimodal* distribution has one peak, and a *multimodal* distribution has more than one peak.

Measures of *central tendency* are indexes, expressed as a single number, that represent the average or typical value of a set of scores. The *mode* is the numerical value that occurs most frequently in the distribution (or with greater frequency than other scores in its vicinity). The *median* is that point on a numerical scale above which and below which 50% of the cases fall. The *mean* is the arithmetic average of all the scores in the distribution. In general, the mean is the preferred measure of central tendency be-cause of its stability and its usefulness in further statistical manipulations.

Variability refers to the spread or disper-sion of the data. Measures of variability include the range, the semiquartile range, and the standard deviation. The *range* is the distance between the highest and lowest score values. The *semiquartile range* indicates one half of the range of scores within which the middle 50% of scores lie. The most commonly used measure of variability is the *standard deviation.* This index is calculated by first computing *deviation scores,* which represent the degree to which the scores of each person deviate from the mean. The standard deviation is designed to indicate how much, on average, the scores deviate from the mean. A related index, *the variance,* is equal to the standard deviation squared.

Bivariate descriptive statistics describe the magnitude and existence of relationships between two variables. A *contingency table* is a two-dimensional frequency distribution in which the frequencies of two variables are cross-tabulated. When the scores have been measured on an ordinal, interval, or ratio scale, it is more common to describe the relationship between two variables with correlational procedures. A *correlation coefficient* can be calculated to express in numerical terms the direction and magnitude of a linear relationship. The values of the correlation coefficient range from -1.00 for a perfect negative correlation, through 0.0 for no relationship, to $+1.00$ for a perfect positive correlation. The most frequently used correlation coefficient is the *product–moment correlation coefficient,* also referred to as *Pearson's r.* The graphic representation of a relationship between two variables is called a *scatter plot* or *scatter diagram.*

❖ *STUDY SUGGESTIONS*

Chapter 17 of the accompanying *Study Guide for Nursing Research: Principles and Methods, 5th ed.,* offers various exercises and study suggestions for reinforcing the concepts presented in this chapter. Additionally, the following study questions can be addressed:

1. Construct a frequency distribution for the following set of scores obtained from a scale to measure attitudes toward primary nursing:

   32 20 33 22 16 19 25 26 25 18 22 30 24 26
   27 23 28 26 21 24 31 29 25 28 22 27 26 30
   17 24

2. Construct a frequency polygon or histogram with the data from above. Describe the resulting distribution of scores in terms of symmetry and modality. How closely does the distribution approach a normal distribution?

3. What are the mean, median, and mode for the following set of data?

   13 12 9 15 7 10 16 8 6 11

   Compute the range and standard deviation.

4. Two hospitals are interested in comparing the tenure rates of their nursing staff. Hospital A finds that the current staff has been employed for a mean of 4.3 years, with an SD of 1.5. Hospital B, on the other hand, finds that the nurses have worked there for a mean of 6.4 years, with an SD of 4.2 years. Discuss what these results signify.

❖ *SUGGESTED READINGS*

METHODOLOGICAL REFERENCES

Judd, C. M., Smith, E. R., & Kidder, L. R. (1991). *Research methods in social relations* (6th ed.). Fort Worth, TX: Holt, Rinehart & Winston.

Knapp, R. G. (1984). *Basic statistics for nurses* (2nd ed.). New York: John Wiley and Sons.

Knapp, T. R. (1970). N vs. N − 1. *American Educational Research Journal, 7,* 625–626.

McCall, R. B. (1990). *Fundamental statistics for behavioral sciences* (5th ed.). Fort Worth, TX: Harcourt Brace Jovanovich College Publishers.

Munro, B. H., & Page, E. N. (1993). *Statistical methods for health-care research* (2nd ed.). Philadelphia: J. B. Lippincott.

Runyon, R. P., & Haber, A. (1984). *Fundamentals of behavioral statistics* (5th ed.). Reading, MA: Addison-Wesley.

Spence, J. T., Underwood, B. J., Dunca, C. P., & Cotton, J. W. (1983). *Elementary statistics* (4th ed.). New York: Appleton-Century-Crofts.

Triola, M. (1992). *Elementary statistics* (5th ed.). Menlo Park, CA: Addison-Wesley.

SUBSTANTIVE REFERENCES

Bernhard, L. A., & Sheppard, L. (1993). Health, symptoms, self-care, and dyadic adjustment in menopausal women. *Journal of Obstetric, Gynecologic, and Neonatal Nursing, 22,* 456–461.

Groër, M., Mozingo, J., Droppleman, P., Davis, M., Jolly, M. L., Boynton, M., Davis, K., & Kay, S. (1994). Measures of salivary secretory immunoglobulin A and state anxiety after a nursing back rub. *Applied Nursing Research, 7,* 2–6.

Ley, S. J., Miller, K., Skov, P., & Preisig, P. (1990). Crystalloid versus colloid therapy after cardiac surgery. *Heart and Lung, 19,* 31–40.

Rudy, S. F., Guckes, A. D., Li, S., McCarthy, G. R., & Brahim, J. S. (1993). Body and orofacial cathexis in edentulous complete-denture-wearing clients. *Clinical Nursing Research, 2,* 296–308.

Thornbury, J. M. (1992). Cognitive performance on Piagetian tasks by Alzheimer's disease patients. *Research in Nursing and Health, 15,* 11–18.

Chapter 18

*I*NFERENTIAL STATISTICS

Descriptive statistics are useful for summarizing empirical information, but usually the researcher wants to do more than simply describe data. *Inferential statistics* provide a means for drawing conclusions about a population, given the data obtained for the sample. Inferential statistics would help us with such questions as, "What do I know about the average 3-minute Apgar score of premature babies (the population) after having learned that a sample of 50 premature babies had a mean Apgar score of 7.5?" or "What can I conclude about the effectiveness of an intervention to promote breast self-examination among women older than 25 years of age (the population) after having found in a sample of 200 women that 50% of the experimental subjects but only 20% of the controls practiced breast self-examination 3 months later?" With the assistance of inferential statistics, researchers make judgments about or generalize to a large class of individuals based on information from a limited number of subjects.

With inferential statistics, the researcher estimates the parameters of a population from the sample statistics. These estimates are based

on laws of probability, and, as we shall see, probabilistic estimates involve a certain degree of error. The difference between estimates based on inferential statistics and estimates arrived at through the ordinary thinking process is that the statistical method provides a framework for making judgments in a systematic, objective fashion. Different researchers working with identical data would be likely to come to the same conclusion after applying inferential statistical procedures.

❖ *SAMPLING DISTRIBUTIONS*

If a sample is to be used as a basis for making estimates of population characteristics, then it is clearly advisable to obtain as representative a sample as possible. As we saw in Chapter 11, random samples (i.e., probability samples) are the most effective means of securing representative samples. Inferential statistical procedures are based on the assumption of random sampling from populations—although this assumption is widely violated and ignored.

Even when random sampling is used, however, it cannot be expected that sample characteristics will be identical to population characteristics. Suppose we had a population of 10,000 freshmen nursing students who had taken the Scholastic Aptitude Test (SAT). Let us say, for the sake of this example, that the mean SAT score for this population is 500 and the standard deviation (SD) is 100. Now, suppose that we do not know these parameters but that we must estimate them by using the scores from a random sample of 25 students. Should we expect to find a mean of exactly 500 and an SD of 100 for this sample? It would be extremely unlikely to obtain the exact population value. Let us say that instead we calculated a mean of 505. If a completely new sample were drawn and another mean computed, we might obtain a value such as 497. The tendency for the statistics to fluctuate from one sample to another is known as *sampling error.*

A researcher actually works with only *one* sample on which statistics are computed and inferences made. However, to understand inferential statistics, we must perform a small mental exercise. With the population of 10,000 nursing students, consider drawing a sample of 25 individuals, calculating a mean, replacing the 25 students, and drawing a new sample. Consider each mean computed in this fashion as a separate piece of data. If we draw 5000 such samples, we will have 5000 means or data points, which could then be used to construct a frequency polygon, such as the one shown in Figure 18-1. This kind of frequency distribution has a special name: it is called a sampling distribution of the mean. A *sampling distribution* is a theoretical rather than actual distribution because one does not in practice draw consecutive samples from a population and plot their means. The concept of a theoretical distribution of sample values is basic to inferential statistics.

Characteristics of Sampling Distributions

When an infinite number of samples are drawn from an infinite population, the sampling distribution of the mean has certain known characteristics. Our example of a population of 10,000 students, and 5000 samples with 25 students each, deals with finite quantities, but the numbers are large enough to approximate these characteristics.

Statisticians have been able to demonstrate that sampling distributions of means follow a normal curve. Furthermore, the mean of a sampling distribution consisting of an infinite number of sample means is always equal to the population mean. In the current example shown in Figure 18-1, the mean of the sampling distribution is 500, the same value as the mean of the population.

In Chapter 17, we discussed the standard deviation in terms of percentages of cases falling within a certain distance from the mean. When data values are normally distributed, 68% of the cases fall between +1 SD and −1 SD from the mean. Because a sampling distribution of means is normally distributed, we can assert that 68 out of 100 randomly drawn sample means will lie within the range of values between +1 SD and −1 SD of the mean on the sampling distribution. Thus, if we knew or could estimate the value of the SD of the sampling distribution, we could then interpret the accuracy of any single sample mean.

Standard Error of the Mean

The standard deviation of a theoretical distribution of sample means is called the *standard error of the mean* (SEM). The word *error* signifies that the various means in the sampling distribution contain some error in their estimates of the population mean. The term *standard* indicates the magnitude of a standard, or average, error. The smaller the standard error—that is, the less variable the sample means—the more accurate are those means as estimates of the population value.

But how can we compute the standard deviation of a sampling distribution without actually constructing such a distribution? Fortunately, there is a formula for estimating the SEM from the data from a single sample. It has been

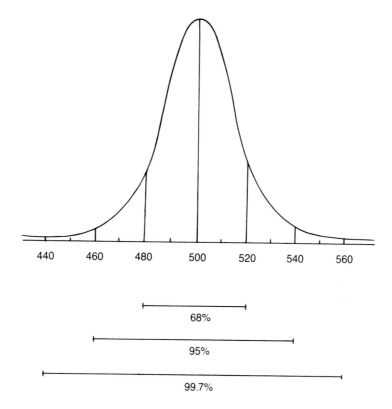

Figure 18–1. *Sampling distribution*

shown that the value of the standard error (often symbolized as $s_{\bar{x}}$) has a systematic relationship to the standard deviation of the population and to the size of the samples drawn from it. The population standard deviation is estimated by the sample standard deviation to yield the following equation:

$$s_{\bar{x}} = \frac{SD}{\sqrt{n}}$$

where SD = the standard deviation of the sample
n = sample size
$s_{\bar{x}}$ = standard error of the mean

If we use this formula to calculate the SEM in our current example, we obtain

$$s_{\bar{x}} = \frac{100}{\sqrt{25}} = 20.0$$

The standard deviation of the sampling distribution is 20, as shown in Figure 18-1. This SEM statistic is an estimate of how much sam-

pling error there is from one sample mean to another.

We can now use these calculations to estimate the probability of drawing a sample with a certain mean. With a sample size of 25, the chances are about 95 out of 100 that any sample mean would fall between the values of 460 and 540. Only five times out of 100 would we draw a sample whose mean exceeded 540 or was less than 460. In other words, only five times out of 100 would we be likely to draw a sample whose mean deviates from the population mean by more than 40 points. Thus, by estimating the SEM, we can estimate the likely accuracy of our sample mean.

From the formula for the SEM, it can be seen that to increase the accuracy of our estimate of the population mean, we need only increase the sample size. Suppose that instead of using a sample of 25 nursing students to estimate the average SAT score, we used a sample of 100 students. With this many students, the SEM would be

$$s_{\bar{x}} = \frac{100}{\sqrt{100}} = 10.0$$

In such a situation, the probability of obtaining a sample mean greater than 520 or less than 480 would be about 5 in 100. The chances of drawing a sample with a mean very different from that of the population is reduced as the sample size increases because large numbers promote the likelihood that extreme cases will cancel each other out.

❖ ESTIMATION OF PARAMETERS

Statistical inference consists of two major types of techniques: estimation of parameters and hypothesis testing. Of the two, hypothesis testing is more commonly encountered in research reports, but estimation plays an important role as well.

Estimation procedures are used to estimate a single population parameter, such as the mean value of some attribute. Suppose a new drug has been developed for people suffering from high blood pressure, and a researcher administers the drug to a sample of patients. The researcher could use estimation procedures to estimate the average blood pressure of a population of people with high blood pressure (or the average reduction in blood pressure) after administration of the drug. Estimation is the method used when no a priori prediction can be made about the attributes of a population, as would probably be the case for the effects of a new drug.

Estimation can take one of two forms: point estimation or interval estimation. *Point estimation* involves the calculation of a single statistic to estimate the population parameter. To continue with the SAT example, if we calculated the mean SAT score for a sample of 25 students and found that it was 510, then this number would represent the point estimate of the population mean.

The problem with point estimates is that they convey no information concerning the accuracy of the estimation. *Interval estimation* of a parameter is more useful because it indicates a range of values within which the parameter has a specified probability of lying. Interval estimates usually are referred to as *confidence intervals,* and the upper and lower limits of the range of values are called *confidence limits.*

The construction of a confidence interval around a sample mean establishes a range of values for a population parameter and also establishes a certain probability of being correct. In other words, we make the estimation with a certain degree of confidence. Although the degree of confidence one wishes to attain is somewhat arbitrary, researchers conventionally use either a 95% or a 99% confidence interval.

The calculation of the confidence limits involves the use of the SEM and the principles associated with the normal distribution. As shown in Figure 18-1, 95% of the scores in a normal distribution lie within about 2 SDs (more precisely, 1.96 SDs) from the mean.

Returning to our example, let us say once again that the point estimation of the mean SAT score is 510, with an SD of 100. The SEM for a sample of 25 would be 20. We can now build a 95% confidence interval by using the following formula:

$$\text{Conf. } (\bar{X} \pm 1.96 \ s_{\bar{x}}) = 95\%$$

That is, the confidence is 95% that the population mean lies between the values equal to 1.96 times the standard error, above and below the sample mean. In the example at hand, we would obtain the following:

$$\text{Conf. } (510 \pm (1.96 \times 20.0)) \ = \ 95\%$$
$$\text{Conf. } (510 \pm (39.2)) \qquad\quad = \ 95\%$$
$$\text{Conf. } (470.8 \leq \mu \leq 549.2) \ \ = \ 95\%$$

The final statement may be read as follows: the confidence is 95% that the population mean (symbolized by the Greek letter mu [μ] by convention) is greater than or equal to 470.8 but less than or equal to 549.2. Another way to interpret the confidence interval concept is in terms of a probabilistic statement. One could say that out of 100 samples with an *n* of 25, 95 out of 100 such confidence intervals would contain the parameter (the population mean).

The confidence interval reflects the degree of risk the researcher is willing to take of being wrong. With a 95% confidence interval, the researcher accepts the probability that she or he will be wrong five times out of 100. A 99% confidence interval sets the risk at only 1% by allowing a wider range of possible values. The formula is as follows:

$$\text{Conf. } (\overline{X} \pm 2.58 \, s_{\overline{x}}) = 99\%$$

The 2.58 reflects the fact that 99% of all cases in a normal distribution lie within ± 2.58 SD units from the mean. In the example, the 99% confidence interval would be:

$$\text{Conf. } (510 \pm (2.58 \times 20.0)) = 99\%$$
$$\text{Conf. } (510 \pm (51.6)) = 99\%$$
$$\text{Conf. } (458.4 \leq \mu \leq 561.6) = 99\%$$

In 99 out of 100 samples with 25 subjects, the confidence interval so constructed would contain the population mean. One accepts a reduced risk of being wrong at the price of reduced specificity. In the case of the 95% interval, the range between the confidence limits was only about 80 points; here the range of possible values is more than 100 points. The risk of error that one is willing to accept depends on the nature of the problem. In research that could affect the well-being of humans, it is not unusual to use stringent 99.9% confidence intervals, but for most research projects, a 95% confidence interval is sufficient.

❖ HYPOTHESIS TESTING

Statistical hypothesis testing is essentially a process of decision making. Suppose a nurse researcher hypothesized that cancer patients' participation in a stress management program would result in lower anxiety. The sample consists of 25 patients in a control group who do not participate in the stress management program and 25 subjects in the experimental group who do. All 50 subjects are administered a self-report scale of anxiety. The researcher finds that the mean anxiety level for the experimental group is 15.8 and that for the control group is 17.5. Should the researcher conclude that the hypothesis has been supported? True, the group differences are in the predicted direction, but the results might simply be the result of sampling fluctuations. Statistical hypothesis testing allows researchers to make objective decisions concerning the results of their studies. Scientists need such a mechanism for helping them to decide which outcomes are likely to reflect only chance differences between sample groups and which are likely to reflect true population differences.

The Null Hypothesis

The procedures used in testing hypotheses are based on rules of negative inference. This logic often seems somewhat awkward and peculiar to beginning researchers, so we try to convey the concepts with a concrete illustration. In the stress management program example, a nurse researcher tested the effectiveness of a special program designed to reduce stress and anxiety in cancer patients. The researcher found that those participating in the program had lower mean anxiety scores than those not participating in the program. There are two possible explanations for this outcome: (1) the experimental treatment was successful in reducing patients' anxiety or (2) the differences resulted from chance factors (such as differences in the anxiety levels of the two groups even before any special treatment). The first explanation corresponds to the researcher's scientific hypothesis, but the second explanation corresponds to the null hypothesis. The *null hypothesis* is a statement that there is no actual relationship between variables and that any such observed relationship is only a function of chance, or sampling fluctuations. The need for a null hypothesis lies in the fact that statistical hypothesis testing is basically a process of rejection. It is impossible to demonstrate directly and conclusively that the first explanation—the scientific hypothesis—is correct. However, it is possible to show that the null hypothesis has a high probability of being incorrect, and such evidence lends support to the scientific hypothesis. The rejection of the null hypothesis, then, is what the researcher seeks to accomplish through *statistical tests.*

The null hypothesis is sometimes stated as a formal proposition, using the following symbols:

$$H_0: \mu_A = \mu_B$$

The null hypothesis (H_0) asserts that the population mean for method A (μ_A) is the same as the population mean for method B (μ_B) with regard to, in this case, anxiety scores. The *alternative,* or research, *hypothesis* may also be stated in similar terms:

$$H_A: \mu_A \neq \mu_B$$

Although null hypotheses are accepted or rejected on the basis of data from a sample, the hypothesis is made about population values. The real interest in testing hypotheses, as in all statistical inference, is to use samples to draw conclusions about relationships within the population.

Type I and Type II Errors

The researcher's decision about whether to accept or reject the null hypothesis is based on a consideration of how probable it is that observed differences are the result of chance alone. Because information concerning the entire population is unavailable, it is not possible to assert flatly that the null hypothesis is or is not true. The researcher must be content with the knowledge that the hypothesis is either probably true or probably false. We make statistical inferences based on incomplete information, so there is always a risk of error.

A researcher can make two types of errors: the rejection of a true null hypothesis or the acceptance of a false null hypothesis. The possible outcomes of a researcher's decision are summarized in Figure 18-2. An investigator makes a *Type I error* by rejecting the null hypothesis when it is, in fact, true. For instance, if we concluded that the experimental treatment was more effective than the control treatment in alleviating patients' anxiety, when in actuality the observed sample differences in anxiety scores resulted only from sampling fluctuations, then we would have made a Type I error. In the reverse situation, if we concluded that the differences in group anxiety levels were the result of chance, when in fact the experimental treatment *did* have an effect on anxiety, we would be committing a *Type II error* by accepting a false null hypothesis.

Level of Significance

The researcher does not know when an error in statistical decision making has been committed. The truth or falseness of a null hy-

	The actual situation is that the null hypothesis is:	
	(1) true	(2) false
The researcher concludes, after applying statistical tests, that the null hypothesis is: (1) true—accepted	correct decision	Type II error
(2) false—rejected	Type I error	correct decision

Figure 18–2. *Outcomes of statistical decision making*

pothesis could only be definitively ascertained by collecting information from the entire population, in which case there would be no need for statistical inference.

The selection of a level of significance determines the chance of making a Type I error. *Level of significance* is the phrase used to signify the probability of committing a Type I error. As in the case of confidence levels, the probability level can be established by the investigator.

The two most frequently used levels of significance (often referred to as α, or alpha) are .05 and .01. If we say we are using a .05 significance level, this means that we are accepting the risk that out of 100 samples, a true null hypothesis would be rejected five times, and accepted 95 times. With a .01 significance level, the risk of a Type I error is *lower:* in only 1 sample out of 100 would we erroneously reject the null hypothesis. By convention, the minimum acceptable level for α generally is .05. A stricter level may be desirable for statistical tests when the decision has important consequences.

Naturally, researchers would like to reduce the risk of committing both types of error. Unfortunately, lowering the risk of committing a Type I error increases the risk of a Type II error. The stricter the criterion we use for rejecting a null hypothesis, the greater the probability that we will accept a false null hypothesis. There is a kind of tradeoff that the researcher must consider in establishing criteria for statistical decision making. Procedures for addressing Type II errors are discussed in Chapter 19.

Tests of Statistical Significance

When a researcher uses quantitative analysis to test a hypothesis, the data collected for the study are used to compute a test statistic. For every test statistic, there is a related theoretical distribution. (The sampling distribution of means discussed previously is an example of a theoretical rather than actual distribution.) Hypothesis testing uses theoretical distributions and the laws of probability to establish probable and improbable values for test statistics, which are in turn used as a basis for accepting or rejecting the null hypothesis.

A simple example illustrates the process. Suppose a researcher wanted to test the hypothesis that the average SAT score for high school students who enter a nursing program is higher than that for all high school students, whose mean score is 500. The null hypothesis is H_0: $\mu_{NURS} = 500$, and the alternate hypothesis is H_A: $\mu_{NURS} \neq 500$. That is, our null hypothesis is that the population mean for students who enter a nursing program is equal to 500; the alternative hypothesis (which is the research hypothesis) is that the nursing student population mean is not equal to 500. To test this hypothesis, we draw a sample of 100 freshmen students in nursing programs. Let us say that the mean score for this sample of students turns out to be 525, with an SD of 100. Using statistical procedures, we can assess the likelihood that a mean score of 525 represents a chance fluctuation from the mean of 500 for all high school students.

In hypothesis testing, one assumes that the null hypothesis is true and then gathers evidence to disprove it. Assuming a population mean of 500, a sampling distribution can be constructed with a mean of 500 and an SD equal to 10 ($s_{\bar{x}} = 100 \div \sqrt{100}$), as shown in Figure 18-3. Based on our knowledge of normal distribution characteristics, we can determine probable and improbable values of sample means drawn from the nursing student population. If, as is assumed, the population mean is actually 500, then 95% of all sample means would fall between 480 and 520. The obtained sample mean of 525 is improbable, given the null hypothesis—if we use as our criterion of improbability a significance level of .05. We would reject, therefore, the null hypothesis that the population mean for nursing students equals 500. We would not be justified in saying that we have *proved* the alternative hypothesis because there is a 5% possibility of having made a Type I error.

Researchers reporting the results of hypothesis tests often say that their findings were (or were not) *statistically significant*. This termi-

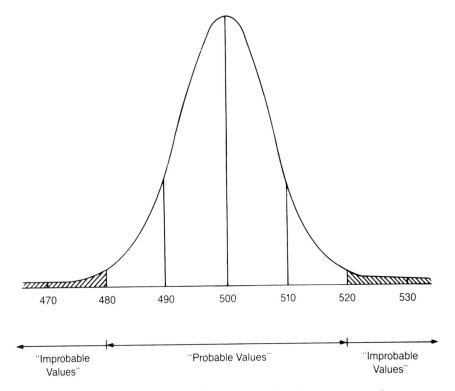

Figure 18–3.   *Sampling distribution for hypothesis test example*

nology has a precise meaning. The word *signif-icant* should not be given the familiar interpretation of important or meaningful. In statistics, significant means that the obtained results are unlikely to have been the result of chance, at some specified level of probability. A nonsignificant outcome means that any difference between an obtained statistic and a hypothesized parameter could have been the result of a chance fluctuation in the sample.

The example used in this section was highly contrived; researchers rarely predict a specific value for a population mean. The use of theoretical distributions to determine probable and improbable values of a test statistic, however, is common to all tests of statistical significance.

One-Tailed and Two-Tailed Tests

In most hypothesis-testing situations, researchers apply what is known as *two-tailed*

tests. This means that both ends, or tails, of the sampling distribution are used to determine the range of improbable values. In Figure 18-3, for example, the critical region that contains 5% of the area of the sampling distribution really involves 2.5% at one end of the distribution and 2.5% at the other. If the level of significance were .01, then the critical regions would involve .5% of the distribution at both tails.

When the researcher has a strong basis for using a directional hypothesis (see Chapter 3), it may be justifiable to use what is referred to as a one-tailed test. For example, if a nurse researcher instituted an outreach program to improve the prenatal practices of low-income rural women, then it might be hypothesized that women in the experimental program would not just be *different* from control women not exposed to the intervention (in terms of outcomes such as pregnancy complications, infant birthweight, and so on). One would expect the experimental subjects to have an *advantage*. It might make little sense to use the tail of the distribution that would signify *worse* outcomes among the experimental than the control mothers. In a one-tailed test, the critical region of improbable values is entirely in one tail of the distribution—the tail corresponding to the direction of the hypothesis, as illustrated in Figure 18-4. When a one-tailed test is used, the critical area of .05 covers a bigger region of the specified tail, and for this reason, one-tailed tests are less conservative. This means that it is easier to reject the null hypothesis with a one-tailed test than with a two-tailed test.

The use of one-tailed tests has been the subject of considerable controversy. Most researchers follow the convention of using a two-tailed test, even if they have stated a directional hypothesis. In reading research reports, one can assume that a two-tailed test has been used, unless the investigator specifically mentions a one-tailed test. However, when there is a strong logical or theoretical reason for using a directional

hypothesis and for assuming that findings opposite to the direction hypothesized are virtually impossible, a one-tailed test may be warranted.

In the remainder of this chapter, the examples use two-tailed tests. If a computer is used to perform statistical analyses, then two-tailed hypothesis testing is almost always assumed.

Parametric and Nonparametric Tests

A distinction is often made between two classes of statistical tests. The bulk of the tests that we consider in this chapter—and also most tests used by researchers—are called parametric tests. *Parametric tests* are characterized by three attributes: (1) they involve the estimation of at least one parameter; (2) they require measurements on at least an interval scale; and (3) they involve several other assumptions about the variables under consideration, such as the assumption that the variables are normally distributed in the population.

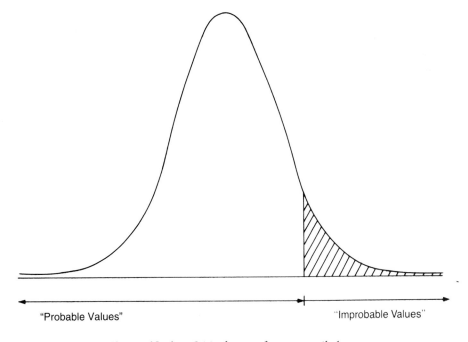

"Probable Values"   "Improbable Values"

Figure 18–4.   *Critical range for a one-tailed test*

Nonparametric tests, by contrast, are not based on the estimation of parameters. They are usually applied when the data have been measured on a nominal or ordinal scale. Nonparametric methods also involve less restrictive assumptions concerning the shape of the distribution of the critical variables than do parametric tests. For this reason, nonparametric tests are sometimes called *distribution-free* statistics.

Statisticians disagree about the utility and virtues of many nonparametric tests. Purists insist that if the strict requirements of parametric tests are not met, then parametric procedures are inappropriate. Many statistical research studies have shown, however, that the violation of the assumptions for parametric tests usually fails to affect statistical decision making or the number of errors made. The more moderate position in this debate, and the one that we think is reasonable, is that nonparametric tests are most useful when the data under consideration cannot in any manner be construed as interval-level measures or the distribution of data is markedly nonnormal. Parametric tests are usually more powerful and offer more flexibility than nonparametric tests and are, for these reasons, generally preferred.

Overview of Hypothesis-Testing Procedures

In the pages that follow, various types of statistical procedures for testing research hypotheses are examined. The discussion emphasizes the applications of statistical tests rather than actual computations. One computational example is worked out to illustrate that numbers are not just pulled out of a hat. However, computers have virtually eliminated the need for manual calculations, and so computational examples have been minimized. Researchers involved in statistical analyses are urged to pursue other references for a fuller appreciation of statistical methods. In this basic text on research methods, our primary concern is to alert researchers to the potential use (or misuse) of statistical tests for different purposes.

Although each of the statistical tests described in the remaining sections of this chapter has a particular application and can be used only with particular kinds of data, the overall process of testing hypotheses is basically the same. The seven steps are essentially as follows:

1. *Determine the test statistic to be used.* The researcher must select an appropriate statistical test, based on a number of factors (e.g., whether a parametric test is justified). Table 18-6, presented later in this chapter, offers assistance in selecting the appropriate test.
2. *Select the level of significance.* An α level of .05 will usually be acceptable. If a more stringent test is required, then α may be set at .01 or .001.
3. *Select a one-tailed or two-tailed test.* In most cases, a two-tailed test should be used, but if the researcher has a firm basis for hypothesizing not only a difference or a relationship but also the *nature* of that difference or relationship, then a one-tailed test may be appropriate.
4. *Compute a test statistic.* Using the values from the collected data, calculate a test statistic using the appropriate computational formulas. Or, alternatively, have the computer calculate the statistic using a program designed for this purpose.
5. *Calculate the degrees of freedom* (symbolized as *df*). *Degrees of freedom* is a concept used throughout hypothesis testing to refer to the number of observations free to vary about a parameter. The concept is too complex for full elaboration here, but fortunately the computation is extremely easy. (The formulas for the *df* vary from one test statistic to another).
6. *Obtain a tabled value for the statistical test.* Theoretical distributions have been developed for all test statistics. These theoretical distributions enable the researcher to discover whether obtained values are beyond the range of what is probable if the null hypothesis is true. That is, at some proba-

bility level specified by the researcher, the obtained value of the test statistic reflects a true relationship between variables (or a reliable estimate of a hypothesized population parameter) and not just a relationship or value that occurred in the sample by chance. The researcher examines a table appropriate for the test used and then obtains the tabled value by entering the table at a point corresponding to the relevant degrees of freedom and level of significance.

7. *Compare the test statistic to the tabled value.* In the final step, the researcher compares the value of the statistic found in the table with the computed value of the statistic. If the absolute value of the test statistic is *larger* than the tabled value, then the results are statistically significant. If the computed value is *smaller,* then the results are nonsignificant.

When a computer program is used to test hypotheses, the researcher really only needs to follow the first step and then make the necessary commands to the computer. The computer will calculate the test statistic, the degrees of freedom, and the *actual* probability that the relationship being tested results from chance. For example, the computer may print that the probability (p) of an experimental group doing better on a measure of postoperative recovery than the control group on the basis of chance alone is .025. This means that fewer than three times out of 100 (or only 25 times out of 1000) would a difference between the two groups as large as the one obtained reflect haphazard sampling differences rather than differences resulting from an experimental intervention. This computed probability level can then be compared with the investigator's desired level of significance. If the significance level desired were .05, then the results would be said to be significant, because .025 is more stringent than .05. If .01 were the significance level, then the results would be nonsignificant (sometimes abbreviated *NS*). Any computed probability level greater

than .05 (e.g., .20) indicates a nonsignificant relationship—that is, one that could have occurred on the basis of chance alone in more than five out of 100 samples.

In the sections that follow, a number of specific statistical tests and their applications are described. Examples of hypothesis tests using computerized computations are provided at the end of the chapter.

❖ TESTING DIFFERENCES BETWEEN TWO GROUP MEANS

A common research situation is the comparison of two groups of subjects with respect to mean values on a dependent variable. For instance, we might wish to compare an experimental and control group of patients on a physiologic measure such as heart rate or blood pressure. Or, perhaps we would be interested in contrasting the average number of school days missed owing to illness among children who had been born preterm versus full-term. This section describes methods for testing the statistical significance of differences between two group means.

The basic parametric procedure for testing differences in group means is the *t-test* (sometimes referred to as *Student's t*). A distinction must be drawn between the case in which there are two independent groups (such as an experimental and control group, or male versus female subjects) and the case in which the sample is paired or dependent (as when a single group yields pretreatment and posttreatment scores). Procedures for handling independent samples are described below to illustrate the computation of the *t*-statistic.

t-Tests for Independent Samples

Suppose that a researcher wanted to test the effect of early discharge of maternity patients on their perceived maternal competence. The researcher administers a scale of perceived maternal competence 1 week after delivery to

10 primiparas who were discharged early (that is, within 24 hours of delivery) and to 10 primiparas who remained in the hospital for longer periods. The researcher finds that the mean scale scores for these two groups are 19 and 25, respectively. The question is, are these differences real (i.e., are they likely to be replicated in other samples of early-discharge and later-discharge mothers?), or are the group differences the result of chance fluctuations? The hypotheses being tested are

$$H_0: \mu_A = \mu_B \qquad H_A: \mu_A \neq \mu_B$$

To test these hypotheses, a *t*-statistic is computed. With independent samples such as in the current example, the formula is

$$t = \frac{\overline{X}_A - \overline{X}_B}{\sqrt{\dfrac{\Sigma_{x_A}^2 + \Sigma_{x_B}^2}{n_A + n_B - 2}\left(\dfrac{1}{n_A} + \dfrac{1}{n_B}\right)}}$$

This formula looks rather complex and intimidating, but it boils down to simple components that can be calculated with elementary arithmetic. Let us work through one example with data shown in Table 18-1.

The first column of numbers presents the scores of the regular-discharge group (group A), whose mean score of 25.0 is shown at the bottom of column 1. In column 4, similar scores are shown for the early-discharge group, whose mean is 19.0. The 20 scores shown in this table vary from one person to another. Some of the variability simply reflects individual differences in perceived maternal competence. Some may also be due to measurement error (i.e., the unreliability of the scale), while some may be the result of the subjects' moods on that particular day, and so forth. The research question is: "Can a significant portion of the 6-point mean group difference be attributed to the independent variable—time of discharge from the hospital?" The calculation of the *t*-statistic allows the researcher to answer this question in an objective fashion.

After calculating mean group scores, deviation scores are obtained for each subject, as shown in columns 2 and 5: 25.0 is subtracted from each score in group A, and 19.0 is subtracted from each score in group B. Then, each deviation score is squared (columns 3 and 6), and the squared deviation scores are added. We now have all the components for the formula presented above, as follows:

$\overline{X}_A = 25.0$ mean of group A
$\overline{X}_B = 19.0$ mean of group B
$\Sigma_{x_A}^2 = 242$ sum of group A squared deviation scores
$\Sigma_{x_B}^2 = 154$ sum of group B squared deviation scores
$n_A = 10$ number of subjects in group A
$n_B = 10$ number of subjects in group B

When these numbers are used in the *t*-equation, the value of the *t*-statistic is computed to be 2.86, as shown in Table 18-1.

To ascertain whether this *t*-value is statistically significant, we need to consult a table that specifies the probability points associated with different *t*-values for the theoretical *t*-distributions. To make use of such a table, the researcher must have two pieces of information: (1) the α level sought—that is, the degree of risk of making a Type I error that one is willing to accept—and (2) the number of degrees of freedom available. For a *t*-test with independent samples, the formula for degrees of freedom is

$$df = n_A + n_B - 2$$

That is, the degrees of freedom is equal to the number of subjects in the two groups, minus 2. Thus, in the present example, the degrees of freedom is equal to 18 [(10 + 10) − 2].

A table of *t*-values is presented in Table B-1, Appendix B. The left-hand column lists various degrees of freedom, and the top row specifies different α values. If we use as our decision-making criterion a two-tailed probability (*p*) level of .05, we find that with 18 degrees of freedom, the tabled value of *t* is 2.10. This value establishes an upper limit to what is probable, if

Table 18-1. *Computation of the* t*-Statistic for Independent Samples*

GROUP A (REGULAR-DISCHARGE GROUP)			GROUP B (EARLY-DISCHARGE GROUP)			
(1)	*(2)*	*(3)*	*(4)*	*(5)*	*(6)*	
X_A	x_A	x_A^2	X_B	x_B	x_B^2	
30	5	25	23	4	16	$t = \dfrac{25 - 19}{\sqrt{\dfrac{242 + 154}{(10 + 10 - 2)}\left(\dfrac{1}{10} + \dfrac{1}{10}\right)}} =$
27	2	4	17	−2	4	
25	0	0	22	3	9	
20	−5	25	18	−1	1	
24	−1	1	20	1	1	
32	7	49	26	7	49	$t = \dfrac{6}{\sqrt{(22)(.2)}} =$
17	−8	64	16	−3	9	
18	−7	49	13	−6	36	
28	3	9	21	2	4	$t = \dfrac{6}{\sqrt{4.4}} =$
29	4	16	14	−5	25	
$\Sigma X_A = 250$ $\overline{X}_A = 25.0$		$\Sigma x_A^2 = 242$	$\Sigma X_B = 190$ $\overline{X}_B = 19.0$		$\Sigma x_B^2 = 154$	$t = \dfrac{6}{2.1} = 2.86$

the null hypothesis were true; values in excess of 2.10 would be considered improbable. Thus, our calculated t of 2.86[*] is improbable, that is, statistically significant. We are now in a position to say that the primiparas discharged early had significantly lower perceptions of maternal competence than those who were not discharged early. The probability that the mean difference of 6 points was the result of chance factors rather than the timing of discharge is less than 5 in 100 ($p < .05$). The null hypothesis is rejected, therefore, and the alternative hypothesis retained.

Paired t*-Tests*

In some studies, the researcher obtains two measures from the same subjects, or measures from paired sets of subjects (such as two siblings). Whenever two sets of scores on the

dependent variable are not independent, then the researcher must use a t-test for paired or dependent samples.

Suppose that we were interested in studying the effect of a special diet on the cholesterol level of adult men older than age 60 years. A sample of 50 men is randomly selected to participate in the study. The cholesterol levels are measured before the start of the investigation and measured again after 2 months on the special diet. The central concern here is the change in the cholesterol levels—the average difference in cholesterol values before and after the treatment. The hypotheses being submitted to a statistical test are

$$H_0: \mu_X = \mu_Y \qquad H_A: \mu_X \neq \mu_Y$$

where X = pretreatment cholesterol levels
Y = postreatment cholesterol levels

As in the previous example, a t-statistic would be computed from the pretest and

---

[*] The tabled t-value should be compared with the absolute value of the calculated t. Thus, if the calculated t-value had been −2.86, then the results would still be significant.

posttest measures (using, however, a different formula).* The obtained *t* would be compared with the *t*-values in Table B-1, Appendix B. For this particular type of *t*-test, the degrees of freedom equals the number of paired observations minus one (*df* = *n* − 1).

Other Two-Group Tests

In certain two-group situations, the *t*-statistic may be inappropriate. If the dependent variable is on an ordinal-level scale, or if the distribution is markedly nonnormal, then a non-parametric test may be preferred. We mention a few such tests here without actually working out examples.

The *median test* involves the comparison of two independent groups on the basis of deviations from the median rather than the mean. In the median test, the scores for both samples are combined and the overall median calculated. Then the number of cases above and below this median is counted separately for each sample, resulting in a 2 × 2 contingency table; (above/below median) × (group A/group B). From such a contingency table, a chi-square statistic (described in a subsequent section) can be computed to test the null hypothesis that the medians are the same for the two populations.

The *Mann-Whitney* U *test* is another non-parametric procedure for testing the difference between two independent samples when the dependent variable is measured on an ordinal scale. The test is based on the assignment of ranks to the two groups of measures. The sum of the ranks for the two groups can be compared by calculating the *U* statistic. The Mann-Whitney *U* test tends to throw away less information than a median test and, therefore, is more powerful.

When ordinal-level data are paired rather than independent, either the sign test or the Wilcoxon signed-rank test can be used. The *sign test* is an extremely simple procedure, involving the assignment of a "+" or "−" to the differences between a pair of scores, depending on whether X is larger than Y, or vice versa. The *Wilcoxon test* involves taking the difference between paired scores and ranking the absolute difference.

Compared with *t*-tests, all these nonparametric tests are computationally easy. Because they are generally less powerful, however, the ease of computation should not be used as the basis for choosing which statistic is most appropriate, especially if a computer is being used to analyze the data.

❖ TESTING DIFFERENCES BETWEEN THREE OR MORE GROUP MEANS

The procedure known as *analysis of variance* (ANOVA) is another commonly used statistical test. Like the *t*-test, ANOVA is a parametric procedure used to test the significance of differences between means. However, ANOVA is not restricted to two-group situations: The means of three or more groups can be compared with ANOVA.

The statistic computed in an ANOVA is the *F-ratio* statistic. Because the statistic is based on more than two groups, it should not be too surprising that the computation of an *F*-ratio is somewhat more complex than that for a *t*-statistic. ANOVA decomposes the total variability of a set of data into two components: (1) the variability resulting from the independent variable and (2) all other variability, such as indi-

---

* The paired *t*-statistic is computed according to the following formula:

$$t = \frac{\bar{D}_{x-y}}{\sqrt{\dfrac{\Sigma d^2}{n(n-1)}}}$$

where D_{x-y} = the difference between two paired scores

$\bar{D}_{x-y}$ = the mean difference between the paired scores

d = the deviation scores for the difference measure

Σd^2 = the sum of the squared deviation scores

n = number of pairs

vidual differences, measurement unreliability, and so on. Variation *between* treatment groups is contrasted with variation *within* groups to yield an *F*-ratio. If the differences between groups receiving different treatments is large relative to fluctuations within groups, then it is possible to establish the probability that the treatment is related to, or has resulted in, the group differences.

One-Way Analysis of Variance

Suppose that we were interested in comparing the effectiveness of different interventions to help individuals stop smoking. One group of smokers will undergo behavior modification therapy, which is based on reinforcement theory (group A). A second group will be treated by hypnosis (group B). A third group will serve as a control and will receive no special treatment (group C). The dependent variable in this experiment will be cigarette consumption during the week that follows completion of the treatments. Thirty subjects who smoke regularly and who wish to stop smoking are randomly assigned to one of the three conditions. The ANOVA will permit a test of the following hypotheses:

$$H_0: \mu_A = \mu_B = \mu_C \qquad H_A: \mu_A \neq \mu_B \neq \mu_C$$

The null hypothesis asserts that the population means for posttreatment cigarette smoking will be the same for all three groups, and the alternative (research) hypothesis predicts inequality of means. Table 18-2 presents some hypothetical data for such a study.

For each of the three groups, the raw score for each subject and the mean group score are shown. The mean numbers of posttreatment cigarettes consumed are 20, 25, and 33 for groups A, B, and C, respectively. These means are different, but are they significantly different—or are the differences attributable to random fluctuations?

The underlying concepts and terms for a one-way ANOVA are briefly explained without working out the computations for this example. Again, the reader is urged to consult a statistics

text for formulas and more detailed explanations. In calculating an *F*-statistic, the total variability within the data is broken down into two sources. The portion of the variance resulting from group membership (i.e., from exposure to different treatments) is determined by calculating a component known as the *sum of squares between groups,* or SS_B. This SS_B represents the sum of squared deviations of the individual group means from the overall mean for all subjects. The SS_B term reflects the variability in individual scores attributable to group membership.

The second component is the *sum of squares within groups,* or SS_W. This is an index of the sum of the squared deviations of each individual score from its own group mean. The SS_W term indicates variability attributable to individual differences, measurement error, and so on.

Recall from Chapter 17 that the formula for calculating a variance is $\text{Var} = \Sigma x^2 \div n - 1$. The two sums of squares described above are analogous to the numerator of this equation. The sums of squares represent sums of squared deviations from means. Therefore, to compute the variance within and the variance between groups, we must divide by a quantity analogous to $(n - 1)$. This quantity is the degrees of free-

Table 18-2. *Fictitious Data for a One-Way ANOVA*

GROUP A	GROUP B	GROUP C
28	22	33
0	31	44
17	26	29
20	30	40
35	34	33
19	37	25
24	0	22
0	19	43
41	24	29
16	27	32
$\Sigma X_A = 200$	$\Sigma X_B = 250$	$\Sigma X_C = 330$
$\bar{X}_A = 20.0$	$\bar{X}_B = 25.0$	$\bar{X}_C = 33.0$

dom associated with each sum of squares. For between groups, $df = G - 1$, which is the number of groups minus one. For within groups, $df = (n_A - 1) + (n_B - 1) + \ldots (n_G - 1)$. That is, degrees of freedom within is found by adding together the number of subjects less 1 for each group.

In an ANOVA context, the variance is conventionally referred to as the *mean square* (MS). The formulas for the mean square between groups and the mean square within groups are

$$MS_B = \frac{SS_B}{df_B} \qquad MS_W = \frac{SS_W}{df_W}$$

The *F*-ratio is the ratio of these mean squares, or

$$F = \frac{MS_B}{MS_W}$$

All these computations for the data in Table 18-2 are presented in the ANOVA summary table shown in Table 18-3. As this table shows, the calculated *F*-statistic for our fictitious example is 3.84.

The last step is to compare the obtained *F*-statistic with the value from a theoretical *F*-distribution. Table B-2, Appendix B, contains the upper limits of probable values for distributions with varying degrees of freedom. The first part of the table lists these values for a significance level of .05, and the second and third parts list those for .01 and .001 significance levels. Let us say that for the current example, we have chosen the .05 probability level. To enter the table, we find the column headed by our between-groups degrees of freedom (2), and go down this column until we reach the row corresponding to the within-groups degrees of freedom (27). The tabled value of *F* with 2 and 27 *df* is 3.35. Because our obtained *F*-value of 3.84 exceeds 3.35, we reject the null hypothesis that the population means are equal. The differences in the number of cigarettes smoked after treatment are beyond chance expectations. In fewer than 5 samples out of 100 would differences of this magnitude be obtained by chance alone. The data support the hypothesis that the interventions affected cigarette-smoking behaviors.

The ANOVA procedure does not allow us to say that each group differed significantly from all other groups. We cannot tell from these results if treatment A was significantly more effective than treatment B. Some researchers incorrectly use *t*-tests to compare the different pairs of means (A versus B, A versus C, B versus C) when this type of information is required. Methods known as *multiple comparison procedures* should be used in such situations. The function of these procedures is to isolate the comparisons between group means that are responsible for the rejection of the ANOVA null hypothesis. Multiple comparison methods are described in most intermediate statistical textbooks.

Multifactor Analysis of Variance

The type of problem described previously is known as a one-way ANOVA because it deals with the effect of one independent variable (the different interventions) on a dependent variable. Chapter 3 pointed out that hypotheses are

Table 18-3.   *ANOVA Summary Table*

SOURCE OF VARIANCE	SS	df	MEAN SQUARE	F	p
Between groups	860.0	2	430.00	3.84	<.05
Within groups	3,022.0	27	111.93		
Total	3,882.0	29			

sometimes complex and make predictions about the effect of two or more independent variables on a dependent variable. The analysis of data from such studies is often performed by means of a *multifactor ANOVA*. In this section, we describe some of the principles underlying a two-way ANOVA. The actual computations, however, are not worked out here.

Suppose that we were interested in determining whether the two smoking cessation treatments were equally effective in helping men and women stop smoking, with no control group in the study. We could design an experiment using a randomized block design, with four groups: Women and men would be randomly assigned, separately, to the two treatment conditions. After the experimental period, each subject would be required to report the number of cigarettes smoked. Some fictitious data for this problem are shown in Table 18-4.

With two independent variables, there are several hypotheses to be tested. First, we are testing whether, for both genders, behavior modification is more effective than hypnosis as a means of reducing smoking, or vice versa. Second, we are testing whether smoking behavior after an intervention is different for men and women, irrespective of the type of treatment. Third, we are examining the differential effect of the two treatments on men and women. This last hypothesis is the *interaction hypothesis*. Interaction is concerned with whether the effect of one independent variable is consistent for every level of a second independent variable. In other words, do the two interventions have the same effect on both genders?

Table 18-4.   *Fictitious Data for a Two-Way (2 × 2) ANOVA*

FACTOR B—GENDER	FACTOR A—TREATMENT			
	BEHAVIOR MODIFICATION (1)		**HYPNOSIS (2)**	
Female (1)	24 28 22 19 27 25 18 21 0 36	Group 1 $\bar{X} = 22.0$	27 0 45 19 22 23 18 20 12 14	Group 2 $\bar{X} = 20.0$	Females $\bar{X}_{B1} = 21.0$
Male (2)	10 21 17 0 33 16 18 13 15 17	Group 3 $\bar{X} = 16.0$	36 31 28 32 25 22 19 30 35 42	Group 4 $\bar{X} = 30.0$	Males $\bar{X}_{B2} = 23.0$
	Treatment 1 $\bar{X}_{A1} = 19$		Treatment 2 $\bar{X}_{A2} = 25$		$\bar{X}_T = 22$

The data in Table 18-4 reveal that, overall, subjects in treatment 1 smoked less than those in treatment 2 (19.0 versus 25.0); that women smoked less than men (21.0 versus 23.0); and that men smoked less when exposed to treatment 1, but women smoked less when exposed to treatment 2. By performing a two-way ANOVA on these data, it would be possible to ascertain the statistical significance of these differences.

Multifactor ANOVA is an extremely important analytic technique. Human behaviors, conditions, and feelings are complex, and the ability to examine the combined effects of two or more independent variables permits this complexity to be incorporated into research designs. Multifactor ANOVA is not restricted to two-way schemes. Theoretically, any number of independent variables is possible, although in practice, studies with more than three or four factors are rare because of the large number of subjects required and the complexity of the design.

Repeated-Measures Analysis of Variance

Repeated-measures ANOVA (sometimes referred to as *within-subjects ANOVA*) is used in several circumstances. First, it is used when there are three or more measures of the same dependent variable for each subject. As discussed in Chapter 8, a repeated-measures experimental design is sometimes used to expose subjects to two or more treatment conditions, with subjects essentially acting as their own controls. When there are only two such conditions—that is, when subjects are exposed to both treatment A and treatment B, with order of exposure determined at random—then a paired *t*-test can be used. However, when there are three or more treatment conditions, a repeated-measures ANOVA is required.

Second, repeated-measures ANOVA is used when multiple measures of the same dependent variable are collected longitudinally at several points in time. For instance, in some studies, physiologic measures such as blood

pressure or heart rate might be collected before, during, and after some medical procedure.

In many applications of repeated-measures ANOVA, there are two or more groups, with two or more measures of the dependent variable collected for each subject. For example, suppose we collected heart rate data before (T1), during (T2), and after (T3) surgery for subjects randomly assigned to an experimental and a control group. Structurally, the ANOVA for analyzing these data would look similar to a multifactor ANOVA, although the calculations would differ. An *F*-statistic would be computed to test for differences in the treatment factor (experimental subjects versus controls), known as the *between-subjects effect*. This statistic would indicate whether, across all time periods, the mean heart rate differed for experimental subjects and controls. Another *F*-statistic would be computed to test for differences across time (T1, T2, T3), known as the *within-subjects effect*. This statistic would indicate whether, across both treatment groups, the mean heart rates differed before, during, and after surgery. Finally, an interaction effect would be tested to determine whether there was a differential treatment effect at different points in time. Given the many situations in which nurse researchers collect data from subjects at multiple time points, repeated-measures ANOVA represents an important analytic tool.

Nonparametric "Analysis of Variance"

Nonparametric tests do not, strictly speaking, analyze variance. There are, however, nonparametric procedures analogous to the parametric ANOVA for use with ordinal-level data or when a markedly nonnormal distribution renders parametric tests inadvisable. When the number of groups is greater than two and a one-way test for independent samples is desired, one may use a statistic developed by statisticians Kruskal and Wallis. The *Kruskal-Wallis test* is a generalized version of the Mann-Whitney *U* test, based on the assignment of ranks to the scores from the various groups. When the researcher is working with paired groups, or when several measures are obtained from a single sample, then the *Friedman test* for "analysis of variance" by ranks may be applied. These tests are described in Hays (1988) and Siegel (1988).

❖ TESTING DIFFERENCES IN PROPORTIONS

The tests we have examined thus far all involve dependent variables measured on an interval or ratio scale, where mean differences between groups are being compared. In this section, we examine procedures for testing group differences when the dependent variable is measured on a nominal scale.

The Chi-Square Test

The *chi-square* statistic is used when we have categories of data and hypotheses concerning the proportions of cases that fall into the various categories. In Chapter 17, we discussed the construction of contingency tables to describe the frequencies of cases falling in different classes. The chi-square (χ^2) statistic is applied to contingency tables to test the significance of different proportions.

Consider the following example. A researcher is interested in studying the effect of planned nursing instruction on patients' compliance with a self-medication regimen. An experimental group of 100 patients is instructed by nurses who are implementing the new instructional approach. A control group of 100 patients is cared for by nurses who continue their usual mode of instruction. The hypothesis being tested is that a higher proportion of subjects in the experimental group will report self-medication compliance than will subjects in the control group.

The chi-square statistic is computed by comparing two sets of frequencies: observed frequencies (i.e., those observed in the data) and expected frequencies. *Observed frequencies* for the example are shown in Table 18-5. As this table shows, 60 out of 100 experimental subjects (60%) but only 40 out of 100 controls (40%) reported self-medication compliance. The chi-square test will enable us to decide whether a difference in proportions of this magnitude is likely to reflect a real experimental effect or only chance fluctuations. *Expected frequencies* are calculated on the basis of the observed total frequencies for the rows and columns of a contingency table: they represent the values in the cells of the contingency table that would be obtained if there were absolutely no relationship between the two variables. In this example, if there were no relationship between treatment group and compliance, the expected frequency would be 50 subjects per cell.

The chi-square statistic is computed* by summarizing differences between observed and expected frequencies for each cell. In our example, there are four cells, and thus χ^2 will be the sum of four numbers. More specifically, $\chi^2 = 8.00$ in the current case. As usual, we need to compare this test statistic with the value from a theoretical chi-square distribution. A table of chi-square values for various degrees of freedom and significance levels is provided in Table B-3, Appendix B. For the chi-square statistic, the degrees of freedom are equal to $(R - 1) \times (C - 1)$, or the number of rows minus 1 times the number of columns minus 1. In the current case, $df = 1 \times 1$, or 1. With 1 degree of freedom, the value that must be exceeded to establish significance at the .05 level is 3.84. The obtained value of 8.00 is substantially larger than would be ex-

---

* The formula for the χ^2 statistic is

$$\chi^2 = \Sigma \frac{(f_O - f_E)^2}{f_E}$$

where f_O = observed frequency for a cell
f_E = expected frequency for a cell
Σ = sum of the $(f_O - f_E)^2/f_E$ ratios for all cells

$$f_E = \frac{f_R f_C}{N}$$

where f_R = observed frequency for the given row
f_C = observed frequency for the given column
N = total number of subjects

Table 18-5. *Observed Frequencies for Chi-Square Example*

PATIENT COMPLIANCE	EXPERIMENTAL GROUP	CONTROL GROUP	TOTAL
Compliant	60	40	100
Noncompliant	40	60	100
TOTAL	100	100	200

pected by chance. Thus, we can conclude that a significantly larger proportion of patients in the experimental group than in the control group complied with self-medication instructions.

Other Tests of Proportions

In certain situations, it may be inappropriate to calculate a chi-square statistic. When the total sample size is small (total *N* of 30 or under) or when there are cells with a value of 0, *Fisher's exact test* is usually used to test the significance of differences in proportions. Also, when the proportions being compared are derived from two dependent or paired groups (e.g., when a pretest–posttest design is used to compare changes in proportions on a nominal-level dichotomous variable), then the appropriate test is the *McNemar test*.

❖ TESTING RELATIONSHIPS BETWEEN TWO VARIABLES

All the procedures we have discussed thus far involve the comparison of two or more *groups;* that is, they involve situations in which the independent variable is a nominal-level variable with a fairly small number of values. In this section, we consider statistical tests for situations in which the independent variable is measured on a higher level of measurement.

Pearson's r

In Chapter 17, the computation and interpretation of the Pearson product–moment correlation coefficient were explained. Pearson's *r*, which is calculated when two variables are measured on at least the interval scale, is both a descriptive and inferential statistic. As a descriptive statistic, the correlation coefficient summarizes the magnitude and direction of a relationship between two variables. As an inferential statistic, *r* is used to test hypotheses concerning population correlations, which are ordinarily symbolized by the Greek letter rho, or ρ. The most commonly tested null hypothesis is that there is no relationship between two variables. Stated formally,

$$H_0: \rho = \phi \qquad H_A: \rho \neq \phi$$

For instance, suppose we were studying the relationship between patients' self-reported level of stress (higher stress scores imply more stress) and the pH level of their saliva. With a sample of 50 subjects, we find that $r = -.29$. This value implies that there was a slight tendency for people who received higher stress scores to have lower pH levels than those with lower stress scores. But we need to question whether this finding can be generalized to the population. Does the coefficient of $-.29$ reflect a random fluctuation, reflecting only the particular group of subjects sampled, or is the relationship significant? The table of significant values in

Table B-4, Appendix B, allows us to make the determination. Degrees of freedom for correlation coefficients are equal to the number of subjects minus 2, or $(n - 2)$. With $df = 48$, the critical value for r (for a two-tailed test with $\alpha = .05$) lies between .2732 and .2875, or about .2803. Because the absolute value of the calculated r is .29, the null hypothesis can be rejected. Therefore, we may conclude that there is significant relationship between a person's self-reported level of stress and the acidity of his or her saliva.

Other Tests of Bivariate Relationships

Pearson's r is a parametric statistic. When the assumptions for a parametric test are violated, or when the data are inherently ordinal-level, then the appropriate coefficient of correlation is either *Spearman's rho* or *Kendall's tau*. The values of these statistics range from -1.00 to $+1.00$, and their interpretation is similar to that of Pearson's r.

Measures of the magnitude of relationships can also be computed with nominal-level data. For example, the *phi coefficient* (ϕ) is an index describing the relationship between two dichotomous variables. *Cramer's V* is an index of relationship applied to contingency tables larger than 2×2. Both of these statistics are based on the chi-square statistic and yield values that range between 0.0 and 1.00, with higher values indicating a stronger association between variables.

❖ THE COMPUTER AND INFERENTIAL STATISTICS

As in Chapter 17, we have stressed the logic and uses of various statistics rather than their computational formulas and mathematic derivations.* Because the computer is increasingly called on to perform the computations for hypothesis test-

---

* Note that this introduction to inferential statistics has necessarily been superficial. We urge novice researchers to undertake further exploration of statistical principles.

ing, and because it is important to be able to make sense of the printed information produced by the computer, we include in this chapter examples of computer-produced information for two statistical tests.

We return to the example described in Chapter 17. A researcher has designed an experiment to test the effect of a special prenatal program on a group of young, low-income women. The raw data for the 30 subjects in this example were presented in Table 17-8 in Chapter 17. Given these data, let us test some hypotheses.

Hypothesis One: t-Test

Let us suppose that our first research hypothesis is as follows:

The babies of the experimental subjects will have higher birthweights than the babies of the control subjects.

In this example, there are two independent groups of subjects, and differences in the mean birthweights are being compared. Therefore, the *t*-test for independent samples is used to test our hypothesis. The null and alternative hypotheses can be stated as follows:

H_0: μ experimental = μ control
H_A: μ experimental $\neq$ μ control

Figure 18-5 presents the computer printout for the *t*-test. The top of the figure presents some basic descriptive statistics for the birthweight variable, separately for the two groups. Thus, the mean birthweight of the babies in group 1 (the experimental group) was 107.53 ounces, compared with 101.87 ounces for the babies in group 2 (the control group). These data, then, are consistent with our research hypothesis—the average weight of the experimental subjects is higher than the average weight of the controls. But do the differences reflect the impact of the experimental intervention, or do they merely represent random fluctuations? To answer this, we examine the results of the *t*-test,

```
t-test for:  WEIGHT    INFANT BIRTH WEIGHT

                Number              Standard    Standard
                of Cases    Mean    Deviation    Error

     Group 1      15      107.5333    13.378     3.454
     Group 2      15      101.8667     7.239     1.869


          Pooled Variance Estimate

           t     Degrees of  2-Tail
         Value    Freedom    Prob.

          1.44      28        .160
```

Figure 18–5. *SPSS Computer Printout:* t-*Test*

shown under the heading "Pooled Variance Estimate." The computer program calculated the value of *t* as 1.44. With 28 degrees of freedom [(15 + 15) − 2], this value is not significant. The two-tailed probability (*p* value) for this *t* statistic is .16. This means that in 16 samples out of 100, one could expect to find a difference in weights at least this large as a result of chance alone. Therefore, since *p* > .05 (a nonsignificant result), we cannot conclude that the special intervention was effective in improving the birthweights of the experimental group.*

Hypothesis Two: Pearson Correlation

A second research hypothesis might involve the relationship between maternal age and the infant's birthweight, and is stated as follows:

Older mothers will have babies of higher birthweight than younger mothers.

In this case, both birthweight and age are measured on the ratio scale, and the appropriate test statistic is the Pearson product–moment correlation. The hypotheses subjected to the statistical test are

H_0: ρ birthweight—age = 0
H_A: ρ birthweight—age $\neq$ 0

The printout for the test of the hypothesis is presented in Figure 18-6. The correlation matrix in Figure 18-6 shows, in row one, the correlation of weight with weight and of weight with age; and in row two, the correlation of age with weight and of age with age. The correlation of interest to us for testing the hypothesis is weight with age (or age with weight—the result is the same). At the intersection of these two variables, we find three numbers. The first is the actual correlation coefficient, and the second shows the number of cases. In our example, $r = .5938$ and $n = 30$. The correlation indicates a moderately strong positive relationship: The older the mother, the higher the baby's weight tends to be, as hypothesized. Again, the data are consistent with the research hypothesis, but does this reflect a true relationship or merely chance fluctuations in the data? The third number at the intersection of age and weight shows the probability that the correlation occurred by chance: S (for significance level) = .000. The printout only shows significance (*p*) levels to the nearest thousandth. In this case, the actual *p* value might be .0004 or .000001, but we do not know the real value. We *do* know, however, that $p < .001$. In other words, a relationship this strong would be found by chance alone in fewer than 1 out of 1000 samples of 30 young mothers. Therefore, the research hypothesis is accepted.

---

*The average difference in birthweights is fairly sizable and in the hypothesized direction. The researcher may wish to pursue this study by increasing the sample size or by controlling some other variables, such as the mother's age, through analysis of covariance (see Chapter 19).

```
Correlations:   WEIGHT       AGE

    WEIGHT      1.0000      .5938
                (   30)     (   30)
                P= .        P= .000

    AGE          .5938     1.0000
                (   30)     (   30)
                P= .000     P= .


(Coefficient / (Cases) / 1-tailed Significance)

" . " is printed if a coefficient cannot be computed
```

Figure 18–6. *SPSS Computer Printout: Pearson Correlation Coefficients*

❖ TIPS FOR USING INFERENTIAL STATISTICS

Most quantitative nursing studies use one of the statistical tests described in this chapter. It is essential for both consumers and producers of research to understand the logic underlying statistical tests and to be familiar with the interpretation of results from such tests. In this section, we offer further guidance relating to the use of inferential statistics.

- Statistical tests are designed to help researchers distinguish "real" relationships from random fluctuations that inevitably occur when data are collected from a sample. Statistical tests use the concept of a standard error to evaluate whether a result is likely to reflect random fluctuations, and all standard errors are directly affected by the size of the sample. Seen in this light, it should be clear that researchers run a risk of a large standard error when they use small samples. Or, put another way, a small sample size increases the likelihood that a Type II error will be committed. That is, when small samples are used, the researcher takes a sizable risk that the test will result in a rejection of the research hypothesis—even when the hypothesis is, in fact, correct. Thus, small samples should generally be avoided in quantitative studies that use inferential statistics.
- When a statistical test indicates that the null hypothesis should be retained (i.e., when the results are nonsignificant), this is sometimes referred to as a *negative result*. Negative results are often disappointing to researchers and may in some cases lead to the rejection of a manuscript by a journal editor. Research reports with negative results are not rejected because editors are prejudiced against certain types of outcomes; they are rejected because negative results are generally inconclusive and therefore difficult to interpret. A nonsignificant result simply indicates that the result *could* have occurred as a result of chance but offers no firm evidence that the research hypothesis is *not* correct.
- The selection and use of a statistical test depends on several factors, such as the measurement level of the variables, the sample size, the number of groups being compared, and the shape of the distribution of the dependent variable. To aid researchers in selecting a test statistic or evaluating statistical procedures used by researchers in the literature, a chart summarizing the major features of several commonly used tests is presented in Table 18-6.
- Among the more important factors to consider in selecting a statistical test is the level of measurement of the independent and dependent variables. Although we have advised that variables should generally be measured on as high a measurement scale as possible, there may be situations when it is appropriate to convert data to a lower level of measurement. For example, Parker and

Table 18-6. *Summary of Statistical Tests*

NAME OF PROCEDURE	TEST STATISTIC	DEGREES OF FREEDOM	PARAMETRIC (P) OR NON-PARAMETRIC (NP)	PURPOSE	LEVELS OF MEASUREMENT Variable 1 (Independent)	LEVELS OF MEASUREMENT Variable 2 (Dependent)
t-Test for independent samples	t	$n_{\text{Group A}} + n_{\text{Group B}} - 2$	P	To test the difference between the means of two independent groups	Nominal	Interval or ratio
t-Test for dependent (paired) samples	t	$n - 1$	P	To test the difference between the means of two related groups or sets of scores	Nominal	Interval or ratio
Median Test	χ^2	$(\text{Rows} - 1) \times (\text{Columns} - 1)$	NP	To test the difference between the medians of two independent groups	Nominal	Ordinal
Mann-Whitney *U* Test	U (Z)	$n - 1$	NP	To test the difference in the ranks of scores of two independent groups	Nominal	Ordinal
Wilcoxon Signed-Rank Test	Z	$n - 2$	NP	To test the difference in the ranks of scores of two related groups or sets of scores	Nominal	Ordinal
ANOVA	F	Between: n of groups $- 1$ Within: n of subjects $- n$ of groups	P	To test the difference among the means of three or more independent groups, or of more than one independent variable	Nominal	Interval or ratio
Kruskal-Wallis Test	H (χ^2)	n of groups $- 1$	NP	To test the difference in the ranks of scores of three or more independent groups	Nominal	Ordinal

Test	Statistic	df	P/NP	Purpose		
Friedman Test	χ^2	n of groups $-$ 1	NP	To test the difference in the ranks of scores for three or more related sets of scores	Nominal	Ordinal
Chi-Square Test	χ^2	(Row $-$ 1) $\times$ (Columns $-$ 1)	NP	To test the difference in proportion in two or more groups	Nominal	Nominal
McNemar's Test	χ^2	1	NP	To test the differences in proportions for paired samples (2 $\times$ 2)	Nominal	Nominal
Fisher's Exact Test	†	†	NP	To test the difference in proportions in a 2 $\times$ 2 contingency table when N $<$ 30	Nominal	Nominal
Pearson Product–moment correlation	r	$n - 2$	P	To test that a correlation is different from zero (i.e., that a relationship exists)	Interval or ratio	Interval or ratio
Spearman's rho	ρ	$n - 2$	NP	To test that a correlation is different from zero (i.e., that a relationship exists)	Ordinal	Ordinal
Kendall's tau	τ	$n - 2$	NP	To test that a correlation is different from zero (i.e., that a relationship exists)	Ordinal	Ordinal
Phi coefficient	ϕ	1*	NP	To examine the magnitude of a relationship between two dichotomous variables (2 $\times$ 2)	Nominal	Nominal
Cramer's V	V	(R $-$ 1) $\times$ (C $-$ 1)*	NP	To examine the magnitude of a relationship between variables in a contingency table (not restricted to 2 $\times$ 2)	Nominal	Nominal

* The test that $\phi \neq 0$ (or $V \neq 0$) is provided by the χ^2 test.
† Fisher's Exact Test computes exact probabilities directly.

her colleagues (1993) studied the incidence of physical and mental abuse among pregnant women, comparing pregnant women who were teenagers to women who were older. In this study, age—a continuous, ratio-level variable—was collapsed into a dichotomous variable (teenaged versus adult). When there is reason to believe that a relationship between variables is not linear, it is often better to transform one of the variables. By *linear*, we mean that changes in one variable are not incrementally affected by changes in the other variable at every point along the measurement scale. In this case, for example, although the researchers hypothesized that very young women might be at especially high risk of abuse, they did not hypothesize differences at older ages (e.g., that 25-year-old women would be at higher risk than 30-year-old women). If age and abuse were linearly related, abuse would diminish at successive ages, but this is clearly an unlikely situation. By collapsing ages into two groups, the researchers were better able to test their hypotheses.

❖ RESEARCH EXAMPLES

The inferential statistics discussed in this chapter have been used in thousands of nursing studies. Some examples illustrating the use of these statistics are presented in Table 18-7. One research example is described in greater detail next.

> Fogel and Martin (1992) studied the mental health of incarcerated women who either were or were not mothers. Data were collected from a sample of 46 women (35 had children) at two points in time: within 1 week of the subjects' imprisonment, and then 6 months later. Two scales were administered to assess mental health: the Center for Epidemiological Studies Depression (CES-D) Scale and the Spielberger State Anxiety Inventory (STAI).
>
> The data were analyzed using two repeated-measures ANOVAs—one for each dependent variable. In these analyses, motherhood status served as one factor, while time of administration of the scales (1 week versus

6 months after imprisonment) was the second factor. For the STAI scores, the analyses revealed a significant main effect for time ($F = 11.35$; $df = 1, 44$; $p = .002$). For the sample as a whole, anxiety levels decreased significantly over the 6 months of imprisonment. A significant interaction effect ($F = 5.06$; $df = 1, 44$; $p = .029$) indicated that, while anxiety declined over time for both groups, the mean STAI scores for the nonmothers declined more than that for the mothers. The main effect comparing mothers and nonmothers on the STAI scale was nonsignificant.

> With respect to depression scores, there were no statistically significant main effects for time or motherhood, and no interaction effects. Levels of depression were found to be high for both groups at both testing points.

❖ SUMMARY

Inferential statistics enable a researcher to make inferences about the characteristics of a population based on data obtained in a sample. The reason that we cannot make such inferences directly from the data is that sample statistics inevitably contain a certain degree of error as estimates of population parameters. Inferential statistics offer the researcher a framework for deciding whether the sampling error is too high to provide reliable population estimates.

The *sampling distribution* of the mean is a theoretical distribution of the means of many different samples drawn from the same population. When an infinite number of samples is drawn from a population, the sampling distribution of means follows a normal curve. Because of this characteristic, it is possible to indicate the probability that a specified sample value will be obtained. The *standard error of the mean* is the standard deviation of the theoretical sampling distribution of the mean. This index indicates the degree of average error in a sample mean as an estimate of the population mean. The smaller the SEM, the more accurate are the estimates of the population value. Sampling distributions are the basis for inferential statistics.

Statistical inference consists of two major types of approaches: estimating parameters and testing hypotheses. When a researcher wants to discover the value of an unknown population

Table 18-7.   *Examples of Statistical Tests Used by Nurse Researchers*

STATISTICAL TEST	RESEARCH HYPOTHESIS	VALUE OF STATISTIC	p VALUE
t-Test, independent samples	Pregnant women who self-administer epidural analgesia will use less total fentanyl than women in the control group with nurse-administered boluses (Gordon, Gaines, & Hauber, 1994)	$t = -2.96$	<.001
t-Test, dependent samples	Nonnutritive sucking in intubated infants will reduce the increase in the heart rate after onset of cry (Miller & Anderson, 1993)	$t = 9.28$	<.0005
Mann-Whitney *U* Test	Colectomy patients who receive a preoperative bolus of epidural morphine will request their first on-demand postoperative analgesic later than patients who do not have a preoperative bolus of epidural morphine (Simpson, Wahl, DeTraglia, Speck, & Taylor, 1993)	$U = 0$	<.005
ANOVA	Perception of the birth experience differs for women with different types of delivery: vaginal, planned cesarean, unplanned cesarean (Fawcett, Pollio, & Tully, 1992)	$F = 8.74$	<.001
Chi-Square Test	Shortness of breath symptoms differ among acute myocardial infarction patients of different ethnicities (Neill, 1993)	$\chi^2 = 9.58$	<.05
Pearson's *r*	Client-focused nursing problems are related to the patient's: • Mental status • Coping ability • Physical abilities (Helberg, 1993)	$r = .14$ $r = -.44$ $r = -.28$	<.01 <.001 <.001
Spearman's rho	Severity of erythema and severity of edema of nipple skin during the first week of breast-feeding are correlated (Ziemer & Pigeon, 1993)	$\rho = .41$	<.01

characteristic, he or she may estimate the value by means of either point or interval estimation. *Point estimation* provides a single numerical value. *Interval estimation* provides the upper and lower limits of a range of values between which the population value is expected to fall, at some specified probability level. The researcher is able to establish the degree of confidence that the population value will lie within this range. Interval estimates are often referred to as *confidence intervals*.

The testing of hypotheses by statistical procedures enables researchers to make objective decisions concerning the results of their studies. The *null hypothesis* is a statement that no relationship exists between the variables and that any observed relationships are the result of chance or sampling fluctuations. In hypothesis testing, failure to reject the null hypothesis means that any observed differences may be due to chance fluctuations. Rejection of the null hypothesis lends support to the research hypothesis.

428 18 · INFERENTIAL STATISTICS

When a researcher fails to reject a null hypothesis that should be rejected, the error is referred to as a *Type II error.* If a null hypothesis is rejected when it should not be rejected, then the error is called a *Type I error.* Researchers are able to control the risk of committing a Type I error by establishing a *level of significance,* which indicates the probability of making a Type I error. The two most commonly used levels of significance (designated as the α level) are .05 and .01. A significance level of .01 means that in only 1 out of 100 samples will the null hypothesis be rejected when, in fact, it should be retained.

Researchers report the results of hypothesis testing as being either statistically significant or nonsignificant. The phrase *statistically significant* means that the obtained results are not likely to be the result of chance fluctuations at the specified level of probability. Although most hypothesis testing involves *two-tailed tests,* in which both ends of the sampling distribution are used to define the region of improbable values, a *one-tailed test* may be appropriate if the researcher has a strong rationale for a directional hypothesis.

Statistical tests are classified as parametric and nonparametric. *Nonparametric tests* require less stringent assumptions than parametric tests and usually are used when the level of data is either nominal or ordinal or when the distribution is not normal. *Parametric tests* involve the estimation of at least one parameter, the use of data measured on an interval or ratio level, and assumptions concerning the variables under consideration. Parametric tests are usually more powerful than nonparametric tests and generally are preferred.

The most common parametric procedures are the *t*-test and *analysis of variance,* both of which can be used to test the significance of the difference between groups means. The *t*-test can only be applied to two-group situations, whereas the ANOVA procedure can handle three or more groups as well as more than one independent variable. Nonparametric analogues of these parametric tests include the *median test,* the *Mann-Whitney U test,* the *sign test,* and

the *Wilcoxon signed-rank test* (two-group situations), and the *Kruskal-Wallis* and *Friedman tests* (three-group or more situations). The nonparametric test that is used most frequently is the *chi-square test,* which is used in connection with hypotheses relating to differences in proportions. Statistical tests to measure the magnitude of bivariate relationships and test whether the relationship is significantly different from zero include Pearson's *r* for interval-level data, *Spearman's rho* and *Kendall's tau* for ordinal-level data, and the *phi coefficient* and *Cramer's V* for nominal-level data.

❖ STUDY SUGGESTIONS

Chapter 18 of the accompanying *Study Guide for Nursing Research: Principles and Methods, 5th ed.,* offers various exercises and study suggestions for reinforcing the concepts presented in this chapter. Additionally, the following study questions can be addressed:

1. A researcher has administered a Job Satisfaction Scale to a sample of 50 primary nurses and 50 team nurses. The mean score on this scale for each group was found to be 35.2 for the primary nurses and 33.6 for the team nurses. A *t*-statistic is computed and is found to be 1.89. Interpret this result, using the table for *t*-values in Appendix B.

2. Compute the chi-square statistic for the following contingency table:

	NUMBER OF COMPLICATIONS FOLLOWING SURGERY		
GROUP	**None**	**One**	**More Than One**
Experimental	38	72	54
Control	29	50	11

How many degrees of freedom are there? At the .05 level of significance, what may be concluded?

3. Given that:
   a. There are three groups of nursing school students, with 50 in each group
   b. Level of significance = .05
   c. Value of test statistic = 4.43
   d. Mean scores on test to measure motivation to attend graduate school: 25.8, 29.3, and 23.4 for groups A, B, and C, respectively

   Specify:
   a. What test statistic was used
   b. How many degrees of freedom there are
   c. Whether the test statistic is statistically significant
   d. What the test statistic means

4. What inferential statistic would you choose for the following sets of variables? Explain your answers. (Refer to Table 18-6.)
   a. Variable 1 represents the weights of 100 patients; variable 2 is the patients' resting heart rate.
   b. Variable 1 is the patients' marital status; variable 2 is the patient's level of preoperative stress.
   c. Variable 1 is whether an amputee has a leg removed above or below the knee; variable 2 is whether or not the amputee has shown signs of aggressive behavior during rehabilitation.

❖ SUGGESTED READINGS

METHODOLOGICAL REFERENCES

Abraham, I. L., Nadzam, D. M., & Fitzpatrick, J. J. (1989). *Statistics and quantitative methods in nursing.* Philadelphia: W. B. Saunders.

Armstrong, G. (1981). Parametric statistics and ordinal data: A pervasive misconception. *Nursing Research, 30,* 60–62.

Brogan, D. R. (1981). Choosing an appropriate statistical test of significance for a nursing research hypothesis or question. *Western Journal of Nursing Research, 3,* 337–363.

Hays, W. L. (1988). *Statistics for the social sciences* (4th ed.). New York: Holt, Rinehart & Winston.

Holm, K., & Christman, N. J. (1985). Post hoc tests following analysis of variance. *Research in Nursing and Health, 8,* 207–210.

Jaccard, J., & Becker, M. A. (1990). *Statistics for the behavioral sciences.* (2nd ed.). Belmont, CA: Wadsworth.

Jacobsen, B. S., Tulman, L., & Lowery, B. J. (1991). Three sides of the same coin: The analysis of paired data from dyads. *Nursing Research, 40,* 359–363.

Kanji, G. K. (1993). *100 statistical tests.* London: Sage Publications.

Liebetrau, A. M. (1983). *Measures of association.* Beverly Hills, CA: Sage.

Marks, R. G. (1982). *Analyzing research data: The basics of biomedical research methodology.* Belmont, CA: Life Long Learning.

Milton, J. S., & Tsokos, J. O. (1983). *Statistical methods in the biological and health sciences.* New York: McGraw-Hill.

Munro, B. H., & Page, E. B. (1993). *Statistical methods for health-care research* (2nd ed.). Philadelphia: J. B. Lippincott.

Sidani, S., & Lynn, M. R. (1993). Examining amount and pattern of change: Comparing repeated measures ANOVA and individual regression analysis. *Nursing Research, 42,* 283–286.

Siegel, S. (1988). *Nonparametric statistics for the behavioral sciences.* (2nd ed.). New York: McGraw-Hill.

Triola, M. (1992). *Elementary statistics* (5th ed.). Menlo Park, CA: Addison-Wesley.

Welkowitz, J., Ewen, R. B., & Cohen, J. (1990). *Introductory statistics for the behavioral sciences* (4th ed.). New York: Academic Press.

Winer, B. J. (1971). *Statistical principles in experimental design* (2nd ed.). New York: McGraw-Hill.

SUBSTANTIVE REFERENCES

Fawcett, J., Pollio, N., & Tully, A. (1992). Women's perceptions of cesarean and vaginal delivery. *Research in Nursing and Health, 15,* 439–446.

Fogel, C. I., & Martin, S. L. (1992). The mental health of incarcerated women. *Western Journal of Nursing Research, 14,* 30–47.

Gordon, S. C., Gaines, S. K., & Hauber, R. P. (1994). Self-administered versus nurse-administered epidural analgesia after cesarean section. *Journal of Obstetric, Gynecologic, and Neonatal Nursing, 23,* 99–103.

Helberg, J. L. (1993). Factors influencing home care nursing problems and nursing care. *Research in Nursing and Health, 16,* 363–370.

Miller, H. D., & Anderson, G. C. (1993). Nonnutritive sucking: Effects on crying and heart rate in intubated infants requiring assisted mechanical ventilation. *Nursing Research, 42,* 305–307.

Neill, K. M. (1993). Ethnic pain styles in acute myocardial infarction. *Western Journal of Nursing Research, 15,* 531–543.

Parker, B., McFarlane, J., Soeken, K., Torres, S., & Campbell, D. (1993). Physical and emotional abuse in pregnancy: A comparison of adult and teenage women. *Nursing Research, 42,* 173–178.

Simpson, T., Wahl, G., DeTraglia, M., Speck, E., & Taylor, D. (1993). A pilot study of pain, analgesia use, and pulmonary function after colectomy with or without a preoperative bolus of epidural morphine. *Heart and Lung, 22,* 316–327.

Ziemer, M. M., & Pigeon, J. G. (1993). Skin changes and pain in the nipple during the first week of lactation. *Journal of Obstetric, Gynecologic, and Neonatal Nursing, 22,* 247–256.

Chapter 19

ADVANCED STATISTICAL PROCEDURES

The phenomena of interest to nurse researchers are generally complex. Patients' preoperative anxieties, nurses' effectiveness in caring for people, the fears of cancer patients, or the abrupt elevation of patients' body temperature are phenomena that have multiple facets and multiple determinants. Scientists, in attempting to explain, predict, and control the phenomena that interest them, have come increasingly to the recognition that a two-variable study is often inadequate for such purposes. The classic approach to data analysis and research design, which consists of studying the effect of a single independent variable on a single dependent variable, increasingly is being replaced by more sophisticated *multivariate** procedures. Whether one structures a study to be multivariate or not, the fact remains that most nursing phenomena are essentially and unalterably multivariate in nature. The modern researcher who is unfamiliar with multivariate

* We use the term *multivariate* in this chapter to refer generally to analyses dealing with at least three variables. Some statisticians reserve the term for problems involving more than one dependent variable.

techniques is at a serious disadvantage both as a designer of research studies and as a consumer of research reports.

Unlike the statistical methods reviewed in Chapters 17 and 18, multivariate statistics are computationally formidable. However, the widespread availability of computers has made complex manual calculations obsolete. Therefore, we make minimal reference to computational formulas. The purpose of this chapter is to provide a general understanding of how, when, and why multivariate statistics are used rather than to explain their mathematic basis. References are available at the end of this chapter for those desiring more comprehensive coverage.

❖ MULTIPLE REGRESSION AND CORRELATION

Multiple regression analysis is a method used for understanding the effects of two or more independent variables on a dependent variable. The terms *multiple correlation* and *multiple regression* will be used almost interchangeably in reference to this technique, given the strong bond between correlation and regression. To comprehend the nature of this bond, we first explain simple regression—that is, bivariate regression—before turning to multiple regression.

Simple Linear Regression

Regression analysis is usually performed with the intention of making predictions about phenomena. In the health care field, as in many other fields, the ability to make accurate predictions has important implications for the quality of services rendered. For example, whenever a costly or scarce resource such as home visitation by nurses is to be allocated, it is important to be able to predict who will most benefit from that resource.

In simple regression, one independent variable (X) is used to predict a dependent variable (Y). For instance, we could use simple regression to predict weight from height, blood pressure from age, nursing school achievement from Scholastic Aptitude Test (SAT) scores, or stress from noise levels. An important feature of regression is that the higher the correlation between the two variables, the more accurate the prediction. If the correlation between diastolic and systolic blood pressure were perfect (i.e., if $r = 1.00$), then one would only need to measure one to be able to know the value of the other. Because most variables of interest to researchers are not perfectly correlated, most predictions made through regression analysis are imperfect.

A simple regression equation is a formula for making predictions about the numerical values of one variable, based on the scores or values of another variable. The basic linear regression equation is

$$Y' = a + bX$$

where Y' = predicted value of variable Y
   a = intercept constant
   b = regression coefficient (slope of the line)
   X = actual value of variable X

Regression analysis solves for a and b, so for any value of X, a prediction about Y can be made. Those readers with recollection of high school algebra may remember that the above equation is the algebraic equation for a straight line. *Linear regression* is essentially a method for determining a straight line to fit the data in such a way that deviations from the line are minimized.

An illustration may help to clarify some of these points. Data for five subjects on two variables (X and Y) are shown in columns 1 and 2 of Table 19-1. Application of the Pearson's r formula to these data reveals that the variables are strongly related, $r = .90$. What we wish to do is develop a way of predicting Y values for a *new* group of subjects from whom we will only have information on the variable X. To do this, we must use the five pairs of values to solve for a and b in the regression equation.

The formulas for these two components are as follows:

$$b = \frac{\Sigma xy}{\Sigma x^2} \qquad a = \bar{Y} - b\bar{X}$$

where b = regression coefficient
   a = intercept constant
   $\bar{Y}$ = mean of variable Y
   $\bar{X}$ = mean of variable X
   x = deviation scores from $\bar{X}$
   y = deviation scores from $\bar{Y}$

The calculations required for the various elements of these equations are worked out for the current example in columns 3 through 7 of Table 19-1. As shown at the bottom of the table, the solution to the regression equation is $Y' = 1.5 + .9X$. What does one do with this information? Suppose for the moment that the X values in column 1 were the only data available for the five subjects and that we wanted to predict the values for variable Y. For the first subject with an X = 1, we would predict that $Y' = 1.5 + (.9)(1)$, or 2.4. Column 8 shows similar computations for each X value. These numbers show that Y' does not exactly equal the actual values obtained for Y. Most of the errors of prediction (e) are small,

Table 19-1.   *Computations for Simple Linear Regression*

(1) X	(2) Y	(3) x	(4) x^2	(5) y	(6) y^2	(7) xy	(8) y'	(9) e	(10) e^2
1	2	−4	16	−4	16	16	2.4	−.4	.16
3	6	−2	4	0	0	0	4.2	1.8	3.24
5	4	0	0	−2	4	0	6.0	−2.0	4.00
7	8	2	4	2	4	4	7.8	.2	.04
9	10	4	16	4	16	16	9.6	.4	.16
$\Sigma X = 25$	$\Sigma Y = 30$		40		40	36		0.0	7.60
$\bar{X} = 5.0$	$\bar{Y} = 6.0$								$\Sigma e^2 = 7.60$

$$r = .90$$

$$b = \frac{\Sigma xy}{\Sigma x^2} = \frac{36}{40} = .90$$

$$a = \bar{Y} - b\bar{X} = 6.0 - (.9)(5.0) = 1.5$$
$$Y' = a + bX$$
$$Y' = 1.5 + .9X$$

as shown in column 9. The errors of prediction result from the fact that the correlation between X and Y is not perfect. Only when $r = 1.00$ or -1.00 does $Y' = Y$. The regression equation solves for *a* and *b* in such a way as to minimize such errors. Or, more precisely, the solution minimizes the sums of squares of the prediction errors, which is why standard regression analysis is said to use a *least-squares principle* (standard regression is sometimes referred to as *ordinary least squares,* or *OLS, regression*). In column 10 of Table 19-1, the error terms—usually referred to as the *residuals*—have been squared and summed to yield a value of 7.60. Any values of *a* and *b* other than those obtained above would have yielded a larger sum of the squared residuals.

The solution to this regression analysis example is displayed graphically in Figure 19-1. The actual X and Y values from the table are plotted on the graph with circles. The line running through these points is the representation of the regression solution. The intercept (*a*) is the point at which the line crosses the Y axis, which in this case is 1.5. The slope (*b*) is the angle of the line, relative to the X and Y axes.

With $b = .90$, the line slopes in such a fashion that for every 4 units on the X axis, we must go up 3.6 units ($.9 \times 4$) on the Y axis. The line, then, embodies the whole regression equation. To find a predicted value for Y, we could go to the point on the X axis for an obtained X score, find the point on the regression line vertically above the score, and read the predicted Y value horizontally from the Y axis. For example, with an X value of 5, we would predict a Y' of 6, as shown by the star designating that point on the figure.

The connection between correlation and regression can be made more evident by pointing out an important aspect of a correlation coefficient. The correlation coefficient, it may be recalled, is an index of the degree to which variables are related. Relationships, from a statistical point of view, are concerned with how variations in one variable are associated with variations in another. The *r* statistic enables us to specify how much variability can be explained or accounted for by two correlated variables. The square of r (r^2) tells us the proportion of the variance in Y that can be accounted for by X. In the previous example, $r = .90$, so $r^2 = .81$. This

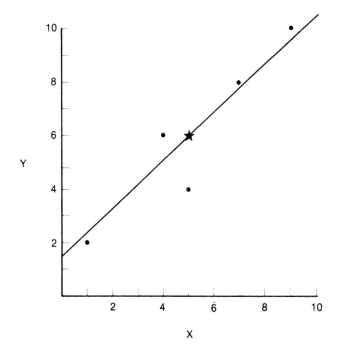

Figure 19-1.   *Example of simple linear regression*

means that 81% of the variability in the Y values can be understood in terms of the variability in the X values. The remaining 19% constitutes variability resulting from other sources.

Returning to the regression problem, it was found that the sum of the squared residuals (error terms) was 7.6. Column 6 of Table 19-1 also informs us that the sum of the squared deviations of the Y values from the mean of Y (Σy^2) was 40. To demonstrate that the residuals constitute 19% of the unexplained variability in Y, we can compute the following ratio:

$$\frac{7.6}{40} = .19 = 1 - r^2$$

Although the computations are not shown, the sum of the squared deviations of the Y′ values from the mean of Y′ $(\Sigma y'^2)$ is equal to 32.4. As a proportion of the variability in the *actual* Y values, this would equal

$$\frac{32.4}{40} = .81 = r^2$$

These calculations reinforce a point made earlier: The stronger the correlation, the better is the prediction. To put this another way, the stronger the correlation, the greater is the percentage of variance explained.

Multiple Linear Regression

Because the correlation between two variables rarely is perfect, it is often desirable to try to improve one's ability to predict a Y value by including more than one X as predictor variables. Suppose that we were interested in predicting graduate nursing students' grade point averages (GPA). Because there are a limited number of students who can be accepted into graduate programs, there is naturally a concern for selecting those individuals who will have the greatest chance of success. Suppose from previous experience it had been found that those students who performed well on the verbal portion of the Graduate Record Examination (GRE) tended to obtain higher grades in graduate school than those with lower GRE scores. The correlation between the GRE verbal scores (GRE-V) and graduate GPAs has been calculated as .50. With only 25% ($.50^2$) of the variance of graduate GPA accounted for, there will be many errors of prediction made: many admitted students will not perform as well as desired, and many rejected applicants would have made successful students. It may be possible, by using additional information about students, to make more accurate predictions. Multiple regression can assist us by developing an equation that provides the best prediction possible, given the correlations among several variables. The basic multiple regression equation is

$$Y' = a + b_1X_1 + b_2X_2 + \ldots b_kX_k$$

where Y' = predicted value for variable Y
   a = intercept constant
   k = number of predictor (independent) variables
   b_1 to b_k = regression coefficients for the k variables
   X_1 to X_k = scores or values on the k independent variables

When the number of predictor variables exceeds two, the computations required to solve this equation are prohibitively laborious and complex. Therefore, we will restrict our discussion to hypothetical rather than worked-out examples.

In the example in which we wished to predict graduate nursing students' GPAs, suppose we decided that information on undergraduate GPA (GPA-U) and scores on the quantitative portion of the GRE (GRE-Q) would improve our ability to predict graduate GPA. The resulting equation might be

$$Y' = .4 + .05(GPA-U) + .003(GRE-Q) + .002(GRE-V)$$

For instance, suppose an applicant had a GRE verbal score of 600, a GRE quantitative score of 550, and an undergraduate GPA of 3.2. The predicted graduate GPA would be

$$Y' = .4 + (.05)(3.2) + .003(550) + .002(600) = 3.41$$

We can assess the degree to which the addition of two independent variables improved our ability to predict graduate school performance through the use of the multiple correlation coefficient. In bivariate correlation, the index expressing the magnitude of a relationship is Pearson's r. When two or more independent variables are used, the index of correlation is the multiple correlation coefficient, symbolized as R. Unlike r, R does not have negative values. R varies only from 0.0 to 1.0, showing the *strength* of the relationship between several independent variables and a dependent variable but not *direction*. It would make no sense to indicate direction, because X_1 could be positively related to Y, and X_2 could be negatively related to Y. The R statistic, when squared, indicates the proportion of variance in Y accounted for by the combined simultaneous influence of the independent variables. Sometimes R^2 is referred to as the *coefficient of determination.*

The calculation of R^2 provides a direct means of evaluating the accuracy of the prediction equation. Let us say that with the three predictor variables used in the current example, the value of $R = .71$. This means that 50% ($.71^2$) of the variability in graduate students' grades can be explained in terms of their verbal and quantitative GRE scores and their undergraduate grades. The addition of two predictors doubled the variance accounted for by the single independent variable, from .25 to .50.

The multiple correlation coefficient cannot be less than the highest bivariate correlation between the dependent variable and one of the independent variables. Table 19-2 presents a correlation matrix that shows the Pearson correlation coefficients for all the variables in this example, taken as pairs. The independent variable that is correlated most strongly with graduate performance is undergraduate grade point average (GPA-U), $r = .60$. The value of R could not have been less than .60.

Another important point is that R tends to be larger when the independent variables have

Table 19-2.   *Correlation Matrix*

	GPA-GRAD	GPA-U	GRE-Q	GRE-V
GPA-GRAD	1.00			
GPA-U	.60	1.00		
GRE-Q	.55	.40	1.00	
GRE-V	.50	.50	.70	1.00

GPA-GRAD, graduate GPA; GPA-U, undergraduate GPA; GRE-Q, GRE quantitative score; GRE-V, GRE verbal score.

relatively low correlations among themselves. In the current case, the lowest correlation coefficient is between GRE-Q and GPA-U ($r = .40$), and the highest is between GRE-Q and GRE-V ($r = .70$). All correlations here are fairly substantial, a fact that helps to explain why R is not much higher than the r between the dependent variable and undergraduate grades alone (.71 compared with .60). This somewhat puzzling phenomenon can be explained in terms of redundancy of information among predictors.

When correlations among the independent variables are high, they tend to add little predictive power to each other because they are redundant. When the correlations among the predictor variables are low, each variable has the ability to contribute something unique to the prediction of the dependent variable.

In Figure 19-2, a Venn diagram illustrates this concept. Each circle represents the total variability inherent in a variable. The circle on the left (Y) is the dependent variable, graduate GPA, whose values we are trying to predict. The overlap between this circle and the other circles represents the amount of variability that the variables have in common. If the overlap were complete—that is, if the entire graduate GPA circle were covered by the other circles—then R would equal 1.00. As it is, only 50% of the circle is covered, because $R^2 = .50$. The hatched area on this figure designates the independent contribution of undergraduate GPA toward explaining graduate performance. This contribution amounts to 36% of Y's variance ($.60^2$). The remaining two independent variables do not con-

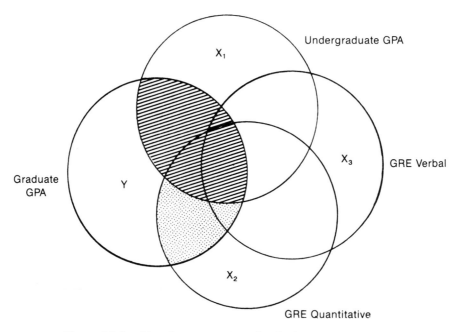

Figure 19-2.   *Visual representation of multiple regression example*

tribute as much as one would anticipate by considering their bivariate correlation with graduate GPA (r for GRE-V $= .50$; r for GRE-Q $= .55$). In fact, their combined additional contribution is only 14% ($.50 - .36 = .14$), designated by the dotted area on the figure. The contribution is small because the two GRE scores have redundant information once the undergraduate grades are taken into account. The implication of this principle is that in selecting predictor variables, the researcher should choose independent variables that are strongly correlated with the dependent variable but moderately correlated with each other.

A related point about multiple correlation is that, as more independent variables are added to the regression equation, the increment to R tends to decrease. It is rare to find many predictor variables that correlate well with a criterion measure and correlate only slightly with one another. Redundancy is difficult to avoid as more and more variables are added to the prediction equation. The inclusion of independent variables beyond the first four or five typically does little to improve the proportion of variance accounted for or the accuracy of prediction.

The dependent variable in multiple regression analysis, as in analysis of variance (ANOVA), should as a rule be measured on an interval or ratio scale. The independent variables, on the other hand, can either be continuous interval-level or ratio-level variables *or* dichotomous variables. A text such as that of Pedhazur (1982) should be consulted for information on how to handle and interpret dichotomous *dummy variables*.

TESTS OF SIGNIFICANCE

In multiple correlation, as in bivariate correlation, researchers wishing to generalize their results must ask: Is the calculated R the result of chance fluctuations, or is it statistically significant? To test the null hypothesis that the population multiple correlation coefficient is equal to zero, we can compute a statistic that

can be compared with tabled values for the F distribution.

We stated in Chapter 18 that the general form for calculating an F-ratio is as follows:

$$F = \frac{SS_{between}/df_{between}}{SS_{within}/df_{within}}$$

In the case of multiple regression, the form is similar:

$$F = \frac{SS_{due\ to\ regression}/df_{regression}}{SS_{of\ residuals}/df_{residuals}}$$

In both cases, the basic principle is the same: The variance resulting from the independent variables is contrasted with variance attributable to other factors or error. To calculate the F-statistic for regression, we can use the following alternative formula:

$$F = \frac{R^2/k}{(1-R^2)(N-k-1)}$$

where $k =$ number of predictor variables
$N =$ total sample size

In the example relating to the prediction of graduate GPAs, suppose that a multiple correlation coefficient of .71 (an R^2 of .50) had been calculated for a sample of 100 graduate students. The value of the F-statistic would be

$$F = \frac{.50/3}{.50/96} = 32.05$$

The tabled value of F with 3 and 96 degrees of freedom for a significance level of .01 is about 4.0. Thus, the probability that the R of .71 resulted from chance fluctuations is considerably less than .01.

Another question that researchers often seek to answer is: Does adding X_k to the regression equation significantly add to the prediction of Y over that which is possible with X_{k-1}? In other words, how effective is, say, a third predictor in increasing our ability to predict Y after two predictors have already been used? An F-statistic can also be computed for answering this question.

Let us number each independent variable in the example at hand, in order according to its correlation with Y: X_1 = GPA-U; X_2 = GRE-Q; and X_3 = GRE-V. We can then symbolize various correlation coefficients as follows:

$R_{y.1}$ = the correlation of Y with GPA-U

$R_{y.12}$ = the correlation of Y with GPA-U *and* GRE-Q

$R_{y.123}$ = the correlation of Y with all three predictors

The values of these *R*s are as follows:

$R_{y.1}$ = .60 $R^2_{y.1}$ = .36
$R_{y.12}$ = .71 $R^2_{y.12}$ = .50
$R_{y.123}$ = .71 $R^2_{y.123}$ = .50

These figures show at a glance that the GRE-V scores made no independent contribution to the multiple correlation coefficient. The value of $R_{y.12}$ is identical to the value of $R_{y.123}$. Figure 19-2 illustrates this point: if the circle for GRE-V were completely removed, then the area of the Y circle covered by X_1 and X_2 would remain the same.

We cannot tell at a glance, however, whether adding X_2 to X_1 *significantly* increases the prediction of Y. What we want to know, in effect, is whether or not X_2 would be likely to improve predictions in a new sample, or if its added predictive power in this particular sample resulted from chance. The general formula for the *F*-statistic for testing the significance of variables added to the regression equation is

$$F = \frac{(R^2_{y.12...k_1} - R^2_{y.12...k_2})/(k_1 - k_2)}{(1 - R^2_{y.12...k_1})/(N - k_1 - 1)}$$

where $R^2_{y.12...k_1}$ = squared multiple correlation coefficient for Y correlated with k_1 predictor variables

k_1 = the larger of the two sets of predictors

$R^2_{y.12...k_2}$ = squared *R* for Y correlated with k_2 predictor variables

k_2 = the smaller of the two sets of predictors

In the current example, the calculated *F*-statistic for testing whether the addition of GRE-Q scores results in significant improvement of prediction over GPA-U alone would be

$$F = \frac{(.50 - .36)/1}{.50/97} = 27.16$$

Consulting Table B-2 in Appendix B, we find that with $df = 1$ and 97 and a significance level of .01, the critical value is about 6.90. Therefore, the addition of GRE-Q to the regression equation significantly improved the accuracy of predictions of GPA-GRAD, beyond the .01 level of significance.

STEPWISE MULTIPLE REGRESSION

If the researcher had 10 independent variables available for use in a regression equation, then the process of testing all possible combinations to determine which set of variables was significant and yielded the highest R^2 would be exceedingly time consuming. *Stepwise multiple regression* is a method by which all potential predictors can be considered and through which the combination of variables providing the most predictive power can be chosen.

The computational aspects of stepwise multiple regression are too involved to discuss here, but some major features of this procedure can be pointed out. In stepwise multiple regression, predictors are stepped into the regression equation sequentially, in the order that produces the greatest increments to R^2. The first step involves the selection of the single best predictor of the dependent variable, which is the independent variable with the highest bivariate correlation coefficient with Y. The second variable to enter the regression equation is the one that produces the largest increase to R^2 when used simultaneously with the variable selected in the first step. The procedure continues until no additional predictor can significantly increase the value of R^2.

The basic principles of stepwise multiple regression are illustrated in Figure 19-3. The first variable to enter the regression, X_1, is correlated

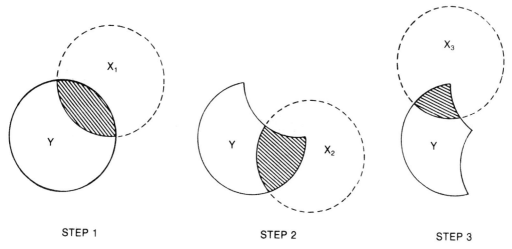

STEP 1   STEP 2   STEP 3

Figure 19-3.   *Visual representation of stepwise multiple regression analysis*

.60 with Y ($r^2 = .36$). No other predictor variable is correlated more strongly with the dependent variable. The variable X_1 accounts for the portion of the variability of Y represented by the hatched area in step 1 of the figure. This hatched area is, in effect, removed from further consideration as far as subsequent predictors are concerned. This portion of Y's variability is explained or accounted for. Therefore, the variable chosen in step 2 is not necessarily the X variable with the second largest correlation with Y. The selected variable is the predictor that explains the largest portion of what *remains* of Y's variability after X_1 has been taken into account. Variable X_2, in turn, removes a second part of Y so that the independent variable selected in step 3 is the variable that accounts for the most variability in Y after *both* X_1 and X_2 are removed.

RELATIVE CONTRIBUTION OF PREDICTORS

Scientists are concerned not only about the prediction of phenomena but also about their explanation. Predictions can be made in the absence of understanding. For instance, in our graduate school example, we could predict

performance moderately well without really understanding how the variables were functioning or what underlying factors were responsible for students' success. For practical applications, it may be sufficient to make accurate predictions, but scientists typically desire to understand phenomena and to make contributions to knowledge.

In multiple regression problems, one aspect of understanding the phenomenon under investigation is the determination of the relative importance of the independent variables. Unfortunately, the problem of determining the relative contributions of various independent variables in predicting a dependent variable is one of the thorniest issues in regression analysis. When the independent variables are correlated, as they usually are, there is no ideal way to untangle the effects of the variables in the equation.

It may appear that a solution can be found by comparing the contributions of the independent variables to R^2. In our graduate school example, GPA-U accounted for 36% of Y's variance, and GRE-Q explained an additional 14% of the variance. Should we conclude that undergraduate grades are about two and one half times as important as GRE quantitative scores in explaining graduate school grades? This conclusion would be inaccurate because the order of entry of variables in a regression equation affects their apparent contribution. If these two predictor variables were entered in reverse order, with GRE-Q first, then the R^2 would remain unchanged at .50; but GRE-Q's share would then be .30 ($.55^2$), and GPA-U's contribution would be .20 ($.50 - .30$). This circumstance results from the fact that whatever variance the independent variables share in common is attributed to the first variable entered in the regression analysis.

Another approach to assessing the relative importance of the predictors is to compare the regression coefficients. Earlier, the regression equation was given as

$$Y' = a + b_1 X_1 + b_2 X_2 + \dots b_k X_k$$

where b_1 to b_k = regression coefficients

These b values are not directly comparable because they are in the units of raw scores, which differ from one X to another. X_1 might be in milliliters, X_2 in degrees Fahrenheit, and so forth. The use of *standard scores* (or *z scores*) eliminates this problem by transforming all variables to scores with a mean of 0.0 and a standard deviation (SD) of 1.00. The formula that accomplishes this standardization* is

$$z_X = \frac{X - \overline{X}}{SD_X}$$

In standard score form, the regression equation is

$$z_{Y'} = \beta_1 z_{X1} + \beta_2 z_{X2} + \dots \beta_k z_{Xk}$$

where $z_{Y'}$ = predicated value of the standard score for Y

β_1 to β_k = standardized regression weights for k independent variables

z_{X1} to z_{Xk} = standard scores for the k predictors

* For a complete discussion of standard scores, an elementary statistical text should be consulted.

With all the βs (referred to as *beta* [β] *weights*) in the same measurement units, is it possible that their relative size could shed light on how much weight or importance to attach to the predictor variables? Many researchers have interpreted beta weights in this fashion, but there are problems in doing so. These regression coefficients will be the same no matter what the order of entry of the variables. The difficulty, however, is that regression weights are highly unstable. The values of beta tend to fluctuate considerably from sample to sample. Moreover, when a variable is added to or subtracted from the regression equation, the beta weights change. Because there is nothing absolute about the values of the regression coefficients, it is difficult to attach much theoretical importance to them.

Another method of disentangling relationships is path analysis. This procedure is an important tool in the testing of theoretical expectations about relationships. Path analysis is described later in this chapter.

❖ ANALYSIS OF COVARIANCE

A significant portion of this chapter has been devoted to multiple regression analysis both because it is the most widely used multivariate technique and because an understanding of it should facilitate comprehension of other related multivariate statistics. Analysis of covariance (ANCOVA) is a good example of a related procedure: it combines features of ANOVA and regression.

Uses of Analysis of Covariance

A central feature of ANCOVA is that it permits statistical control of extraneous variables, as indicated in Chapter 10. ANCOVA is especially appropriate in certain types of research situations. For example, when random assignment to treatment groups is not feasible, a quasi-experimental design is often adopted. The initial equivalence of the comparison groups in such studies is always questionable; therefore, the researcher has to consider whether the obtained results were influenced by preexisting differences between the experimental and comparison groups. When experimental control such as the ability to randomize is lacking, ANCOVA offers the possibility of post hoc statistical control. Even in true experiments, ANCOVA can play a role in permitting a more precise estimate of group differences. This is because even when randomization procedures are used, there are typically slight differences between groups. ANCOVA can adjust for initial differences so that the final analysis will reflect more precisely the effect of an experimental intervention.

In both these situations, the researcher is concerned with the possibility that the comparison groups differ in some respect at the beginning of the study. That is, the groups may differ with regard to an attribute or attributes that affects the dependent variable and thereby obscure the relationship between the independent and dependent variables.

Strictly speaking, ANCOVA should not be used with intact groups because one of the underlying assumptions of ANCOVA is randomization. However, this assumption is frequently violated because no other alternative analysis works as effectively. Random assignment should always be done when possible, but in many situations in which randomization is not feasible, ANCOVA could make an important contribution to the internal validity of a study.

Analysis of Covariance Procedures

To use ANCOVA, a researcher must anticipate the extraneous variables to be controlled and must measure them at the outset of the study. For instance, suppose a researcher wanted to test the effectiveness of biofeedback therapy on patients' anxiety. An experimental group in one hospital is exposed to the treatment, and a comparison group of patients in another hospital is not. If the researcher wanted to test the initial equivalence of the two groups, then the anxiety levels of all subjects could be measured both before and after the intervention. The initial anxiety score could be statistically controlled through ANCOVA. In such a situation, the posttest anxiety score is the dependent variable, experimental/comparison group status is the independent variable, and the pretest anxiety score is referred to as the *covariate*. Covariates can either be continuous variables (e.g., anxiety test scores) or dichotomous variables (male/female). However, in ANCOVA, the independent variables are always categorical, that is, nominal-level variables.

ANCOVA tests the significance of differences between group means after first adjusting the scores on the dependent variable to eliminate the effects of the covariate. The adjustment of scores uses regression procedures. In essence, the first step in ANCOVA is the same as the first step in a stepwise multiple regression analysis. The variability in the dependent measure that can be explained by the covariate is removed from further consideration. ANOVA is performed on what remains of Y's variability to see whether, once the covariate is controlled, significant differences between the groups remain. Figure 19-4 illustrates this two-step process. Pursuing the example just cited, Y would be patients' posttest anxiety scores, the covariate X* would be the pretest anxiety scores, and the independent variable X would designate whether or not the patients were exposed to the biofeedback therapy.

Another example may help to further explore aspects of the ANCOVA procedure. Suppose that we wanted to test the effectiveness of three different types of diets on overweight individuals. Although the sample of 30 subjects is randomly assigned to one of the three treatment groups, an ANCOVA, using pretreatment weights as the covariate, permits a more sensitive analysis of weight change than a simple ANOVA. Some hypothetical data for such a study are displayed in Table 19-3.

Two aspects of the weight scores in this table are immediately discernible. First, despite

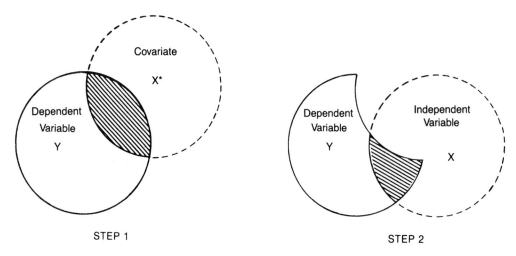

STEP 1   STEP 2

Figure 19-4. *Visual representation of analysis of covariance*

random assignment to the treatment groups, the initial group means are different. Subjects assigned to diet B differ from those assigned to diet C by an average of 10 pounds (175 versus 185 pounds). This difference is not significant* but rather reflects chance sampling fluctuations. Second, the posttreatment means are similarly different by a maximum of only 10 pounds. However, the mean number of pounds *lost*

ranged from 10 pounds for diets A and B to 25 pounds for diet C.

An ordinary ANOVA for group differences in posttreatment means results in a nonsignificant *F*-value. The ANOVA summary table is presented in part A of Table 19-4. Based on the

* Calculations demonstrating nonsignificance are not shown. The calculated $F = .45$. With 2 and 27 *df*, $p > .05$.

Table 19-3. *Fictitious Data for ANCOVA Example*

DIET A (X_A)		DIET B (X_B)		DIET C (X_C)	
X_A^*	Y_A	X_B^*	Y_B	X_C^*	Y_C
195	185	205	200	175	160
180	170	150	140	210	165
160	150	145	135	150	130
215	200	210	190	185	170
155	145	185	185	205	180
205	195	160	150	190	165
175	165	190	175	160	135
180	170	165	150	165	140
140	135	180	165	180	160
195	185	160	160	230	195
1800	1700	1750	1650	1850	1600
$\bar{X}_A^* = 180.0$	$\bar{Y}_A = 170.0$	$\bar{X}_B^* = 175.0$	$\bar{Y}_B = 165.0$	$\bar{X}_C^* = 185.0$	$\bar{Y}_C = 160.0$

X, independent variable (diet); X*, covariate (pretreatment weight); Y, dependent variable (posttreatment weight)

Table 19-4. *Comparison of ANOVA and ANCOVA Results*

SOURCE OF VARIATION	SUM OF SQUARES	df	MEAN SQUARE	F	p
A. SUMMARY TABLE FOR ANOVA					
Between groups	500.0	2	250.0	0.55	>.05
Within groups	12,300.0	27	455.6		
Total	12,800.0	29			
B. SUMMARY TABLE FOR ANCOVA					
Step 1 { Covariate	10,563.1	1	10,563.1	132.23	<.01
Residual	2236.9	28	79.9		
Total	12,800.0	29			
Step 2 { Between groups	1284.8	2	642.4	17.54	<.01
Within groups	952.1	26	36.6		
Total	2236.9	28			

ANOVA results, we would conclude that all three diets were equally effective in influencing weight loss.

Part B of Table 19-4 presents the summary table for the ANCOVA. The first step of the analysis breaks the total variability of the post-treatment weights into two components: (1) variability that can be accounted for by the covariate, the pretreatment weights; and (2) residual variability. As the table shows, the covariate accounted for a significant amount of the variance, which is not surprising in light of the strong relationship between the pretreatment and posttreatment weights ($r = .91$). This merely indicates that people who started out especially heavy (or light) tended to stay that way, relative to others in the sample. In the second phase of the analysis, the residual variance is broken down to reflect the between-group and within-group contributions. With 2 and 26 degrees of freedom, the F of 17.54 is significant beyond the .01 level. The conclusion is that, after controlling for the initial weight of the subjects, there is a significant difference in weight loss resulting from exposure to different diets.

This fictitious example was deliberately contrived so that a result of "no difference" could be altered by the addition of a covariate to yield a significant difference. Most actual results are less dramatic than this example might suggest. Nonetheless, it is true that if the researcher can select meaningful covariates, then a more sensitive statistical test will always be made than if an ordinary ANOVA were performed. The increase in sensitivity results from the fact that the covariate reduces the error term (the within-group variability), against which treatment effects are compared. In part A of Table 19-4, it can be seen that the within-group term is extremely large, thereby masking the contribution made by the experimental treatments.

Theoretically, it is possible to use any number of covariates. It is probably unwise to use more than five or six in practice, however. For one thing, the inclusion of more than five or six covariates is probably unnecessary because of the typically high degree of redundancy beyond the first few variables. Moreover, it may be to the researcher's disadvantage to add covariates that do not explain a statistically significant portion of the variability of a dependent variable. Each covariate uses up a degree of freedom, leaving the balance for the within-group term. Fewer degrees of freedom means that a higher computed F is required for significance. For instance, with 2 and 26 *df*, an F of 5.53 is required for significance at the .01 level, but with 2 and 23 *df* (i.e., adding three covariates), an F of 5.66 is needed.

Multiple Classification Analysis

As shown in part B of Table 19-4, an ANCOVA table provides information relating to significance testing. The table indicates that at least one of the three groups had a posttreatment weight that is significantly different from the overall grand mean, after adjusting for pretreatment weights. Sometimes it is extremely useful to examine *adjusted means*, that is, mean values on the dependent variable by group, after adjusting for (i.e., removing the effect of) covariates.*

Multiple classification analysis (MCA) is a versatile supplement to ANCOVA and multiple regression that produces information about the mean value of a dependent variable, *after* adjustment for covariates, for every level of one or more independent variables. MCA is versatile because it allows for dichotomous or continuous covariates, correlated independent variables or covariates, and nonlinear relationships between dependent and predictor variables. MCA can be performed on some standard statistical programs, such as the Statistical Package for the Social Sciences (SPSS; see Chapter 20). A subsequent section of this chapter, which discusses computer examples of multivariate statistics, provides more information about MCA.

❖ FACTOR ANALYSIS

Factor analysis is a somewhat controversial multivariate procedure because it involves a higher degree of subjectivity than one ordinarily finds in a statistical technique. It is, nevertheless, a highly powerful and widely applied procedure and, therefore, merits attention. The major purpose of *factor analysis* is to reduce a large set of variables into a smaller, more manageable set of measures. Factor analysis disentangles complex interrelationships among variables and identifies which variables go together as unified concepts. The underlying dimensions thus identified are called *factors*. As an example, consider a researcher who has prepared 100 Likert-type items aimed at measuring women's attitudes toward menopause. Suppose that the research goal was to compare the attitudes of premenopausal and postmenopausal women. If the researcher does not combine some of the items to form a scale, it would be necessary to calculate 100 chi-square statistics. The formation of a scale is preferable, but it involves adding together the scores from several individual items. The problem is, which items are to be combined? Would it be meaningful to combine all 100 items? Probably not, because the 100 questions are not all asking exactly the same thing. There are various aspects or themes to a woman's attitude toward menopause. One aspect may relate to the aging process, and another aspect is concerned with a loss of the ability to reproduce. Other questions may touch on the general issue of sexuality, and yet others may concern avoidance of monthly pain or bother. There are, in short, multiple dimensions to the issue of attitudes toward menopause, and each dimension should be captured by a separate scale. The identification of these dimensions can be made a priori by the researcher, but the difficulty is that different researchers may read different concepts into the items. Factor analysis offers an empirical method of elucidating the underlying dimensionality of a large number of measures.

A factor, mathematically, is a linear combination of the variables in a data matrix. A data matrix contains the scores of N people on k different measures. For instance, a factor might be defined by the following equation:

$$F = b_1X_1 + b_2X_2 + b_3X_3 + \ldots b_kX_k$$

where F = a factor score
X_1 to X_k = values on the k original variables
b_1 to b_k = weights

---

*It is possible to compute such adjusted means from information provided from regression analyses, as described in Pedhazur (1982). When several covariates are used to control extraneous variables statistically, however, manual computations become laborious.

The development of such an equation for a factor permits the reduction of the X_k scores to one or more factor scores.

Factor Extraction

Most factor analyses consist of two separate phases. The first step is to condense the variables in the data matrix into a smaller number of factors. Sometimes this first phase is referred to as the *factor extraction* phase. The factors usually are derived from the intercorrelations among the variables in the correlation matrix. The general goal is to seek clusters of highly interrelated variables within the matrix. There are various methods of performing the first step, each of which uses different criteria for assigning weights to the variables. Probably the most widely used method of factor extraction is called *principal components* (or principal factor or principal axes), but other methods that a researcher may come across are the image, alpha, centroid, maximum likelihood, and canonical techniques.

The result of the first step of the factor analysis is a *factor matrix* (sometimes labeled as the unrotated factor matrix), which contains coefficients or weights for each variable in the original data matrix on each extracted factor. Because unrotated factor matrixes are difficult to interpret, we will postpone a detailed discussion of factor matrixes until the second factor analysis phase is described. In the principal components method, weights for the first factor are defined such that the average squared weight is a maximum, thereby permitting a maximal amount of variance to be extracted by the first factor. The second factor, or linear combination, is formed in such a way that the highest possible amount of variance is again extracted from what *remains* after the first factor has been taken into account. The factors thus delineated represent independent sources of variation in the data matrix.

In extracting factors in this fashion, some criterion must be applied to delimit the number of factors or underlying dimensions. Factoring should continue until there is no further meaningful variance left. There are several criteria available from which the researcher can choose to specify when factoring should cease. It is partly the availability of so many different criteria or justifications for halting factor extraction that makes factor analysis a semisubjective process. Several of the most commonly used criteria can be described by illustrating information that is usually output from factor analysis programs. Table 19-5 presents hypothetical values for eigenvalues, percentages of variance accounted for, and cumulative percentages of variance accounted for, for 10 factors. *Eigenvalues* are values equal to the sum of the squared

Table 19-5.   *Summary of Factor Extraction Results*

FACTOR	EIGENVALUE	PERCENTAGE OF VARIANCE EXPLAINED	CUMULATIVE PERCENTAGE OF VARIANCE EXPLAINED
1	12.32	29.2	29.2
2	8.57	23.3	52.5
3	6.91	15.6	68.1
4	2.02	8.4	76.5
5	1.09	6.2	82.7
6	.98	5.8	88.5
7	.80	4.5	93.0
8	.62	3.1	96.1
9	.47	2.2	98.3
10	.25	1.7	100.0

weights for each factor. Many researchers establish as their cutoff point for factor extraction eigenvalues greater than 1.00. In the example in the table, this would mean that the first five factors or dimensions would meet this criterion. Another cutoff rule that is adopted sometimes is a minimum of 5% of explained variance, in which case six factors would qualify for inclusion in our current example. Yet another criterion is based on a principle of discontinuity. According to this procedure, a sharp drop in the percentage of explained variance indicates the appropriate termination point. In Table 19-5, one might argue that there is considerable discontinuity between the third and fourth factors. The general consensus appears to be that it is probably better to extract too many factors than too few.

Factor Rotation

The factor matrix produced in the first phase of factor analysis usually is rather difficult to interpret. For this reason, a second phase known as *factor rotation* is almost invariably performed on those factors that have met one or more of the criteria for inclusion. The concept of rotation is complex and can be best explained graphically. Figure 19-5 shows two coordinate systems, marked by axes A1 and A2 and B1 and B2. The primary axes (A1 and A2) represent factors I and II, respectively, as they are defined before rotation. The points 1 through 6 represent six variables in this two-dimensional space. The weights associated with each variable can be determined in reference to the appropriate axis. For instance, before rotation, variable 1 is assigned a weight of .80 on factor I and .85 on factor II, and variable 6 has a weight of −.45 on factor I and .90 on factor II. The unrotated axes are designed to account for a maximum of variance but rarely provide a structure that has conceptual meaning. However, by rotating the axes in such a way that clusters of variables are distinctly associated with a factor, interpretability is enhanced. In the figure, B1 and B2 represent the rotated factors. The rotation has been performed in such a way that variables 1, 2, and 3 would be assigned large weights on factor I and small weights on factor II, and the reverse would be true for variables 4, 5, and 6.

The researcher must choose from two general classes of rotation procedures. Figure 19-5 illustrates *orthogonal rotation,* in which the factors are kept at right angles to one another. Orthogonal rotations maintain the independence of factors. That is, orthogonal factors are uncorrelated with one another. *Oblique rotations,* on the other hand, permit the rotated axes to depart from a 90-degree angle. In our figure, an oblique rotation would have put axis B1 between variables 2 and 3 and axis B2 between variables 5 and 6. This placement of the axes strengthens the clustering of variables around an associated factor. The result is that oblique rotation produces correlated factors. Some researchers insist that orthogonal rotation leads to greater theoretical clarity; others claim that it is unrealistic. Those advocating oblique rotation point out that if the concepts *are* correlated, then the analysis should be permitted to reflect this fact. In practice, studies have revealed that similar conclusions are often reached by both rotational procedures.

The rotated factor matrix is what the researcher normally works with in interpreting the factor analysis. An example of such a matrix is displayed in Table 19-6 for discussion purposes. To make this discussion less abstract, let us say that the 10 variables listed in the table are the first 10 of the 100 items measuring attitudes toward menopause. The entries under each factor are the weights on that factor, which are called *factor loadings.* For orthogonally rotated factors, factor loadings can be readily interpreted. Like correlation coefficients, they range from −1.00 to +1.00. In fact, they can be interpreted in much the same way as a correlation coefficient. Factor loadings express the correlations between individual variables and factors (underlying dimensions). In this example, variable 1 is fairly highly correlated with factor 1, .75.

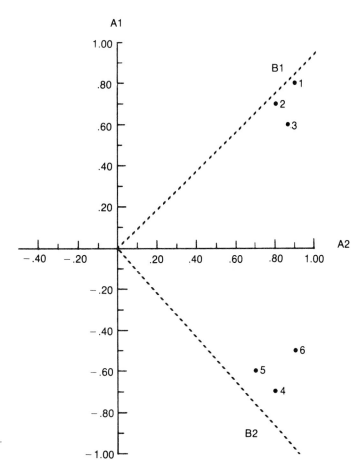

Figure 19-5.   *Illustration of factor rotation*

Therefore, it is possible to find which variables "belong" to a factor. For factor I, variables 1, 3, 8, and 10 have fairly sizable loadings. Normally, a cutoff value of about .40 or .30 is used for such determinations. The researcher is now in a position to interpret the underlying dimensionality of the data. By inspecting items 1, 3, 8, and 10, it is usually possible to find some common theme that makes the variables go together. Perhaps these four questions have to do with the link between menopause and infertility, and perhaps items 2, 5, and 6 (i.e., the items with high loadings on factor II) are related to sexuality. The naming of factors is essentially a process of identifying theoretical constructs.

Factor Scores

In some cases in which the main purpose of factor analysis is to delineate the conceptual makeup of a set of measures, the analysis may end at this point. Frequently, however, the researcher wants to use the information obtained to develop *factor scores* for use in subsequent analyses. For instance, the factor analysis of the 100 menopause items might demonstrate that there are five principal dimensions or concepts being tapped. By reducing 100 variables to five variables, the analysis of differences between premenopausal and postmenopausal women using some procedure such as *t*-tests or ANCOVA will be greatly simplified.

Table 19-6.   *Rotated Factor Matrix*

VARIABLE	FACTOR I	FACTOR II	FACTOR III
1	.75	.15	.23
2	−.02	.61	.18
3	−.59	−.11	.03
4	.05	.08	.48
5	.21	.79	.02
6	−.07	−.52	−.29
7	.08	.19	.80
8	.68	.12	−.01
9	−.04	.08	−.61
10	−.43	−.13	.06

Several methods can be used to form factor scores. One procedure is to weight the variables according to their factor loading on each factor. For example, a factor score for the first factor in Table 19-6 could be computed for each subject by the following formula:

$$F_1 = .75X_1 - .02X_2 - .59X_3 + .05X_4 + .21X_5$$
$$- .07X_6 + .08X_7 + .68X_8 - .04X_9 - .43X_{10} \ldots b_{100}X_{100}$$

where the X values* = subject's scores on the 100 items

Some factor analysis computer programs can directly compute this type of factor score.

A second method of obtaining factor scores is to select certain variables to represent the factor and to combine them with unit weighting. This composite estimate method would produce a factor score on the first factor of our example in the following fashion:

$$F_1 = X_1 - X_3 + X_8 - X_{10} \pm \ldots$$

The variables here are those with high loadings on factor I (the "± . . ." indicates the inclusion of any of the other 90 variables with high loadings). This procedure is both computationally and conceptually simpler than the first approach; both have been found to yield similar results.

*Standardized (*z*) scores are often used in lieu of raw scores in computing factor scores when the means and standard deviations of the variables differ substantially.

To illustrate the composite estimate approach more concretely, consider the rotated factor matrix in Table 19-6 and assume that factor scores were to be computed on the basis of this 10-item analysis, omitting for the sake of simplicity the remaining 90 items on the menopause scale. Suppose that two respondents had the following scores on these 10 items:

Subject 1: 7, 1, 1, 5, 1, 6, 7, 6, 3, 2
Subject 2: 2, 5, 6, 3, 7, 3, 2, 3, 4, 4

Factor I has fairly high loadings on variables 1, 3, 8, and 10. Thus, the two subjects' factor scores on factor 1 would be

$$7 - 1 + 6 - 2 = 10$$

$$2 - 6 + 3 - 4 = -5$$

The minus signs reflect the negative loadings on variables 3 and 10.[†] The same procedure would be performed for all three factors, yielding the following factor scores:

Subject 1: 10, −3, 9
Subject 2: −5, 9, 1

Factor scores would similarly be computed for all respondents, and these scores could then be used in the subsequent analyses as measures of different dimensions of attitudes toward menopause.

❖ OTHER LEAST-SQUARES MULTIVARIATE TECHNIQUES

In addition to ANCOVA, several other multivariate techniques are closely related to least-

[†]Researchers forming scale scores with Likert items often reverse the direction of the scoring on negatively loaded items before forming the factor score to eliminate negative scores. Direction of an item can be reversed by subtracting the raw score from the sum of 1 + the maximum item value. For example, in a 7-point scale, a score of 2 would be reversed to 6 [(1 + 7) − 2]. When such reversals have been done, all raw scores can be added in forming factor scores.

squares multiple regression analysis. In this section, the methods known as discriminant function analysis, canonical correlation, and multivariate analysis of variance are introduced. The introduction is brief and computations are entirely omitted because these procedures are exceedingly complex. The intent of this review is to acquaint the reader with the types of research situations for which these methods are appropriate. Advanced statistical texts such as the ones listed in the references may be consulted for additional information.

Discriminant Analysis

In multiple regression, the dependent variable being predicted is normally a measure on either the interval or ratio scale of measurement. The regression equation makes predictions about scores that take on a large range of values, such as heart rate, weight, or scores on a depression scale. *Discriminant analysis,* in contrast, makes predictions about membership in categories or groups. The purpose of the analysis is to distinguish groups from one another on the basis of available independent variables. For instance, we may wish to develop a means of predicting membership in or affiliation with such groups as complying versus noncomplying cancer patients, graduating nursing students versus drop-outs, or normal pregnancies versus those terminating in a miscarriage.

Discriminant analysis develops a regression equation—called a *discriminant function*—for a categorical dependent variable, with independent variables that are either categorical or continuous. The researcher begins with data from subjects whose group membership is known. The intent is to develop an equation that can be used to predict membership for new subjects for whom only measures of the independent variables are available. The discriminant function indicates to which group each subject will probably belong.

Discriminant analysis that is used to predict membership into only two groups (e.g., nursing school drop-outs versus graduates) is

relatively simple and can be interpreted in much the same fashion as a multiple regression. When there are more than two groups or categories, the calculations and interpretations are more complicated. With three or more groups (e.g., very-low-birthweight, low-birthweight, and normal-birthweight infants), the number of discriminant functions is either the number of groups minus one or the number of independent variables, whichever is smaller. The first discriminant function is the linear combination of predictors that maximizes the ratio of between-group variance to within-group variance. The second function derived is the linear combination that maximizes this ratio, after the effect of the first function is removed. Because the independent variables are assigned different weights on the various functions, it is possible to develop theoretical interpretations based on the knowledge of which predictors are important in discriminating among different groups.

Discriminant analysis has several features in common with multiple regression analysis, aside from the fact that prediction equations based on a linear combination of independent variables are developed. For one thing, it is possible to use a stepwise approach in entering predictors into the equation. Also, the analysis produces an index designating the proportion of variance in the dependent variable accounted for by the predictor variables. The index is known as *Wilks' lambda* (λ). Actually, λ indicates the proportion of variance *unaccounted for* by predictors, or $\lambda = 1 - R^2$. In sum, discriminant analysis has potential for being useful to researchers, particularly those with practical problems of classification or diagnosis.

Canonical Correlation

Canonical correlation is the most general multivariate technique, of which other procedures are special cases. *Canonical correlation* analyzes the relationship between two or more independent variables and two or more dependent variables. Conceptually, one can think of this technique as an extension of multiple regression to more than one dependent variable. Mathematically and interpretatively, the gap between multiple regression and canonical correlation is greater than this statement suggests.

Like other techniques described thus far in this chapter, canonical correlation uses the least-squares principle to partition and analyze variance. Basically, two linear composites are developed, one of which is associated with the dependent variables, the other of which is for the independent variables. The relationship between the two linear composites is expressed by the canonical correlation coefficient, R_C. As in the case of the coefficient of determination (R^2), R_C^2 indicates the proportion of variance accounted for in the analysis. When there is more than one source or dimension of covariation in the two sets of variables, more than one canonical correlation can be found.

Examples of research utilizing canonical correlation are relatively rare. Perhaps the method is not well known, and it requires a higher degree of mathematic sophistication than is needed for most statistical techniques. Still, when a study involves multiple dependent and independent variables, canonical correlation may be the most suitable way to analyze the data.

Multivariate Analysis of Variance

Multivariate analysis of variance, sometimes abbreviated MANOVA, is the extension of ANOVA procedures to more than one dependent variable. This procedure is used primarily to test the significance of differences between the means of two or more dependent variables, considered simultaneously. Like ordinary ANOVA, MANOVA was developed for use in experimental situations in which at least one independent variable was manipulated. For instance, if we wanted to examine the effect of two methods of exercise (A_1 and A_2) and two lengths of exercise treatment (B_1 and B_2) on both diastolic and systolic blood pressure (Y_1 and Y_2), then a MANOVA would be appropriate. Researchers often analyze such data by per-

forming two separate univariate ANOVAs. Strictly speaking, this practice is incorrect. Separate ANOVAs imply that the dependent variables have been obtained independently of one another. In fact, the dependent measures have been obtained from the same subjects and are, therefore, correlated. MANOVA takes the intercorrelations of the dependent variables into account in computing the test statistics. However, ANOVA is a more widely understood procedure than MANOVA, and thus results may be more easily communicated to a broad audience.

MANOVA can be readily extended in ways analogous to ANOVA. For example, it is possible to perform *multivariate analysis of covariance* (MANCOVA), which allows for the control of extraneous variables (covariates) when there are two or more dependent variables. MANOVA can also be used in situations when there are repeated measures of the dependent variables (sometimes abbreviated *RMANOVA*).

Links Among Least-Squares Multivariate Techniques

The analogy might be made that multiple regression is to canonical correlation what ANOVA is to MANOVA. This analogy, although correct, obscures a point that the astute reader has perhaps already suspected, and that is the close affinity between multiple regression and ANOVA.

In fact, ANOVA and multiple regression are virtually identical. Both techniques are concerned with analyzing the total variability in a dependent measure and contrasting the proportion of the variability attributable to one or more independent variables with that attributable to unexplained sources of variation, or error. Multiple regression and ANOVA use a different approach and use different symbols and terminology, but both analyses boil down to a final *F*-ratio. By tradition, experimental data are typically analyzed by ANOVA, and ex post facto data are analyzed by regression procedures. Nevertheless, it should be realized that any data for which ANOVA is appropriate could also be analyzed by multiple regression, although the reverse is not true. In many cases, multiple regression is preferable because it can be used with a broader range of data and because it provides more information, such as a prediction equation and an index of association, *R*. However, with respect to the index of association issue, it should be noted that a formula can easily be applied to ANOVA results to derive the statistic known as *eta-squared* (η^2), which indicates the strength of association between variables and, like R^2, the proportion of variance in the dependent variable explained by the independent variables. Eta-squared is simply the sum of squares between groups divided by the total sum of squares. The value of η^2 is computed routinely by most ANOVA computer programs.

❖ PATH ANALYSIS

Path analysis is a regression-based method for studying patterns of causation among a set of variables in ex post facto studies. As discussed in Chapter 8, path analysis usually begins with a theory or causal model that dictates the type of data to be collected. It is not a method for discovering causes; rather, it is a method applied to a prespecified model formulated on the basis of prior knowledge and theory.

Path analysis is a complex topic to which entire books have been devoted. Therefore, we briefly describe some of the key concepts without discussing actual analytic procedures. Path analytic reports often use a *path diagram* to display their results; we use such a diagram (Figure 19-6) here to illustrate important concepts. This model postulates that the dependent variable, patients' length of hospitalization (V4), is the result of their capacity for self-care (V3); this, in turn, is affected by nursing actions (V1) and the severity of their illness (V2).

In path analysis, a distinction is often made between exogenous and endogenous variables. An *exogenous variable* is a variable whose determinants lie outside the model. In Figure 19-6, nursing actions (V1) and illness severity (V2) are exogenous; no attempt is made in the model to elucidate what causes different nursing actions or different degrees of illness. An *endogenous variable,* by contrast, is one whose variation is determined by other variables in the model. In our example, self-care capacity (V3) and length of hospitalization (V4) are endogenous.

In path analysis, causal linkages are illustrated by arrows, drawn from the presumed causes to the presumed effects. In our illustration, severity of illness is hypothesized to affect length of hospitalization both directly (path p_{42}) and indirectly through the *mediating variable* self-care capacity (paths p_{32} and p_{43}). Correlated exogenous variables are indicated by curved lines, as shown by the curved line between nursing actions and illness severity.

Ideally, the model would totally explain the outcome of interest, which in this case is length of hospitalization. In practice, this almost never happens because causal theories are rarely comprehensive when dealing with human phenomena. There are usually other determinants, which are generally referred to as *residual variables.* In Figure 19-6, there are two boxes labeled *e*, which denote a composite of all determinants of self-care capacity and hospital stay that are not in the model. The residuals summarize our lack of understanding of other determinants of endogenous variables. If we can identify and measure additional causative forces and incorporate them into the overarching theory, then they should be in the model.

Figure 19-6 represents what is referred to as a *recursive* model. This means that the causal flow is unidirectional and without feedback loops. In other words, it is assumed that variable 2 is a cause of variable 3, and that variable 3 is *not* a cause of variable 2.

In Figure 19-6, causal paths are indicated by symbols denoting that a given variable (e.g., V3) is caused by another (e.g., V2), yielding a path labeled p_{32}. In research reports, the path symbols would be replaced by actual numbers developed by applying regression procedures.

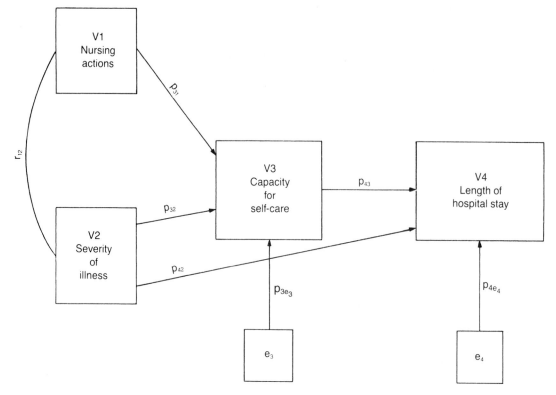

Figure 19-6.   *Path diagram*

The numbers shown are called *path coefficients,* which are standardized partial regression slopes. For example, path p_{32} is equal to $\beta_{32.1}$—the beta weight between variables 2 and 3, holding variable 1 constant. Because path coefficients are in standard form, they indicate the proportion of a standard deviation difference in the caused variable that is directly attributable to a 1.00 SD difference in the specified causal variable. Thus, the path coefficients give us some indication of the relative importance of various determinants.

Path analysis involves estimation of the path coefficients through the use of *structural equations.* The structural equations for Figure 19-6 are as follows:

$$z_1 = e_1$$
$$z_2 = e_2$$

$$z_3 = p_{31}z_1 + p_{32}z_2 + e_3; \text{ and}$$
$$z_4 = p_{43}z_3 + p_{42}z_2 + e_4$$

These equations indicate that z_1 and z_2 (standard scores for variables 1 and 2) are determined by outside variables; that z_3 depends directly on z_1 and z_2 plus outside variables; and that z_4 depends directly on z_2, z_3, and outside variables. In our example, the structural equations could be solved to yield path coefficients by performing two multiple regressions: by regressing variable 3 on variables 1 and 2; and by regressing variable 4 on variables 2 and 3.

The model presented in Figure 19-6 may or may not be a reasonable construction of the hospitalization process. Path analysis involves a number of procedures for testing causal models and for determining effects. Ped-hazur (1982) provides a good overview of path analytic techniques, and the advanced student should refer to books such as that by Blalock (1972).

❖ *POWER ANALYSIS*

Many published (and even more unpublished) nursing studies result in nonsignificant findings; that is, one or more of the researcher's hypotheses are not supported. Although standard statistical texts pay considerable attention to the problem of Type I errors (wrongly rejecting a *true* null hypothesis), little attention has been paid to Type II errors (wrongly accepting a *false* null hypothesis). *Power analysis* represents a method for reducing the risk of Type II errors and for estimating their occurrence.

As indicated in Chapter 18, the probability of committing a Type I error is established by the investigator as the level of significance, or alpha (α). The probability of a Type II error is beta (β). The complement of $(1 - \beta)$ is the *probability of obtaining a significant result* and is referred to as the *power* of a statistical test. It has been shown that many nursing studies have insufficient power (Polit & Sherman, 1990) and are therefore at high risk of committing a Type II error.

In performing a power analysis, there are four components, at least three of which must be known to or estimated by the researcher; power analysis solves for the fourth component. The four major factors are as follows:

1. *The significance criterion,* α. Other things being equal, the more stringent this criterion, the lower is the power.
2. *The sample size, n.* As sample size increases, power increases.
3. *The population effect size, gamma* (γ). Gamma is a measure of how wrong the null hypothesis is, that is, how strong the

effect of the independent variable is on the dependent variable in the population.
4. *Power, or* $1 - \beta$. This is the probability of rejecting the null hypothesis.

Researchers typically use power analysis for two purposes: (1) to solve for the sample size needed in a study to increase the likelihood of demonstrating significant results and (2) to determine the power of a statistical test, after it has been applied. In this section, which is only a brief summary of power analysis, we focus on the first of these purposes.

To solve for an estimate of the needed sample size, the researcher must specify α, γ, and $1 - \beta$. Usually, the researcher establishes α, the risk of a Type I error, as .05; in some cases, a lower (stricter) criterion such as .01 may be required. Just as .05 has been adopted as the standard for the α criterion, a conventional standard for $1 - \beta$ is .80. With power equal to .80, there is a 20% risk of committing a Type II error. Although this risk may seem high, a stricter criterion would require sample sizes much larger than most nurse researchers could manage. Most nursing studies being conducted have a power well below .80, making it difficult to avoid a Type II error.

With α and $1 - \beta$ specified, the only other piece of information needed to solve for *n* is γ, the population effect size. The *effect size* is an estimate of the magnitude of the relationship between the research variables. When relationships are strong, large samples are not needed to detect the effect at statistically significant levels. When the relationships are modest, then large sample sizes are needed to avoid Type II errors.

The value of γ is arrived at differently depending on the nature of the data and the statistical test to be performed. However, the principles for arriving at the estimate of γ are the same for all tests. The researcher needs to use available evidence to estimate the magnitude of the effect size. Sometimes this evidence comes from the researcher's own pilot study, a procedure that is highly recommended when the main study is likely to be costly. More often, the researcher uses evidence from other published studies on the same or a similar problem. That is, an effect size is calculated (through procedures that follow) based on other researchers' data.* When there are *no* data that could reasonably be construed as relevant, the researcher may be forced to use conventions based on whether the effect size is expected to be small, medium, or large. In using these conventions, it is wise to be conservative because most nursing studies have modest effect sizes.

The procedures for estimating effects and the relevant power tables vary from one statistical test to another. We provide formulas for four situations that are especially common in nursing research: (1) testing the difference between two group means (i.e., situations requiring a *t*-test); (2) testing the difference between three or more group means (i.e., situations requiring an ANOVA); (3) testing the significance of a bivariate linear relationship (i.e., situations requiring Pearson's *r*); and (4) testing the significance of differences in proportions between two groups (i.e., situations requiring a chi-square test). Cohen (1977) and Jaccard and Becker (1990) discuss power analysis in the context of many other situations.[†]

Sample Size Estimates for Test of Difference Between Two Means

Suppose we were interested in testing the hypothesis that cranberry juice reduces the uri-

---

*Usually, a researcher will be able to find more than one piece of research from which the effect size can be estimated. In such a case, the estimate should be based on the study that yields the most stable and reliable results or whose design most closely approximates that of the new study. In some cases in which equally good (or equally bad) prior research is available, it may be desirable to combine information from multiple studies (through averaging or weighted averaging) to develop an effect size estimate.

[†] Computer software for performing power analyses is available for personal computers (Borenstein & Cohen, 1988).

nary pH of diet-controlled patients. In our study, we plan to randomly assign some subjects to a control condition (no cranberry juice) and others to an experimental condition in which they would be given 200 milliliters of cranberry juice with each meal for 5 days. How large a sample is needed for this study, given an α of .05 and power equal to .80?

To answer this question, we must first estimate γ. In a two-group situation in which the difference of means is of interest, the formula for the effect size is

$$\gamma = \frac{\mu^1 - \mu^2}{\sigma}$$

That is, γ is the difference between the two population means, divided by the population standard deviation. But how can the researcher know this information in advance? If we knew, for example, the mean urinary pH of all subjects who had or had not ingested cranberry juice, there might not be any point in doing the study. Nevertheless, as explained above, the researcher must *estimate* the population means and standard deviation, based on whatever information is available. In our present example, suppose we found an earlier ex post facto study that compared the urinary pH of subjects who had or had not ingested cranberry juice in the previous 24 hours. The earlier and current studies are different. In the ex post facto study, the diets are uncontrolled; there may be selection biases in who drinks or does not drink cranberry juice, the length of ingestion is only one day, and so on. However, this study is a reasonable starting point. Suppose the results of the earlier study were as follows:

$\bar{X}_1$ (no cranberry juice) = 5.70

$\bar{X}_2$ (cranberry juice) = 5.50

σ (pooled SD) = .50

Thus, the value of γ would be .40:

$$\gamma = \frac{5.70 - 5.50}{.50} = .40$$

Table 19-7 presents approximate sample size requirements for various effect sizes and powers, and two values of α (for two-tailed tests), in a two-group mean-difference situation. In part A of the table for α = .05, we find that the estimated *n* needed for an effect size of .40 and a power of .80 is 98 subjects per group. That is, assuming that the earlier study provided a roughly accurate estimate of the population effect size, the total number of subjects required in the new study would be about 200, with half assigned to the control group (no cranberry juice) and the other half assigned to the experimental group. A sample size smaller than 200 would have a greater than 20% chance of resulting in a Type II error.

If there is *no* prior relevant research (which is rarely the case), then the researcher can, as a last resort, estimate on the basis of readings or experience whether the expected effect is small, medium, or large. By a conven-tion developed by Cohen (1977), the value of γ in a two-group test of mean differences is esti-mated at .20 for small effects, .50 for medium ef-fects, and .80 for large effects. With an α value of .05 and power of .80, the *total* sample size (number of subjects in both groups) for studies with expected small, medium, and large effects would be 784, 126, and 50, respectively. Most nursing studies cannot expect effect sizes in excess of .50, and those in the range of .20 to .40 are especially common. In Polit and Sherman's (1990) analysis of effect sizes for all studies appearing in *Nursing Research* and *Research in Nursing and Health* in 1989, the average ef-fect size for *t*-test situations was .35. Cohen noted that in new areas of research inquiry, effect sizes are likely to be small. A medium effect should be estimated only when the ef-fect is so substantial that it can be detected by the naked eye (i.e., without formal research procedures).

Table 19-7.   *Approximate Sample Sizes* Necessary To Achieve Selected Levels of Power as a Function of Estimated Effect Size for Test of Difference of Two Means*

	ESTIMATED EFFECT†									
POWER	*.10*	*.15*	*.20*	*.25*	*.30*	*.40*	*.50*	*.60*	*.70*	*.80*
PART A: α = .05										
.60	977	434	244	156	109	61	39	27	20	15
.70	1230	547	308	197	137	77	49	34	25	19
.80	1568	697	392	251	174	98	63	44	32	25
.90	2100	933	525	336	233	131	84	58	43	33
.95	2592	1152	648	415	288	162	104	72	53	41
.99	3680	1636	920	589	409	230	147	102	75	58
PART B: α = .01										
.60	1602	712	400	256	178	100	64	44	33	25
.70	1922	854	481	308	214	120	77	53	39	30
.80	2339	1040	585	374	260	146	94	65	48	37
.90	2957	1324	745	477	331	186	119	83	61	47
.95	3562	1583	890	570	396	223	142	99	73	56
.99	4802	2137	1201	769	534	300	192	133	98	

* Sample size requirements for *each* group; total sample size would be twice the number shown.

† Estimated effect (γ) is the estimated population mean group difference, divided by the estimated population standard deviation or:

$$\gamma = \frac{\mu_1 - \mu_2}{\sigma}$$

Sample Size Estimates for Test of Difference Between Three or More Means

Suppose we wanted to study the effectiveness of three different modes of stimulation—auditory, visual, and tactile—on preterm infants' sensorimotor development. The dependent variable will be a standardized scale of infant development, such as the Denver Scale. With an α of .05 and power of .80, how many infants should be randomly assigned to the three groups?

There are alternative approaches to doing a power analysis in an ANOVA context, but the simplest approach is to calculate or estimate eta-squared, based on information from either other relevant studies or a pilot study. As noted earlier in this chapter, η^2 is the index indicating the proportion of variance explained in ANOVA and is equal to the sum of squares between (SS_B) divided by the total sum of squares (SS_T). Eta-squared can be used directly as an estimate of the effect size.

In the modes of stimulation example, suppose we were able to find an earlier study that tested the same or a similar hypothesis, and that study yielded an η^2 of .05. Table 19-8 presents approximate sample size requirements for various ANOVA situations. Note that, for the sake of economy and practicality, this table presents much more limited information in terms of power (the power ranges between .70 and .95) and α (only .05) than was true for the two-group situation because of the increased complexity: here, the sample size requirements vary as a function of the number of groups in the study. The table presents sample size estimates only for the most common group sizes: 3, 4, and 5. Jaccard and Becker (1990) provide expanded tables for different αs, powers, and group sizes.

Assuming that we desire a power of .80 and an α level of .05 in the hypothetical example, the number of subjects needed in each of

Table 19-8. *Approximate Sample Sizes* Necessary To Achieve Selected Levels of Power for α = .05 as a Function of Estimated Population Values of Eta-Squared*

POWER	.01	.03	.05	.07	.10	.15	.20	.25	.30	.35
GROUPS = 3										
.70	255	84	50	35	24	16	11	9	7	6
.80	319	105	62	44	30	19	14	11	9	7
.90	417	137	81	57	39	25	18	14	11	9
.95	511	168	99	69	47	30	22	16	13	11
GROUPS = 4										
.70	219	72	43	30	21	13	10	8	6	5
.80	272	90	53	37	26	17	12	9	7	6
.90	351	115	68	48	33	21	15	12	9	8
.95	426	140	83	58	40	25	18	14	11	9
GROUPS = 5										
.70	193	64	38	27	18	12	9	7	6	5
.80	238	78	46	33	23	15	10	8	7	5
.90	306	101	59	42	29	18	13	10	8	7
.95	369	121	72	50	34	22	16	12	10	8

POPULATION ETA-SQUARED

* The values are the number of subjects *per group.*

the three stimulation groups would be 62 infants. If the experiment were undertaken with only 50 infants per group, there would be a 30% chance (power = .70) of finding nonsignificant results, even if the null hypothesis were false.

If no estimates of eta-squared can be developed on the basis of prior research, then the researcher would have to predict whether effects are likely to be small, medium, or large. For ANOVA-type situations, Cohen's conventional values of small, medium, and large effects would be values of η^2 equal to .01, .06, and .14, respectively. This would correspond to sample size requirements of approximately 319, 53, or 22 subjects *per group* (in a three-group study), assuming an α of .05 and power of .80.*

Sample Size Estimates for Bivariate Correlation Tests

Suppose we wanted to study the relationship between social support and primiparas' acceptance of the motherhood role. We plan to administer two scales to women who have had a normal vaginal delivery of full-term infants. One scale measures the amount of social support available to the mother in her family and community; the other scale measures the woman's positive and negative reactions to her new role. The hypothesis is that women who have more social support available to them are more accepting of the role transition to motherhood. How many women should be included in the study, given an α of .05 and power of .80?

As in the previous cases, we need an estimate of γ. In this situation, we have two measures on an interval scale, and the relationship between them would be tested using Pearson's *r*. The estimated value of γ here is actually ρ, that is, the expected population correlation coefficient.

Suppose we found an earlier study that correlated a simple measure of social support

(the number of people subjects felt they could count on in times of stress) with an observational measure of maternal warmth. Neither of these measures perfectly captures the variables in the new study, but they are conceptually close, and if no better information were available, they would provide a useful approximation. Suppose the completed study found $r = .18$, which we will use as our estimate of ρ and hence of γ. Table 19-9 shows sample size requirements for various powers and effect sizes in situations in which Pearson's *r* is used. With an α of .05 and power of .80, the sample size needed in the study would lie between 197 (for an effect size of .20) and 349 (for an effect size of .15). Extrapolating for an effect size of .18, we would need a sample of about 250 subjects to achieve a power of .80 with an α of .05. With a sample this size, we would wrongly reject the null hypothesis only 5 times out of 100 and wrongly retain the null hypothesis 20 times out of 100. To increase the power to .95 (wrongly retaining the null hypothesis only 5 times out of 100), we would need a sample of about 400 women.

When prior estimates of effect size are unavailable, the conventional values of small, medium, and large effect sizes in a bivariate correlation situation are .10, .30, and .50, respectively. In Polit and Sherman's (1990) study, the average correlation found in nursing studies was in the vicinity of .20.

Sample Size Estimates for Testing Differences in Proportions

Estimating sample size requirements when differences in proportions between groups are being studied is more complex than in the previously described situations. For this reason, we present only a partial discussion of this topic here and recommend that other references such as Cohen (1977) or Jaccard and Becker (1990) be consulted. We restrict our coverage to 2 × 2 contingency tables.

Suppose we were interested in comparing the rates of breastfeeding in two groups of

---

*When ANCOVA is used in lieu of *t*-tests or ANOVA, the sample size requirements are smaller—sometimes appreciably so—because of reduced error variance.

Table 19-9.   *Approximate Sample Sizes Necessary To Achieve Selected Levels of Power as a Function of Estimated Population Value of* ρ

POWER	\multicolumn{10}{c}{POPULATION CORRELATION COEFFICIENT}
	.10	.15	.20	.25	.30	.40	.50	.60	.70	.80
PART A: $\alpha = .05$										
.60	489	218	123	79	55	32	21	15	11	9
.70	616	274	155	99	69	39	26	18	14	11
.80	785	349	197	126	88	50	32	23	17	13
.90	1050	468	263	169	118	67	43	30	22	17
.95	1297	577	325	208	145	82	53	37	27	21
.99	1841	819	461	296	205	116	75	52	39	30
PART B: $\alpha = .01$										
.60	802	357	201	129	90	51	33	23	17	14
.70	962	428	241	155	108	61	39	28	21	16
.80	1171	521	293	188	131	74	48	33	25	19
.90	1491	663	373	239	167	94	61	42	31	24
.95	1782	792	446	286	199	112	72	50	37	28
.99	2402	1068	601	385	267	151	97	67	50	39

women: 1) those receiving a special intervention—home visits by nurses during the third trimester, in which the advantages of breast-feeding would be described—and 2) those in a control group not receiving any home visits. How many subjects should be randomly assigned to the two groups?

The effect size for this type of situation is not arrived at in a straightforward fashion. This is because the effect size is influenced not only by expected differences in proportions (e.g., 60% in one group versus 40% in another, a 20 percentage point difference) but also by the absolute values of the proportions. In other words, the effect size for 60% versus 40% is *not* the same as that for 30% versus 10%. In general, the effect size is *larger* (and consequently sample size needs are *smaller*) at the extremes than near the midpoint: A 20 percentage point difference is easier to detect when the two percentages are 10% and 30% (or 70% and 90%) than when they are near the middle, such as 40% and 60%.

The computation of the effect size index involves a complex transformation (the arcsine transformation) that we do not fully elaborate on here. Rather than present sample size estimates based on effect size, Table 19-10 presents the approximate sample size requirements for detecting differences in various proportions, assuming an α of .05 and a power of .80. To use this table, we would need to have estimates of the proportions for both groups. Then we would find the proportion for one group in the first column and the proportion for the second group in the top row. The approximate sample size requirement *for each group* would be found at the intersection of the two appropriate proportions. Thus, in our example, if we had reason to expect (on the basis of a pilot study, say), that 20% of the control group mothers and 40% of the experimental group mothers would breast-feed their infants, then the sample size needed in the study (to keep the risk of a Type II error down to 20%) would be 80 subjects per group.

Because we have not presented information on the computationally complex effect size for the situation involving a 2 × 2 contingency table, we cannot conveniently identify Cohen's convention for small, medium, and large effects.

Table 19-10. *Approximate Sample Sizes* Necessary To Achieve a Power of .80 for α = .05 for Estimated Population Difference Between Two Proportions*

GROUP II PROPORTIONS	GROUP I PROPORTIONS														
	.10	.15	.20	.25	.30	.35	.40	.45	.50	.55	.60	.70	.80	.90	1.00
.05	421	133	69	44	31	24	19	15	13	11	9	7	5	4	2
.10		689	196	97	59	41	30	23	18	15	12	9	6	5	4
.15			901	247	118	71	48	34	26	21	16	11	8	5	3
.20				1090	292	137	80	53	38	28	22	14	10	6	3
.25					1252	327	151	87	57	40	30	18	12	8	4
.30						1371	356	161	93	60	42	23	14	9	4
.35							1480	374	169	96	61	31	18	10	5
.40								1510	385	172	97	42	22	12	5
.45									1570	393	173	60	28	15	6
.50										1570	389	93	38	18	6
.55											1539	162	53	23	7
.60												356	80	30	8
.70													292	59	12
.80														195	18
.90															38

* The values are the number of subjects *per group.*

We can, however, give *examples* of differences in proportions (i.e., the proportions in group 1 versus group 2) that conform to the conventions:

Small: .05 versus .10, .20 versus .29, .40 versus .50, .60 versus .70, .80 versus .87

Medium: .05 versus .21, .20 versus .43, .40 versus .65, .60 versus .82, .80 versus .96

Large: .05 versus .34, .20 versus .58, .40 versus .78, .60 versus .92, .80 versus .996

Thus, if the researcher expected a medium effect in which the proportion for group 1 could be expected to be in the vicinity of .40, then the number of subjects in each of the two groups would need to be about 70 to 75. As in other situations, researchers are encouraged to avoid the use of the conventions, if possible, in favor of more precise estimates based on prior empirical evidence; when the use of the conventions is unavoidable, conservative estimates should be used to minimize the risk of finding nonsignificant results.

❖ OTHER STATISTICAL PROCEDURES

The statistical procedures described in this chapter and in Chapters 17 and 18 cover most of the techniques for analyzing quantitative data used by nurse researchers today. However, the widespread use of computers and new developments in statistical analysis have combined to give researchers more options for analyzing their data than were available in the past. Although a full exposition of other sophisticated statistical procedures is beyond the scope of this book, we briefly describe a few of these advanced techniques and provide references for readers interested in more comprehensive discussions.

Life Table and Event History Analysis

Life table analysis is a procedure that is widely used by epidemiologists and medical researchers. It is used when the dependent variable represents the time interval between an initial event and a termination event. Life table analysis is often applied to situations in which mortality is the termination event—such as when the initial event is the onset of a disease or the initiation of treatment for the disease, and death is the end event. Because of this fact, life table analysis is also referred to as *survival analysis*. Life table analysis involves the calculation of a survival score, which compares the survival time for one subject with that for all other subjects. When the researcher is interested in group comparisons—for example, comparing the survival function of subjects in a special treatment versus a control group—a statistic can be computed to test the null hypothesis that the groups are samples from the same survival distribution.

Life table analysis can be applied to many situations that are unrelated to mortality. For example, a life table analysis could be used to analyze such time-related phenomena as length of time in labor, length of time elapsed between release from a psychiatric hospital and reinstitutionalization, duration of pain after surgery, and length of time between the termination of a first pregnancy and the onset of a second one. Further information about life table analysis may be found in Gross and Clark (1975), and Lee (1980).

More recently, extensions of life table analysis have been developed that allow researchers to examine the determinants of survival-type transitions in a multivariate framework. In these analyses, independent variables are used to model the risk (or hazard) of experiencing an event at a given point in time, given that one has not experienced the event before that time. The most common specification of the hazard is known as the *proportional hazards model*. These *event history* methodologies are likely to prove useful to nurse researchers in the 1990s. A relatively straightforward explanation and illustration of this technique is presented in Teachman (1982), and further discus-

sion may be found in Allison (1984), Gross and Clark (1975), or Tuma and Hannan (1984).

Logistic Regression

Most of the analyses we have discussed thus far have been based on a single approach to estimating parameters, the least-squares approach. There are, however, alternative estimation procedures that are being used increasingly by researchers in certain situations. In particular, *maximum likelihood estimation* has gained in popularity and use in analyzing complex multivariate data. Although a full elaboration is beyond the scope of this text, we note that maximum likelihood estimators are ones that estimate the parameters most likely to have generated the observed measurements. For further discussions of maximum likelihood theory, the reader is urged to consult Hanushek and Jackson (1977).

Logistic regression (sometimes referred to as *logit analysis*) is a procedure that uses maximum likelihood estimation for analyzing relationships between multiple independent variables and a dependent variable that is categorical (i.e., a nominal-level measure). Logistic regression transforms the probability of an event occurring (e.g., that a woman will practice breast self-examination or not) into its odds, that is, into the ratio of one event's probability relative to the probability of a second event. As a result, probabilities that range between zero and one in actuality are transformed into continuous variables that range between zero and infinity. Because this range is still restricted, a further transformation is performed, namely calculating the logarithm of the odds. The range of this new variable (known as the *logit of the decision*) is now transformed from minus to plus infinity. Using the logit as a continuous dependent variable, maximum likelihood approaches are then used to estimate the coefficients of the independent variables. These techniques can also be used in the case of a categorical dependent variable that has more than two categories.

Logistic regression is often used in preference to discriminant function analysis for several reasons. First, as Cleary and Angel (1984) noted, logistic models are considered to be more theoretically appropriate than models based on the least-squares approach for exact model fitting. Second, logistic regression is concerned more with modeling the probability of an outcome than with just the prediction of group membership. Also, logistic regression enables the researcher to generate odds ratios that can be meaningfully interpreted and graphically displayed, and therefore may promote better understanding of the underlying relationships of the variables. Although logit analysis was avoided by researchers for many years because of the unavailability of convenient computer programs, that is no longer the case. We expect that logistic regression will be used increasingly by nurse researchers in the upcoming years.

Linear Structural Relation Analysis

Another statistical procedure that is based on maximum likelihood estimation is *linear structural relation analysis,* more commonly referred to as *LISREL.* LISREL is a versatile, but complex, approach used in the analysis of multivariate data. It is most frequently used as a method of testing causal models, much the same as path analysis, but it is also used as an approach to factor analysis.

One of the drawbacks of using ordinary least-squares regression in doing path analysis is that the validity of the method is based on a set of restrictive assumptions, most of which are virtually impossible to meet. First, it is assumed that the variables are measured without error. As we discussed in Chapter 16, most measures used by nurse researchers contain some degree of error. Second, it is assumed that any of the residuals (error terms) in the different regression equations are uncorrelated. However, because error terms often represent untapped sources of individual differences—differences that are not

entirely random—this assumption is seldom tenable. Third, traditional path analysis assumes that the causal flow is unidirectional or recursive. In reality, causes and effects are often reciprocal or iterative.

LISREL avoids all these problems. LISREL can be used for the analysis of models with multiple indicators,* reciprocal causation, measurement errors, and correlated residuals. Because of its versatility, LISREL is a highly complex procedure, and one whose computer program (LISREL 7) is not easy to learn. Readers interested in further information on LISREL are urged to consult Jöreskog and Sörbom (1989) or Hayduk (1987).

❖ THE COMPUTER AND MULTIVARIATE STATISTICS

Multivariate analyses are invariably done by computer because the computations are laborious. To illustrate computer analyses for two multivariate techniques, we return to the example described in Chapters 17 and 18, involving the implementation of a special prenatal intervention for low-income young women. All the data for the examples below were presented in Table 17-8.

Example of Multiple Regression

In Chapter 18, we tested the hypothesis that older mothers in the sample would have infants with higher birthweights than younger mothers, using Pearson's *r.* The computer calculated the value of *r* to be .5938, which was highly significant, thereby supporting the research hypothesis.

---

* LISREL generally involves the use of multiple indicators designed to tap complex latent (unobservable) variables, such as anxiety or motivation. Within LISREl, a measurement model is developed to specify the relations between unobserved and observed (i.e., latent and manifest) variables.

Suppose now that we want to test whether we can significantly improve our ability to predict infant birthweight by adding two other variables to the equation by means of multiple regression: whether or not the mother smoked during the pregnancy (SMOKE), and the number of prior pregnancies (NPREGS). Figure 19-7 presents a part of the SPSS printout for a stepwise multiple regression in which WEIGHT is the dependent variable, and AGE, SMOKE, and NPREGS are the predictor variables. We will explain some of the most noteworthy aspects of this printout.

Figure 19-7 shows (under Equation Number 1) that the first variable stepped into the regression equation is AGE and that the multiple $R = .59383$—the same value shown in Figure 18-6 in Chapter 18 for the bivariate correlation. The value of R^2 is .35264 ($.59383^2$), which represents the amount of variance in birthweight accounted for by the mother's age.* AGE was the first of the three available predictor variables stepped into the equation because it had the highest bivariate correlation with WEIGHT. (As shown in the correlation matrix at the top of Fig-

* The adjusted R^2 of .32925 is the R^2 after it has been adjusted to reflect more closely the goodness of fit of the regression model in the population, through a formula that involves sample size and number of independent variables.

```
        * * * *   M U L T I P L E   R E G R E S S I O N   * * * *

Correlation:

              WEIGHT      AGE      NPREGS      SMOKE

WEIGHT        1.000      .594       .324       -.244
AGE            .594     1.000       .522       -.301
NPREGS         .324      .522      1.000       -.054
SMOKE         -.244     -.301      -.054       1.000

Equation Number 1    Dependent Variable..    WEIGHT   INFANT BIRTH WEIGHT

Block Number  1.  Method:  Stepwise     Criteria   PIN  .0500   POUT  .1000

Variable(s) Entered on Step Number
   1..     AGE       AGE OF MOTHER

Multiple R          .59383
R Square            .35264
Adjusted R Square   .32952
Standard Error     8.97022

Analysis of Variance
                    DF      Sum of Squares      Mean Square
Regression           1         1227.28336       1227.28336
Residual            28         2253.01664         80.46488

F =      15.25241       Signif F =  .0005


------------------ Variables in the Equation ------------------

Variable             B         SE B        Beta        T   Sig T

AGE            3.118890     .798603     .593833     3.905   .0005
(Constant)    48.040159   14.600097                 3.290   .0027


------------ Variables not in the Equation ------------

Variable     Beta In  Partial  Min Toler      T  Sig T

NPREGS       .019634  .020811   .727277     .108  .9147
SMOKE       -.072164 -.085540   .909592    -.446  .6591

End Block Number    1    PIN =      .050 Limits reached.
```

Figure 19-7. SPSS Computer Printout: Multiple Regression ure 19-7, the *r* between WEIGHT and NPREGS is .324, and the *r* between WEIGHT and SMOKE is −.244).

The next panel (under the Analysis of Variance) shows the calculation of the *F*-ratio in which the variability due to regression (i.e., to the relationship between WEIGHT and AGE) is contrasted with residual variability. The value of *F*(15.25241) with 1 and 28 *df* is significant at the .0005 level, consistent with the information from Figure 18-6.

The actual regression equation is presented in the next panel under Variables in the Equation. If we wanted to predict new values of WEIGHT from the same population as this sample based on maternal age at birth, the equation would be:

WEIGHT′ = (3.118890 × AGE) + 48.040159

That is, predicted values of WEIGHT would be equal to the regression coefficient (*b*) times values of AGE, plus the value of the intercept constant.

In regression, a statistical test can be performed for each regression coefficient by dividing *b* by the standard error for *b*; this is shown here under the columns T and Sig T. The value of T for the AGE coefficient is 3.905, which is significant at the .0005 level.

The final panel shows the predictor variables not yet in the equation (NPREGS and SMOKE). Among other pieces of information shown here, the T values for the regression coefficients for these two predictors are both nonsignificant (*p* = .9147 and .6591, respectively), once variation due to AGE is taken into account. Because of this fact, the stepwise regression procedure ends at this point, without adding either of the two additional predictors. Given the significance level of .05 (shown as PIN = .050, i.e., the *P* value for variables going *IN* the equation), the inclusion of either of the two predictor variables would not have significantly added to the prediction of WEIGHT, over and above that which was already achieved with AGE alone.

It is, of course, possible to *force* the two additional predictors into the regression equa-

tion by conducting a nonstepwise regression. When this is done (this is not shown in the table), the value of *R* increases from .59383 to .59836, a negligible and nonsignificant increase. Thus, we must conclude that we cannot improve our ability to predict infant birthweight in this sample, based on the two additional predictors available here.

Example of Analysis of Covariance

In Chapter 18, we tested the hypothesis that infants in the experimental group would have higher birthweights than infants in the control group, using a *t*-test. The computer calculated the value of *t* to be 1.44 which, with 28 *df*, was nonsignificant. The research hypothesis was therefore rejected.

Now that more sophisticated statistical procedures are available to us, we can test the same hypothesis using ANCOVA. Through ANCOVA, we can control for the effect of AGE, which, as we have just seen, is significantly correlated with WEIGHT. Figure 19-8 presents the printout for both ANCOVA and MCA for this analysis, with WEIGHT as the dependent variable, AGE as the covariate, and GROUP (experimental versus control) as the independent variable. At the top of the first panel, we see that the *F*-value for the covariate AGE is 19.457, significant at the .000 level (i.e., beyond the .001 level). After controlling for the effect of AGE, the *F*-value for the independent variable GROUP (the main effect) is 8.719, which is significant at the .006 level. In other words, once AGE is controlled, our research hypothesis about experimental versus control differences is supported rather than rejected. The total amount of variability explained with the two variables, when contrasted with residual variability, is also significant (*F* = 14.088, *p* < .000).

The next panel shows the results of the MCA. For the sample as a whole, the overall mean (grand mean) is 104.700. The original, unadjusted means for the experimental and control groups can be calculated by taking the unad-

```
* * *   A N A L Y S I S   O F   V A R I A N C E   * * *

            WEIGHT    INFANT BIRTH WEIGHT
       BY   GROUP
       WITH AGE       AGE OF MOTHER


                            Sum of                Mean              Signif
Source of Variation         Squares     DF       Square       F      of F

Covariates                 1227.283      1      1227.283    19.457   .000
  AGE                      1227.283      1      1227.283    19.457   .000

Main Effects                549.945      1       549.945     8.719   .006
  GROUP                     549.945      1       549.945     8.719   .006

Explained                  1777.228      2       888.614    14.088   .000

Residual                   1703.072     27        63.077

Total                      3480.300     29       120.010


   30 Cases were processed.
    0 Cases (   .0 PCT) were missing.

 * * *   M U L T I P L E   C L A S S I F I C A T I O N   A N A L Y S I S   * * *

            WEIGHT    INFANT BIRTH WEIGHT
       By   GROUP
       With AGE       AGE OF MOTHER


Grand Mean =       104.700                                       Adjusted for
                                              Adjusted for      Independents
                                Unadjusted    Independents      + Covariates
Variable + Category       N     Dev'n  Eta    Dev'n   Beta     Dev'n    Beta

GROUP
   1 EXPERIMENTAL         15      2.83                           4.38
   2 CONTROL              15     -2.83                          -4.38
                                        .26                              .41

Multiple R Squared                                                      .511
Multiple R                                                              .715
```

Figure 19-8. *SPSS Computer Printout: Analysis of Covariance and Multiple Classification Analysis*

justed deviations from the grand mean. For example, the original mean for the experimental group was 107.53 (104.70 + 2.83), consistent with the information presented earlier in Figure 18-5 in Chapter 18. After adjusting for maternal age, however, the experimental mean is 109.08 (104.70 + 4.38), and the control mean is 100.32 (104.70 − 4.38), a much more sizable difference. The multiple R^2 for predicting birthweight, based on both AGE and GROUP, is .511—substantially more than the R^2 between AGE and WEIGHT alone (.352).

❖ TIPS FOR USING MULTIVARIATE STATISTICS

With the widespread availability of computers and user-friendly programs for performing statistical analysis, multivariate statistics have become increasingly common in nursing studies. In this section, we offer a few suggestions with regard to multivariate statistics.

• If you are using a computer to analyze data, you should definitely consider the use of a multivariate procedure in lieu of a bivariate one for testing your hypotheses because the commands to the computer are not appreciably more complicated. As we have seen, researchers can come to the wrong conclusions about their hypotheses (i.e., commit Type I errors) when extraneous variables are not controlled. Moreover, because the power of statistical tests is enhanced with multivariate procedures, sample size requirements are usually lower.

- With regard to the previous point, ANCOVA is a particularly good technique for researchers without extensive statistical training to use as a substitute for ANOVA and *t*-tests. ANCOVA is relatively easy to run on the computer, and the output is also relatively easy to interpret. Covariates are almost always available: at a minimum, you can use important background characteristics, such as age, gender, and so on. The covariates should be ones that the researcher suspects are correlated with the dependent variable, and demographic characteristics are usually related to a wide variety of other attributes and behaviors. A pretest measure is an excellent choice for a covariate, if one is available. A *pretest* is simply a measure of the dependent variable, taken before the occurrence of the independent variable.

- One of the difficulties with using a multivariate procedure is that the findings may be less readily accessible to statistically unsophisticated readers, such as many practicing nurses or undergraduate nursing students. Thus, in some instances, you may opt to use a simpler analysis to enhance the utilizability of the findings. For example, three separate ANOVAs might be used in lieu of a single MANOVA. However, if the primary reason for *not* using the appropriate multivariate procedure is for communication purposes—rather than your own discomfort with complex procedures—you may want to consider some alternatives. For example, you could describe

the bivariate analyses (e.g. ANOVA) in the report, but also perform the appropriate procedure (e.g. MANOVA) and note in the report that the results remained the same with the multivariate tests (if this is true). Another strategy is to make an extra effort to explain multivariate results in terms that are readily comprehensible. Complex analyses can often be boiled down to relatively straightforward statements about the research hypotheses.

- It is strongly recommended that power analysis be performed to estimate needed sample sizes during the design phase of the study. Once the study has been completed, however, power analysis is a useful tool for interpreting findings, especially when the statistical tests yield nonsignificant results that are often ambiguous.

❖ RESEARCH EXAMPLES

Table 19-11 illustrates some of the applications of multivariate statistics within recent nursing studies. The following study, which used multiple regression, is described in greater detail.

> Dibble, Bostrom-Ezrati, and Rizzuto (1991) conducted a study to describe the frequency of intravenous (IV) site symptoms among patients with an IV placement and to develop a predictive model to explain the number of such symptoms. The 514 research subjects were recruited from four hospitals in the San Francisco area. All patients were adults whose IV placement was distal to the antecubital fossa and whose placement was anticipated for more than 24 hours. The occurrence of IV site symptoms was assessed using a checklist with five symptoms: pain, redness, swelling, induration, and a venous cord. The dependent variable for the analyses was the total number of symptoms observed, which could range from 0 to 5. Additional data consisted of demographic characteristics as well as information about

Table 19-11.   *Examples of Nursing Studies Using Multivariate Statistics*

RESEARCH QUESTION	STATISTICAL PROCEDURE
What are the factors associated with fatigue among older adults with rheumatoid arthritis? (Belza, Henke, Yelin, Epstein & Gilliss, 1993)	Multiple regression
What are the effects of gender and six different types of verbal and tactile stimuli on the arousal of infants hospitalized for congenital heart disease, controlling for age and baseline arousal? (Weiss, 1992)	ANCOVA
What are the primary dimensions of patients' satisfaction with nursing care during hospitalization? (Larson & Ferketick, 1993)	Factor analysis
What are the predictive factors that distinguish between college freshmen who practice safer sex behaviors and those who do not? (DiIorio, Parsons, Lehr, Adame, & Carlone, 1993)	Discriminant function analysis
What are the relationships among the components of perceived health status and various positive health practices in adolescents? (Mahon, 1994)	Canonical correlation
What are the effects of guided imagery and maximal inspiratory muscle training on functional status, fatigue, dyspnea, and inspiratory muscle strength among patients with chronic bronchitis or emphysema? (Moody, Fraser, & Yarandi, 1993)	MANOVA
What are the causal influences on psychological adaptation in dying patients? (Dobratz, 1993)	Path analysis
What is the duration of infection-free catheter days for cancer patients undergoing bone marrow transplantation versus those not undergoing bone marrow transplantation? (Kelly, Dumenko, McGregor, & McHutchion, 1992)	Life table analysis
What are the pathway and gatekeeper variables most predictive of hospital readmission for psychiatric patients? (Polk-Walker, Chan, Meltzer, Goldapp, & Williams, 1993)	Logistic regression
How successful is Pender's Health Promotion Model in predicting selected health-promoting behaviors? (Johnson, Ratner, Bottorff, & Hayduk, 1993)	LISREL

the insertion, maintenance, and removal of the IV.

The analyses revealed that 40% of the patients developed one or more site symptom; the number of symptoms ranged from 0 to 4. Pain was the most common symptom, experienced by 65% of those with a symptom. Multiple regression was used to predict the total number of symptoms experienced, based on both clinical and demographic independent variables. The multiple regression analysis revealed that the most significant predictor was the duration of the IV placement: the longer the placement, the greater the number of symptoms ($p < .001$). Even with placement duration statistically controlled, however, other variables contributed significantly to the prediction of symptoms. For example, having no tape placed over the insertion site to anchor the device ($p < .05$) and receiving an IV solution with higher osmolarity ($p < .05$) tended to result in a significantly greater number of symptoms. Even with all these factors controlled, women had significantly more symptoms than men ($p < .01$). Other variables in the regression analyses (e.g., the gauge of the needle, the use of ointment at the IV site) were not significant predictors. Overall, the various independent variables taken together did only a modest job in explaining individual differences in the number of symptoms: the R^2 was only .18, meaning that 82% of the variability in the number of symptoms could not be explained in terms of the demographic and clinical factors used in the regression analysis. Thus, although several important predictive variables were identified in this study, the researchers concluded that further research is needed to explore other potential causes for IV site symptoms.

❖ SUMMARY

The *multivariate* statistical procedures explored in this chapter are used to untangle complex relationships among three or more variables. One of the most versatile multivariate procedures is *multiple correlation or regression,* which is a statistical method for understanding the effects of two or more independent variables on a dependent variable. A simple regression equation is a formula for making predictions about the numerical values of one variable based on the values of a second variable. The researcher can often improve the precision of the predictions by including more than one predictor (independent) variable in the regression equation. The multiple correlation coefficient is symbolized by R. The multiple correlation coefficient, when squared (R^2), indicates the proportion of the variance of the dependent variable that is ex-

plained or accounted for by the combined influences of the independent variables. R^2 is sometimes referred to as the *coefficient of determination.* The versatility of multiple regression analysis is demonstrated by its various related analyses and special options. For example, in *stepwise multiple regression,* the researcher can identify from a pool of potential predictor variables those variables that in combination have the greatest predictive power.

Analysis of covariance (ANCOVA) is a procedure that permits the researcher to control extraneous or confounding influences on dependent variables. The effect of one or more variable (called the *covariate*) is statistically controlled or removed before testing for group differences by way of traditional ANOVA procedures. ANCOVA is often used in ex post facto or quasi-experimental designs to control for potential pretreatment differences but can also be used in experimental designs to provide more precise estimates of experimental effects. *Multiple classification analysis* (MCA) is a supplement to ANCOVA that yields information about a dependent variable after adjusting for covariates. The information is usually provided in the form of *adjusted means* of each group.

Factor analysis is used to reduce a large set of variables into a smaller set of underlying dimensions, called *factors.* Mathematically, each factor represents a linear combination of the variables contained in a data matrix. The first phase of factor analysis, called *factor extraction,* identifies clusters of variables with a high degree of communality, and condenses the larger set of variables into a smaller number of factors. The second phase of factor analysis involves *factor rotation,* which enhances the interpretability of the factors by aligning variables more distinctly with a particular factor. The *factor loadings* shown in a rotated factor matrix can then be examined to identify and name the underlying dimensionality of the original set of variables and to compute *factor scores.*

Discriminant analysis is essentially a multiple regression analysis in which the dependent variable is categorical (i.e., nominal level of measurement). This procedure is useful for making predictions about membership in groups on the basis of two or more predictor variables. *Canonical correlation* is the most general of all the multivariate procedures: it analyzes the relationship between two or more independent *and* two or more dependent variables. *Multivariate analysis of variance* (*MANOVA*) is the extension of ANOVA principles to cases in which there is more than one dependent variable.

Path analysis is a regression-based procedure for testing causal models. The researcher first prepares a *path diagram* that stipulates hypothesized causal linkages among variables. Using regression procedures applied to a series of *structural equations,* a series of *path coefficients* are developed. These path coefficients represent weights associated with a causal path in standard deviation units. The simplest form of a causal model is one that is *recursive*, that is, one in which causation is presumed to be unidirectional.

Power analysis refers to techniques for estimating either the likelihood of committing a Type II error or sample size requirements. Power analysis involves four components: 1) a desired significance level (α); 2) power ($1 - \beta$); 3) sample size, (n); and 4) an estimated *effect size* (γ). To calculate needed sample size, all three other components must be specified by the researcher. The most difficult part is estimating the effect size, but there is usually at least one existing study that can provide rough guidelines for the estimate. The application of power analysis would probably greatly reduce the number of nonsignificant findings reported in the nursing literature.

New statistical methodologies are likely to gain in popularity among nurse researchers in the 1990s. These include such techniques as *life table analysis, event history analysis, logistic regression,* and *linear structural relation analysis* (*LISREL*).

❖ STUDY SUGGESTIONS

Chapter 19 of the accompanying *Study Guide for Nursing Research: Principles and Methods, 5th ed.,* offers various exercises and study suggestions for reinforcing the concepts presented in this chapter. Additionally, the following study questions can be addressed:

1. Refer to Figure 19-1. What would the value of Y′ be for the following X values: 8, 1, 3, 6?

2. A researcher has examined the relationship between preventive health care attitudes on the one hand and the person's educational level, age, and gender on the other. The multiple correlation coefficient is .62. Explain the meaning of this statistic. How much of the variation in attitudinal scores has been explained by the three predictors? How much is *unexplained*? What other variables might improve the power of the prediction?

3. Which multivariate statistical procedures would you recommend using in the following situations:
   a. A researcher wants to test the effectiveness of a nursing intervention for reducing stress levels among surgical patients, using an experimental group of patients from one hospital and a control group from another hospital.
   b. A researcher wants to predict which students are at risk of venereal disease by using background information such as sex, socioeconomic status, religion, grades in sex education course, and attitudes toward sex.
   c. A researcher wants to test the effects of three different diets on blood sugar levels and blood pH.

4. Estimate the required total sample sizes for the following situations:
   a. Comparison of two group means: α = .01; power = .90; γ = .35.

b. Comparison of three group means: $\alpha = .05$; power $= .80$; $\eta^2 = .07$.

c. Correlation of two variables: $\alpha = .01$; power $= .85$; $\rho = .27$.

d. Comparison of two proportions: $\alpha = .05$; power $= .80$, $P_1 = .35$; $P_2 = .50$.

❖ SUGGESTED READINGS

METHODOLOGICAL REFERENCES

Aaronson, L. S. (1989). A cautionary note on the use of stepwise regression. *Nursing Research, 38,* 309–311.

Aaronson, L. S., Frey, M., & Boyd, C. J. (1988). Structural equation models and nursing research: Part II. *Nursing Research, 37,* 315–318.

Allison, P. D. (1984). *Event history analysis: Regression for longitudinal event data.* Beverly Hills, CA: Sage.

Blalock, H. M., Jr. (1972). *Causal inferences in nonexperimental research.* New York: W. W. Norton.

Borenstein, M., & Cohen, J. (1988). *Statistical power analysis: A computer program.* Hillsdale, NJ: Erlbaum Associates.

Boyd, C. J., Frey, M. A., & Aaronson, L. S. (1988). Structural equation models and nursing research: Part I. *Nursing Research, 37,* 249–253.

Brown, B., Walker, H., Schimeck, M., & Wright, P. (1979). A life table analysis package for SPSS. *American Sociological Review, 33,* 225–227.

Cleary, P. D., & Angel, R. (1984). The analysis of relationships involving dichotomous dependent variables. *Journal of Health and Social Behavior, 25,* 334–348.

Cohen, J. (1977). *Statistical power analysis for the behavioral sciences.* New York: Academic Press.

Cohen, J., & Cohen, P. (1983). *Applied multiple regression: Correlation analysis for behavioral sciences* (2nd ed.). New York: Halsted Press.

Cox, D. R., & Oakes, D. (1984). *Analysis of survival data.* London: Chapman and Hall.

Goodwin, L. D. (1984a). Increasing efficiency and precision of data analysis: Multivariate vs. univariate statistical techniques. *Nursing Research, 33,* 247–249.

Goodwin, L. D. (1984b). The use of power estimation in nursing research. *Nursing Research, 33,* 118–120.

Gross, A. J., & Clark, V. (1975). *Survival distributions: Reliability applications in the biomedical sciences.* New York: John Wiley and Sons.

Hanushek, E., & Jackson, J. (1977). *Statistical methods for social scientists.* New York: Academic Press.

Hayduk, L. A. (1987). *Structural equation modeling with LISREL: Essentials and advances.* Baltimore: Johns Hopkins University Press.

Jaccard, J., & Becker, M. A. (1990). *Statistics for the behavioral sciences.* (2nd ed.). Belmont, CA: Wadsworth.

Jöreskog, K. G., & Sörbom, D. (1989). *LISREL® 7: User's reference guide.* Mooresville, IN: Scientific Software.

Kerlinger, F. N. (1986). *Foundations of behavioral research* (3rd ed.). New York: Holt, Rinehart & Winston.

Knapp, T. R. (1994). Regression analysis: What to report. *Nursing Research, 43,* 187–189.

Knapp, T. R., & Campbell-Heider, N. (1989). Numbers of observations and variables in multivariate analyses. *Western Journal of Nursing Research, 11,* 634–641.

Lee, E. T. (1980). *Statistical methods for survival data analysis.* Belmont, CA: Lifelong Learning.

Mason-Hawkes, J., & Holm, K. (1989). Causal modeling: A comparison of path analysis and LISREL. *Nursing Research, 38,* 312–314.

Maxwell, A. E. (1978). *Multivariate analysis in behavioral research: For medical and social science students* (2nd ed.). New York: Methuen.

Pedhazur, E. J. (1982). *Multiple regression in behavioral research* (2nd ed.). New York: Holt, Rinehart & Winston.

Polit, D. F., & Sherman, R. (1990). Statistical power in nursing research. *Nursing Research, 39,* 365–369.

Tatsuoka, M. (1970). *Discriminant analysis: The study of group differences.* Champaign, IL: Institute for Personality and Ability Testing.

Tatsuoka, M. (1987). *Multivariate analysis: Techniques for educational and psychological research.* (2nd ed.). New York: John Wiley and Sons.

Teachman, J. D. (1982). Methodological issues in the analysis of family formation and dissolution.

Journal of Marriage and the Family, 44, 1037–1053.

Tuma, N. B., & Hannan, M. T. (1984). *Social dynamics: Models and methods.* New York: Academic Press.

Volicer, B. J. (1981). *Advanced statistical methods with nursing applications.* Bedford, MA: Merestat Press.

Weisberg, S. (1985). *Applied linear regression* (2nd ed.). New York: John Wiley and Sons.

Welkowitz, J., Ewen, R. B., & Cohen, J. (1982). *Introductory statistics for the behavioral sciences* (3rd ed.). New York: Academic Press.

Wu, Y. B., & Slakter, M. J. (1989). Analysis of covariance in nursing research. *Nursing Research, 38,* 306–308.

SUBSTANTIVE REFERENCES

Belza, B. L., Henke, C. J., Yelin, E. H., Epstein, W. V., & Gilliss, C. L. (1993). Correlates of fatigue in older adults with rheumatoid arthritis. *Nursing Research, 42,* 93–99.

Dibble, S. L., Bostrom-Ezrati, J., & Rizzuto, C. (1991). Clinical predictors of intravenous site symptoms. *Research in Nursing and Health, 14,* 314–420.

DiIorio, C., Parsons, M., Lehr, S., Adame, D., & Carlone, J. (1993). Factors associated with use of safer sex practices among college freshmen. *Research in Nursing and Health, 16,* 343–350.

Dobratz, M. C. (1993). Causal influences of psychological adaptation in dying. *Western Journal of Nursing Research, 15,* 708–724.

Johnson, J. L., Ratner, P. A., Bottorff, J. L., & Hayduk, L. A. (1993). An exploration of Pender's Health Promotion Model using LISREL. *Nursing Research, 42,* 132–138.

Kelly, C., Dumenko, L., McGregor, S. E., & McHutchion, M. E. (1992). A change in flushing protocols of central venous catheters. *Oncology Nursing Forum, 19,* 599–605.

Larson, P. J., & Ferketich, S. L. (1993). Patients' satisfaction with nurses' caring during hospitalization. *Western Journal of Nursing Research, 15,* 690–703.

Mahon, N. E. (1994). Positive health practices and perceived health status in adolescents. *Clinical Nursing Research, 3,* 86–103.

Moody, L. E., Fraser, M., & Yarandi, H. (1993). Effects of guided imagery in patients with chronic bronchitis and emphysema. *Clinical Nursing Research, 2,* 478–486.

Polk-Walker, G. C., Chan, W., Meltzer, A. A., Goldapp, G., & Williams, B. (1993). Psychiatric recidivism prediction factors. *Western Journal of Nursing Research, 15,* 163–173.

Weiss, S. J. (1992). Psychophysiological and behavioral effects of tactile stimulation on infants with congenital heart disease. *Research in Nursing and Health, 15,* 93–101.

Chapter 20

COMPUTERS AND SCIENTIFIC RESEARCH

Computers have evolved and expanded at a tremendous rate since their development in the 1940s. Few aspects of American society have remained untouched by the impact of computers: bills are sent out, weather is predicted, literature sources are retrieved, classroom schedules are determined, production machines are controlled, medical records are maintained, and diagnoses are made—all with the assistance of computers. With the advent of personal computers, computers have become ubiquitous.

The use of computers in scientific research, as one might suspect, is substantial. Computers have, in fact, revolutionized research by making possible certain operations that could not have been attempted with human labor alone. Computers are now used by researchers throughout the research process—to conduct bibliographic searches, to collect and store data of all types, to maintain administrative research records, to analyze data, and to produce research reports and other documents. Although there are numerous applications of computer technology in scientific investigations, the discussion here focuses primarily on the use of computers to analyze quantitative research data.

One of the most striking features of modern computer technology is that computer users do not need to understand in detail how a computer works to benefit from its labor-saving computations. Computers have become accessible to broader and broader classes of users. It is hoped that an acquaintance with some of the basic characteristics of computers will be sufficient to demonstrate that computer analysis is within the reach of all readers of this book.

❖ POWERS AND LIMITATIONS OF COMPUTERS

Computers are machines of tremendous power. Without any doubt, they have become indispensable to modern scientists. Computers are not, however, on the verge of making human intelligence obsolete. Respect for the potency of computers must be balanced by a recognition of their limitations.

Computer Capabilities

The most noteworthy characteristic of computers is unquestionably their remarkable speed. The fact that computers are fast probably is familiar to everyone, but it is difficult to grasp how incredibly speedy computers actually are. Some computers can perform more arithmetic in 1 second than a human could perform working 40-hour weeks for several years. The speed of computers, therefore, removes the drudgery and delays of doing computations manually and can increase researcher productivity.

Not only are computers fast, but they also are accurate. Highly complex calculations can be performed without error. By contrast, humans are fallible. The person who spends an hour calculating a statistic such as a correlation coefficient would probably have to spend at least as much time checking for computational errors. A computer could perform the same calculation, error-free, in less than 1 second. An additional advantage of computers is that they are *dependably* accurate. They can work hour after hour without making a mistake.

The memory capacity of large computers is impressive. The memory of a computer can store immense files of symbols to which it can gain access in a fraction of a second. Some memory devices can store millions of digits. What is even more impressive is that the information stored in memory is not permanent but can be erased and replaced with new information. In other words, the memory can be used over and over again to solve new problems.

Another noteworthy aspect of computers is their flexibility. Most computers have been built for a variety of purposes. A university computer, for instance, does the payroll, produces income tax forms, keeps track of scholarship monies, bills students, produces grade reports, analyzes data from faculty research, and so forth.

Finally, although computers do break down, they behave for the most part as our faithful servants. They do exactly what they are told to do, day in and day out, no matter how boring or repetitive the task might be.

Computer Limitations

One of the most conspicuous limitations of computers is their utter and complete stupidity. Computers are sometimes referred to as giant brains, but computers have no innate intelligence. They do only those operations that they are told to do by humans. The computer's inability to think sometimes can result in frustrating experiences for its users. Unlike humans, a computer is unable to make even the simplest of inferences.

Computer time for the analysis of complex data sets on a large computer can be costly, although computer costs have decreased dramatically over the past 10 years. However, although computer costs for complex analyses may be high, they are really a bargain in comparison with the costs of human labor. Moreover, there is often no cost when more routine analyses are performed on smaller computers.

Another limitation of computers is the detail with which instructions must be described. When a human is confronted with the task 2 + 2 = ?, the solution is (at the conscious level at least) straightforward and simple. A computer normally requires several instructions to process such computations. Every logical and arithmetic operation must be explained to the computer in detail, a feature that makes most tasks seem more complex than they would to humans. Fortunately, the average researcher does not have to worry about such matters. The detailed instructions are developed by experts who have taken pains to simplify the use of computers.

❖ TYPES OF COMPUTERS

Broadly speaking, computers are either special-purpose or general-purpose machines. A *special-purpose computer* is dedicated to a single function: controlling the machines in which they are embedded. Many pieces of hospital equipment contain special-purpose computers. A *general-purpose computer* can be used for a wide variety of applications. *Applications* are the things that computers can be used to do.

There are four major types of general purpose computers: 1) microcomputers, 2) minicomputers, 3) mainframes, and 4) supercomputers. These four types vary with respect to speed, memory capacity, cost, size, and direct accessibility to researchers. For the most part, nurse researchers are most likely to use either mainframes or microcomputers.

Many universities, hospitals, and other large institutions own what is referred to as a *mainframe computer,* which is a large multiuser system that usually can be accessed from multiple locations. Mainframes typically have huge memory capacities and operate at very high rates of speed. Figure 20-1 presents a picture of the major components of such a mainframe computer. Specialized mainframes that are needed to perform highly complex operations (such as the management of a space launch) are sometimes referred to as *supercomputers.*

Minicomputers are moderate-sized computers that operate at intermediate speeds. Such computers have most frequently been used for mid-sized applications, such as the storage and analysis of laboratory data. However, minicomputers are becoming less common with the advent of powerful microcomputers.

Microcomputers or *personal computers* (*PCs*) are becoming increasingly popular both in institutions and in private homes and offices. PCs are slower and have less memory than mainframes, yet PCs are inexpensive and generally easy to use and are useful for many research applications, such as word processing and the analysis of most data sets. Personal computers vary in size from hand-held and laptop models with rather restricted uses to desktop models with many possible uses. Figure 20-2 shows an example of a desktop PC.

❖ OVERVIEW OF COMPUTER COMPONENTS

A computer system consists of numerous components that perform specialized functions. The components of a computer system can be classiﬁed as either hardware or software. *Hardware* refers to the physical equipment that stores, processes, and controls information. *Software* refers to the instructions and procedures required to operate the computer. In this section, the major aspects of both hardware and software are reviewed.

Computer Hardware

A schematic diagram of computer hardware is presented in Figure 20-3. Essentially, the

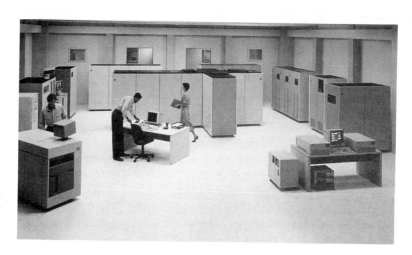

Figure 20-1. *Computer hardware, mainframe computer (Courtesy of International Business Machines Corporation).*

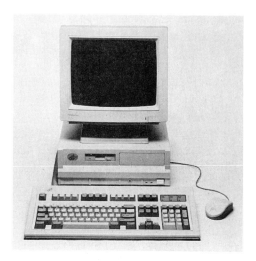

Figure 20-2. *A personal computer (Courtesy of International Business Machines Corporation).*

computer consists of five types of components. Information is fed into the computer through some type of *input device*—the device that allows you to "talk to" the computer. The information read in through an input device for statistical analysis comprises data, on the one hand, and instructions concerning how the data are to be processed, on the other. A keyboard or terminal frequently serves as the primary input device. After the computer has performed its necessary calculations, the resulting information comes out through an *output device*—the device that allows the computer to "talk back" to you. The most common output device is a printer. In a mainframe environment, input/output devices (sometimes abbreviated *I/O devices*) are generally the only parts of the machine with which a researcher comes in direct physical contact.

The information that is read into the computer is stored in a device called *memory*. One way to conceptualize memory is as a series of pigeon holes or post office boxes. Each mailbox can store either an instruction or a numerical value. The cells are organized into a series and assigned a number so that any piece of information stored in memory can be located by its "address." The memory unit of a computer is de-

signed to store large amounts of information and to allow rapid access to any specific portion of that information. Memory capacity is measured in *kilobytes* (K) or *megabytes* (MB). A *byte* is equivalent to a single character, such as a number, letter, or specialized symbol, such as a "+" sign. One kilobyte equals 1000 bytes, and 1 megabyte equals 1 million bytes.

From the memory, the instructions are sent to the *control unit*. This component coordinates the functions of the other components. The control unit interprets the instructions, determines the sequence of operations of the computer, and controls the movements of information from one component to another. The *arithmetic/logic unit* is the component in which arithmetic operations are accomplished. The control unit and arithmetic/logic unit are together referred to as the *central processing unit* (CPU), which is where all the decisions are made and calculations are performed.

Computer Software

The software components of a computer include the instructions for performing operations (referred to as a *program*) and the documentation for those instructions. The ability of a computer to solve problems depends on computer programs, which specify clearly and precisely what operations the machine is to perform and how to perform them.

To give the computer a set of commands, people must be able to communicate with the machine. Computers, unfortunately, do not directly understand natural languages such as English. Direct machine language that a computer *can* comprehend is extremely complex and accessible to only programming experts. Happily, various *programming languages* have been developed that are reasonably easy to learn and that are structured in a manner comfortable to human communicators. The instructions to the computer can be written in a programming language, and then another program called a *compiler* (or, in some cases, an *interpreter*) translates the instructions into an equiv-

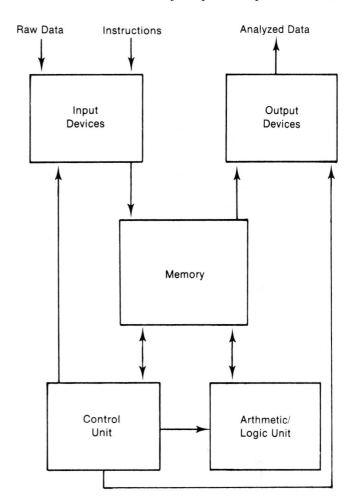

Figure 20-3. *Scheme of computer components and interrelationships*

alent *machine language* program that the computer can comprehend and execute.

Various programming languages are available. Many of these languages have been developed for a specific type of application. The languages most often used in scientific and engineering applications are *FORTRAN* (an acronym for FORmula TRANslation) and *PL/1* (Programming Language 1). One of the simplest languages for beginning programmers to learn is *BASIC* (Beginners All-purpose Symbolic Instruction Code). *PASCAL* is another language that is especially popular in introducing programming to students.

Most researchers can easily use computers without ever having to learn a programming language. This is because there are standard programs available for widely used applications. The applications software most commonly used by nurse researchers include the following:

• *Word processing*—software used for composing, revising, storing, and printing written documents, such as research reports, questionnaires, or research proposals
• *Desktop publishing*—software for printing documents, charts, and graphs at near-typeset quality

- *Spreadsheets*—interactive programs that perform a variety of mathematic calculations and organize numeric information
- *Data base management*—programs used for storing, retrieving, and manipulating large collections of data or information
- *Communications*—programs that allow computers to talk to one another over telephone lines by means of a special piece of equipment known as a *modem*
- *Statistical analysis*—software for organizing and analyzing data and performing statistical tests

Various statistical software packages are discussed later in this chapter.

❖ *PERSONAL COMPUTERS*

Most nurse researchers today enter and analyze their research data (and perform other functions as well) on PCs rather than on mainframes. Therefore, we devote this section to a discussion of the main features of PCs.

The Two Personal Computer Camps

Most PCs currently used by researchers fall into two camps: 1) IBM PCs and compatible computers; and 2) Apple Macintosh computers (Macs). The IBM line of PCs have been widely imitated by other manufacturers. The terms *IBM clone* and *IBM compatible* indicate a computer not made by IBM, but one that uses similar components and a similar design and that can use the same programs as IBM PCs. Clones of Macintosh computers are, by contrast, rare.

The main difference between IBM PCs and Macs concerns their *user interface*—the software that passes information to and from the person using the computer. Macs have traditionally had a more comfortable-looking *user-friendly* interface, centered around pictures, graphic symbols, and *menus* (lists of options). The Mac's interface also uses *windows*—a method for dividing the display screen into rectangles for viewing two or more applications or parts of a single application at the same time. Traditional IBM interfaces tend to be more text-oriented. However, special windows programs are now available for IBMs, in effect making IBMs and their clones look and function more like a Mac. Figure 20-4 shows a PC screen with a windows program. Because most sophisticated statistical software for PCs have been designed for use on IBM-type computers, some of the discussion in this section is more relevant to IBM PCs than to Macs.

Personal Computer Systems

The basic hardware components of a PC system consist of the following: a keyboard for inputting information; a display device; the systems unit; the disk drives and disks; and a printer.

A *keyboard*, an example of which is shown in Figure 20-5, is a device that converts keystrokes into codes that are intelligible to the computer. A PC keyboard looks like a typewriter but has a number of additional keys, including *function keys* (labeled F1 to F12) that perform special functions idiosyncratic to the application. The keyboard also includes a set of keys marked with arrows that control the movement of a visual aid—the *cursor*—on the display screen. Many keyboards also include a numerical keypad arranged like a calculator, for entering large amounts of numerical information. Although keyboards are usually the primary input device, some PCs have additional input devices, such as a pointing device—a *mouse*—that allows you to point to words or objects on the computer screen.

The *display* (sometimes called a *monitor* or *computer screen*) is one of the output devices of a PC. A display is a device that gives you immediate feedback while you operate the computer (e.g., by displaying your keystrokes as you enter them) and that is sometimes used for viewing the computer's output, such as the results of a statistical analysis.

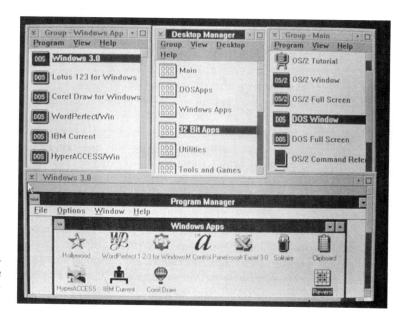

Figure 20-4. *A computer monitor showing a Windows program (Courtesy of International Business Machines Corporation).*

The PC's *systems unit* houses the memory and CPU. The memories in PCs generally have between 1 and 4 megabytes, and they are expandable. In a PC, the CPU is the *microprocessor chip.* Microprocessors vary considerably in processing speed, measured in *megahertz* (MHz). One MHz represents 1 million cycles per second, so that in a 20-MHz microprocessor, there are 20 million cycles per second.

Disks are flat spinning objects, analogous to records, typically with magnetizable surfaces and concentric tracks. Disks are used to store information and can be used as either an input or output device, or for *external storage**. The device that operates the disk is called a *disk drive.* There are two types of magnetic disks—floppy disks and hard disks. *Hard disks* are large-capacity storage devices that are housed within

---

* New I/O and external storage devices are constantly under development. One of the most noteworthy advances in recent years is the *CD-ROM* (compact disk, read-only memory). CD-ROM represents a microcomputer application of the technology responsible for the highly popular audio compact disks. A single CD-ROM can hold more than 550 MB of information, the equivalent of 1500 floppy disks.

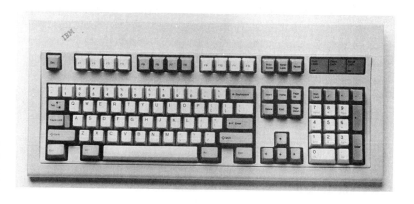

Figure 20-5. *A keyboard for a personal computer (Courtesy of International Business Machines Corporation).*

the systems unit case, invisible to the computer user. *Floppy disks* have lower storage capacity and need to be inserted into the appropriate disk drive by the user before use. The two most common sizes for floppies are 3½ inches and 5¼ inches; the smaller floppies generally have much higher storage capacity. Most PCs have a hard disk drive and one or two disk drives for floppies. The floppy drives are sometimes referred to as the *A drive* (and the *B drive* if there are two floppy drives), and the hard disk drive is the *C drive*. Both hard disks and floppy disks can be erased and used over and over again.

For many applications, the primary output device is a *printer*, which produces paper-copy output from a computer program. Printers are connected to the computer by a cable through a *port*, typically located on the back of the systems unit case. Printers come in a variety of types, from relatively inexpensive *dot-matrix* printers that form characters with a pattern of dots, to *laser-jet* printers that create highly professional-looking output. Statistical output produced by printers is usually called a *printout*.

Operating System

An *operating system* is the software that controls the overall operation of the computer system. The operating system allows various parts of the computer system to talk to one another, and it also supports applications programs by managing the flow of information and keeping track of everything in memory. Applications software is designed for use with specific operating systems.

One part of the operating system is the *boot program*—the instructions that help the computer "pull itself up by its boot straps" by loading the rest of the operating system into memory. The first thing a computer does when you turn it on is to look for this boot program, usually located on the C (hard disk) drive. Note that if you have a floppy disk inserted in your A drive or B drive when you turn on the computer—and if this floppy does not contain the operating system software—the computer will

typically display some message such as "Disk error." Thus, floppies should generally not be inserted until the computer has finished booting.

There are two basic types of operating systems: single-tasking and multitasking. A *single-tasking* operating system runs one application program or task at a time. *Multitasking* operating systems allow more than one application program or task to be active simultaneously.

Several different operating systems are currently in use. If you are running an IBM-type PC, you will probably be using a single-tasking operating system called *MS-DOS* (*M*icro*s*oft *d*isk-*o*perating *s*ystem). A noteworthy advantage of MS-DOS is that an extensive number of application programs have been written for it. Users of MS-DOS who want to create a windows environment can obtain the software extension known as Microsoft Windows.

Statistical software is increasingly becoming available for *OS/2* (Operating Systems/2), a multitasking operating system designed for the current generation of IBM-type computers. The latest version of OS/2 provides a window-based user interface for the operating system's file management functions. A noteworthy advantage of OS/2 for some statistical programs is that it imposes fewer restrictions on the number of variables that can be handled. For large data sets (e.g., many longitudinal data sets), this is a distinct advantage.

Networks

Networks are groups of computers and related equipment that are linked together by communication devices. There are several reasons for networking computers. First, networking allows multiple computers to share expensive peripheral equipment, such as laser-jet printers. Second, people connected by means of a computer network can exchange messages through the process of *electronic mail* (E-mail). Finally, networks allow computers to share data and programs. For example, students taking a statistics course can share the same data base when the computers they are using are networked.

The term *local-area network* (*LAN*) refers to a network in which the computers are connected with wire cables. LANs are usually installed in relatively close proximity in a single building. If the computer you are using is part of a network, you may see a prompt after the booting process is completed that asks for you to *log on* by giving your *user name*. You may also be asked to enter a *password* as well. The user name and password are security features that limit access to the computer or to certain files stored in the network.

In *wide-area networks* (*WANs*), some of the links in the networking chain are connected by modems. A *modem* (short for *mo*dulate and *dem*odulate) is a hardware device that enables two computers to exchange information over standard telephone lines. Modems are sometimes external devices, separate from the computer, but in other cases, they may be built into the computer's system unit case. Through a modem and appropriate communications software, intercity (and even intercountry) communication between computers is possible. For example, researchers can exchange data or reports with a colleague located in another city. WANs are also used to tap into online information services (e.g., CompuServe and Prodigy) and to access electronic bulletin boards.

❖ *MAINFRAME COMPUTERS*

Many universities and hospitals are replacing their mainframe computers with clusters of powerful PCs that are networked. However, mainframes continue to be available in some environments. Many of the concepts introduced in the previous section on PCs are also relevant to users of mainframes.

The only components of mainframes with which researchers typically interact are input and output devices. The input devices are generally terminals or keyboards that are similar to the PC keyboards. The keyboard is connected to a display screen or monitor that serves as an important output device and gives the user instant access to information entered on the keyboard.

Researchers can communicate with a mainframe computer in one of several modes. For many mainframe applications, instructions to the computer are processed in the batch-processing mode. *Batch processing* refers to a method in which a batch of programs is assembled for execution during the same machine run. The data and instructions regarding the analysis of the data are entered into the computer (sometimes through more than one input device if the data are being stored on an external storage device such as a hard disk), and the program is processed without any further intervention. The researcher must normally wait some time before getting the output from a batch processing job. The delay between the input of the job and the availability of the output, which is referred to as the *turnaround time*, may be several minutes or several hours.

Most computer systems and software packages offer users the capability of interacting directly with the computer, in what is called the *interactive mode*. In this mode, a researcher may be able to type in information and receive feedback essentially immediately, either on the monitor or on a printed copy, similar to how processing occurs with a PC. On large computer systems, direct communication between the computer and numerous users concurrently is made possible by a concept known as time sharing. *Time sharing* is a method of operation by means of which several different programs are interleaved, giving the users the impression that the jobs are being processed simultaneously. Time sharing usually operates on a round-robin system. The computer spends a small amount of time (perhaps only 1/100th of a second) on each program, passing onto the next user. Because an entire cycle takes only seconds, it appears to all users as though they are getting instantaneous, personal service. The slowness of the keyboard and the rapidity of the CPU have combined to make time sharing feasible. Interactive terminals operate through networks connected to the computer by telephone lines, and thus the terminals need not be in the same building or even the same city as the computer.

A variety of printer options are often available for mainframes. The *line printer* is typically one of the principal output devices. These printers create an entire line of print at once and can print more than 1000 lines per minute.

Each mainframe computer installation has developed its own idiosyncratic procedures by which users gain access to computer facilities. If you are a first-time user of a system, you will need to learn exactly what steps must be taken to make use of the equipment. You may obtain such information from your instructors or from one of the many computer assistants who are generally available to guide you. Generally, you will need to provide the computer with some administrative information that allows the computer to determine whether you should have access to it, such as a user ID and a password.

Mainframe computers often have several options for interacting with the system and creating files. Two common options in university settings are TSO (Time-Sharing Option) and CMS (Conversational Monitoring System). You will need to learn which monitoring system is available at your institution and how to gain access to and use it.

❖ AVAILABLE PROGRAMS FOR STATISTICAL ANALYSIS

A great boon to researchers in all disciplines is the widespread availability of ready-made programs for the analysis of quantitative research data. The computer centers at universities are particularly likely to have a variety of software packages available to their users. Most computer centers have a professional staff that is accessible for consultation concerning the computer's library of programs. Sophisticated programs for performing statistical analysis are available for both mainframes and PCs. As we will discuss in Chapter 22, various programs also are available for the analysis of qualitative

data. The main statistical software packages currently available are discussed in this section.

Major Statistical Software Packages

The most widely used statistical software packages for use on mainframe and PCs include the Statistical Package for the Social Sciences (SPSS); Statistical Analysis System (SAS); and the Biomedical Computer Programs—P Series (BMD-P). Each of these packages contains programs to handle a broad variety of statistical analyses. The reference section at the end of this chapter identifies the major statistical capabilities available for each of these packages. Because these packages are updated, refined, and expanded frequently, readers are advised to check with personnel at their computer facility for any modifications to the description and listings provided in this chapter.

SPSS

SPSS was developed by researchers at the University of Chicago and National Opinion Research Center to assist researchers in the analysis of social science data. SPSS represents a highly flexible program with a syntax that is not technically oriented. For people with limited statistical and computer backgrounds, SPSS is relatively easy to learn. Among its many strong features, SPSS provides excellent capabilities for labeling variables and includes all of the most commonly used parametric and nonparametric statistical procedures, and many less frequently used ones, including survival analysis. On mainframes, this software is sometimes called SPSSX. SPSS is also available in a microcomputer version, SPSS/PC+. SPSS for PCs is particularly powerful in the version that has been designed for use with the OS/2 operating system.

SAS

SAS is a computer package that was developed at North Carolina State University for use in research. It has evolved into a widely used and flexible package. It is generally considered to be somewhat more sophisticated, from a statistical point of view, than SPSS. Like SPSS, the syntax of SAS is fairly easy to learn, even for those without a strong statistical or computer background. One disadvantage of SAS, in comparison with SPSS, is that SAS uses a more cumbersome approach for the labeling of variables (e.g., labeling the variable GENDER) and for categories within variables (e.g., MALE/FEMALE). However, SAS uses a less rigid format in syntax than SPSS and contains a more complete set of sophisticated statistical procedures. Like SPSS, SAS is also available in both a mainframe and a PC version.

BMD-P

The programs referred to as Biomedical Programs were originally developed in the 1960s at the Health Sciences Computer Facility of the University of California, Los Angeles. The package has been vastly improved and simplified since its original development, and the current P series (BMD-P) is now widely used. The BMD-P package contains a large variety of elementary and advanced statistical procedures and uses a highly flexible syntax. One major way in which BMD-P differs from SPSS and SAS is that the particular BMD-P program to be accessed must be indicated at the outset. Thus, only one program can be used for any given computer run (although the program may contain numerous statistical methods as options). In SPSS and SAS, the various statistical procedures are all incorporated as separate steps or subprograms. BMD-P also has a counterpart available for PCs.

Using a Packaged Program

Researchers using packaged programs do not need to know a programming language, but they still must be able to communicate to the computer some basic information about what their variables are and how the data are to be

analyzed. This is accomplished by means of certain commands that are unique to each software package. To illustrate the kinds of commands the researcher would need to know, an example of a set-up for an analysis using the SPSS-PC software is presented. First, however, we need to explain a bit about computer files.

A *file* is a named collection of information that can be accessed by the computer. Computer programs like SPSS are stored on disk files that are accessed through a set of commands to the computer. In running a statistical software package, you are likely to have to create several different types of files.

- *Command file.* First, you will need to create a command file that communicates specific information about your data set (for example, what variables are in the data set) and instructions regarding the analyses you want to perform.
- *Data files.* The actual research data are usually stored in a separate data file. Data files are generally organized as a series of fields and records. In data files, a *field* designates the column or set of consecutive columns in which a piece of information is stored; a *record* represents a line or row of information. The data for each subject or *case* may require more than one record if there are many variables. (When the amount of data is very small, the data can be included in the command file rather than in a separate data file, as in the example we present below.)
- *Output files.* The results of the analyses are often written to a separate output file for subsequent printing.
- *Systems files.* If you have a large data set, you may also want to create special systems files that integrate your command and data files and make them more efficient to run.

Each file that you create must be named. Naming conventions and rules vary somewhat from one type of computer to the next, but often file names are restricted to eight characters—with an optional extension of up to three characters that are separated from the rest of the file name by a period. File names must begin with an alphabetical letter. For example, a command file might be named RESEARCH.COM, the data file might be named RESEARCH.DAT, and the output file might be named RESEARCH.OUT.

Now we can proceed with our example. Suppose that we wanted to analyze the data that we used as an example in Chapters 17 through 19 concerning an intervention for low-income pregnant young women. The data for 30 subjects are shown in Table 17-8 in Chapter 17. The six variables, it may be recalled, are as follows: 1) group—experimental versus control; 2) weight of the infant; 3) repeat pregnancy; 4) mother's age; 5) number of prior pregnancies; and 6) whether or not the mother smoked during pregnancy. Because there are only six variables, these data would be entered onto the computer file with one record for each subject. Thus, the data would be entered onto 30 lines, with each line containing information on these six variables.

On each record, the information for the research variables would have to be entered into fields according to some plan. Suppose, for example, the data were to be entered as follows: an arbitrary identification number would be assigned and entered in columns 1 and 2; designation of group status (column 3); the infant's birthweight in ounces (columns 4 to 6); whether the mother had a repeat pregnancy (column 7); the mother's age (columns 8 and 9); number of pregnancies (column 10); and smoking status (column 11). A subsequent section of this chapter explains how such formatting decisions are made.

To use SPSS to analyze the data, we must tell the computer how we have set up our data, just as we had to communicate this information to you in the preceding paragraph. Figure 20-6 presents the command file—the SPSS instructions and the data. The first line (DATA LIST) is an SPSS command that tells the computer that we are about to define the variables that are in the data file. The next two lines contain all the variable definition and variable location information. The first entry on the second line (/) tells the computer to start reading one line of

data. If we had collected information on 50 variables for each subject, we might have used two lines per subject, in which case the second line would have begun with another slash (/). Next, each variable is specified by a name, followed by the designation of the columns in which data for that variable will appear. In SPSS, variable names can be up to eight alphanumeric characters. In this example, we have called our variables ID, GROUP, WEIGHT, REPEAT, AGE, NPREGS, and SMOKE. Then, to the right of each variable name, we have designated the appropriate field or column numbers. For example, the data for mothers' age (AGE) are in columns 8 and 9.

The next line instructs the computer to begin reading the data (BEGIN DATA), which follow immediately. There are 30 records here, one for each of the 30 subjects. (If these data had been in a separate data file rather than in the command file, we would have had to tell the computer where to find the data using a GET FILE command, such as GET FILE = 'RESEARCH.DAT'.) After indicating to the computer that there are no more data (END DATA), the final two lines indicate the SPSS commands that tell the computer what statistical analysis to perform. These instructions will produce, for every variable in the data set except ID, a frequency distribution and many basic descriptive statistics, such as the mean, median, and standard deviation. The printout produced by this program for the WEIGHT variable was presented in Figure 17-10 in Chapter 17. If we wanted more complex statistics, such as those described in Chapters 18 and 19, we would need only to replace the FREQUENCIES/STATISTICS instructions with other instructions.

We hope that this simple example has made it clear that a researcher need not be a computer whiz or statistical expert to make use of a computer. SPSS has many features that were not described here, but these features are not difficult to understand either. Similarly, other packaged programs have commands that are designed to be easy to learn by people with limited computer skills.

```
DATA LIST
/ID 1-2 GROUP 3 WEIGHT 4-6 REPEAT 7 AGE 8-9
 NPREGS 10 SMOKE 11.
BEGIN DATA.
01110711711
02110101400
03111902130
04112812020
051 8901511
061 9901901
07111101910
08111711811
09110211700
10112002000
111 7601301
12111601801
13110011600
14111501800
15111302121
16211111900
17210802110
182 9501921
192 9901701
20210311900
212 9401501
22210111710
23211402120
242 9702010
252 9911801
26211301801
272 8901910
282 9802000
29210201700
30210501911
END DATA.
FREQUENCIES VARIABLES=WEIGHT, REPEAT, AGE, NPREGS, SMOKE
 /STATISTICS=ALL.
```

Figure 20-6. *Instructions for an SPSS program*

❖ CODING OF DATA FOR COMPUTER ANALYSIS

When a computer is to be used to perform statistical analyses, the information must be converted to a form amenable to such analyses. Computers cannot process verbatim responses to open-ended questions. It is similarly difficult for a computer to read and analyze information with verbal labels such as male or female, agree or disagree. *Coding* is the process by which basic research information is transformed into symbols compatible with computer analysis. It is possible to code information using alphabetic symbols. For example, the code for females could be F, and the code for males could be M. However, we strongly urge that a completely numerical coding scheme be developed to facilitate statistical analysis.

Inherently Quantitative Variables

Although most data collected in the course of a project will need to be coded, there are certain variables that are inherently quantitative and therefore directly amenable to computer analysis. For example, variables such as age, weight, body temperature, and diastolic blood pressure do not normally require coding—the data are already in a form that statistical programs can use. Sometimes the researcher may ask for information of this type in a way that *does* call for the development of a coding plan. If a researcher asks respondents to indicate whether they are younger than 30 years of age, between the ages of 31 and 49, or older than 50 years of age, then the responses would have to be coded before being entered into a computer file. When the responses to questions such as age, height, income level, and so forth are given in their full, natural form, the researcher should *not* reduce the information to coded categories for data entry purposes.

Information that is naturally quantitative thus may need no coding whatsoever, but the researcher should inspect and edit the data before entering them. It is important that all the responses be of the same form and precision. For instance, in entering a person's height, the researcher would need to decide whether to use feet and inches or to convert the information entirely to inches. Whichever method is adopted, it must be used consistently for all subjects. There must also be consistency in the method of handling information reported with different degrees of precision.

Precategorized Data

Much of the data from questionnaires, interviews, observation schedules, and psychological scales can be coded easily through precategorization. Closed-ended questions that provide for response alternatives can easily be preassigned a numerical code, as in the following example:

> From what type of program did you receive your basic nursing preparation?
> 1. Diploma school
> 2. Associate degree program
> 3. Baccalaureate degree program

Thus, if a nurse received his or her nursing preparation from a diploma school, the response to this question would be coded 1.

In many cases, the codes will be arbitrary, as in the case of a variable such as gender. Whether a female is coded 1 or 2 will have no bearing on the subsequent analysis as long as females are consistently assigned one code and males another. Other variables will appear to have a more obvious coding scheme, as in the following example:

> How often do you suffer from insomnia?
> 1. Almost never
> 2. Once or twice a year
> 3. Three to 11 times a year

> 4. At least once a month but not weekly
> 5. Once a week or more

Sometimes respondents may have the option of checking off more than one answer in reply to a single question, as in the following illustration:

> To which of the following journals do you subscribe?
> ( ) *American Journal of Nursing*
> ( ) *Nursing Forum*
> ( ) *Nursing Outlook*
> ( ) *Nursing Research*

With questions of this type, it is incorrect to adopt a 1-2-3-4 code because subjects may check several, or none, of the responses. The most appropriate procedure for questions such as this one is to treat each journal on the list as a separate question. In other words, the researcher would code the responses as though the item were four separate questions asking, "Do you subscribe to the *American Journal of Nursing?* Do you subscribe to *Nursing Forum?*" and so on. A check mark beside a journal would be treated as though the reply were yes. In effect, the question would be turned into four dichotomous variables, with one code (perhaps 1) signifying a yes response and another code (perhaps 2) signifying a no response.

Uncategorized Data

Qualitative data from open-ended questions, unstructured observations, and other narrative forms are not readily amenable to direct statistical analysis. When this type of information is to be statistically analyzed by the computer, it is necessary to categorize and code it. Sometimes it is possible for the researcher to develop a coding scheme in advance of data collection. For instance, a question might ask, "What is your occupation?" If the researcher knew the sample characteristics, he or she could probably predict such major categories as Professional, Managerial, Clerical, and so forth.

Usually, however, unstructured formats for data collection are adopted specifically because it is difficult to anticipate the kind of information that will be obtained. In such a situation, it is necessary to code responses after the data are collected. The researcher typically begins by scanning a sizable portion of the data to get a feel for the nature of the content. The researcher can then proceed to develop a scheme to categorize the material. The categorization scheme should be designed to reflect both the researcher's theoretical and analytic goals as well as the substance of the information. The amount of detail in the categorization scheme can vary considerably, but the researcher should keep in mind that too much detail is better than too little detail. In developing a coding scheme for unstructured information, the only rule is that the coding categories should be both mutually exclusive and collectively exhaustive.

Precise instructions should always be developed for the coders and documented in a coding manual. Coders, like observers and interviewers, must be properly trained. Intercoder reliability checks are strongly recommended.

Coding Missing Data

A code should be designated for every question or variable for every subject, even if in some cases no response or information is available. *Missing data* can be of various types. A person responding to an interview question may be undecided, refuse to answer, or say "Don't know." And, when a skip pattern is used, there is usually missing information for those questions that are irrelevant to a portion of the sample. In observational studies, an observer coding behavior may get distracted during a 10-second sampling frame, may be undecided about an appropriate categorization, or may observe behavior not listed on the observation schedule. In some studies, it may be important to distinguish between various types of missing data by specifying separate codes (e.g. distinguishing refusals and "don't knows"), and in other cases a single missing data code may suffice. This decision must be made with the conceptual aims of the research in mind. A person

who replied "Don't know" to a question seeking to understand the public's familiarity with health maintenance organizations should probably be distinguished from the person who refused to answer the question.

Insofar as possible, it is desirable to code missing data in the same manner for all variables. If a nonresponse is coded as a 4 on variable 1, a 6 on variable 2, a 5 on variable 3, and so forth, there is a greater risk of error than if a uniform code is adopted. The choice of what number to use as the missing data code is fairly arbitrary, but the number must be one that has not been assigned to an actual piece of information. Many researchers follow the convention of coding missing data as 9 because this value is normally out of the range of codes for true information. Others use blanks, zeros, or negative values to indicate missing information.

Some software packages require a specific handling of missing information. For example, SAS uses periods (.) for missing values. Therefore, the researcher should decide what software will be used for data analysis before finalizing coding decisions.

❖ ENTERING CODED DATA

For most types of computer analysis, the coded data are transferred onto a data file through a keyboard or a computer terminal. Coded data are transferred to files in accordance with a predesignated plan. The next section discusses the considerations in designing and implementing such a plan.

Preparing Data for Data Entry

In many cases, data files are set up to store 80 columns of information on a single record. This is because data were originally input onto computer files using punch cards that contained 80 columns; also, display screens can usually show 80 columns at a time. In this section, we illustrate data preparation activities based on an 80-column scheme, but it is sometimes desirable to use longer record lengths.

The researcher should plan in advance of the actual data entry the layout of information within the 80 columns. It is often preferable to adopt what is known as a *fixed format,* which places the values for any specific variable in the same column for every case. We used a fixed format for entering the data for the example with 30 subjects in Figure 20-6. Some packaged programs also permit data to be entered in a *free format,* in which there is no necessary correspondence between the variables entered in any particular column from one case to the next, although the variables are always in the same order. In free format, the values for different values are separated by a *delimiter,* such as a comma or a blank space. We recommend using a fixed format because checking for errors is often easier.

With a fixed format, the researcher must specify in which columns all the data are to be entered. For many variables, the field width is a single column. If a variable has a code whose maximum value is one digit, then the variable can be assigned to one column. Examples include variables whose responses are agree/disagree and yes/no/maybe. Other variables, such as age, weight, and blood pressure measures, must occupy more than one column. Anytime the maximum value of a variable exceeds 9, the researcher must be sure to reserve two (or more, if the number is larger than 99) columns.

The researcher must be careful in dealing with a variable whose values may be of different widths for different subjects. For example, when we recorded infant birthweight in the example used earlier, we needed only two digits for infants weighing less than 100 ounces but three digits for those weighing 100 ounces or more. Because the maximum value was three digits long, three columns on the record were required for all subjects. To record the weight of an 89-ounce infant, for example (data record number 5 of Figure 20-6), it was necessary to enter 89 preceded by a blank space (or by a zero, as 089). This procedure is known as *right-justifying* the data. Whenever a number smaller than the corresponding field is entered in fixed format, the number should be entered as far to the right as possible in the designated field. In the example, columns 4, 5, and 6 were reserved for the weight measurement, so 89 was entered in columns 5 and 6. If, instead, 89 were entered in columns 4 and 5, then the value would be read as 890.

In designing the layout for the data, the researcher should allocate space for recording an *identification (ID) number.* Each individual case (i.e., the information from a single questionnaire, test, observation, and so forth) should be assigned a unique ID number, and this number should be entered along with the actual data. This procedure permits the investigator to go back to the original source if there are any difficulties with the data file. The numbering is completely arbitrary and is used only as a label. Usually, a consecutive numbering scheme is used, running from number 1 to the number of actual cases. The ID number normally is entered in the first columns of the record. If there are fewer than 100 subjects, then the first two columns are used, starting with subjects 01, 02, and so on. As in the case of other variables, the field width is determined by the maximum value of the ID number.

The researcher will often find that a single 80-column format is insufficient for recording all the information obtained from a single case. There is no restriction on the number of records (lines) that may be used for a given case or subject. In fact, it is common to require multiple records to enter all the data for each subject. When multiple records are needed, the ID number for a particular case should be entered onto all records for that case. The researcher often enters a number identifying the order of the records within a case. That is, the first record of a case would be identified with a 1, the second card with a 2, and so forth. The record sequence number is often entered either immediately after the ID number or in column 80.

Various procedures are available to facilitate the actual data entry process. The simplest is to have the data recorded on special sheets that can be optically scanned, but this is usually expensive and requires subjects essentially to code their own data—as on a standardized test. A commonly used procedure is to use a margin on the original source to write the appropriate numerical codes for the data entry person to follow, which is referred to as *edge-coding*. An example of edge coding is presented in the next section.

Data Entry and Verification

Once the data are coded and a scheme has been developed for the data file, the process of entering data onto the file can begin. Various types of software can be used for data entry. On a PC, data can be entered onto a data file using spreadsheet programs, database programs, or many word processing programs, with the data saved in *ASCII format*. (ASCII, which stands for *A*merican *S*tandard *C*ode for *I*nformation *I*nterchange, is a set of standardized codes used to represent keyboard characters.) Alternatively, you may want to use the *editor program* that is included with most statistical software packages. On a mainframe, data are often entered using an editor program.

Data entry is a tedious and exacting task that is usually subject to numerous errors. Therefore, it is necessary to verify or check the entries to correct the mistakes that are inevitably made. Several verification procedures exist. The first is to compare visually the numbers printed on a printout of the data file with the codes on the original source. A second possibility is to enter all the data twice and to compare the two sets of records. The comparison can be done either visually or with the assistance of the computer. Finally, there are special verifying programs that are designed to perform comparisons during direct data entry. The use of such verification is recommended as the best method for eliminating data entry inaccuracies.

Data Cleaning

Even after the records are verified, the data usually contain a few errors. These errors could be the result of data entry mistakes but could also arise from coding or reporting problems. Data are not ready for analysis until they have been cleaned. *Data cleaning* involves two types of checks. The first is a check for *outliers* or wild codes. One procedure involves using a computer printout of the frequency counts associated with every value for every variable, and checking for undefined code values. The variable gender might have the following three defined code values: 1 for female, 2 for male, and 9 for not reported. If it were discovered that a code of 5 were entered in the column designated for the gender variable, then it would be clear that an error had been made. The computer could be instructed to list the ID number of the culpable record, and the error could be corrected by checking the appropriate code on the original source. Another procedure is to use a program for data entry that automatically performs range checks.

Editing of this type, of course, will never reveal mistakes that look respectable or plausible. If the gender of a male is entered incorrectly as a 1, then the mistake may never be detected. Because errors can have a profound effect on the analysis and interpretation of data, it is naturally important to perform the coding, entering, verifying, and cleaning with great care.

The second data-cleaning procedure involves performing *consistency checks,* which focus on internal data consistency. In this task, the researcher looks for data entry or coding errors by testing whether data in one part of a record are compatible with data in another part. For example, one question in a questionnaire might ask respondents their current marital status and another might ask how many times they had been married. If the data were internally consistent, then the subjects who responded "Single, never married" to the first question should have a zero entered in the field for the second. As another example, if the respondent's gender were entered with the code for male and there was an entry of 2 for the variable "Number of pregnancies," then one of those two fields would contain an error. The researcher should identify as many opportunities for checking the consistency of entered data as possible.

Once the data have been cleaned to the researcher's satisfaction, a backup copy of the data file should be made immediately as a protection against loss or damage. The duplicate copy should be stored in a safe place.

Documentation

The decisions that a researcher makes concerning coding, field width, placement of data in columns, and so on should be documented in full. Documentation is essential for the proper handling of any data set. The researcher's own memory should not be trusted to store all the required information. Several weeks after coding, the researcher may no longer remember if males were coded 1 and females 2, or vice versa. Moreover, colleagues may wish to borrow the data set to perform a secondary analysis. Whether one anticipates a secondary analysis or not, documentation should be sufficiently thorough so that a person unfamiliar with the original research project could use the data.

A major portion of the documentation involves the preparation of a codebook. A *codebook* is essentially a listing of each variable, the column or columns in which the variable has been entered, and the codes associated with the various values of the variable. The codebook is often prepared before coding so that it can be used as a guide by coders. A codebook can be generated by the statistical software programs, but these codebooks may not be sufficiently detailed for coders. In the next section, we present an example of a codebook.

A Hypothetical Example of Coding and Cleaning

The concepts and recommendations presented thus far in this chapter can be best understood by reference to a detailed example. Figure 20-7 presents a questionnaire that was contrived to illustrate many of the points made in the preceding sections. This hypothetical instrument should not be taken as an example of good questionnaire design. The intent was to include a variety of item types to demonstrate how different coding problems could be handled.

On the left-hand margin of the questionnaire are the numerical codes to be transferred to a computer file. The first code—001—represents the ID number assigned to the respondent who completed the questionnaire. The three-digit number implies that at least 100 (but fewer than 1000) respondents participated in the study. Following the ID number are the codes corresponding to the subject's responses. In the second part of question 2, the missing values code of 9 signifies that the subject skipped over the question. With regard to question 5, each individual symptom is treated for data analysis purposes as a separate question, with a check or X being coded as 1 and no check coded as 2. Note that the subject's height, reported in question 10, has been converted into inches.

The data entry person using edge-coded questionnaires such as this would simply follow the numbers in the left margin, entering them in consecutive columns. The total number of columns required to store the information from this fictitious questionnaire is 31. If there were 150 respondents, then there would be 150 records, each with information in the first 31 columns.

The example presented here involves a simple and straightforward coding scheme. Because all the questions are closed-ended, there is little confusion or ambiguity concerning how to code the various responses. Even for uncomplicated data, it is a good practice to develop a codebook. An example of a codebook setup is shown in Figure 20-8, which includes the information for questions 1 to 4 of this example only.

The example can also be used to illustrate data cleaning. Figure 20-9 presents a computer listing of the frequency counts corresponding to all values entered for question 3, "Do you smoke cigarettes?" Of the 150 cases, 76 responses were entered as 1, or yes, and 68 responses were entered as 2, or no. Three respondents apparently failed to answer the question (entered as 9). The printout tells us that, in two cases, a 3 was incorrectly entered

001 This questionnaire is part of a study on health-related habits and attitudes. We hope you will help us by answering the following questions.

1. Overall, how would you describe your health in comparison with that of others your **age**?

2
( ) above average health
(χ) average health
( ) below average health

2. Have you been hospitalized within the past two years?

2
( ) yes ⎯⎯⎯⎯⎯⎯⎯
(×) no

If yes: how many times have you been hospitalized?
( ) once
9
( ) two times
( ) more than two times

3. Do you smoke cigarettes?

1
(×) yes ⎯⎯⎯⎯⎯⎯⎯
( ) no

If yes, how many cigarettes do you usually smoke per day?
1
(×) 1 pack or less
( ) between one and two packs
( ) two packs or more

4. How often do you drink alcoholic beverages?

4
( ) never   (×) 2 or 3 times a month
( ) 10 times a year or less   ( ) about once a week
( ) about once a month   ( ) several times a week
                                   ( ) nearly every day

5. Below is a list of some common somatic complaints. Please check off those symptoms which have bothered you within the past month or so.

1 (×) headache
2 ( ) indigestion
1 (×) constipation
2 ( ) diarrhea
2 ( ) insomnia
2 ( ) lower back pains
2 ( ) lack of appetite

6. Which of the following statements best describes your health care practices?

2
( ) I go for regular physical checkups as a preventive health care measure.
(×) I see a health care professional only when I have a specific complaint.
( ) I have to be extremely ill before I will see a health care professional.

7. Please indicate how important the following things are to you by placing an "X" under the appropriate column:

		Extremely important	Somewhat important	Not too important
1	Abundant leisure time	×		
3	A long life			×
2	Financial success and security		×	
1	Good family relationships	×		
2	Good health		×	
2	Lots of friends, popularity		×	

38 8. What is your present age? ___38___ years.
135 9. How much do you weigh? ___135___ pounds.
66 10. How tall are you? ___5___ feet, ___6___ inches.
1 11. What is your sex?
(×) female
( ) male

Figure 20-7. *Example of a questionnaire with edge coding* for question 3, and in one case, an 8 was entered. This computer listing has informed us that there are errors on three records in column 7. We could now go through the data file—either manually with a printout or by using the computer—to find the three records in question. The records would indicate the ID number of the questionnaires to be rechecked, and the necessary corrections could then be made.

❖ TIPS FOR USING COMPUTERS

Unless your data set is very small and your analyses are very simple, we urge you to learn enough about computers to use a statistical program. Here are a few suggestions regarding the use of a computer.

- You should *assume* that you have the capability of using the computer for statistical

Card Column	Variable Description and Codes	Question Number
1-3	Respondent Identification Number (001 to 150)	
4	"Overall, how would you describe your health in comparison with that of others your age?" 1. above average health 2. average health 3. below average health 9. no response	1
5	"Have you been hospitalized within the past two years?" 1. yes 2. no 9. no response	2
6	"If yes: how many times have you been hospitalized?" 1. once 2. two times 3. more than two times 9. no response	2
7	"Do you smoke cigarettes?" 1. yes 2. no 9. no response	3
8	"If yes: how many cigarettes do you usually smoke per day?" 1. 1 pack or less 2. between one and two packs 3. two packs or more 9. no response	3
9	"How often do you drink alcoholic beverages?" 1. never 2. 10 times a year or less 3. about once a month 4. 2 to 3 times per month 5. about once a week 6. several times a week 7. nearly every day 9. no response	4

Figure 20-8. *Example of a section of a codebook*

```
SMOKE        DO YOU SMOKE CIGARETTES?


                                                      VALID      CUM
     VALUE LABEL              VALUE   FREQUENCY  PERCENT  PERCENT  PERCENT

 YES                           1          76     50.7     51.7     51.7
 NO                            2          68     45.3     46.3     98.0
                               3           2      1.3      1.4     99.3
                               8           1       .7       .7    100.0
                               9           3      2.0    MISSING
                                        -------  -------  -------
                     TOTAL                150    100.0    100.0

 MEAN          1.537     STD ERR        .062     MEDIAN        1.000
 MODE          1.000     STD DEV        .752     VARIANCE       .565
 KURTOSIS     36.298     S E KURT       .397     SKEWNESS      4.428
 S E SKEW       .200     RANGE         7.000     MINIMUM       1.000
 MAXIMUM       8.000     SUM         226.000


 VALID CASES     147     MISSING CASES       3
```

Figure 20-9. *Hypothetical data for data cleaning example*

analysis. You do not need to know anything about electronic circuits. You do not need to learn any programming language. You will need to learn a few fairly simple procedures. You can probably learn to produce simple statistical output, like frequency distributions, with a few hours of training. As you become more comfortable on the computer, you can increase the repertoire of statistical procedures available to you.

- When learning a new software package, find out if there is a tutorial available. *Tutorials* are special programs that contain step-by-step instructions on how to use a software package and that make learning easier through real hands-on experience. Many applications software have tutorials. For example, SPSS-PC has a separate tutorial disk that can be used on most PCs, even those without a hard disk.

- If someone is teaching you how to use a particular computer and software package through a demonstration, take very specific and detailed notes about every step in the process. Often people who are adept at computers do a lot of things automatically, with-

out giving much thought to the individual steps because the steps have become so routine to them. If the person instructing you has done something that you do not understand, ask him or her to slow down and back up. Also, be sure that your notes are precise. For example, if you were making a backup copy of your data file on a PC from the hard disk (drive C) onto a floppy disk in drive A, the command might be:

COPY C:RESEARCH.DAT A:

This is the MS-DOS command that instructs the computer to make a duplicate copy of the data file RESEARCH.DAT and to store it on the floppy in drive A under the same file name. In entering this command, it is important that there is *no* space between the colon and the name of the file, and that there *is* a space between the name of the file and the designated drive A. Thus, you must be sure that your notes are sufficiently clear that instructions can be followed precisely.

- *Always* remember to make backup copies of the files you create, and store them in a secure place. It is a good protection against accidental erasures and also against computer *viruses* that occasionally infect some machines.

- Do not be afraid to make mistakes—especially if you have all your files backed up! If you make a mistake, it can usually be corrected easily. For example, data files and control files can readily be edited. If you make a mistake using the statistical software package, the computer will send you an *error message*, usually giving you some clues about what is wrong. If you cannot decipher an error message by yourself, ask someone who knows the software for help.

❖ SUMMARY

The advantages of computers to researchers include their speed, accuracy, and flexibility. On the other hand, computers require considerable attention to detail on the part of users, because computers have no capacity to think.

Large, multiuser computer systems are often referred to as *mainframe computers* or, for certain *applications, supercomputers*. Mid-sized computers (*minicomputers*) are increasingly being replaced by powerful *microcomputers,* also known as *personal computers* or *PCs*. The components of a computer system are broadly categorized as either hardware or software. *Hardware* refers to the physical equipment that stores, processes, and controls information. *Software* refers to the instructions and procedures required to operate the computer.

There are five components of computer hardware. The *input device* is the means by which the researcher feeds information into the computer. The *memory* is the device that stores the information. The *control unit* coordinates the functions of the other components. The *arithmetic/logic unit* performs the arithmetic or logic operations requested. Finally, the *output device* produces the resulting information. The control unit and the arithmetic/logic unit are collectively called the *central processing unit (CPU)*.

A *program*—the main part of a computer's software—is a set of instructions informing the computer what to do. *Programming languages* make it possible for humans to communicate with computers. Many packaged software programs exist for the researcher who is not greatly skilled in a programming language. Researchers are most likely to use several of the following types of applications software: *word processing, desktop publishing, spreadsheets, data base managers, communications software*, and *statistical analysis software.*

Researchers can now rely on PCs for most applications. PCs fall into two camps: IBMs (and their *clones*) and MacIntosh computers (Macs). These two types differ primarily with regard to their *user interface*—the software that passes information to and from the user of the computer. The availability of special *windows* programs for IBM-type PCs has made these computers look more like a Mac, whose interface has traditionally been considered more *user-friendly*. The main input devices for PCs are the *keyboard* and the *mouse*, and the main output devices are the *display screen* (*monitor*) and *printers* that provide hard-copy *printouts*. Magnetic *disks* are used for both input and output as well as for *external storage*. Most PCs have both *hard disks*, embedded in the *systems unit* case, and *floppy disks*. The *operating system* is the software that controls the overall operation of the computer system, and for IBM-type PCs, the most frequently used operating systems are *MS-DOS* and *OS/2*. PCs are often linked together in a *network*, either in the same building through cables (a *local-area network*) or through telephone lines by means of a *modem* (a *wide-area network*).

In a mainframe environment, users generally communicate with the computer through a terminal or keyboard, in either an interactive mode or batch processing mode. *Batch processing* refers to a process in which a batch of programs is assembled for execution during the same computer run. The delay between feeding the information in and receiving output is referred to as the *turnaround time*. The *interactive mode*, in which the user interacts conversationally with the computer, uses the concept of *time sharing*, a method by which the computer spends a small amount of time with multiple users in a round-robin fashion.

Computer programs and data are stored in *files*, which are named collections of information. In using a statistical package, the instructions of the researcher are stored in *command files* and the data are usually stored in *data files*. Data files are organized into *fields* (a column or set of consecutive columns where a piece of information is stored) and *records* (a line or row of information). The statistical results are often stored in *output files* for later review and printing.

Researchers generally do not need to learn programming to analyze their data by computer because of the widespread availability of sophisticated statistical packages. The most widely used packages, for both mainframes and PCs, are *SPSS*, *SAS*, and *BMD-P*.

When a computer is used for statistical analysis, research data must be converted to machine-readable form. *Coding* is the procedure of transforming research data into symbols (preferably numbers) compatible with computer analysis. Special codes need to be developed to signify *missing data*.

The researcher usually must plan in advance the layout of information on each record, whose length is often 80 columns. In a *fixed-format* arrangement, which is commonly used for research data, variables are entered onto the same column for every case. The width of the field for a variable is determined by the maximum numerical value for that variable. The data should always be *right-justified*, or entered as far to the right as possible in the designated field. The researcher may use an *edge-coding* scheme, in which the numerical codes to be entered are written onto the margin of the original source, to help with data entry. The researcher should document the decisions made concerning the coding, field placement, and naming of variables. A fairly standard procedure is the preparation of a *codebook* that serves as a comprehensive, permanent record of the researcher's data processing decisions.

The next step is *data entry* onto an input medium (usually a disk file), a task that is susceptible to a high error rate. Entered data, therefore, should be checked or *verified* for errors. Even after the data are verified, they almost inevitably contain a few errors. Because of this fact, data should be *cleaned* before proceeding with any analyses. The cleaning process is primarily a check for *outliers* or numerical values that are not part of the coding scheme and *consistency checks* to determine if the data are internally consistent.

❖ STUDY SUGGESTIONS

Chapter 20 of the accompanying *Study Guide for Nursing Research, 5th ed.*, offers various exercises and study suggestions for reinforcing the concepts presented in this chapter. Additionally, the following study questions can be addressed:

1. If you have access to a PC, find out how much memory is available on your computer. Also, find out the speed of the microprocessor. Which operating system does it use?

2. Suppose you had data from 50 subjects on the following four variables: 1) age; 2) sex (coded 1 for females, 2 for males); 3) number of cigarettes smoked per day; and 4) number of days absent from work in the past year. Write out SPSS instructions that would produce a frequency listing for these four variables. (Note: first determine in which columns the data would be entered.)

3. What field width would you need for the following variables: marital status, annual income, body temperature, number of children, white blood cell count, religious

affiliation, days absent from work, Apgar score, time to first voiding, and pulse rate?

❧ SUGGESTED READINGS

GENERAL REFERENCES

Ball, M. J., & Hannah, K. J. (1984). *Using computers in nursing.* Reston, VA: Reston Publishing.

Barcikowski, R. S. (Ed.). (1983). *Computer packages and research design, with annotations of input and output from the BMD-P, SAS, and SPSSx* statistical packages. New York: University of America Press.

Barhyte, D., & Bacon, L. D. (1985). Approaches to cleaning data sets. *Nursing Research, 34,* 62–65.

Biow, L. (1993). *How to use your computer.* Emeryville, CA: Ziff-Davis Press.

Blissmer, R. H. (1993) *Introducing computers: Concepts, systems, and applications.* New York: John Wiley & Sons.

Brownell, B. A. (1985). *Using microcomputers: A guidebook for writers, teachers, and researchers in the social sciences.* Beverly Hills, CA: Sage.

Capron, H. L., & Williams, B. K. (1984). *Computers and data processing* (2nd ed.). Menlo Park, CA: Benjamin/Cummings.

Chang, B. L. (1985). Computer use and nursing research. *Western Journal of Nursing Research, 7,* 142–144.

Cox, H., Harsanyi, B., & Dean, L. (1988). *Computers and nursing: Applications to practice, education and research.* Norwalk, CT: Appleton & Lange.

Grobe, S. J. (1984). *Computer primer and resource guide for nurses.* Philadelphia: J. B. Lippincott.

Jacobsen, B. S., Tulman, L., Lowery, B. J., & Garson, C. (1988). Experiencing the research process by using statistical software on microcomputers. *Nursing Research, 37,* 56–59.

Lobo, M. L. (1993). Code books—a critical link in the research process. *Western Journal of Nursing Research, 15,* 377–385.

Nicoll, L. H. (1987). The microcomputer: An alternative for data analysis. *Nursing Research, 36,* 320–323.

Saba, V. K., & McCormick, K. A. (1986). *Essentials of computers for nurses.* Philadelphia: J. B. Lippincott.

Turley, J. P. (1989). Transferring data files between microcomputer statistical packages. *Nursing Research, 38,* 315–317.

Walker, G., Pullam, J., & Farmer, G. (1990). *Introduction to data analysis* (2nd ed.). Dubuque, IA: Kendall/Hunt Publishing Co.

REFERENCES ON SOFTWARE PACKAGES

Dixon, W. J. (Ed.). (1992). *BMD-P statistical software manual.* Berkeley, CA: University of California Press. Major programs include summary statistics, correlations, analysis of variance (ANOVA), analysis of covariance (ANCOVA), multiple regression analysis, cluster analysis, factor analysis, canonical correlation, and discriminant analysis.

SAS Institute. (1989). *SAS language and procedures: Usage, version 6.* Cary, NC: SAS Institute. (See also SAS Institute. (1992). *SAS-STAT users' guide.* (4th ed.). Cary, NC: SAS Institute.) This package includes all basic descriptive and inferential statistics, plus additional programs for cluster analysis, Guttman scalogram analysis, multiple regression, factor analysis, discriminant function analysis, canonical correlation, logit/probit analysis, and spectral analysis.

SPSS, Inc. (1993). *SPSS base system syntax reference guide.* Old Tappans, NJ: Prentice-Hall Publishers. (See also SPSS, Inc. (1992). *SPSS PC+ base system users' guide.* Old Tappans, NJ: Prentice-Hall Publishers.) Major programs include descriptive statistics, frequency distributions, contingency tables and related measures of association, bivariate correlation and scatter diagrams, partial correlation, multiple regression analysis, *t*-tests, ANOVA, ANCOVA, multivariate ANOVA, discriminant analysis, factor analysis, canonical analysis, survival analysis, logistic regression, loglinear analysis, LISREL, reliability analysis, and various nonparametric procedures.

Chapter 21

DESIGNING AND IMPLEMENTING AN ANALYSIS STRATEGY

The successful analysis of quantitative data requires considerable planning and attention to detail. This chapter provides an overview of the steps that normally have to be taken in designing and implementing an analytic plan. The final phase of analyzing quantitative data involves the interpretation of the findings, and the interpretive process is discussed at some length.

❖ PHASES IN THE ANALYSIS OF QUANTITATIVE DATA

The analysis of quantitative data normally proceeds through a number of different phases. The phases and the steps within the phases may vary from one project to another. For example, if a computer is not used, or if the data set is an extremely simple one, then the researcher may be able to proceed fairly quickly from the collection to the analysis of the data. However, in most cases, a number of intermediary steps are necessary.

Figure 21-1 summarizes what the flow of tasks might look like when a researcher uses a computer, and when the final analyses involve the use of multivariate statistical procedures. Progress in the analysis of data may not always be as linear as this figure suggests. For example, some backtracking may be required if data anomalies are discovered during the final analyses. However, the figure provides an adequate framework for discussing various steps in the analytic process.

The first set of steps, shown in the figure as Pre-analysis Steps, involves a variety of clerical and administrative tasks that were discussed in Chapter 20. The remainder of this section describes the tasks that typically might be undertaken in the other three phases of the data analysis.

Preliminary Analysis Steps

Researchers typically undertake a number of preliminary analyses before they proceed

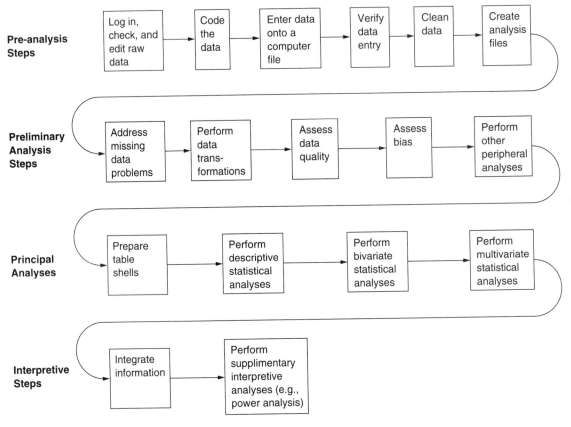

Figure 21-1. *Flow of tasks in analyzing quantitative data*

with the testing of their hypotheses. Several of these preparatory activities are discussed next.

ADDRESSING MISSING DATA PROBLEMS

Researchers almost always find that their data set has missing information on some variables for some subjects. If the sample is large and the number of missing values is small, then the missing data should not cause problems. However, because many samples in nursing studies are small, missing data are often of considerable concern. The best overall strategy is to take steps to minimize data loss during the design and implementation of the data collection plan. However, because it is usually inevitable to have some missing data—regardless of the vigilance of the researcher—various approaches

have been used to deal with this situation after it has occurred.

In selecting one or more of these approaches, the researcher should first determine the distribution and patterning of the missing data. The appropriate solution will depend on such factors as the extensiveness of the missing data; the role that the variable with missing data plays in the analytic scheme (i.e., whether the missing values are in the dependent, independent, or descriptive variables); and the randomness of the missing data (i.e., whether missing values are related in any systematic way to important variables in the study). Obviously, the problem differs if only 2% of the values for a relatively minor variable are missing, as opposed to 20% of the values for the primary dependent variable. Also, if the missing values disproportionately come from subjects with certain characteristics, there is likely to be some bias. A simple procedure for determining whether missing values are occurring at random is to divide the sample into two groups—those with missing data on a variable and those without missing data. These two groups can then be compared in terms of the other variables in the data set to determine if the two groups are comparable. Thus, before adopting a solution such as those described below, the researcher must undertake some preliminary descriptive analyses to examine the distribution of variables and cases with missing values.

1. *Delete the missing cases.* One simple strategy is to delete a case (i.e., a subject) entirely if there is any missing information. However, particularly when samples are small, it is irksome to throw away an entire case—especially if information is missing for only one or two variables. If a subject has extensive missing information, however, the deletion of this case is advisable. Also, if the missing information is for key dependent variables, it may be necessary to remove the entire case. This strategy is sometimes referred to as *listwise deletion* of missing values.

2. *Delete the variable.* Another option is to throw out information on a particular variable for all subjects. This option is especially suitable when a high percentage of cases have missing values on a specific variable. (This may occur if, for example, a question is objectionable and is left unanswered, or if there were problems in understanding directions and a question was inadvertently skipped by many). When missing data on a variable are extensive, there may be systematic biases with regard to those subjects for whom data *are* available. Obviously, this approach is not attractive if the variable is a critical independent or dependent variable.

3. *Substitute the mean value.* When the missing values are reasonably random (and when the problem is not extensive), it is often useful to substitute real data values for the missing value codes. In essence, such a substitution represents a best guess as to what the value of the variable would have been, had the data actually been collected. Because of this fact, researchers generally substitute a value that is typical for the sample, and typical values generally come from the center of the distribution. For example, if data for a subject's age were missing and if the average age of subjects in the sample were 45.2, the researcher might substitute the value 45 in place of the missing values code for subjects whose age is unknown.

This approach is especially useful when there are missing values for variables that comprise a multiple-item scale, such as a Likert scale. Suppose, for example, that we have a 20-item scale that measures anxiety, and that one subject answered only 18 of the 20 items. It would be inappropriate to score the scale by adding together responses on the 18 items only; and it would be a waste of information on the 18 answered items to code the entire scale as missing. Thus, for the two missing items, the researcher could substitute the most typical responses (based on either the mean, median, or mode, depending on the distribution of scores) so that a scale score on the full 20 items could be computed. Needless to say, this approach only makes sense when a small proportion of scale items are missing. And, if the scale is a test of knowledge rather than a measure of a psychosocial characteristics, it usually is more appropriate to consider a missing value as a "don't know," and to mark the item as incorrect.

4. *Estimate the missing value.* When a researcher substitutes a mean value for a missing value, there is always the risk that the substitution is erroneous, perhaps dramatically so. For example, if the mean value of 45 is substituted for a missing

value on a subject's age, but the range of ages in the sample is 25 to 70, then the substituted value could be wrong by 20 years or more. When only a couple of cases have missing data for the variable age, an error of even this magnitude is unlikely to alter the findings. However, if missing values are more widespread, it is often worthwhile to substitute values that have a greater likelihood of being accurate.

Various procedures can be used to derive estimates of what the missing value should be. The simplest procedure is to use the mean for a subgroup that is most like the case that has the missing value, if there are subgroup differences with regard to the variable that has missing data. For example, suppose the mean age for women in the sample were 42.8 and the mean age for men were 48.9. The researcher could then substitute 43 for women with missing age data and 49 for men with missing age data. This would likely result in improved accuracy, in comparison with the use of the overall mean of 45 for all subjects with missing age data.

Sometimes multiple regression procedures are used to "predict" the correct value of the missing data. To continue with the example used previously, suppose that subjects' age was correlated with gender, heart rate, and length of hospital stay in this research sample. Using subjects that have no missing data, these three variables could be used to develop a regression equation that could predict age for subjects whose age information is missing but whose values for the three other variables are not missing.

5. *Delete cases selectively and pairwise.* Perhaps the most widely used (but not necessarily the best) approach is to delete cases selectively, on a variable-by-variable basis. For example, in describing the characteristics of the sample, the researcher might use whatever information is available for each characteristic, resulting in a fluctuating number of cases across the range of descriptors. Thus, the mean age might be based on 95 cases, the gender distribution might be based on 102 cases, and so on. However, if the number of cases fluctuates widely across characteristics, the information is difficult to interpret because the sample of subjects is essentially a "moving target."

The same strategy is sometimes used to handle missing information for dependent variables. For example, an evaluation of an intervention to reduce patient anxiety might have blood pressure, self-reported anxiety, and an observational measure of stress-related behavior as the dependent variables. Suppose that 10 subjects out of a sample of 100 failed to complete the anxiety scale. The researcher might base the analyses of the anxiety data on the 90 subjects who completed the scale but use the full sample of 100 subjects in the analyses of the other dependent variables. The problem with this approach is that it can cause interpretive problems, especially if there are inconsistent findings across outcomes. For example, if there were experimental versus control group differences on all outcomes except the anxiety scale, one possible explanation is that the anxiety scale sample is simply not the same set of subjects as the full sample. Researchers generally strive for what is referred to as a *rectangular matrix* of data: data values for all subjects on all relevant and important variables. In the example just described, the researcher should, at a minimum, perform supplementary analyses using the rectangular matrix—that is, rerun all analyses using only the 90 subjects for whom complete data are available. If the results are different from when the full sample was used, the researcher would at least be in a better position to interpret the findings.

In analyses involving a correlation matrix, researchers sometimes use what is referred to as *pairwise deletion* of cases with missing values. Figure 21-2 illustrates a

```
Correlations:   AGE          WEIGHT       HEIGHT       HARTRATE     STRESS

   AGE         1.0000        .0453       -.0227        .2925        .4456
              (     0)      (    23)     (    25)     (    24)     (    20)
              P= .          P= .419      P= .457      P= .083      P= .024

   WEIGHT       .0453       1.0000        .8304        .3502        .0737
              (    23)      (     0)     (    23)     (    22)     (    18)
              P= .419       P= .          P= .000      P= .055      P= .386

   HEIGHT      -.0227        .8304       1.0000        .2197       -.0293
              (    25)      (    23)     (     0)     (    24)     (    20)
              P= .457       P= .000      P= .          P= .151      P= .451

   HARTRATE     .2925        .3502        .2197       1.0000        .5335
              (    24)      (    22)     (    24)     (     0)     (    19)
              P= .083       P= .055      P= .151      P= .          P= .009

   STRESS       .4456        .0737       -.0293        .5335       1.0000
              (    20)      (    18)     (    20)     (    19)     (     0)
              P= .024       P= .386      P= .451      P= .009      P= .


(Coefficient / (Cases) / 1-tailed Significance)

" . " is printed if a coefficient cannot be computed
```

Figure 21-2. Correlation matrix with pairwise deletion of missing values

correlation matrix with five variables in which pairwise deletion of missing values was used on a nonrectangular data matrix. As this figure shows, the correlations between pairs of variables are based on varying numbers of cases (shown in parentheses below the correlation coefficients), ranging from 18 subjects for the correlation between WEIGHT and STRESS to 25 subjects for the correlation between AGE and HEIGHT. Pairwise deletion is a tolerable procedure for descriptive purposes if the missing values are missing totally at random. But it is a risky procedure because data are often missing in some systematic fashion. It is especially imprudent to use this procedure for any multivariate analyses because the criterion correlations (i.e., the correlations between the dependent variable and the various predictors) are based on nonidentical subsets of subjects.

Each of these solutions has accompanying problems, so care should be taken in deciding how the missing data are to be handled. Procedures for dealing with missing data are discussed at greater length in Cohen and Cohen (1983) and Little and Rubin (1990).

PERFORMING DATA TRANSFORMATIONS

Raw data entered directly onto a computer file often need to be modified or transformed before the hypotheses can be tested using statistical analysis. *Data transformations* can be of various types and can easily be handled directly through instructions to the computer. The software packages described in Chapter 20 all have the ability to create totally new variables through arithmetic manipulations of variables in the original data set. We present several examples of such transformations in this section.*

• *Item reversals.* Sometimes response codes to certain items need to be completely reversed (i.e., high values becoming low, and vice versa), often for the purposes of combining items in the construction of a composite scale. For example, the widely used Center for Epidemiological Studies Depression (CES-D) scale consists of 20 items, 16 of which are statements indicating respondents'

* Throughout this chapter, SPSS commands are used to illustrate data manipulations. If other statistical software were used, the commands for performing transformations would be somewhat different.

negative feelings in the prior week (e.g., item 9 states, "I thought my life had been a failure"), and four of which are statements worded positively (e.g., item 8 states, "I felt hopeful about the future"). To score the scale, the positively worded items must be reversed before all items can be added together, as discussed in Chapter 13. CES-D items have four response options, from 1 (rarely felt that way) to 4 (felt that way most days). To reverse an item (i.e., to convert a 4 to a 1, and so on), the raw value of the item is subtracted from the maximum possible value, plus 1. The Statistical Package for the Social Sciences (SPSS) instruction to perform this transformation is as follows:

COMPUTE CESD8NEW = 5 − CESD8

This command instructs the computer to create a new variable (CESD8NEW) that is set equal to 5 minus the value of the original variable for item 8 on the CES-D (CESD8). Thus, a person who had an original score of 4 on item 8 (indicating hopefulness about the future on most days) would get a score of 1 on the new variable.

- *Scale construction.* Transformations are also needed for the construction of composite scales or indexes, using responses to individual items. Commands in statistical software packages for creating such composite indexes are generally straightforward, using algebraic conventions. For example, using SPSS, a 6-item Likert scale could be created with the following command:

COMPUTE SELFCARE = Q1+Q2+Q3 +Q4+Q5+Q6

In this example, the original values of the six items (Q1 through Q6) would be added together to form a new variable, labeled SELFCARE.

Item reversals can be done directly within the command to create a scale, as in the following example (in which items 3 and 5 needed reversing, and the scale item responses could range from 1 to 7):

COMPUTE COPING=Q1+Q2+(8 − Q3) + Q4+(8 − Q5)

In this example, a scale labeled COPING is created by adding together 5 variables (Q1 through Q5); the coding on Q3 and Q5 is reversed before the addition is performed.

- *Counts.* Sometimes composite indexes are created when the researcher is interested in a cumulative tally of the occurrence of some behavior or attribute. For example, suppose a researcher asked subjects to indicate which contraceptive methods they had used in the past 12 months, from a list of 10 different contraceptive options. Each question would be answered independently in a yes (coded 1) or no (coded 2) fashion. The researcher may want to create a variable indicating the total number of contraceptive methods used. The SPSS command would be as follows:

COUNT NMETHODS=METH1 TO METH10(1)

This command instructs the computer to create a new variable (NMETHODS) that represents a count of the number of different contraceptive methods to which the respondent answered yes (1), from the 10 individual contraceptive variables, named METH1 to METH10.

- *Recodes.* Other transformations involve recoded values that change the nature of the original data. For example, in some analyses, an infant's original birthweight (entered on the computer files in grams) might be used as a dependent variable. In other analyses, however, the researcher might be interested in comparing the subsequent morbidity of low-birthweight versus normal-birthweight infants. In SPSS, a command such as the following could be used to recode the original variable (BWEIGHT) into a dichotomous variable with a code of 1 for a low-birthweight infant and a code of 2 for a normal-birthweight infant, based on whether the baby weighed less than 2500 grams:

RECODE BWEIGHT (LOWEST THRU 2499=1)(2500 THRU HIGHEST=2)

Recodes are also used to substitute values for missing data. For example, in an example described earlier, female and male sample members with missing values for age would have the values of 43 and 48, respectively, substituted. The commands in SPSS for recoding the missing data, conditional on the subject's gender, would be as follows:

IF (GENDER EQ 1 AND AGE EQ 99) AGE=43

IF (GENDER EQ 2 AND AGE EQ 99) AGE=48

Here, a code of 1 for GENDER signifies female, a code of 2 for GENDER signifies male, and a code of 99 for AGE signifies missing data. These commands indicate that the value of the recode depends on the gender of the subject and that the value for age should be recoded if, and only if, the original value for age is missing.

- *Standard scores.* Sometimes data transformations that involve the creation of standard scores are necessary so that the data can be meaningfully interpreted. For example, children's raw scores on a test or scale may be uninterpretable unless the scores are standardized by age. In this situation, the researcher would need to transform the raw scores into standard scores (see Chapter 19) by using the means and standard deviations (SDs) for children of different ages. For example, the following SPSS commands would create standard scores with a mean of 0 and an SD of 1 on a scale of hospitalization fear, for children in three different age groups with different means and standard deviations:

IF (CHILDAGE EQ 6) FEARSS=(FEAR 15.0)/2.0

IF (CHILDAGE EQ 7) FEARSS=(FEAR 18.0)/2.5

IF (CHILDAGE EQ 8) FEARSS=(FEAR 20.5)/3.0

where FEAR is the original score on the hospitalization fear scale, FEARSS is a newly created age-standardized fear score, and CHILDAGE is a variable indicating the child's age.

The researcher previously determined that the mean score on FEAR is 15.0 (with an SD of 2.0) for children 6 years of age, the mean is 18.0 (with an SD of 2.5) for children 7 years of age, and the mean is 20.5 (with an SD of 3.0) for children 8 years of age. Thus, if a 6-year-old child's raw score on the FEAR scale were 18.0, then the value of FEARSS for this child would be 1.5 (i.e., $18 - 15 = 3$; $3 \div 2.0 = 1.5$). However, if the child were 7 years old, a raw score of 18.0 would yield a standard score of 0 (i.e., $18 - 18 = 0$; $0 \div 2.5 = 0$).

- *Meeting statistical assumptions.* Transformations are also undertaken to render data appropriate for certain statistical tests. For example, most parametric statistical tests assume that the distribution of values on a variable is normal. Parametric tests are fairly robust and can tolerate mild violations to the underlying assumptions. However, if a distribution is markedly nonnormal, then a transformation may be needed to make the use of powerful parametric procedures appropriate.[*] A logarithmic transformation, for example, often tends to normalize the distribution. In SPSS, the command that would be used to normalize the distribution of values on family income (which is often highly skewed) would be

COMPUTE INCLOG=LN(INCOME)

The new variable, INCLOG, is actually the natural log of the original values on the INCOME variable; INCLOG would then be used in statistical tests in place of INCOME. Discussions of the use of transformations for changing the characteristics of a distribution may be found in Dixon and Massey (1983).

---

[*] Criteria for determining whether a distribution deviates significantly from a normal distribution are discussed in most statistical textbooks (e.g., Munro & Page, 1993).

- *Dummy variables.* Multivariate statistical procedures usually require data transformations for variables measured on the nominal scale. For example, for dichotomous variables, it is advisable to use a 0 versus 1 code to facilitate interpretation of the regression coefficients. Thus, if the original codes for gender were 1 for women and 2 for men, the variable should be recoded, as in the following example using SPSS:

  RECODE GENDER (2=0)

  In this recode, the women in the sample continue to be coded as 1 on the GENDER variable, but the men are recoded from 2 to 0.

  When nominal variables have three or more different categories, the researcher usually creates a series of dummy variables for use in multivariate analyses. *Dummy variables* are dichotomous, indicating the presence or absence of some attribute. For example, suppose we have a variable indicating subjects' blood type (BLOODTYP), and the original codes are 1 for Type A, 2 for Type B, 3 for Type AB, and 4 for Type O. Four dummy variables could be created to designate whether or not a person is or is not of any given blood type:

  ```
  COMPUTE TYPEA=0
  COMPUTE TYPEB=0
  COMPUTE TYPEAB=0
  COMPUTE TYPEO=0
  IF (BLOODTYP EQ 1) TYPEA=1
  IF (BLOODTYP EQ 2) TYPEB=1
  IF (BLOODTYP EQ 3) TYPEAB=1
  IF (BLOODTYP EQ 4) TYPEO=1
  ```

  The first four commands simply initialize the four new dummy variables by setting them equal to zero for everyone in the sample. The next four commands indicate the conditions for setting the new variables equal to 1: a person with code 1 for BLOODTYP would have a code 1 for TYPEA, a person with code 2 for BLOODTYP would have code 1 for TYPEB, and so on. Thus, a person

with Type O blood would have the following codes on the five variables:

  ```
  BLOODTYP = 4
  TYPEA = 0
  TYPEB = 0
  TYPEAB = 0
  TYPEO = 1
  ```

  Clearly, we have not described all possible types of transformations, but these examples cover a wide range of realistic situations. Researchers can rarely analyze raw data that have been input directly onto a computer file, so the analysis plan must take into consideration the types of transformations that will be required to produce the most meaningful results.

ASSESSING DATA QUALITY

Steps are often undertaken to assess the quality of data in the early stage of the analyses. For example, when psychosocial scales or composite indexes are used, the researcher should generally assess the reliability of the measures, using either test–retest methods or, more commonly, internal consistency methods (see Chapter 16).

The distribution of data values for key variables also should be examined to determine any anomalies, such as limited variability, extreme skewness, or the presence of ceiling or floor effects. For example, the use of a vocabulary test appropriate for 10-year-olds likely would yield a clustering of high scores for a sample of 11-year-olds, creating a *ceiling effect* that would tend to reduce correlations between test scores and other characteristics of the children. Conversely, there likely would be a clustering of low scores on the test for 9-year-olds, resulting in a *floor effect* with similar consequences. As described previously, the data may need to be transformed to meet the requirements for certain statistical tests.

ASSESSING BIAS

Before proceeding to the main analyses, researchers often undertake preliminary analyses designed to assess the direction and extent of any biases. A few examples illustrate the types of analysis that the researcher should consider.

- *Nonresponse bias.* Researchers are often interested in determining whether a biased subset of the population volunteered to participate in a study. If there is information available about the characteristics of all people who were asked to participate in a study (e.g., demographic information from hospital records), the researcher should compare the characteristics of those who did and did not volunteer to participate in the study to determine the nature and direction of any biases. This means, of course, that the data file for the study has to include a case for each respondent and each nonrespondent. Additionally, the data file should contain a variable that indicates the response status of each person (e.g., a variable named RESPONSE could be coded 1 for participating subjects and 2 for those who declined to participate).

    Nonresponse bias should also be analyzed within the sample of participating subjects when there is extensive missing data for certain variables, to determine if the missing data are occurring at random. In this case, the researcher would compare the characteristics of subjects who have actual data on the relevant variable with those of subjects who have missing data on that variable.

- *Selection bias.* When a nonequivalent control group design is used (in a quasi-experimental or ex post facto study), the researcher should always check for selection biases by comparing the background characteristics of the groups. It is particularly important to be aware of any possible group differences on variables that are strongly related to the dependent variable. These variables can (and should, if possible) then be controlled—for example, through analysis of covariance.

    Even when a true experimental design has been used, the researcher should check

the success of the random assignment procedure. Random assignment does not guarantee equivalent groups across all characteristics, and the researcher should be aware of characteristics for which the different groups are not, in fact, comparable.

- *Attrition bias.* In longitudinal studies, it is always important to check for attrition biases, which involves a comparison of people who did and did not continue to participate in the study in later waves of data collection, based on characteristics of these two groups at the initial wave.

    In performing any of these analyses, significant group differences are an indication of bias, and such bias must be taken into consideration in interpreting the results. Whenever possible, the biases should be controlled in testing the main hypotheses. Any detected biases should be discussed in the research report.

Performing Additional Peripheral Analyses

Depending on the research project, additional peripheral analyses may need to be undertaken before proceeding to the substantive analyses. It is impossible to catalog all such peripheral analyses, but a few examples are provided to alert readers to the kinds of issues that need to be given some thought.

- *Manipulation checks.* In testing an experimental intervention, the primary research question is whether the treatment is effective in achieving the intended outcome. However, the researcher sometimes also wants to know whether the intended treatment was, in fact, received; this is an especially important question if the results indicate that the treatment had no effect. Subjects may perceive a treatment, or respond to it, in unanticipated ways, and this can influence the extent of the treatment's effectiveness. Therefore, researchers sometimes build in mechanisms to test whether the treatment was actually in place. For example, suppose we were testing the effect of noise levels on stress, exposing two groups of subjects to two different noise levels in a laboratory setting. As a *manipulation check*, we could ask subjects to rate how noisy they perceived the settings to be. If the subjects did not rate the noise levels in the two settings differently, it would probably affect our interpretation of the results—particularly if the stress in the two groups was not significantly different.

- *Data pooling.* Researchers sometimes obtain data from more than one source or from more than one type of subject. For example, to enhance the generalizability of their studies, researchers sometimes draw subjects from multiple sites; or they may recruit subjects with several different types of medical conditions. The risk in doing this is that the subjects may not really be drawn from the same population. Therefore, it is wise in such a situation to determine whether *pooling* of the data (combining data for all subjects) is warranted. This involves comparing the different subsets of subjects (i.e., the subjects from the different sites, and so on) in terms of key research variables. There are specific statistical tests that can be applied to evaluate whether pooling is justifiable (e.g., *Chow tests*); these tests are described in advanced textbooks on statistics.

- *Cohort effects.* Nurse researchers sometimes need to gather data over an extended period of time to achieve the sample sizes required to test the research hypotheses adequately. If sample members are recruited over a lengthy time period, it is possible that there will be *cohort effects*, that is, that relationships between research variables will vary over time. This might occur because the characteristics of the sample evolve over time, or because of changes in the community, in families, in health care, and so on. If the research involves an experimental treatment, it may also be that the treatment itself is modified over time—for example, if early program experience is used to improve the treatment or if those administering the treatment simply get

better at doing it. Thus, researchers with a long period of sample intake should consider testing for cohort effects because such effects can confound the results, or even mask existing relationships. This activity usually involves splitting the sample into two or three groups based on the date of entry into the sample and comparing the cohorts on key research variables.

Principal Analyses

At this point, the researcher should have a data set that has been cleaned, has missing data problems resolved, and includes any needed transformed variables. The researcher should also at this point have some understanding of data quality and the extent of any biases. The researcher can now proceed with more substantive analyses of the data.

PREPARING TABLE SHELLS

In many research projects, the researcher collects data on dozens, and often hundreds, of variables. The researcher cannot realistically analyze every variable in relation to all others, and so a plan to guide data analysis must be developed. The researcher's hypotheses and research questions provide only broad and general direction.

One approach to analytic planning is to develop a list of the analyses to be undertaken, specifying both the variables and the statistical test to be used. Another approach (which can be used in conjunction with a list of analyses) is to develop table shells. *Table shells* are layouts of how the researcher envisions presenting the research findings in a report, without any numbers in the table. Once a table shell has been prepared, the researcher can undertake whatever analyses are necessary to fill in the table entries.

Table 21-1 presents an example of an actual table shell created for an evaluation of an intervention for low-income women. This table guided a series of analyses of covariance that compared the experimental and control groups

Table 21-1. *Example of a Table Shell: Program Impacts on Indicators of Emotional Well-Being at the Time of the Follow-up Interview**

OUTCOME	EXPERIMENTAL GROUP	CONTROL GROUP	DIFFERENCE	p
Mean Score on the CES-D (depression) scale				
Percentage at risk of clinical depression (Scores of 16 and above on the CES-D)				
Mean Score, Master (self-efficacy) scale				
Mean score, Difficult Life Circumstances scale				
Percentage who cited no one as available as a social support				
Mean number of categories of social support cited as available				
Mean level of satisfaction with available social support				

* Note: Analyses to be performed using ANCOVA, controlling for 51 baseline characteristics.

in terms of several indicators of emotional well-being, after controlling for various characteristics that were measured at random assignment. The completed table that eventually appeared in the research report was somewhat different than this table shell. For example, another outcome variable was eventually added (a variable indicating the amount of change in depression scores between random assignment and follow-up). Thus, a researcher does not need to be rigid in adhering to the table shells, but they provide an excellent mechanism for organizing the analysis of vast amounts of data.

SUBSTANTIVE ANALYSES

Once the researcher has developed an analytic plan, the next step involves performing the actual substantive analyses designed to answer the research questions. Typically, the task begins with descriptive analyses. For example, the researcher generally develops a descriptive profile of the sample and examines the distribution of values on all key variables. Also, the researcher often looks, in a descriptive fashion, at the correlations among the variables. These descriptive analyses may help to suggest further analyses (or further data transformations) that

initially had not been envisioned. They also give the researcher an opportunity to become familiar with the data.

In the final stages of the substantive analyses, the researcher typically performs several statistical analyses to test the research hypotheses. In some cases, the researcher whose data analysis plan calls for multivariate analyses (e.g., MANOVA) will proceed directly to that procedure, but often the researcher will first perform various bivariate analyses (e.g., a series of ANOVAs). The primary statistical analyses are complete when all the research questions are addressed and, if relevant, when all the table shells have the applicable numbers in them.

The final phase of the data analysis task involves the interpretation of the findings and the conduct of any supplementary analyses that can aid in that endeavor. The interpretative phase is discussed in the next section.

❖ INTERPRETATION OF RESULTS

The analysis of research data provides what are referred to as the *results* of the study. These results need to be evaluated and interpreted by the researcher with due consideration to the overall aims of the project, its theoretical underpinnings, the specific hypotheses being tested, the existing body of related research knowledge, and the limitations of the adopted research methods.

The interpretive task primarily involves a consideration of five aspects of the study findings: (1) their accuracy, (2) their meaning, (3) their importance, (4) the extent to which they can be generalized, and (5) their implications. In this section, we review issues relating to each of these five aspects.

Accuracy of the Results

One of the first tasks that the researcher faces in interpreting the results is assessing whether the findings are likely to be accurate. This assessment, in turn, requires a careful analysis of the study's methodological and conceptual limitations. Whether one's hypotheses are supported or not, the validity and meaning of the results depend on a full understanding of the study's shortcomings.

Such an assessment relies heavily on the researcher's critical thinking skills as well as on an ability to be reasonably objective about one's own decisions. The researcher should carefully evaluate (e.g., using criteria such as those that we present in Chapter 25) all the major methodological decisions made in planning and executing the study to determine whether alternative decisions might have yielded different results.

The assessment of accuracy, however, also depends on the ability of the researcher to assemble different types of evidence. One type of evidence is the body of prior research on the topic. The investigator should examine whether his or her results are consistent with those of other studies; if there are discrepancies, a careful analysis of the reasons for any differences should be undertaken.

Other types of evidence can often be developed through peripheral data analyses, some of which were discussed earlier in this chapter. For example, the researcher needs to assess carefully the quality of the data collected, the re-

liability of measures used, and the presence or absence of any biases.

Another highly recommended strategy in quantitative studies is the conduct of a power analysis. In Chapter 19, we described how power analysis is often used before a study is undertaken to estimate sample size requirements. The researcher can also determine the actual power of his or her own analyses to evaluate the likelihood of having committed a Type II error. It is especially useful to perform a power analysis when the results of the main hypothesis tests were not statistically significant.

For example, suppose we were testing the effectiveness of an intervention to reduce patients' perception of pain. The sample of 200 subjects (100 subjects each in an experimental and control group) are compared in terms of pain scores, using a t-test. Suppose further that the mean pain score for the experimental group was 7.8 (SD = 1.3), while for the control group, the mean pain score was 8.2 (SD = 1.3), indicating lower reported pain among the experimental subjects. Although the results are in the hypothesized direction, the t-test was nonsignificant. We can provide a context for interpreting the accuracy of the nonsignificant results by performing a power analysis. First, we must estimate the effect size, using the formula presented in Chapter 19:

$$\gamma = \frac{8.2 - 7.8}{1.3} = .31$$

Table 19-7 in Chapter 19 shows us that, with an effect size of about .30, α = .05, and a sample size of 100 per group (which is close to the N of 109 under the column headed .30 in the table), the power of the statistical test is about .60. This means that we had a 40% risk of committing a Type II error—that is, the incorrect retention of the null hypothesis. The power analysis also tells us that the next researcher testing the effectiveness of this intervention should use a sample of about 175 per group to reach power = .80, which is the conventional standard for acceptable risk with Type II errors.

A critical analysis of the research methods and conceptualization and an examination of various types of external and internal evidence will almost inevitably indicate some limitations. These limitations must be taken into account in interpreting the results.

Meaning of the Results

In qualitative studies, interpretation and analysis occur virtually simultaneously. In quantitative studies, however, the results are in the form of test statistic values and probability levels. It is the researcher's role to imbue these results with meaning. Sometimes this involves supplementary analyses that were not originally planned. For example, if research findings are not what the researcher hypothesized, often other types of information in the data set can be examined to help the researcher understand what the findings mean.

In this section, we discuss the interpretation of various types of research outcomes within a hypothesis testing context. If the research was conceived on the basis of a theory or conceptual model, then it is important to relate the findings to that theoretical framework. That is, if a theoretical framework was truly the basis for the study, then it should also provide a basis for trying to understand the data.

INTERPRETING HYPOTHESIZED RESULTS

When the tests of statistical significance support the original research hypotheses, the task of interpreting the results is somewhat easier than when the hypotheses are challenged. In a sense, the interpretation has been partly accomplished beforehand in such a situation because the researcher has already had to bring together prior research findings, a theoretical framework, and logical reasoning in the development of the hypotheses. This groundwork can then form the context within which more specific interpretations are made.

Naturally, researchers are gratified when the results of many hours of effort offer support for their predictions. There is a decided preference on the part of individual researchers, advisers, and journal reviewers for studies whose hypotheses have been supported. This preference is understandable, but it is important not to let personal predilections interfere with the critical appraisal that is appropriate in all interpretive situations. A few cautionary suggestions should be kept in mind.

First, it is preferable to be somewhat conservative in drawing conclusions from the data. The intrusion of personal viewpoints and subjective judgments is inevitable in making sense of research results, but they must be held in check as much as possible. It is sometimes tempting to go far beyond the data in developing explanations for what the results mean, but conscientious scientists avoid doing so. A simple example might help to explain what is meant by "going beyond" the data. Suppose a nurse researcher hypothesized that a relationship existed between a pregnant woman's level of anxiety about the labor and delivery experience and the number of children she has already borne. The data reveal that a negative relationship between anxiety levels and parity ($r = -.40$) does indeed exist. The researcher, therefore, concludes that increased experience with childbirth causes decreasing amounts of anxiety. Is this conclusion supported by the data? The conclusion appears to be logical, but in fact, there is nothing within the data that leads directly to this interpretation. An important, indeed critical, research precept is: *Correlation does not prove causation*. The finding that two variables are related offers no evidence suggesting which of the two variables—if either—caused the other. In the example, perhaps causality runs in the opposite direction, that is, that a woman's anxiety level influences how many children she bears. Or perhaps a third variable not examined in the study, such as the woman's relationship with her husband, causes or influences both anxiety and number of children.

Alternative explanations for the findings should always be considered and, if possible, tested directly. If these competing interpretations can be ruled out on the basis of the data or previous research findings, so much the better. However, every angle should be examined to see if one's pet explanation has been given adequate competition. Any evidence from the researcher's assessment of bias and data quality should be brought to bear at this point.

Empirical evidence supporting the research hypotheses never constitutes proof of their veracity. Hypothesis testing, as we have seen, is probabilistic. There always remains a possibility that the obtained relationships resulted from chance or from some artifact of the research methods. Therefore, one must be tentative about both the results and the interpretations given to those results. In summary, even when the findings are in line with expectations, the researcher should exercise restraint in drawing conclusions and should give due consideration to any limitations identified in the assessment of the accuracy of the results.

INTERPRETING NONSIGNIFICANT RESULTS

Failure to reject a null hypothesis is particularly problematic from an interpretative point of view. The statistical procedures currently prevalent are geared toward disconfirmation of the null hypothesis. The failure to reject a null hypothesis could occur for one or more reasons, and the researcher does not usually know which of these reasons pertains. The null hypothesis could actually be true. The nonsignificant result, in this case, would accurately reflect the absence of a relationship among the research variables. On the other hand, the null hypothesis could be false, in which case a Type II error would have been committed.

The retention of a false null hypothesis can be attributed to several things, such as internal validity problems, the selection of a deviant sample, the use of a weak statistical procedure, or the use of too few subjects. Unless the researcher has special justification for attributing the nonsignificant findings to one of these factors, interpreting such results is a tricky

business. However, we suspect that in most of cases, the failure to reject the null hypothesis is the consequence of insufficient power (usually reflecting too small a sample size). For this reason, the conduct of a power analysis can often come to the researcher's aid in interpretation when nonsignificant results are obtained, as indicated earlier.

In any event, there is never justification for interpreting a retained null hypothesis as proof of a *lack* of relationship among variables. *The safest interpretation is that nonsignificant findings represent a lack of evidence for either truth or falsity of the hypothesis.* Thus, one can see that if the researcher's actual research hypothesis states that no differences or no relationships will be observed, traditional hypothesis testing procedures will not permit the required inferences.

When no significant results are found, there is sometimes a tendency to be overcritical of one's research strategy and methods and undercritical of the theory or logical reasoning on which the hypotheses were based. This is understandable: it is easier to say "My ideas were sound, I just didn't use the right approach to demonstrate this" than to admit that one has reasoned incorrectly. It is important to look for and identify flaws in the research methods, but it is equally important to search for theoretical shortcomings. The result of such endeavors should be recommendations for how the methods, the theory, or perhaps an experimental intervention could be improved.

INTERPRETING UNHYPOTHESIZED SIGNIFICANT RESULTS

Unhypothesized significant results can occur in two situations. The first involves findings about relationships that were not even considered in the design of the study. For example, in examining correlations among variables, the researcher might notice that two variables that were not central to the hypotheses or research question were nevertheless significantly correlated—and interesting. In determining how to interpret this finding, the researcher should try to evaluate whether the relationship is real or spurious. Sometimes there are other indications within the data set that shed light on this issue, but in other cases, the researcher may need to consult the literature to determine if other investigators have observed similar relationships.

The second situation is more perplexing: obtaining results *opposite* to those hypothesized. For instance, a nurse researcher might hypothesize that individualized patient teaching of breathing techniques is more effective than group instruction, but the results might reflect that the group method was better. Or a positive relationship might be predicted between a nurse's age and level of job satisfaction, but a negative relationship might be found.

It is, of course, unethical to alter the hypothesis after the results are in. Although some researchers may view such situations as awkward or embarrassing, there is really little basis for such feelings. The purpose of research is not to corroborate the scientist's notions, but to arrive at truth and enhance understanding. There is no such thing as a study whose results "came out the wrong way," if the "wrong way" is the truth.

In the case of significant findings opposite to what was hypothesized, it is less likely, though not impossible, that the methods are flawed than that the reasoning or theory is incorrect. As always, the interpretation that the researcher gives to the findings should involve comparisons with other research, a consideration of alternate theories, and a critical scrutiny of the data collection and analysis procedures. The final result of such an examination should be a tentative explanation for the unexpected findings, together with suggestions for how such explanations could be tested in other research projects.

INTERPRETING MIXED RESULTS

The interpretive process is often confounded by mixed results. The investigator may find some hypotheses supported by the data and others that cannot be supported. Or a hypothesis may be accepted when one measure of the dependent variable is used but rejected when using a separate measure of the same variable. Of all the situations mentioned, mixed results are probably the most prevalent.

When only some results run counter to a theoretical position or conceptual scheme, the research methods are probably the first aspect of the study that deserve scrutiny. Differences in the validity and reliability of the various measures could account for such discrepancies, for example. On the other hand, mixed results could indicate how a theory needs to be qualified or how certain constructs within the theory need to be reconceptualized. Mixed results often present opportunities for making conceptual advances because close scrutiny and attempts to make sense of disparate pieces of evidence may lead to breakthroughs that otherwise might have been impossible. This point is elaborated on more fully in Chapter 23, which covers integrating qualitative and quantitative data.

In summary, the interpretation of research findings is a demanding task, but it offers the possibility of unique intellectual rewards. The researcher must in essence play the role of a scientific detective, trying to make pieces of the puzzle fit together so that a coherent picture emerges.

Importance of the Results

In quantitative studies, results in support of the researcher's hypotheses are described as being significant. A careful analysis of the results of a study involves an evaluation of whether, in addition to being statistically significant, they are important.

The fact that statistical significance was attained in testing the hypothesis does not necessarily mean that the results were of value to the nursing community and their clients. Statistical significance indicates that the results were unlikely to be a function of chance. This means that the observed group differences or observed relationships were probably real but not necessarily important. With large samples, even modest relationships are statistically significant. For instance, with a sample of 500, a correlation coefficient of .10 is significant at the .05 level, but a relationship of this magnitude may have little practical value. Researchers, therefore, must pay attention to the numerical values obtained in an analysis in addition to the significance level when assessing the implications of the findings.

The absence of statistically significant results does not mean that the results are unimportant—although because of the difficulty in interpreting nonsignificant results, the case is more complex. However, let us suppose that the study involved testing two alternative procedures for making a clinical assessment (e.g., body temperature). Suppose that a researcher retained the null hypothesis, that is, found no statistically significant differences between the two methods. If a power analysis revealed an extremely low probability of a Type II error (e.g., power = .99, a 1% risk of a Type II error), then the researcher might be justified in concluding that the two procedures yield equally accurate assessments. If one of these procedures was more efficient or less painful than the other, then the nonsignificant findings could indeed be clinically important.

Generalizability of the Results

Another aspect of the results that the researcher should carefully assess is their generalizability. Researchers are rarely interested in discovering relationships among variables for a specific group of people at a specific point in time. The aim of research is typically to reveal enduring relationships, the understanding of which can be used to improve the human condition. If a nursing intervention under investigation is found to be successful, others will want to adopt the procedure. Therefore, an important interpretive question is whether the intervention will "work" or whether the relationships will "hold" in other settings, with other people. Part of the interpretive process involves asking the question: To what groups, environments, and conditions can the results of the study be applied?

Implications of the Results

Once the researcher has formed conclusions about the accuracy, meaning, importance, and generalizability of the results, he or she is in a good position to draw inferences about the implications of the results and to make recommendations for how best to use and build on the study findings. The researcher should consider the implications with respect to future research endeavors, theory development, and nursing practice.

The results of one study are often used as a springboard for additional research, and the investigator is typically in a good position to recommend "next steps." Armed with a comprehensive understanding of the study's limitations and strengths, the researcher can pave the way for studies that avoid the same pitfalls or that capitalize on known strengths. Moreover, the researcher is in a good position to assess how a new study could move a topic area forward. Is a replication needed, and, if so, with what groups? If observed relationships are significant, what do we need to know next for the information to be maximally useful?

If the study was based on a theoretical framework or conceptual model, then the researcher should also consider the implications of the study results for the theory. If the analysis of the study methods leads the researcher to conclude that the study had many flaws, then it may be difficult to make any inferences about the validity of the theory. However, if the study was reasonably rigorous methodologically, then the results should be used to either document support for the theory, suggest ways in which the theory ought to be modified, or discredit the theory as a useful approach for studying the topic under investigation.

Finally, the researcher should carefully consider the implications of the findings for nursing practice and nursing education. How can client outcomes or the nursing process be improved, based on the findings of the study? Specific suggestions for implementing the results of the study in a real nursing context are extremely valuable in the utilization process, as we discuss in Chapter 26. Of course, if the study is seriously flawed, it may be that the results are not usable within the nursing profession. But they will probably be useful, nevertheless, in designing an improved new study for the same research question.

❖ TIPS FOR DEVELOPING AND IMPLEMENTING THE ANALYTIC PLAN

This chapter was designed to provide practical advice about the development and implementation of a data analysis plan. A few additional suggestions are offered next.

• Whenever you create transformed or recoded variables, it is important to check that the computer is performing the intended manipulation by examining a sample of values for the original and transformed variables. For instance, in an example used earlier in this chapter, a set of computer instructions was developed to create four dichotomous variables for the four major blood types, based on a single four-category blood type variable. The computer could be instructed to display

a subset of values so that we could manually verify that the calculations were correct. The SPSS commands would be as follows:

> LIST VARIABLES=ID, BLOODTYP, TYPEA,
>   TYPEB, TYPEAB, TYPEO
>   /CASES = FROM 1 TO 20

This command would cause the computer to list the actual values of the data for the six specified variables (both the original variables—the identification number and the four-category blood type—and the four created dichotomous variables). The third line of the command instructs that the computer list only the first 20 cases rather than the entire data set. A sample of about 20 cases is usually sufficient to detect errors in recodes and transformations. The printout from this command is shown in Figure 21-3. With this listing, the researcher can check that each value for the four created variables is correct.

Indeed, this printout shows that there is an error. For the subject with ID number 03, data for the BLOODTYP variable was missing (coded 9). In creating the four dummy variables, no instruction was given regarding how to handle missing values. As a consequence,

ID	BLOODTYP	TYPEA	TYPEB	TYPEAB	TYPEO
1	4	.00	.00	.00	1.00
2	2	.00	1.00	.00	.00
3	9	.00	.00	.00	.00
4	1	1.00	.00	.00	.00
5	4	.00	.00	.00	1.00
6	3	.00	.00	1.00	.00
7	2	.00	1.00	.00	.00
8	4	.00	.00	.00	1.00
9	1	1.00	.00	.00	.00
10	1	1.00	.00	.00	.00
11	2	.00	1.00	.00	.00
12	3	.00	.00	1.00	.00
13	4	.00	.00	.00	1.00
14	4	.00	.00	.00	1.00
15	1	1.00	.00	.00	.00
16	2	.00	1.00	.00	.00
17	4	.00	.00	.00	1.00
18	3	.00	.00	1.00	.00
19	2	.00	1.00	.00	.00
20	4	.00	.00	.00	1.00

Figure 21-3. *Listing to check variable creation*

all four variables were set equal to zero, which is incorrect: This coding signifies that subject 03 is *not* of each specified blood type, and so at least one of the four dummy variables is erroneous. When there are missing data, the transformation instructions have to indicate how to handle these cases. Thus, additional commands would be needed to properly complete the creation of the four dichotomous blood type variables in this example.

- When transformed and recoded variables become an integral part of your data set, you should remember to document the transformations in the codebook carefully. This will make secondary analysis by other researchers much more feasible. It will also facilitate your own use of the data set at some later date.

- When you begin to undertake analyses designed to acquaint you with your data set, you should resist the temptation to go on a fishing expedition, that is, to hunt for *any* interesting relationships between variables, even if they were not anticipated or even contemplated. The facility with which computers can generate statistical information certainly can free you from laborious (and error-prone) manual calculations. But it also permits you to run analyses in a rather indiscriminate fashion. The risk is that you will serendipitously find significant correlations between variables that are simply a function of chance. It is important to remember that if you adopt the conventional .05 probability level for a Type I error, there is a strong possibility that there will be some significant correlations that do not reflect true relationships in the population. To make this more concrete, in a correlation matrix with 10 variables (which will result in 45 nonredundant correlations), there are likely to be two or three spurious significant correlations (.05 × 45 = 2.25.)

- In formulating your interpretation of the data, you should remember that others will be reviewing your interpretation with a critical and perhaps even a skeptical eye. Part of your job will be to convince others, in a fashion not dissimilar to convincing a jury in a judicial proceeding. Your hypotheses and interpretations are, essentially, on trial—and it must be remembered that the null hypothesis is considered "innocent" until proven "guilty." The evidence for your interpretation may come primarily from the statistical tests of the hypotheses, but you should look for opportunities to gather and present supplementary evidence in support of your conclusion. This includes evidence from other studies as well as internal evidence from your own study. You should scrutinize your data set and ask if there are any further analyses that could support your tentative explanation of the findings.

❖ RESEARCH EXAMPLES

Researchers typically undertake many of the steps depicted in Figure 21-1 without reporting on them in their research reports. Thus, the research literature does not offer many examples that fully describe the design and implementation of an analysis plan. A few examples of the types of analyses described in this chapter are presented in Table 21-2.

Considerable analytic detail is provided in a study published by Davis, Maguire, Haraphongse, and Schaumberger (1994), which we describe at some length here.

> Davis and her colleagues examined whether the type of preparatory information provided to cardiac catheterization (CC) patients was equally effective in reducing anxiety for patients with different coping styles. The coping styles of the 145 patients who served as the subjects in this study were first assessed, and patients were then categorized as either "monitors" (i.e., people who coped through information-seeking strategies) or "blunters" (i.e., people who coped through an information-avoiding strategy). Using a randomized block design, the two coping style groups were then randomly assigned to one of three preparatory information treatment condi-

Table 21-2.   *Examples of Analyses Undertaken in Research Projects*

RESEARCH QUESTION	TYPE OF ANALYSIS
What is the relationship between family stress, maternal conflict resolution tactics, and children's behavior problems in low-income inner-city families? (Murata, 1994)	Analysis of data quality (reliability); analysis of differences between those participating in the study and those refusing
What is the relationship between stress appraisal, coping, and characteristics of individuals responsible for older adults recently placed in nursing homes? (Kammer, 1994)	Comparison of subjects from two sites on key variables to determine if the data could be pooled
What is the validity and reliability of the Prenatal Psychosocial Profile? (Curry, Campbell, & Christian, 1994)	Listwise deletion to remove cases with missing data on key variables (for supplementary analyses performed on data merged from two studies)
To what extent do demographic variables and attachment predict quality of life in community-dwelling older men? (Rickelman, Gallman, & Parra, 1994)	Analysis of data quality (internal consistency reliability); recoding of variables for multiple regression
What is the effect of alternative types of information on coping with unplanned child hospitalization? (Melnyk, 1994)	Analysis of questions to determine whether subjects processed information they received—a manipulation check
What are the effects of ambulation at 3 versus 6 hours after cardiac angiogram on delayed bleeding, pain, and anxiety? (Barkman & Lunse, 1994)	Comparison of experimental and control group members on pretreatment variables to test the integrity of randomization
Do the partners of women with a low-risk pregnancy differ from those of women with a high-risk pregnancy in terms of paternal role competence? (Ferketich & Mercer, 1994)	Analysis of the characteristics of men in both the high-risk and low-risk groups who dropped out of the study compared with those who remained, to test for attrition bias

tions: (1) procedural information presented on videotape, (2) procedural–sensory information presented on videotape, and (3) procedural–sensory information presented in a booklet. Anxiety was measured at four points in time: preintervention, postintervention, pre-CC procedure, and post-CC procedure.

The central hypothesis regarding effects on patient anxiety was tested with a 2 × 3 × 4 ANOVA (coping style × preparatory treatment × time period). In addition, the researchers undertook the following analyses:

- The six treatment groups (2 coping styles × 3 treatment groups) were compared in terms of basic demographic character-

istics (age and education) and preintervention anxiety—an analysis aimed at assessing potential selection effects. One significant difference emerged: monitors reported more preintervention anxiety than blunters.

- The researchers then wondered whether gender might be implicated in the observed preintervention anxiety differences. A 2 × 3 × 2 ANOVA (coping style × treatment group × gender) yielded a significant gender effect on preintervention anxiety scores (women were significantly more anxious than men). The researchers concluded that gender should be taken into account in their analyses but realized that they had too few women in the sample to analyze results for women separately.

- A subgroup analysis was, however, undertaken with the 107 men in the sample. This analysis revealed a significant coping style by treatment interaction in terms of preintervention anxiety. The male blunters randomly assigned to the three treatment groups were found to be comparable in terms of pretreatment anxiety, while the male monitors were not. This analysis, then, indicated that the random assignment did not result in the sought-after anxiety equivalency among the subgroup of male blunters. (A further analysis was performed to determine whether the nonequivalence among groups was the result of only one or two extreme scores on the preintervention anxiety measure, but this proved not to be the case).

- The investigators then examined whether it made sense to use preintervention anxiety as a covariate in subsequent analyses, which would allow them to statistically control for the differences in preintervention anxiety among male blunters. However, they found that the correlations between preintervention anxiety and postintervention anxiety varied both across time and across groups, which precluded using preintervention anxiety as a covariate. Therefore, the researchers used ANOVA (rather than ANCOVA) for the main analyses. However, their knowledge of the pretreatment differences was taken into consideration in interpreting the results.

- The investigators calculated effect sizes as a means of assessing effects that were both statistically and clinically significant. They determined that any mean difference on the anxiety scale of 3 points or greater constituted an effect size of .30, which they established as their criterion for clinical significance.

As hypothesized, the researchers found that there was a significant three-way ANOVA interaction. Essentially, the results indicate that the procedural–sensory videotape treatment was especially beneficial for the monitors. The procedural modeling video was the optimal treatment for blunters. Over time, the monitors and blunters in each treatment group reported decreases in anxiety.

The researchers' results, then, include both expected and unexpected findings, which they addressed in the Discussion section of their report. The finding that coping styles moderated the effects of the preparation strategies was predicted on the basis of theory and prior research. The finding that women were significantly more anxious than their male counterparts in both coping style groups led the researchers to recommend that gender be considered as a primary rather than an incidental variable in CC preparatory intervention research.

The nonequivalence among male monitors led the researchers to consider the following theoretical implications:

> From a theoretic standpoint, it was determined that the observed nonequivalence in state anxiety among the male monitor groups might reflect an important and heretofore unexamined aspect of coping style: the relationship between subjects' monitoring and blunting repertoires and their procedural anxiety levels. (p. 136)

The researchers then pursued the implications of this suggestion with several supplementary analyses.

In summary, the researchers appear to have implemented a thorough and thoughtful analysis plan that took unexpected findings and design quality issues into account in interpreting the findings.

❖ SUMMARY

Researchers who have collected quantitative data typically must progress through a series of steps in the analysis and interpretation of their data. The careful researcher lays out an analysis plan in advance to guide that progress.

The focus of much of this chapter was on the preliminary analysis steps that pave the way for substantive statistical analysis. An important early step is the implementation of procedures to address missing data problems. These steps include the deletion of cases with missing values (i.e., *listwise deletion*), the deletion of variables with missing values, substitution of mean values, estimation of missing values, and selective and *pairwise deletion* of cases. Researchers strive to achieve a *rectangular matrix* of data (valid information on all variables for all cases), and several of these strategies can help the researcher to reach this goal.

Raw data entered directly onto a computer file often need to be modified for analysis. *Data transformations* can be of many types and are usually handled directly through commands to the computer. Examples of transformations include reversals of the coding of items, combining individual variables to form a composite scale, recoding the values of a variable, obtaining standardized scores on a variable, performing mathematical transformations for the purpose of meeting statistical assumptions, and creating dichotomous *dummy variables* for multivariate analyses.

Before the main analyses can proceed, the researcher usually has to undertake a number of additional steps to assess data quality and to maximize the value of the data. These steps include evaluating the reliability of measures, examining the distribution of values on key variables for any anomalies, and analyzing the magnitude and direction of any biases. Sometimes peripheral analyses involve *manipulation checks*, tests to determine whether *pooling* of subjects is warranted, or tests for *cohort effects.*

Once the data are fully prepared for the substantive analysis, the researcher should develop a formal plan to reduce the temptation to go on a "fishing expedition." One of the mechanisms that researchers sometimes use in the planning process is the development of *table shells*, that is, fully laid-out tables that do not yet have any numbers in them.

The interpretation of research findings basically represents the researcher's attempts to understand the research results. The interpretation typically involves five subtasks: (1) analyzing the accuracy of the results, (2) searching for the meaning underlying the results, (3) considering the importance of the findings, (4) analyzing the generalizability of the findings, and (5) assessing the implications of the study regarding future research, theory development, and nursing practice.

❖ STUDY SUGGESTIONS

Chapter 21 of the accompanying *Study Guide for Nursing Research: Principles and Methods, 5th ed.*, offers various exercises and study suggestions for reinforcing the concepts presented in this chapter. Additionally, the following study questions can be addressed:

1. Read the study by Coffman, Levitt, and Brown (1994) entitled "Effects of clarification of support expectations in prenatal couples" (*Nursing Research, 43*, 111–116). Indicate which steps in the process shown in Figure 21-1 are described in this report.

2. Using the SPSS commands illustrated in this chapter, undertake the following:
   a. Create four dummy variables for a person's marital status, coded originally on the variable MARITAL as 1 = married; 2 = single, never married; 3 = divorced or separated; and 4 = widowed.
   b. Reverse a seven-point Likert item measuring attitudes toward breastfeeding, whose variable name is BFATT.
   c. Create a variable indicating the total number of different types of drugs an adolescent has used, from a list of 10 different drug types whose variable names are DRUG01, DRUG02, . . . DRUG10.

3. Suppose you were studying gender differences in physical health 6 months after loss of a spouse. Create a fictitious table shell for such a study.

❖ SUGGESTED READINGS

METHODOLOGICAL REFERENCES

Cohen, J., & Cohen, P. (1983). *Applied multiple regression/correlation analysis for the behavioral sciences*. (2nd ed.). New York: John Wiley and Sons.

Dixon, W. J., & Massey, F. J. (1983). *Introduction to statistical analysis* (4th ed.). New York: McGraw-Hill.

Harris, M.L. (1991). *Introduction to data processing* (3rd ed.). New York: John Wiley and Sons.

Jacobsen, B. S. (1981). Know thy data. *Nursing Research, 30,* 254–255.

Kim, J., & Curry, J. (1977). The treatment of missing data in multivariate analysis. In D. F. Alwin (Ed.), *Survey design and analysis.* Beverly Hills, CA: Sage.

Little, R. J. A., & Rubin, D. B. (1990). The analysis of social science data with missing values. In J. Fox & J. S. Long (Eds.), *Modern methods of data analysis.* Newbury Park, CA: Sage.

Munro, B. H., & Page, E. B. (1993). *Statistical methods for health care research* (2nd ed.). Philadelphia: J. B. Lippincott.

Norusis, M. J. (1991). *The SPSS guide to data analysis.* (2nd ed.). Chicago, IL: SPSS, Inc.

Tabachnick, B. G., & Fidell, L. S. (1989). *Using multivariate statistics.* (2nd ed.). New York: Harper & Row.

SUBSTANTIVE REFERENCES

Barkman, A., & Lunse, C. P. (1994). The effect of early ambulation on patient comfort and delayed bleeding after cardiac angiogram. *Heart and Lung, 23,* 112–117.

Curry, M. A., Campbell, R. A., & Christian, M. (1994). Validity and reliability testing of the Prenatal Psychosocial Profile. *Research in Nursing and Health, 17,* 127–135.

Davis, T. M. A., Maguire, T. O., Haraphongse, M., & Schaumberger, M. R. (1994). Preparing adult patients for cardiac catheterization: Informational treatment and coping style interactions. *Heart and Lung, 23,* 130–139.

Ferketich S. L., & Mercer, R. T. (1994). Predictors of paternal role competence by risk status. *Nursing Research, 43,* 80–85.

Kammer, C. H. (1994). Stress and coping of family members responsible for nursing home placement. *Research in Nursing and Health, 17,* 89–98.

Melnyk, B. M. (1994). Coping with unplanned childhood hospitalization: Effects of informational interventions on mothers and children. Nursing Research, *43,* 50–55.

Murata, J. (1994). Family stress, social support, violence, and sons' behavior. *Western Journal of Nursing Research, 16,* 154–168.

Rickelman, B. L., Gallman, L., & Parra, H. (1994). Attachment and quality of life in older, community-residing men. *Nursing Research, 43,* 68–72.

Chapter 22

THE ANALYSIS OF QUALITATIVE DATA

An ever-growing number of nurse researchers are engaging in qualitative research, which is sometimes referred to as *naturalistic inquiry.* Qualitative data generally take the form of loosely structured, narrative materials, such as verbatim dialogue between an interviewer and a respondent in a phenomenological study, the field notes of a participant observer in an ethnographic study, or diaries used by historical researchers. These data are generally not amenable to the type of analyses we discussed in the chapters on statistical analysis. This chapter describes methods for analyzing such qualitative data.

❖ *INTRODUCTION TO QUALITATIVE ANALYSIS*

Qualitative analysis is a very labor-intensive activity that requires insight and ingenuity. Before describing actual analytic procedures, we briefly discuss the arguments often made in

favor of qualitative analysis as well as its major applications.

Aims of Qualitative Research

Qualitative research was described by Benoliel (1984) as "modes of systematic inquiry concerned with understanding human beings and the nature of their transactions with themselves and with their surroundings" (p. 3). Qualitative research is often described as holistic, that is, concerned with humans and their environment in all of their complexities. Many qualitative studies are based on the premise that gaining knowledge about humans is impossible without describing human experience as it is lived and as it is defined by the actors themselves.

Because of its emphasis on the subjects' realities, qualitative studies typically require a minimum of researcher-imposed structure and a maximum of researcher involvement, as the researcher tries to comprehend those people whose experiences are under study. Imposing structure on the research situation (e.g., by deciding in advance exactly what questions to ask and how to ask them) necessarily restricts the portion of the subjects' experiences that will be revealed.

There is an ongoing debate over whether qualitative or quantitative studies are better suited for advancing nursing science (e.g., Munhall, 1982; Webster, Jacox, & Baldwin, 1981), but there is a growing recognition that both approaches are needed (Bargagliotti, 1983; Goodwin & Goodwin, 1984; Gorenberg, 1983). The most balanced perspective appears to be that the degree of structure a researcher imposes should be based on the nature of the research question. For example, if the question under investigation is, "What are the processes by which infertile couples resolve their infertility?" then the investigator is really seeking to understand how men and women make sense of an experience that is complex, interpersonal, and dynamic. It would be possible to investigate this problem with structured instruments, but it is likely that the investigator would never really come to understand the *process* that is the focus of the inquiry.

On the other hand, if the research question is, "What is the effect of alternative topical gels applied during wound debridement on the patient's level of pain and extent of debridement accomplished?" then it would be appropriate to seek specific, concrete data in a structured format. Both these hypothetical questions have a place in nursing research because both can contribute to the improvement of nursing practice.

Benoliel (1984) identified four broad areas in which unstructured, qualitative approaches appear most promising:

- Environmental influences on caregiving systems
- Decision-making processes
- People's adaptation to critical life experiences, such as chronic illness or developmental changes
- The nature of nurse–client social transactions in relation to stability and change

Applications of Qualitative Analysis

Qualitative methods, as suggested in the previous section, are more appropriately applied to certain types of research problems than others. There is a fair amount of agreement that qualitative methods are less suitable than quantitative approaches for establishing cause-and-effect relationships, for rigorously testing research hypotheses, or for determining the opinions, attitudes, and practices of a broad population. The unsuitability of qualitative methods for these purposes is based in part on the difficulties of analyzing qualitative data, as we discuss later. Another problem, however, is that qualitative research tends to yield vast amounts of intensive narrative data—consequently, it is impractical (and in many cases, not even necessary or desirable) for the researcher to use large, representative samples for obtaining the data. Moreover, qualitative research generally makes no attempt to control extraneous variation—the kind of control that enables researchers to establish causal relationships. Qualitative research, with its holistic emphasis, seeks to understand human experience within its full context rather than attempting to isolate a small portion of it through research design or statistical control.

Although qualitative research has some disadvantages when applied to certain research problems, it offers important advantages. In particular, highly structured methods can never yield the rich and potentially insightful material that is generated using an unstructured approach. Among the important purposes of qualitative research are the following:

- *Description*. When little is known about a group of people, an institution, or a phenomenon of interest, in-depth interviewing or participant observation are good ways to learn about them. For example, suppose we wanted to learn about the experiences of deinstitutionalized mental patients. How do they cope with the transition to a new environment? What kinds of supports are available to them? What factors facilitate or impede improved mental health? For this type of study, a survey approach might be unfeasible or unprofitable.

- *Hypothesis generation.* A researcher using qualitative techniques often has no explicit a priori hypotheses. The collection of in-depth information about some phenomenon might, however, lead to the formulation of hypotheses that could be tested more formally in subsequent research. For example, a researcher may be investigating by means of in-depth interviews the reasons for discontinued use of oral contraceptives among teenaged girls. Open-ended discussion with a sample of girls might lead the researcher to observe that girls whose boyfriends have complained about the birth control pill's side effects on the girls (e.g., weight gain, moodiness, or headaches) appear to be substantially more likely to stop using the pill than girls whose boyfriends have not made such complaints. This hypothesis could be tested systematically in another study.

- *Theory development.* Qualitative researchers often analyze their data with an eye toward developing an integrated explanatory scheme. The term *grounded theory* is frequently used in connection with a certain approach to analyzing qualitative data, as developed by two sociologists, Glaser and Strauss (1967). This approach involves the generation of theory on the basis of comparative analysis between or among groups within a substantive area, using methods of field research for data collection. The term grounded theory refers to the fact that a theorization does not spring from the investigator's preconceived hypotheses about a social situation but rather is discovered by being *grounded* in the data.

Qualitative data can also serve a number of additional functions when combined with quantitative data. These purposes are discussed in Chapter 23.

Qualitative Data: To Quantify or Not

One of the decisions a qualitative researcher must make is whether the narrative materials that compose the data will be quantified to some extent. After all, most quantitative measurement methods involve ascribing numbers to *qualities* of people or objects, for example, their self-esteem, their degree of compliance, or their level of preoperative anxiety. In quantitative research, decisions about how to translate qualities of phenomena into numerical expression are generally made before data collection. However, researchers who collect qualitative materials sometimes develop schemes for quantifying their narrative materials after the data have been gathered.

Qualitative materials can be quantified to varying degrees. At one extreme, the researcher can convert all the narrative information to a numerical system and subject the data to quantitative analysis through statistical procedures. The technique known as content analysis, described in Chapter 9, often involves the complete quantification of narrative personal communications. At the other extreme, all the narrative materials can be left intact and can be analyzed through procedures that are described in this chapter. In between these extremes are quantitative methods for introducing some checks and balances into qualitative analysis. For example, a procedure referred to as *quasi-statistics,* which resembles an accounting system more than a method of statistical analysis, is sometimes used in conjunction with qualitative analysis.

Qualitative materials can be quantified in a variety of ways. For example, suppose we asked patients to discuss, in their own words, the quality of nursing care they received during a long-term hospitalization. Suppose each patient's response was tape-recorded and then transcribed, yielding descriptions ranging from 5 to 10 typewritten pages. How could the material be quantified? We could *count* the number of specific complaints mentioned; we could *count* the number of lines devoted to negative versus positive comments; we could *code* for the presence or absence of specific patient concerns, such as complaints about the time required for the nurse to respond to a call; or we could *rate* the description in terms of overall favorableness toward the care received. The researcher who wants to quantify qualitative material can be extremely creative and ingenious in developing a meaningful approach. The trick is to develop a system that is consistent with the aims of the research and faithful to the message conveyed in the qualitative materials.

Whether qualitative data *should* be quantified is a different issue. Some investigators argue that everything can be measured (quantified) and that quantitative analysis is the best way to determine objectively whether relationships between variables exist. This argument aside, it is sometimes useful to quantify qualitative materials purely as a way of coping with the volume of data that is typically produced in qualitative research. Other researchers argue against any quantification, asserting that qualitative materials are substantially richer than numbers and offer greater potential for understanding relationships and meanings. They also argue that because data collection and coding procedures are not immune to subjectivity, the use of numbers merely disguises potential bias and gives the illusion of objectivity. We are inclined to disagree with either extreme. We believe that an understanding of human behaviors, problems, and characteristics is best advanced by the judicious use of both qualitative and quantitative data. Sometimes, as we discuss in Chapter 23, that combination is appropriate in a single study. Ultimately, the decision about whether to quantify any aspect of qualitative data must be based on the nature of the research question and the philosophical orientation of the researcher.

Qualitative Analysis: General Considerations

The purpose of data analysis, regardless of the type of data one has and regardless of the tradition that has driven its collection, is to impose some order on a large body of information so that some general conclusions can be reached and communicated in a research report. Although the overall aim of both qualitative and quantitative analysis is to organize, synthesize, provide structure to, and elicit meaning from research data, an important difference is that data collection and data analysis often occur simultaneously in qualitative studies. Because qualitative researchers tend to use an intuitive approach to sampling and gathering information, they must be prepared to redirect the research as new insights emerge from the analysis.

The data analysis task is almost always a formidable one, but it is particularly challenging for the qualitative researcher, for three major reasons. First, there are no systematic rules for analyzing and presenting qualitative data. It is at least partly because of this fact that qualitative methods have been described by some critics as "soft." The absence of systematic analytic procedures makes it difficult for the researcher engaged in qualitative analysis to present conclusions in such a way that their validity is patently clear. And, the absence of well-defined and universally accepted procedures makes replication difficult. Some of the procedures described in Chapter 16 (e.g., member checking and investigator triangulation) are extremely important tools for enhancing the trustworthiness not only of the data themselves but also of the analyses and interpretation of those data.

The second aspect of qualitative analysis that makes it challenging is the sheer amount of work that is required. The qualitative analyst must organize and make sense of pages and pages of narrative materials. In a qualitative study directed by one of the authors (Polit), the data consisted of transcribed, unstructured interviews with more than 100 women who had recently divorced. The transcriptions ranged from 40 to 80 pages in length, resulting in more than 6000 pages that had to be read, organized, integrated, and synthesized. It is this labor-intensive aspect of qualitative research, combined with the fact that samples must necessarily be rather small, that sometimes makes it difficult to obtain funding for qualitative studies; they are expensive but may be of limited generalizability.

The final challenge comes in reducing the data for reporting purposes. The major results of quantitative research can often be summarized in two or three tables. However, if one compresses qualitative data too much, the very point of maintaining the integrity of narrative materials during the analysis phase becomes lost. If one merely summarizes the conclusions reached without including numerous supporting excerpts directly from the narrative materials, then the richness of the original data disappears. As a consequence, it is challenging to present the results of qualitative research in a format that is compatible with space limitations in professional journals. Qualitative researchers often find that the best medium for disseminating their results is books rather than journal articles.

Despite the fact that there are no universally accepted rules for the analysis of qualitative materials, numerous systems have evolved. It is beyond the scope of this book to describe all the major systems in detail, but we present some guidelines that should provide a basic understanding of the general process. We also describe the major features of two different strategies: (1) analytic induction and (2) grounded theory. However, we strongly encourage readers interested in performing qualitative analysis to consult several of the references listed at the end of this chapter.

❖ DATA MANAGEMENT AND ORGANIZATION

Data management tasks involve activities that prepare the data for subsequent analysis. Whether you are working with field notes from a participant observation study, verbatim transcriptions from unstructured interviews, historical documents, or some other narrative materials, you will need to prepare carefully for the analysis of data by imposing some structure on the mass of information. Both manual and computerized techniques for data management are discussed in this section.

Preliminary Activities

As in quantitative studies, there are some preliminary steps that should be undertaken. It is usually important to check that the data are all there, are of reasonably good quality, and are in a format that facilitates organization. For example, you should confirm that the verbatim transcripts really *are* verbatim (some well-meaning typists are often tempted to edit or clean up dialogue). As another example, you should also ensure that all the field notes have been written up and that there are no glaring holes in the data.

The data organization task can be done either manually or with the assistance of a computer. If it is being done manually, it is best to have all the data typed or printed with double-spacing and with wide margins so that notes and codes can be inserted into them. Whether using a manual or computerized approach to organize the data, you should always be sure to have at least one backup copy of all the data, and in some cases multiple copies may be needed.

Finally, you should set up administrative files for storing the data. These files usually contain the master copy of the material and are arranged in some administratively relevant manner, such as by chronologic date or by subject identification number. These files may also contain other types of cross-referenced materials, such as listings that link subject identification numbers with other types of information, such as the dates and locations of data collection or forms with the informant's background information.

Developing Categories and Codes

The main task in organizing qualitative data is developing a method to index the materials. That is, the researcher must design a mechanism for gaining access to parts of the data, without having to repeatedly reread the set of data in its entirety. This phase of data management is essentially a reductionistic activity—data must be converted to smaller, more manageable, and more manipulatable units that can easily be retrieved.

The most widely used procedure is to develop a category scheme and to then code the data according to these categories. There are, unfortunately, no straightforward or easy guidelines for this task. The development of a high-quality categorization scheme for qualitative data involves a careful reading of a portion of the data, with an eye to identifying underlying concepts and clusters of concepts. Depending on the aims of the study, the nature of the categories may vary in level of detail or specificity as well as in level of abstraction.

Researchers whose aims are primarily descriptive tend to use categories that are fairly concrete. For example, the category scheme may focus on differentiating various types of actions or events or different phases in a chronologic unfolding of an experience. The topical coding scheme used in Gagliardi's (1991) study of the family's experience of living with a child with Duchenne muscular dystrophy is presented in Figure 22-1. (Gagliardi's study was presented as a research example in Chapter 16.) This is an example of a category system that is fairly concrete and descriptive. For example, it allows the coders to code for specific relationships among family members and for events occurring in specific locations.

Studies that are designed to develop a theory are more likely to develop highly abstract and conceptual categories. In designing conceptual categories, the data should be broken into segments, closely examined, and compared to other segments for similarities and dissimilarities to determine what type of phenomena are reflected in the data and what the meaning of those phenomena are. The researcher asks questions about discrete events, incidents, or thoughts that are indicated in an observation or statement, such as the following:

- What is this?
- What is going on?
- What does it stand for?
- What else is like this?
- What is this distinct from?

Important concepts that emerge from close examination of the data are then given a name or label that forms the basis for a category system. These category names are necessarily abstractions, but ideally the labels should be sufficiently graphic that you can readily remember the nature of the material to which it refers.

In developing a category scheme, related concepts are often grouped together to facilitate the coding process. As shown in Figure 22-1, Gagliardi's system involved five major clusters of categories. For example, all the excerpts illustrating how family members feel about living with a child with Duchenne muscular dystrophy are clustered under Feeling Codes.

Once a category scheme has been developed, all the data are then reviewed for content and coded for correspondence to the identified categories. The codes corresponding to the category system can be an abbreviation of the category (e.g., B-ACT for Boy's Activities in Gagliardi's category system), a code corresponding to an outline structure (e.g., Boy's Ac-

Activity Codes	Strategy Codes	Feeling Codes
• Boy's Activities	• Physical Difference	• Feelings
• Family's Activities	• Life's Reality	• Support
• Physical Therapy/Exercises		• Silence
		• Ambivalence
Relationship Codes	**Events Codes**	• Normalcy/Autonomy
• Father	• School	
• Mother	• Physical Environment	
• Siblings	• School Bus	
• Extended Family		

Figure 22-1. *Gagliardi's (1991) Coding Scheme of Families' Experiences (Reprinted with permission)*

tivities might be A.1 and Family's Activities might be A.2), or some other type of symbolic configuration. When a computer is used to index the data, the software being used should be reviewed to determine requirements for labeling the codes.

This process of coding qualitative material is seldom an easy one, for several reasons. First, the researcher may have difficulty in deciding which code is most appropriate or may not fully comprehend the underlying meaning of some aspect of the data. It may take a second reading of the material to grasp the nuances contained in some portions of the data.

Second, the researcher often discovers in going through the data that the initial category system was incomplete or otherwise inadequate. In some cases, this might mean going back and starting from scratch. For this reason, it is usually necessary to review a large portion of the data before an adequate coding scheme can be developed. It is not unusual for some topics to emerge that were not initially conceptualized. When this happens, it is sometimes risky to assume that the topic failed to appear in materials that have already been coded. That is, a topic might not be identified as important until it has emerged three or four times in the data. In such a case, it would be necessary to reread all previously coded material to have a truly complete grasp of that category.

Another problem stems from the fact that narrative materials are generally not linear. For example, paragraphs from transcribed interviews may contain elements relating to three or four different categories, embedded in a complex fashion. An example of a multitopic segment of an interview from Polit's study of divorced women mentioned earlier, with codes in the margin, is shown in Figure 22-2.*

---

* Figure 22-2 does not show the categories that the alphanumeric codes in the margin represent. The code categories used in the figure are as follows: 2b—General psychologic state during the divorce; 9—Finances; 5c—Feelings about single parenting; and 1b—Perceived advantages of divorce.

Manual Methods of Organizing Qualitative Data

A variety of procedures have traditionally been used to organize and manage qualitative data. When the amount of data is small, or when a category system is fairly simple, it may be possible to use color paper clips or color Post-It Notes to code the content of the narrative materials. For example, if we were analyzing responses to a single open-ended question about women's attitudes toward menopause, we might use blue paper clips for positive comments, red clips for negative comments, yellow clips for neutral comments, and green clips for comments that are mixed. Then the researcher could pull out all the responses coded with a blue clip to examine women's negative reactions to menopause.

Before the advent of computer programs for managing qualitative data, the most usual procedure was the development of *conceptual files*. In this approach, a physical file is developed for each of the various categories, and all the materials relating to that topic are cut out and inserted into the file. To create conceptual files, the researcher must first go through all the data and write the relevant codes in the margins, as in Figure 22-2. Then the researcher cuts up a copy of the material by category area, and places the cut-out excerpt into the file for that category. In this fashion, all the content on a particular topic can be retrieved by going to the applicable file folder.

The creation of such conceptual files is clearly a cumbersome and labor-intensive task. This is particularly true when segments of the narrative materials have multiple codes, as is true in the excerpt shown in Figure 22-2. In such a situation, there would need to be four copies of the paragraph—one for each file corresponding to the four codes. The researcher must also be sensitive to the need to provide enough context that the cut-up material can be understood. For example, it might be necessary to include material preceding or following the directly relevant materials. Finally, the researcher must

```
Subject 025
June 25, 1980
Page 32

Int:      How did you feel right after the separation?  Will you tell
          me a little more about that?

025:      Well, you know, when I look back...I mean I think anybody
          would have felt hopeless and helpless...because of, you
          know, emotionally...I think maybe it's a little easier if
          you've got more security...more money.  I was really stuck.
          I caught myself thinking..."Oh, if it wasn't for the
          kids..."  I love them both dearly, but...I mean there have
          been times when I've said to myself--I think a lot of women
          go through this too--I really had thought of giving them
          up.  In the beginning I used to think, too, they'd be so
          much better off with somebody that could, you know...When I
          was really struggling--I was on welfare----I used to think,
          "My God, how am I going to educate them?  What are they
          going to have?  I can't make ends meet now."  It's kinda
          projecting the unknown...fear of the unknown.  I think you
          can get mixed up.
```

2b
9
5c
1b.

Figure 22-2. *Coded excerpt from an unstructured interview*

usually include pertinent administrative information on each item in the conceptual files. For example, if the data consisted of transcribed interviews, each informant would ordinarily be assigned an identification number. Each excerpt filed in the conceptual file should also include the appropriate identification number so that the researcher could, if necessary, obtain additional information from the master copy.

In lieu of conceptual files, some researchers use qualitative sort cards for indexing their data. These index cards have holes on all sides that can be used for easy retrieval of information on a given topic or concept. That is, the researcher places notches in the holes corresponding to coded topical categories or concepts. Then, when information relating to a particular topic or theme is needed, all the cards notched for that category can easily be pulled from the deck of index cards. Some researchers directly paste their data on these cards, when the data set is of a manageable size, and then directly code each data segment using the notched holes to indicate a code. Others write an abstract of an entire case (e.g., one interview or one observational session) onto the card, and

then indicate on the card the page numbers (e.g., pages of the observational notes or transcribed interview) where different codes may be found. An example of the latter procedure from the study of divorced women is shown in Figure 22-3.

Computer Programs for Managing Qualitative Data

The traditional manual methods of organizing qualitative data have a long and respected history, but they are becoming increasingly outmoded as a result of the widespread availability of personal computers (PCs) that can be used to perform the filing and indexing of qualitative material. The early attempts to computerize qualitative data involved numbering all paragraphs of the researcher's field notes or interviews, coding each paragraph for topical codes, and then entering the information into computer files. This is essentially an automated version of the manual indexing and retrieval systems described previously.

Sophisticated computer programs for managing qualitative data are now available and

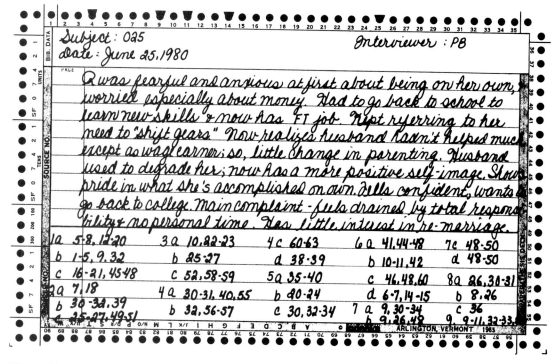

Figure 22-3. *Example of interview abstract with code and page summary*

are becoming widely used. These programs permit the entire data file to be entered onto the computer, each portion of an interview or observational record coded and categorized, and then portions of the text corresponding to specified codes retrieved and printed (or shown on a screen) for analysis. The current generation of programs also has features that go beyond simple indexing and retrieval—they offer possibilities for actual analysis and integration of the data.

Computer programs remove the drudgery of cutting and pasting pages and pages of narrative material and are fast becoming indispensable research tools. However, some people argue that beginning researchers should gain at least some experience with manually organizing qualitative data. Part of this argument stems from the sentiment that manual indexing provides a more hands-on type of experience that allows the researcher to get closer to the data. Other concerns have been expressed about the use of computers with qualitative data. For example, one potential pitfall is that the researcher might develop an overly elaborate coding system, resulting from the fact that retrieval of information is vastly simplified with a computer. The advent of sophisticated programs that aid in the analysis of data has also given rise to objections to having a process that is basically cognitive turned into an activity that is mechanical and technical. Despite these concerns, most qualitative researchers have switched to computerized management of their data, and this trend is unlikely to be reversed. Computerized data management frees up the researcher's time so that greater attention can be paid to more important conceptual issues. Moreover, a more comprehensive analysis may be possible by using computers because there is less of a risk that certain parts of the data set will be overlooked.

The most widely used computer programs for qualitative data have been designed for PCs, and most are for use on IBM-compatible computers rather than on MacIntosh computers (Macs). There are mainframe programs for managing qualitative data sets that are too large to handle on a PC (e.g., QUAL), but PCs now have sizable memories and operate at fast enough speeds that most qualitative data sets can be managed on a PC. The most widely used programs include the following: Ethnograph, GATOR, MARTIN, QUALPRO, Textbase Alpha, Text Analysis Package (all for use with IBM-type PCs), and HyperQual (for use with Macs). These programs have been debugged for computer problems and have user manuals that are relatively straightforward. The program NUDIST (*N*onnumerical *U*nstructured *D*ata *I*ndexing, *S*earching, and *T*heorizing) is an example of a program designed to support analysis and theory-building. Undoubtedly other similar (and even more sophisticated) programs will become available in the years ahead, and many of the programs already available will offer enhancements that make them even more attractive.

It is beyond the scope of this text to describe the main features of all the available programs—and, in any event, the description would likely be quickly outdated because new releases of these programs become available almost yearly. However, we can describe some attractive features of programs for qualitative analysis so that such programs can be more readily appraised.

Typically, the researcher begins by entering the qualitative data onto a computer file using a word processing program (e.g., WordPerfect). The data are then imported into the analysis program in ASCII format. When a file is saved in ASCII, it is stripped of any proprietary codes specific to the word-processing programming, leaving only "plain vanilla" text. A few qualitative data management programs (e.g., QUALPRO, HyperQual) allow text to be entered directly rather than requiring an ASCII import file from a word processor.

Next, the researcher marks the boundaries (i.e., the beginning and end) of a segment of data, and then codes the data according to the previously developed category system. In some programs (e.g., Textbase Alpha), this step can be done directly on the computer screen in a one-step process, but others require two steps. The first step involves the numbering of lines of text and the subsequent printing out of the text with the line numbers appearing in the margins. Then, after coding the paper copy, the researcher tells the computer which codes go with which lines of text. Most (but not all) programs permit overlapping codings and the nesting of segments with different codes within one another.

All the major qualitative analysis programs permit proofreading and editing. That is, codes can be altered, expanded, or deleted, and the boundaries of segments of text can be changed. All programs also provide screen displays or printouts of collated segments—however, some programs do this only on a file-by-file basis (e.g., one interview at a time) rather than allowing the researcher to retrieve all the segments with a given code across files.

Beyond these basic features, the available programs vary considerably in the enhancements they offer the researcher. The following is a nonexhaustive list of features that are available in some programs but not in others:

- Automatic coding according to words or phrases found in the data
- Compilation of a master list of all codes used
- Selective searches (i.e., restricted to cases with certain characteristics, such as searching for a code only in interviews with women)
- Searches for co-occurring codes (i.e., retrieval of data segments to which two or more specific codes are attached)
- Retrieval of information on the sequence of coded segments (i.e., on the order of appearance of certain codes)
- Frequency count of the occurrence of codes
- Calculation of code percentages, in relation to other codes
- Calculation of the average size of data segments
- Listing and frequency count of specific words in the data files
- Searches for relationships among coded categories

Several of these enhancements have lead to a blurring in the distinction between qualitative data management and data analysis.

❖ ANALYTIC PROCEDURES

Data management tasks in qualitative research are typically reductionist in nature because they convert large masses of data into smaller, more manageable segments. By contrast, qualitative data analysis tasks are constructionist in nature: they involve putting together segments into a meaningful conceptual pattern. Although different approaches to qualitative data analysis have been advocated, there are some elements that are common to several of them. We provide the following general guidelines, together with a description of the steps undertaken by one research team in performing a qualitative study.

The analysis of qualitative materials generally begins with a search for *themes* or recurring regularities. In some cases, the thematic analysis occurs in the field, as the data are being collected. In other situations, the thematic analysis occurs after the data have been collected, during a reading (or rereading) of the data set. Themes often develop within categories of data (i.e., within categories of the coding scheme used for indexing materials) but sometimes cut across them. For example, in Gagliardi's (1991) study, six themes describing the families' experiences were identified, and these themes were further grouped under three headings corresponding to the stages in the process of adapting to the child's disability. The first theme, disillusionment, embraced content that had been coded under several topical codes (see Figure 22-1), primarily the topic of feeling.

The search for themes involves not only the discovery of commonalities across subjects but also a search for natural variation in the data. Themes that emerge from unstructured observations and interviews are never universal. The researcher must attend not only to what themes arise but also to how they are patterned. Does the theme apply only to certain subgroups? In certain types of communities or or-

ganizations? In certain contexts? At certain periods? What are the conditions that precede the observed phenomenon, and what are the apparent consequences of it? In other words, the qualitative analyst must be sensitive to *relationships* within the data.

The analyst's search for themes, regularities, and patterns in the data can sometimes be facilitated by charting devices that enable the researcher to summarize the evolution of behaviors, events, and processes. For example, for qualitative studies that focus on dynamic experiences—such as decision making—it is often useful to develop flow charts or timelines that highlight time sequences, major decision points and events, and factors affecting the decisions. An example of such a flow chart from a study of decision making among infertile couples is presented in Figure 22-4. The construction of such flow charts for all subjects would help to highlight certain regularities in the subjects' evolving behaviors.

A further step frequently taken involves the *validation* of the understandings that the thematic exploration has provided. In this phase, the concern is whether the themes inferred are an accurate representation of the perspectives of the people interviewed or observed. Several procedures can be used in this validation step, some of which were discussed in Chapter 16. If there is more than one researcher working on the study, debriefing sessions in which the themes are reviewed and specific cases discussed can be highly productive. Multiple perspectives—what we referred to in Chapter 16 as *investigator triangulation*—cannot ensure the validity of the themes, but it can minimize any idiosyncratic biases. Using an iterative approach is almost always necessary. That is, the researcher derives themes from the narrative materials, goes back to the materials with the themes in mind to see if the materials really do fit, and then refines the themes as necessary. It is generally useful to undertake member checks—that is, to present the preliminary thematic analysis to some of the subjects or informants, who can be encouraged to offer suggestions that might support or contradict this analysis.

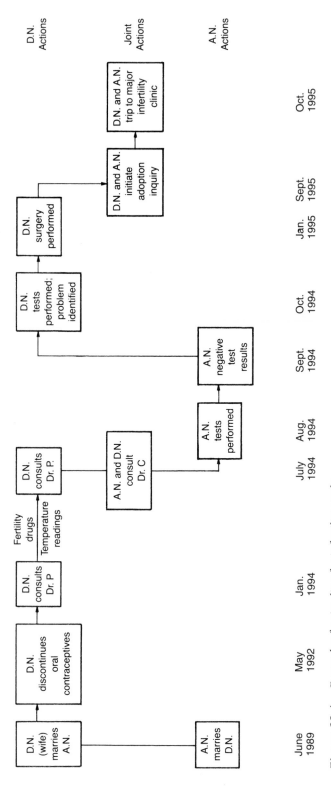

Figure 22-4. *Example of a timeline for infertility study*

It is at this point that some researchers introduce what is referred to as quasi-statistics. *Quasi-statistics* involve a tabulation of the frequency with which certain themes, relationships, or insights are supported by the data. The frequencies cannot be interpreted in the same way as frequencies generated in survey studies because of imprecision in the sampling of cases and enumeration of the themes. Nevertheless, as Becker (1970) pointed out,

> Quasi-statistics may allow the investigator to dispose of certain troublesome null hypotheses. A simple frequency count of the number of times a given phenomenon appears may make untenable the null hypothesis that the phenomenon is infrequent. A comparison of the number of such instances with the number of negative cases—instances in which some alternative phenomenon that would not be predicted by his theory appears—may make possible a stronger conclusion, especially if the theory was developed early enough in the observational period to allow a systematic search for negative cases. Similarly, an inspection of the range of situations covered by the investigator's data may allow him to negate the hypothesis that his conclusion is restricted to only a few situations, time periods, or types of people in the organization or community. (p. 81)

In the final stage of analysis, the researcher strives to weave the thematic pieces together into an integrated whole. The various themes need to be interrelated in a manner that provides an overall structure (such as a theory or integrated description) to the entire body of data. The *integration* task is an extremely difficult one because it demands creativity and intellectual rigor if it is to be successful. A strategy that sometimes helps in this task is to cross-tabulate dimensions that have emerged in the thematic analysis. For example, Barton (1991), in her study of parents' adaptations to their adolescent children's drug abuse problems, found that parental power and parental responsibility were two important dimensions that, when cross-tabulated, reflected important coping patterns among the parents in her sample. Her diagram displaying the cross-tabulated schema is presented in Figure 22-5.

Qualitative researchers seldom discuss in any detail the ways in which they analyze their data. However, the steps undertaken by a research team that studied how the role of clinical nurse researchers was being defined, enacted, and evaluated was described by Knafl and Webster (1988). This study involved in-depth telephone interviews with 34 clinical nurse researchers (CNRs) and their corresponding chief nurse executives (CNEs). The data consisted of about 1000 pages of interview transcripts. The researchers undertook six major tasks during

	+ **POWER** **−**	
+ **RESPONSIBILITY** **−**	The parents feel guilty despite professionals' attempts to eliminate guilt Style is "committed"/ "correcting the flaw"	The parents are especially "fused" to the child Style is "stuck"/"secondary gains" or "protection from social responsibility"
	The parents accept not feeling responsible and have power. Style is "successful"/ "mastery"	The parents accept not feeling responsible but let go of power. Style is "letting go"/"new meaning"

Figure 22-5.   *Barton's (1991) schema describing parental adaptation to adolescent drug abuse (Reprinted with permission)*

the data management phase and five major tasks during the data analysis phase:

PHASE I: DATA MANAGEMENT

1. Independent reading of a sample of interview transcripts by team members; collaborative development of six major descriptive coding categories; development of a codebook to ensure consistent application of final coding categories
2. Independent coding of all interviews in margins of transcripts by two coders; collaborative review of codes and resolution of differences in coding
3. Cut-and-paste transfer of all data onto color-coded 5- × 8-inch index cards, with colors corresponding to the six major categories
4. Identification of subcategories reflecting narrower topical areas within the major categories
5. Coding of the index cards according to the subcategories identified
6. Construction of descriptive summary grids for each subcategory across all subjects, with each cell of the grid containing a brief summary of pertinent content

PHASE II: DATA ANALYSIS

1. Description of the content of each subcategory and identification of major themes; preparation of a written analysis summary
2. Description of the content of each major category, constructed from the subcategory summary
3. Description of the CNR group, synthesizing and integrating relevant material
4. Description of the CNE group, synthesizing and integrating relevant material
5. Description of CNR–CNE pairs, contrasting of within-pair themes

Analytic Induction

The general procedures and steps previously described provide a general outline of how qualitative researchers make sense of their data and distill from them their understandings of processes and behaviors operating in naturalistic settings. However, there are some variations in the goals and underlying philosophies of qualitative researchers that also lead to variations in how the analytic task is handled. One of the major strategies for analyzing qualitative data is referred to as *analytic induction,* an approach that was developed in the 1930s.

The analytic induction approach requires a careful scrutiny of all the researcher's data, usually according to the following six steps:

1. Define the phenomenon to be studied and explained.
2. Based on a review of the data, formulate a hypothetical explanation of the phenomenon; that is, develop an inductively derived hypothesis.
3. Conduct an intensive analysis of individual cases to see whether the hypothesis fits particular cases.
4. Search for negative cases that, if found, lead to a reformulation of the hypothesis *or* a redefinition of the phenomenon to exclude the particular case.
5. Continue the examination of cases, redefinition of the phenomenon, and reformulation of hypotheses until a universal pattern of relationships is established.
6. Create a higher level of abstraction or conceptualization through comparison with other settings or groups.

In practice, the use of analytic induction results in a procedure that alternates back and forth between tentative explanation and tentative definition, each refining the other so that a sense of closure can be achieved when an integral relation between the two is established.

Grounded Theory

A second major strategy is Glaser and Strauss's (1967) method of generating theories from data, using a procedure that they described as the discovery of *grounded theory.* This approach, which has been widely used by nurse researchers, is more than just a method of data analysis; it is an entire philosophy about how to conduct field research. For example, a study that truly follows Glaser and Strauss's precepts does not begin with a highly focused research problem; the problem itself emerges from the data.

One of the fundamental features of the grounded theory approach is that data collection and data analysis occur simultaneously. A procedure referred to as *constant comparison* is used to develop and refine theoretically relevant categories. The categories elicited from the data are constantly compared with data obtained earlier in the data collection so that commonalities and variations can be determined. As data collection proceeds, the inquiry becomes increasingly focused on emerging theoretical concerns. In contrast to analytic induction, this approach requires data saturation rather than the consideration of all data. *Saturation* refers to the sense of closure that the researcher experiences when data collection ceases to yield any new information.

Glaser and Strauss identified the following four stages in the constant comparative method:

1. Establish categories based on similarity of content in incidents and dissimilarity of content with other categories, with the aim of elucidating the theoretical properties of each category.
2. Compare each incident within each category with the dimensions of the category for integration into a unified whole that reflects the relationships of the dimensions or properties of the category.
3. Examine categories and their properties for underlying uniformities that may reduce the number of categories. Look for theoretical saturation of content, and add only new incidents to categories when they explicate a new dimension.
4. Produce analytic memos to summarize the theoretical explanations; the memos provide the basis for the writing of publications and reports.

There are some obvious similarities between the grounded theory and analytic induction approaches, but there are also some important differences. Of particular importance is their overall aims. Analytic induction is concerned with the testing of inductively derived hypotheses; it is purported to be a method for coming to terms with the problem of causal inference while remaining faithful to qualitative, naturalistic data. The grounded theory method is concerned with the generation of categories, properties, and hypotheses rather than with testing them. The product of many grounded theory studies is a conceptual or theoretical model that endeavors to explain the phenomenon under study. As an example, Figure 22-6 presents the model developed by King and Jensen (1994) in their grounded theory study that conceptualized the process of women's "preserving the self" during cardiac surgery.

Qualitative Analysis and Qualitative Research Traditions

There is considerable diversity in the way that qualitative researchers refer to their studies. Qualitative research, as we saw in Chapter 9, is often designed to address certain types of questions; for example, ethnographic studies focus on specific cultures and their world views, and phenomenological studies inquire about the essence of phenomena as experienced by people. In research reports, researchers sometimes describe their study in terms of the research tradition on which the research was based (e.g., ethnography); others refer to their study in terms of the overall analytic approach that was used (e.g., grounded study); others refer to both the tradition and the analytic approach (e.g., an ethonographic study that used a grounded theory approach); and still others simply say that they have undertaken a qualitative study or a naturalistic inquiry, without any reference to a research tradition or analytic approach.

Qualitative researchers sometimes report that a content analysis was performed in analyz-

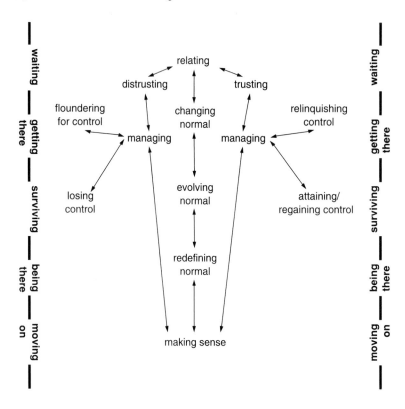

Figure 22-6. *King and Jensen's (1994) Model of Preserving the Self During Cardiac Surgery (Reprinted with permission)*

ing the data. In most cases, the researcher is not referring to a classic content analysis involving the quantification of aspects of written materials. *Qualitative content analysis* involves an analysis of the content of narrative data to identify prominent themes and patterns among the themes. Here again, a researcher may use the term content analysis either with a reference to the research tradition (e.g., a phenomenological study in which the data were content analyzed) or without such a reference.

Many other terms are used in connection with qualitative research that are beyond the scope of this textbook to describe fully but that students may encounter in the research literature. For example, *hermeneutical analysis* is sometimes used in conjunction with phenomenological studies as a means of analyzing and interpreting commonalities in the meanings of lived experiences (Packer and Addison, 1989). An approach known as *typological analysis* is sometimes used in connection with ethnographic and other qualitative studies to categorize activity phenomena by meaning, antecedents, and consequences (Lofland & Lofland, 1984). Researchers interested in studying cognitive processes often apply *protocol analysis* to verbal transcripts (Fonteyn, Kuipers, & Grobe, 1993). Language within its social context is sometimes analyzed through *sociolinguistic microanalysis* (Green & Wallat, 1980). Finally, some researchers use the *responsive reader method* in analyses of moral orientations, motivations, and justifications of informants (Brown & Gilligan, 1991).

❖ TIPS FOR ANALYZING QUALITATIVE DATA

Qualitative analysis is a challenging—but often a very rewarding—enterprise. In this section, we offer a few additional tips to beginning students regarding the conduct of a qualitative analysis.

- In developing a category system for coding qualitative data, a substantial sample of the data should be carefully read before the scheme is finalized. To the extent possible, the researcher should try to read materials that vary along important dimensions, in an effort to capture the full range of content. The dimensions might include informant characteristics (e.g., transcripts of men versus women, articulate versus less articulate informants), or aspects of the data collection experience (e.g., shorter versus longer interviews, observations in different types of settings). If the researcher can identify in advance what the important dimensions might be, methods should be used to facilitate identification of good exemplars (e.g., by appending written comments on the relevant dimensions at the end of an interview).
- Even when a category system is "finalized," the researcher should be prepared to amend or even totally revise it. Even simple changes may mean rereading all previously coded material. Making changes midway is often painful and frustrating, but without a highly effective category system, the researcher will be unable to identify and integrate important themes adequately.
- In most studies, it is wise to develop a codebook, that is, written documentation describing the exact definition of the various categories used to code the data. Good qualitative codebooks usually include two or three actual excerpts that typify materials coded in each category.
- Even if you have little experience using a computer, the available programs for qualitative data management are relatively easy to learn and should not be a cause for anxiety. In selecting a program, try to discuss the merits of various programs with other researchers who have experience using them. They may have suggestions for which program to select and may also be helpful in answering questions once you have begun using the program.
- Many researchers engage in qualitative studies on their own rather than with a co-investigator. However, collaborative efforts are becoming more common, as journal editors and peers have come to demand that greater attention be paid to validating qualitative data and the meanings associated with them. Having one or more team member ensures that the data will not be analyzed and interpreted in a totally subjective and biased fashion.

❖ RESEARCH EXAMPLES

The number of qualitative studies that have been published in nursing journals over the past decade has risen dramatically. Table 22-1 lists some of the research problems that have been addressed through qualitative methods. An additional example of a grounded theory study is described in greater detail below.

Bright (1992) studied the birth of a first child as an intergenerational experience with the aim of discovering the basic social process associated with this event and generating a theory on normative family process. She collected in-depth interview and observational data over a 15-month period from three families: three first-born infants and their parents and six sets of grandparents. Data collection began during the last trimester of pregnancy and continued until the child's first birthday. The families differed in terms of whether the pregnancy was planned and wanted.

Within each family, the interviews were initially conducted in a group setting, which allowed the researcher to observe family interactional patterns and to learn about family beliefs and customs as well as expectations about the anticipated birth event. Subsequent interviews were conducted with individual family members, with dyads, and with small groups as deemed needed on the basis of the developing hypotheses. Interviews and observations occurred in parental and grandparental homes, on the hospital mater-

Table 22-1.   *Examples of Nursing Studies Involving Qualitative Analysis*

RESEARCH QUESTION	NUMBER OF SUBJECTS	RESEARCH OR ANALYSIS TRADITION
How do nurses cope with their concerns about acquiring HIV infection when caring for people with AIDS? (Reutter & Northcott, 1994)	13	Grounded theory
What are the lifelong patterns of physical activity and processes of managing physical activity among African American working women? (Mayo, 1992)	51	Ethnography, analytic induction
What are the processes through which public health nurses develop rapport with and strengthen the resources of high-risk families? (Zerwekh, 1992)	30	Phenomenology, grounded theory
What types of communication pattern do nurses use when interacting with elderly patients during hospital admission interviews? (VanCott, 1993)	20 dyads	Sociolinguistic microanalysis
How do family caregivers experience loss and grief after the death of a relative with dementia? (Collins, Liken, King, & Kokinakis, 1993)	82	Qualitative content analysis
What are parents' caring practices that evolve in response to the demands of living with a schizophrenic offspring? (Chesla, 1991)	21	Hermeneutics
How do experienced nurses reason when they are formulating a plan of care for their clients? (Grobe, Drew, & Fonteyn, 1991)	7	Protocol analysis
What are the moral concerns of nurses during the process of ethical decision making? (Sherblom, Shipps, & Sherblom, 1993)	31	Responsive reader method

nity ward, and at other locations such as baptismal ceremonies. Telephone interviews were used to clarify data and to check on the validity of the emerging hypotheses.

The analysis of data was done as an ongoing process, integrated with data collection and coding. Interviews were audiotaped, transcribed, and then coded line by line. One three-generation family interaction was videotaped to provide recorded nonverbal as well as verbal data for coding. Coded data were grouped into related categories and then compared with one another and with new data to refine and discard emerging hypotheses continually. Memoranda were prepared concurrently to record the researcher's theoretical analysis of the data. Several methods were used to validate the themes emerging from the analysis, including review by members of the families.

The analysis resulted in the identification of an evolutionary family process that reflected reorganized interpersonal patterns. "Making place," the central social process that emerged from Bright's analysis, was defined as the family process through which a newborn individual receives recognition as a member of that family. The family made place both physically and socially for the new and expanded relationships created by the child's birth.

❖ SUMMARY

Qualitative research typically involves the collection and analysis of loosely structured information regarding people in naturalistic settings. Qualitative nursing research has become an increasingly attractive method of inquiry, complementing more quantitative approaches in advancing nursing science. Qualitative research is especially well suited to description, hypothesis generation, and theory development. However, qualitative approaches are less suitable for establishing cause-and-effect relationships, for rigorously testing research hypotheses, and for determining the opinions, practices, and attitudes of a large population. Although narrative data *can* be quantified and subsequently analyzed with statistical procedures, most qualitative researchers prefer to analyze their data through qualitative analysis.

The first major step in analyzing qualitative data is to organize the materials according to some plan, so that portions of the data can be readily retrieved. Typically, qualitative researchers develop a category system (based on a reading of a portion of the data) and then code the content of the data based on this system. Traditionally, researchers have developed *conceptual files* for organizing their data. In using this system, researchers first code their data in the margins of the printed narrative materials (e.g., observational notes or transcripts of interviews); cut out the coded excerpts; and finally place each excerpt into a file corresponding to each of the topics covered in the coding scheme. Then the researcher can retrieve all the information on a topic by going to a single file.

The widespread availability of PCs and appropriate software has lessened the burden of indexing, organizing, and retrieving qualitative materials. There are now a wide variety of programs that not only perform basic indexing functions but also offer various enhancements that can facilitate analysis of the data. Most qualitative programs require that the data first are typed into a word processing file and then imported in ASCII format into the data management program.

The actual analysis of data begins with a search for *themes*. The search for themes involves the discovery not only of commonalities across subjects but also of natural variation in the data. The next step generally involves a *validation* of the thematic analysis. Some researchers use a procedure known as *quasi-statistics,* which involves a tabulation of the frequency with which certain themes or relations are supported by the data. In a final step, the analyst tries to weave the thematic strands together into an integrated picture of the phenomenon under investigation.

Although this overview summarizes some of the major steps, there are a number of different philosophies underlying qualitative analysis. *Analytic induction* refers to an approach in which the researcher alternates back and forth between tentative definition of emerging hypotheses and tentative explanation, with each iteration making refinements. *Grounded theory* is a term used to describe field investigations, the purpose of which is to discover theoretical precepts grounded in the data. This approach makes use of a technique called *constant comparison*: Categories elicited from the data are constantly compared with data obtained earlier so that commonalities and variations can be determined.

There is no direct correspondence between the underlying qualitative research tradition, which is the basis for certain research questions, and the analytic approach. Some researchers identify neither a specific approach nor a specific research tradition; and some researchers say that they used *qualitative content analysis* as their analytic method. Other terms that sometimes appear in the qualitative research literature include *hermeneutical analysis, typological analysis, protocol analysis, sociolinguistic microanalysis*, and the *responsive reader method*.

❖ *STUDY SUGGESTIONS*

Chapter 22 of the accompanying *Study Guide for Nursing Research: Principles and Methods, 5th ed.*, offers various exercises and study suggestions for reinforcing the concepts presented in this chapter. Additionally, the following study questions can be addressed:

1. Suggest a research problem amenable to qualitative research. Explain why you think the problem is better suited to a qualitative than to a quantitative approach.

2. Read a qualitative nursing study (several are suggested under Substantive References). Do you think that if a different investigator had gone into the field to study the same problem, the conclusions would have been the same? How generalizable are the researcher's findings? What did the researcher learn that he or she would probably not have learned with a more structured and quantified approach?

3. As a class assignment, have each student ask two people to describe their conception of preventive health care and what it means in their daily lives. Pool all the narrative descriptions, and develop a coding scheme to organize the reasons. What are the major themes that emerge?

❖ *SUGGESTED READINGS*

METHODOLOGICAL REFERENCES

Artinian, B. A. (1988). Qualitative modes of inquiry. *Western Journal of Nursing Research, 10*, 138–149.

Bargagliotti, L. A. (1983). The scientific method and phenomenology: Toward their peaceful coexistence in nursing. *Western Journal of Nursing Research, 5*, 409–411.

Becker, H. S. (1970). *Sociological work*. Chicago: Aldine.

Benoliel, J. Q. (1984). Advancing nursing science: Qualitative approaches. *Western Journal of Nursing Research, 6*, 1–8.

Brown, L., & Gilligan, C. (1991). Listening for self and relational voices: A responsive/resisting reader's guide. *Harvard Project on the psychology of women and the development of girls.* Cambridge, MA: Harvard University Graduate School of Education.

Carey, M. A., & Smith, M. W. (1994). Capturing the group effect in focus groups: A special concern in analysis. *Qualitative Health Research, 4*, 123–127.

Chenitz, W. C., & Swanson, J. M. (1986). *From practice to grounded theory: Qualitative research in nursing.* Menlo Park, CA: Addison-Wesley.

Fielding, N. G., & Fielding, J. L. (1985). *Linking data.* Beverly Hills, CA: Sage.

Fonteyn, M. E., Kuipers, B., & Grobe, S. J. (1993). A description of Think Aloud method and protocol analysis. *Qualitative Health Research, 3*, 430–441.

Gephart, R. P., Jr. (1988). *Ethnostatistics: Qualitative foundations for quantitative research.* Newbury Park, CA: Sage.

Glaser, B. G., & Strauss, A. L. (1967). *The discovery of grounded theory: Strategies for qualitative research.* Chicago: Aldine.

Goodwin, L. D., & Goodwin, W. L. (1984). Qualitative vs. quantitative research or qualitative *and* quantitative research. *Nursing Research, 33*, 378–380.

Gorenberg, B. (1983). The research tradition of nursing: An emerging issue. *Nursing Research, 32*, 347–349.

Green, J., & Wallat, C. (1980). Mapping instructional conversations: A sociolinguistic ethnography. In J. Green and C. Wallat (Eds.), *Ethnography and language in educational settings.* Norwood, NJ: Ablex.

Knafl, K. A., & Webster, D. C. (1988). Managing and analyzing qualitative data: A description of tasks, techniques, and materials. *Western Journal of Nursing Research, 10*, 195–218.

Leininger, M. M. (Ed.). (1985). *Qualitative research methods in nursing.* New York: Grune & Stratton.

Lofland, J., & Lofland, L. H. (1984). *Analyzing social settings: A guide to qualitative observation and analysis* (2nd ed.). Belmont, CA: Wadsworth.

Miles, M. B., & Huberman, A. M. (1984). *Qualitative data analysis.* Beverly Hills, CA: Sage.

Morgan, D. L. (1993). Qualitative content analysis: A guide to paths not taken. *Qualitative Health Research, 3,* 112–121.

Morse, J. M., & Morse, R. M. (1989). QUAL: A mainframe program for qualitative data analysis. *Nursing Research, 38,* 188–189.

Munhall, P. L. (1982). Nursing philosophy and nursing research: In apposition or opposition? *Nursing Research, 31,* 176–177.

Oiler, C. (1982). The phenomenological approach in nursing research. *Nursing Research, 31,* 178–181.

Packer, M. J., & Addison, R. B. (1989). *Entering the circle: Hermeneutic investigation in psychology.* Albany, NY: SUNY Press.

Parse, R. R., Coyne, A. B., & Smith, M. J. (1985). *Nursing research: Qualitative methods.* Bowie, MD: Brady.

Pfaffenberger, B. (1988). *Microcomputer applications in qualitative research.* Newbury Park, CA: Sage.

Taft, L. B. (1993). Computer-assisted qualitative research. *Research in Nursing and Health, 16,* 379–383.

Tesch, R. (1991). Computer programs that assist in the analysis of qualitative data: An overview. *Qualitative Health Research, 1,* 309–325.

Walker, B. L. (1993). Computer analysis of qualitative data: A comparison of three packages. *Qualitative Health Research, 3,* 91–111.

Webster, G., Jacox, A., & Baldwin, B. (1981). Nursing theory and the ghost of the received view. In H. Grace & B. McCloskey (Eds.), *Contemporary issues in nursing.* Boston: Blackwell Scientific Publications.

SUBSTANTIVE REFERENCES

Barton, J. A. (1991). Parental adaptation to adolescent drug abuse: An ethnographic study of role formulation in response to courtesy stigma. *Public Health Nursing, 8,* 39–45.

Bright, M. A. (1992). Making place: The first birth in an intergenerational family context. *Qualitative Health Research, 2,* 75–78.

Chesla, C. A. (1991). Parents' caring practices with schizophrenic offspring. *Qualitative Health Research, 1,* 446–466.

Collins, C., Liken, M., King, S., & Kokinakis, C. (1993). Loss and grief among family caregivers of relatives with dementia. *Qualitative Health Research, 3,* 236–253.

Gagliardi, B. A. (1991). The family's experience of living with a child with Duchenne muscular dystrophy. *Applied Nursing Research, 4,* 159–164.

Grobe, S. J., Drew, J. A., & Fonteyn, M. E. (1991). A descriptive analysis of experienced nurses' clinical reasoning during a planning task. *Research in Nursing and Health, 14,* 305–314.

King, K. M., & Jensen, L. (1994). Preserving the self: Women having cardiac surgery. *Heart and Lung, 23,* 99–105.

Mayo, K. (1992). Physical activity practices among American black working women. *Qualitative Health Research, 2,* 318–333.

Reutter, L. I., & Northcott, H. C. (1994). Achieving a sense of control in a context of uncertainty: Nurses and AIDS. *Qualitative Health Research, 4,* 51–71.

Sherblom, S., Shipps, T. B., & Sherblom, J. C. (1993). Justice, care, and integrated concerns in the ethical decision making of nurses. *Qualitative Health Research, 3,* 442–464.

VanCott, M. L. (1993). Communicative competence during nursing admission interviews of elderly patients in acute care settings. *Qualitative Health Research, 3,* 184–208.

Zerwekh, J. V. (1992). Laying the groundwork for family self-help. *Public Health Nursing, 9,* 15–21.

Chapter 23

INTEGRATION OF QUALITATIVE AND QUANTITATIVE ANALYSIS

Until recently, nursing research was dominated by quantitatively oriented studies. However, consistent with the overall expansion of nursing research inquiry, qualitative studies gained considerable ground during the 1980s. An emerging trend, and one that we believe will gain momentum in the years to come, is the integration of qualitative and quantitative data within single studies or coordinated clusters of studies. This chapter discusses the reasons for such integration and strategies for accomplishing it.

❖ RATIONALE FOR INTEGRATION

The dichotomy between quantitative and qualitative data analysis represents the key epistemological and methodological distinction within the social and behavioral sciences. Some argue that qualitative and quantitative research are based on fundamentally incompatible paradigms. Thus, there undoubtedly are people who will disagree with the fundamental premise of this chapter, namely that many areas of inquiry can be enriched through the judicious blending

of qualitative and quantitative data. It would be imprudent to argue that all (or even most) research problems could be enhanced by such integration or that all (or most) researchers should strive to collect and integrate both types of data. However, we believe that there are many noteworthy advantages of combining various types of data in a single investigation and that these advantages increasingly will come to be recognized by nurse researchers in the years ahead. Some of the major advantages are reviewed in the following sections.

Complementarity

One argument in support of blending qualitative and quantitative data in a single project is that they are complementary; they represent words and numbers, the two fundamental languages of human communication. Webster's* defines *complementary* as "mutually supplying each other's lack," and this characterizes the two

* From Webster's Ninth New Collegiate Dictionary © 1985 by G. & C. Merriam Company, publishers of the Merriam-Webster® Dictionaries, with permission.

methodological strategies well. As we have noted repeatedly in this text, researchers address their problems with methods and measures that are invariably fallible. By integrating different methods and modes of analysis, the weaknesses of a single approach may be diminished or overcome.

Quantitative data derived from relatively large or representative samples have many strengths. Quantitative studies are often strong in terms of generalizability, precision, control over extraneous variables, and reliability of measurement. However, a major problem with quantitative research is that its validity is sometimes called into question. By introducing tight controls, quantitative studies may fail to capture the full context of a situation. Moreover, by reducing complex human experiences, behavior, and characteristics to numbers, such analyses sometimes suffer from superficiality. Another issue is that the use of tightly structured questions or observational instruments may lead to biases in capturing constructs under study. All these weaknesses are aspects of the study's ability to yield valid and meaningful answers to the research questions.

Qualitative research, by contrast, has strengths and weaknesses that are diametrically opposite. The strength of qualitative research lies in its flexibility and its potential to yield insights into the true nature of complex phenomena through a wealth of in-depth information. However, such insights are not gratuitous. Because qualitative research is almost always based on small and unrepresentative samples and is often engaged in by a solitary researcher or small team of researchers using data collection and analytic procedures that rely on subjective judgments, qualitative research may suffer in terms of reliability and generalizability.

This discussion suggests that *neither of the two styles of research can fully deliver on its promise to establish the truth about phenomena of interest to nurse researchers*. However, the strengths and weaknesses of quantitative and qualitative data are complementary. Haase and Myers (1988) also noted the complementarity

of the assumptions underlying the two approaches. Combined judiciously in a single study, qualitative and quantitative data can "supply each other's lack." By using multiple methods, the researcher can allow each method to do what it does best, with the possibility of avoiding the limitations of a single approach. In essence, this argument in favor of integration represents an extension of the argument for methodological triangulation discussed in Chapter 16.

Enhanced Theoretical Insights

Most theories do not have paradigmatic or methodological boundaries. As discussed in Chapter 5, the major nursing theories embrace four broad concepts: 1) person; 2) environment; 3) health; and 4) nursing. There is nothing inherent in these concepts that demands (or excludes) a qualitative or quantitative orientation.

The world in which we live is complex and multidimensional, as are most of the theories we have developed to make sense of it. Qualitative and quantitative research constitute alternative ways of viewing and interpreting the world. These alternatives are not necessarily correct or incorrect; rather, they reflect and reveal different aspects of reality. To be maximally useful, nursing research should strive to understand these multiple aspects. We believe that the blending of quantitative and qualitative data in a single analysis can lead to insights on these multiple aspects that might be unattainable without such integration. Denzin (1989), who has been a staunch advocate of methodological triangulation, captured this notion eloquently:

Each method implies a different line of action toward reality—and hence each will reveal different aspects of it, much as a kaleidoscope, depending on the angle at which it is held, will reveal different colors and configurations of objects to the viewer. Methods are like the kaleidoscope: depending on how they are approached, held, and acted toward, different observations will be revealed. This is not to imply that reality has the shifting qualities of the colored prism, but that it too is an object that moves and that will not permit one interpretation to be stamped upon it. (p. 235)

Incrementality

It is sometimes argued that different approaches are especially appropriate for different phases in the evolution of a theory or problem area. In particular, it has been said that qualitative methods are well suited to exploratory or hypothesis-generating research early in the development of a research problem area, and quantitative methods are needed as the problem area matures for the purposes of verification.

It is certainly true that in-depth qualitative research can be highly productive in revealing theoretically relevant aspects of a phenomenon and suggesting lines for further inquiry. It is also true that statistical analysis provides a useful framework for the testing of hypotheses. However, the fact remains that the evolution of a theory or problem area is rarely linear and unidirectional. The need for exploration and in-depth insights is rarely confined to the beginning of an area of research inquiry, and subjective impressions may need to be checked for accuracy early and continuously.

Thus, progress in a developing area tends to be incremental and to rely on multiple feedback loops. It therefore could be productive to build a loop into the design of a single study, potentially speeding the progress toward understanding. This point is illustrated by inquiry in the area of work-related stress and coping. Bargagliotti and Trygstad (1987) conducted two separate studies of job stress among nurses, one using quantitative procedures and the other using qualitative procedures. The quantitative study identified discrete events as sources of stress, and the qualitative study revealed stress-related processes over time. The discrepant findings, because they were derived from different samples of nurses working in different settings, could not be easily integrated and reconciled. The investigators noted, "Comparison of findings from the two studies suggests that the questions raised by the findings in each study might have been more fully addressed by using a combined quantitative/qualitative methodology" (p. 172).

Enhanced Validity

Another advantage of combining quantitative and qualitative data lies in the potential for enhancements to the validity of the study findings. When a researcher's hypothesis or model is supported by multiple and complementary types of data, the researcher can be much more confident about the validity of the results. Scientists are basically skeptics, constantly seeking evidence to validate their theories and models. Evidence derived from different approaches can be especially persuasive. As Brewer and Hunter (1989) noted, "Although each type of method is relatively stronger than the others in certain respects, none of the methods is so perfect even in its area of greatest strength that it cannot benefit from corroboration by other methods' findings" (p. 51).

In Chapters 10 and 16, we discussed various types of validity problems—such problems as rival hypotheses to explain the data, difficulties of generalizing beyond the study circumstances, and measures that fail to capture the constructs under investigation. The use of a single approach leaves the study vulnerable to at least one (and often more) of these problems. The integration of qualitative and quantitative data can provide better opportunities for testing alternative interpretations of the data, for examining the extent to which the context helped to shape the results, and for arriving at convergence in tapping a construct. For example, Hinds (1989), in her study of adolescents' change in hopefulness as they progressed through a program for substance abuse, used qualitative findings as a means of validating her quantitative findings. As Hinds noted, "Using both methods together results in an increased ability to rule out rival explanations of observed change and reduces skepticism of change-related findings" (p. 442).

Creating New Frontiers

Inevitably, researchers will sometimes find that qualitative and quantitative data are inconsistent with each other. This lack of congruity—when it happens in the context of a single investigation—can actually lead to insights that can push a line of inquiry further than would otherwise have been possible.

When separate investigations yield inconsistent results, the differences are difficult to reconcile and interpret because they may reflect differences in subjects and circumstances rather than theoretically meaningful distinctions that merit further study. In a single study, any discrepancies that emerge can be tackled head on. By probing into the reasons for any observed incongruities, the researchers can help to rethink the constructs under investigation and possibly to redirect the research process. The incongruent findings, in other words, can be used as a springboard for the investigation of the reasons for the discrepancies and for a thoughtful analysis of both the methodological and theoretical underpinnings of the study.

❖ APPLICATIONS OF INTEGRATED ANALYSES

Researchers make decisions about the types of data to collect and analyze based on the specific objectives of their investigation. In this section, we illustrate how the integration of qualitative and quantitative data can be used in addressing a variety of research goals.

Instrumentation

One of the most frequent uses of an integrated approach in nursing research involves the development of instruments. When a researcher becomes aware of the need for a new measuring tool, where do the items come from? The item pool is sometimes generated by the researcher based on theory, his or her clinical experience, readings in the field, or prior research. However, when a construct is new, these mechanisms may be inadequate to capture its full complexity and dimensionality. No matter how rich the researcher's experience or knowledge base, the fact remains that this base is highly personal and inevitably biased by the researcher's values and world view.

In recognition of this situation, many nurse researchers have begun to use data obtained from qualitative inquiries as the basis for generating items for quantitative instruments that are subsequently subjected to rigorous psychometric assessment. For example, Gulick (1991) developed the Work Assessment Scale to evaluate situations that impede or enhance the work capabilities of people with multiple sclerosis. The items for her scale were developed on the basis of a qualitative analysis of responses to open-ended questions regarding the conditions and situations that make the performance of tasks easy or difficult for multiple sclerosis patients. This approach essentially represents a mechanism for building content validity into the instrument from its inception.

Qualitative data have also been used as a means of assessing the validity of a quantitative instrument at later stages in the development process. For example, Nyamathi and Flaskerud (1992) developed an instrument designed to document the concerns of highly disadvantaged groups of women. After a pilot testing of the initial 50 items, which were derived on the basis of the literature, a qualitative focus-group study was undertaken to verify the concerns and stresses experienced by low-income women. The focus group discussion validated 34 of the initial 50 concerns and suggested 6 others that needed to be added to the instrument.

These examples illustrate the important role that the integration of qualitative and quantitative data can play in enhancing the measurement of constructs important to nurse researchers.

Illustration

Qualitative data are sometimes combined with quantitative data to illustrate the meaning of descriptions or relationships. Such illustrations help to clarify important concepts, and they serve further as a method of corroborating the understandings gleaned from the statistical analysis. In this sense, these illustrations often help to illuminate the analyses and give guidance to the interpretation of results.

As an example, Hough and her colleagues (Hough, Lewis, & Woods, 1991; Lewis, Woods, Hough, & Bensley, 1989) conducted a study on family coping and adaptation to a mother's chronic illness. Using structured self-report information, the researchers performed a path analysis to test a theoretical model of family functioning under stress. The quantitative analyses suggested that the mother's illness had an impact on the spouse and on the quality of his relationship with his wife. Qualitative data were also gathered in the course of the same study (through observations and unstructured interview). The following excerpt illustrating a family that adjusted poorly after the mother's diagnosis of breast cancer adds a perspective that the quantitative results alone could not provide:

> It was a tremendous surprise how I felt about myself after losing part of my body. The fact that this is a life-threatening disease and you could die is quite sobering. The relationships within the family have been difficult. My husband's a denier—he can't understand why I can't forget about it. He left the house when he knew I was going to get a call regarding the lab results. The denial and the sexuality change is a strain on our relationship. (Hough, et al., 1991, p. 577)

Qualitative materials can be used to illustrate specific statistical findings or to provide more global and dynamic views of the phenomena under study, often in the form of illustrative case studies. For example, Polit and her colleagues (1989, 1990), in their study of the sexual and contraceptive behavior of teenagers who had been abused as children, used quantitative data to model statistically the probability of a premarital pregnancy in this high-risk sample. In addition, their report included several case studies illustrating the emotional and social problems these teenagers faced and the evolution and resolution of these problems over time.

The case studies were based on interviews with the teenagers, their parents or foster parents, and their social workers as well as on information available in their case records.

Understanding Relationships and Causal Processes

Quantitative methods often demonstrate that variables are systematically related to one another, but they often fail to provide insights about *why* the variables are related. This situation is especially likely to occur with ex post facto research.

Typically, the discussion section of research reports is devoted to an interpretation of the findings. In quantitatively oriented studies, the interpretations are often speculative, representing the researcher's best guess (a guess that may, of course, be built on solid theory or prior research) about what the findings mean. In essence, the interpretations represent a new set of hypotheses that could be tested in another study. When a study integrates both qualitative and quantitative data, however, the researcher may be in a much stronger position to derive meaning immediately from the statistical findings. Suppose, for example, that we found that single men and women had significantly poorer health (based on a variety of quantitative indexes) than married people. What is the meaning of this relationship? Are single people less healthy because they lack an important source of social support? Or are single people less financially able to obtain adequate health care? Or are single people less healthy to begin with, and do their health problems make them less "marriageable"? Qualitative methods might yield some understanding about the mechanisms underlying this relationship.

A collaborative study by a group of researchers (Meleis, Norbeck, & Laffrey, 1989; Hall, Stevens, & Meleis, 1992) provides a good illustration of this application of blended data collection methods. These researchers examined how married, low-income working women from different cultural backgrounds integrate their multiple roles on a daily basis. The data were collected by means of lengthy interviews that included both structured questions and in-depth, probing questions that focused on role integration. In the quantitative analysis, these researchers learned that role integration was important in predicting health outcomes—but not *why* this was so. By means of an analysis of the qualitative data, the researchers developed a theoretical understanding of the construct of role integration. The theoretical framework identified and related the aspects, processes, and patterns of role integration as they are experienced in women's everyday lives. The framework provided insights into how health could be affected by role integration.

Quantitative analyses can also help to clarify and give shape to findings obtained in qualitative analyses. For example, a thematic analysis of interviews with infertile couples could reveal various aspects of the emotional consequences of infertility and shed light on the meaning of those consequences to individuals; the administration of a standardized scale (such as the Center for Epidemiological Studies Depression, or CES-D, Scale) to the same subjects could indicate more precisely the distribution of depressive symptoms and their magnitude among the infertile couples. A study by Lipson (1992) illustrates this approach. Lipson conducted an in-depth field study to investigate the health and adjustment of Iranians who had immigrated to the United States. The primary data were qualitative, gathered by means of participant observation and in-depth interviews. After a dozen interviews, Lipson observed that many of the immigrants reported various stress-related physical symptoms. Thereafter, interview respondents were also asked to complete a structured scale (the Health Opinion Survey, or HOS) that measured in a more systematic fashion the symptoms that are common reactions to stress.

The integration of qualitative and quantitative materials for the purpose of enhancing the interpretability of study results is essentially a mechanism of substantive validation. In some studies, it may be useful to use multiple data sources as a methodological check. For exam-

ple, if a researcher is concerned with biases that could result from attrition in a longitudinal survey, it might be profitable to undertake a small number of in-depth interviews with nonrespondents (if feasible) to evaluate the direction and magnitude of such biases.

Theory Building, Testing, and Refinement

The most ambitious application of an integrated approach is in the area of theory development. As we have pointed out repeatedly, a theory is never proved nor confirmed but rather is supported to a greater or lesser extent. A theory gains acceptance as it escapes disconfirmation. The use of multiple methods provides greater opportunity for potential disconfirmation of the theory. If the theory can survive these assaults, it can provide a substantially stronger context for the organization of our clinical and intellectual work. Brewer and Hunter (1989), in their discussion of the role of multimethod research in theory development, made the following observation:

> Theory building and theory testing clearly require variety. In building theories, the more varied the empirical generalizations to be explained, the easier it will be to discriminate between the many possible theories that might explain any one of the generalizations. And in testing theories, the more varied the predictions, the more sharply the ensuing research will discriminate among competing theories. (p. 36)

Salazar and Carter (1993) conducted a study that promotes the development of theory in the area of decision making. These researchers sought to identify the factors that influence the decision of working women to practice breast self-examination (BSE). The first phase of the study involved in-depth interviews with 19 women, purposively selected on the basis of how frequently the women said they practiced BSE. The transcribed interviews were qualitatively analyzed and led to the development of a hierarchical scheme of factors influencing the BSE decision. This scheme is presented in Figure 23-1. In the next phase of the research, the researchers used the hierarchy as the basis for developing a survey questionnaire, which was administered to 52 women. BSE performers and nonperformers were compared, and a discriminant function analysis was used to identify factors in the decision hierarchy that best distinguished the two groups.

❖ STRATEGIES FOR INTEGRATION

The ways in which a researcher might choose to integrate qualitative and quantitative methods in a single study are almost limitless—or rather, are limited only by the ingenuity of the investigator. Therefore, it is impossible to develop a catalog of integration strategies. However, some of the following scenarios are apt to be especially common.

Embedding Qualitative Approaches Within a Survey

By far the most common form of data collection method currently used by nurse researchers is structured self-reports, either in the form of a structured interview or questionnaire or the administration of social–psychological scales. Once the researcher has gained the cooperation of the sample for the structured portion of a study, he or she is in an ideal position to move into a second in-depth stage with a subset of the initial respondents. The second stage might involve such approaches as in-depth or focus group interviews, unstructured observations in a naturalistic environment such as a hospital or nursing home, or the use of health diaries.

From a practical point of view, it is efficient to have the two forms of data collection occurring simultaneously. For example, the re-

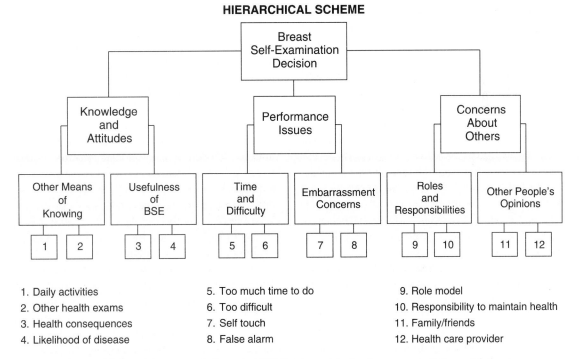

HIERARCHICAL SCHEME

1. Daily activities
2. Other health exams
3. Health consequences
4. Likelihood of disease
5. Too much time to do
6. Too difficult
7. Self touch
8. False alarm
9. Role model
10. Responsibility to maintain health
11. Family/friends
12. Health care provider

Figure 23-1. *Salazar and Carter's (1993) hierarchical scheme on beliefs and behaviors related to breast self-examination (Reprinted with permission)* searcher could administer social–psychological scales and an in-depth interview on the same day for a subset of the entire sample. In some studies, this procedure is likely to work well. However, a two-stage approach has two distinct advantages. First, if the second-stage data collection can be postponed until after the quantitative data have been collected and analyzed, then the researcher will have greater opportunity to probe deeply into the reasons for any obtained results. This is especially likely to be beneficial if the quantitative analyses did not confirm the researcher's hypotheses or if there were any inconsistencies in the results. The second-stage respondents, in other words, can be used as informants to help the researcher interpret the outcomes.

A second reason for using a two-stage approach is that the researcher can use information from the first stage to select a useful subsample for the second. One strategy might be to use a stratified design so that the subset participating in the second stage will be roughly comparable to that in the larger sample. Alternatively, the researcher might want to use information from the first round to hand-pick respondents with certain characteristics, for example, respondents who are most knowledgeable about the phenomena under investigation, who represent "typical" cases, or who are at opposite extremes with regard to the key constructs.

Murphy's longitudinal study of the consequences and processes relating to a natural disaster (the eruption of Mt. St. Helens in southwestern Washington state in 1980) provides an example of multimethod research in which qualitative interviews were embedded within a larger survey (Murphy, 1989). In the study, the bulk of the data were collected by way of structured self-report instruments administered to three groups of individuals: 1) a bereaved group (individuals who experienced the loss of a family member or close friend); 2) a property-loss group (individuals who experienced serious damage or destruction to their homes); and 3) a matched no-disaster-loss group for com-

parison purposes. Complex multivariate analyses of the quantitative data were undertaken to test alternative theories regarding disaster-related effects. In addition, in-depth interviews were conducted with stratified subsets of the study group participants to obtain richer information regarding disaster-induced stress, coping strategies, and processes of recovery.

Embedding Quantitative Measures Into Field Work

Field research, more than other types of research, has a long history of using multiple methods of data collection. Generally, the methods used in field studies yield data amenable to qualitative analysis, such as field notes from participant observation, unstructured interviews, and narrative documents such as diaries and letters. However, field researchers can in some cases profit from the collection of more structured information from a larger or more representative sample than is possible in collecting the qualitative data. The secondary data might be in the form of structured self-reports from a survey, or quantifiable records. For example, if the researcher's field work focused on family violence, police and hospital records could be used to gather systematic data amenable to statistical analysis.

As field work progresses, researchers typically gain considerable insight into the communities, organizations, or social groups under study. With this knowledge, the researcher can generate hypotheses that can be subjected to more systematic scrutiny through structured data collection methods. Alternatively, the quantitative portion of the study could be used to gather descriptive information about the characteristics of the community or group so that the qualitative findings could be understood in a broader context. In either case, having already gained entrée into the community and the trust and cooperation of its members, the field researcher may be in an ideal position to pursue a survey or a record-extraction activity.

A study by Grau and Wellin (1992) provides an example of a field study that included the use of structured, quantitative data. Their ethnographic study focused on the question of how nursing homes cope with the demands of government regulation for state licensure and Medicaid and Medicare certification. Two skilled-care nursing facilities were studied over a 6-month period. The field work included participant observation in the two nursing homes and in-depth interviews with the nursing home staff, residents, and residents' families. The researchers provided a context for interpreting the qualitative data by administering structured interviews to all administrative personnel, social workers, registered nurses, and licensed practical nurses working in the two facilities. The structured interviews obtained information on the employees' backgrounds, daily work routines, knowledge of regulatory strategies, and experience with regulatory surveys.

Qualitative and Quantitative Data in Experimental Research

Because experimental research involves highly controlled designs and the testing of causal hypotheses, it is easy to get the impression that only quantitative data are appropriate. However, qualitative data can greatly enrich studies that use an experimental or quasi-experimental design. Through in-depth, unstructured approaches, the researcher can better understand qualitative differences between groups, including differences in the reactions of subjects to the experimental conditions and in experiences and processes underlying experimental effects.

Qualitative data collection methods may be especially useful when the researcher is evaluating complex interventions. When an experimental treatment is simple and straightforward (e.g., a new drug), it might be relatively easy to interpret the results. Any posttreatment group differences (assuming that sufficient controls have been instituted) can be attributed to the intervention. However, many nursing interventions are not so straightforward. They may involve new ways of interacting with patients or new approaches to organizing the delivery of care. Sometimes the intervention is multidimensional, involving several different components. At the end of the experiment, even when hypothesized results are obtained, people may ask, What *is* it that really caused the group differences? (If there were no group differences, then the important question would be, *Why* was the intervention unsuccessful?) In-depth qualitative interviews with subjects could help to address these questions. In other words, qualitative data may help researchers to address the *black box* question—understanding what it is about the complex intervention that is driving any observed effects. This knowledge can be helpful for theoretical purposes, and can also help to streamline an intervention and make it more efficient and cost-effective.

Another reason for gathering qualitative data in evaluations of complex interventions is that there is often a need to understand exactly what the intervention was like in practice and how people reacted to it. Unstructured observations and interviews with people with different perspectives (e.g., nurses, physicians, hospital administrators, patients, or patients' family members) are especially well-suited for such process evaluations.

A study in which one of the authors was a co-investigator (Quint, Polit, Bos, & Cave, 1994; Quint, Fink, & Rowser, 1991; Quint & Musick, 1994) provides an example of using both qualitative and quantitative data collection and analysis in an experimental study. The study was a multifaceted evaluation of a comprehensive program for poor teenaged mothers, implemented in 16 sites nationwide. The intervention, known as New Chance, included educational, health, employment, parenting, and social services for participating young mothers and their children. Data were collected over a 4-year period from a sample of over 2000 young mothers. The quantitative data were obtained through several structured interviews with young mothers in the experimental and control groups, various psychosocial scales and tests administered to the mothers and their young children, and structured observations of the home environment. The evaluation also involved in-depth ethnographic interviews with a small sample of the mothers, unstructured observations of program operations, and unstructured interviews with program staff and participants.

❖ OBSTACLES TO INTEGRATION

Throughout this chapter, we have stressed the advantages of blending qualitative and quantitative data in a single investigation. We believe that the potential for advancing nursing science through such integration is great and is as yet relatively untapped. We also believe that integration efforts such as those proposed are inevitable because, at the level of the problem, almost all research questions are inherently multimethod.

Nevertheless, we recognize that there are various obstacles that may constrain the gathering of qualitative and quantitative data in a single investigation. Among the most salient are the following:

- *Epistemological biases.* Qualitative and quantitative researchers often operate with a different set of assumptions about the world and ways of learning about it. For those with a hard-line view, these assumptions may be seen as mutually and inevitably irreconcilable. According to a survey of nurses with doctorates, however, extreme biases of this type are atypical among nurse researchers (Damrosch & Strasser, 1988).
- *Costs.* A major obstacle facing researchers who would like to gather qualitative and quantitative data is that such integrated research is usually expensive. Agencies that sponsor research activities may need to be "educated" about the contribution that integrated data collection efforts can make. In addition to the many substantive advantages

that integration offers, it can also be argued that blending qualitative and quantitative data in a single study is actually less costly and more efficient than two discrete research projects on the same topic.

- *Researcher training.* Most researchers obtain graduate-level training that stresses either qualitative or (more typically) quantitative research methods. According to a survey by Damrosch and Strasser (1988), only about one-third of doctorally prepared academic nurses have training in both qualitative and quantitative methods. Thus, investigator skills may pose an obstacle to integration. However, there is nothing about the integration model that suggests that all phases of the investigation must be done by a single researcher. Collaboration among researchers might, indeed, be an important byproduct of the decision to use an integrated approach. Such collaboration provides opportunities for both methodological and investigator triangulation.
- *Publication biases.* Some journals have a distinct preference for studies that are qualitative, and others lean toward quantitative studies. Because of this fact, researchers might be concerned that they would need to write up the qualitative and quantitative results separately, foregoing many of the advantages of an integrated analysis. However, publication biases are much less evident today than they were a decade ago. All the major nursing journals devoted to research publish qualitative and quantitative studies, and they are increasingly publishing reports of integrated analyses.

In conclusion, although it is recognized that there are various obstacles to integrated analyses, we believe that the simultaneous use of qualitative and quantitative data to address problems of interest to the nursing profession represents a powerful methodological strategy. We are confident that nurse researchers will develop mechanisms for dealing with the obstacles.

❖ TIPS FOR INTEGRATING QUALITATIVE AND QUANTITATIVE DATA

The integration of qualitative and quantitative data in a single study is not always feasible, nor necessarily desirable. However, we offer the following suggestions for those contemplating the possibility of a multimethod study.

- In many situations, a researcher comes to the final stage of a study—the interpretation of the findings—realizing that the interpretation is hampered by the absence of information on some issues. In some cases, this "if only" situation involves the wish that additional information were available using the same data collection method already used (e.g., the addition of another structured scale or question). However, in many other cases, the researcher's interpretation would be enhanced by data of a different sort, such as in-depth questioning. This suggests that many studies would benefit from additional planning. It is often wise to consider in advance a wide variety of scenarios with regard to the findings (especially in studies that are primarily quantitative, which tend to be somewhat less flexible once the study is underway). For example, if you knew in advance that the hypotheses would *not* be supported, what else might you want to ask respondents? If you knew that the hypotheses were supported only for certain types of people, or in certain types of conditions, what kinds of data would you like to have to help explain this pattern? In many situations, the information you will want will not be of the same type used to test the hypotheses. Integrated methods may be the obvious and natural strategy among researchers who use their imagination—and who are thoughtful in anticipating alternative findings.
- If you are considering the possibility of doing an integrated study, try to find someone whose research skills complement yours to collaborate with you. It is almost always useful to have two (or more) minds working on a common problem, and this is especially true when the methods are varied. Top-notch qualitative researchers are rarely top-notch quantitative researchers, and vice versa. It is usually wise to do what you do best and to brainstorm with a person whose talents are different.
- Many multimethod studies are conducted in two or more phases, for example, conducting in-depth interviews with a subsample of patients from whom biophysiologic data were obtained after analysis of those data has been done. If there is a possibility that you *might* go back to research subjects to obtain more data, be sure to structure your consent form in such a way that subjects are aware of any potential future demands on their time. Also, be sure to obtain contact information to facilitate finding the subjects at a later date.

❖ RESEARCH EXAMPLES

We have provided examples of studies using integrated analyses throughout this chapter in an effort to demonstrate the advantages of such an approach as well as to illustrate different applications to which such integration has been put. Table 23-1 identifies some additional studies in which qualitative and quantitative data were blended, and one additional example is described in greater detail.

> Reed (1991) studied the link between developmental resources on the one hand and mental health on the other among the oldest-old (those over 80 years of age). Specifically, Reed was interested in a resource that she labeled "self-transcendence"—the expansion of one's conceptual boundaries inwardly through introspective activities, outwardly through concerns about the welfare of others, and temporally by integrating perceptions of one's past and future.
>
> Reed collected a variety of both quantitative and qualitative data from a sample of 55 older adults living independently. Several

Table 23-1. *Examples of Integrated Studies*

RESEARCH QUESTION	DATA SOURCES
What is the effect of a neonate's breastfeeding competence on the mother's satisfaction with and perception of the experience? (Matthews, 1993)	Hospital records, structured scales; open-ended questions, unsolicited comments
What is the perception of loneliness among adults receiving treatment in a psychiatric facility? (Lee, Coenen, & Heim, 1994)	In-depth interviews; structured psychological scales
What is the effect of cannabis consumption during pregnancy and lactation on offspring from birth to school age? (Dreher & Hayes, 1993)	Structured scales; participant observation, in-depth interviews
What are the informational needs of patients undergoing submucous resection, in comparison to the needs of patients undergoing other surgical procedures? (Oberle, Allen, & Lynkowski, 1993)	Structured questionnaire; in-depth interviews
What are the nurses' judgments of pain in newborns, and what cues do they use to assess the possible presence of pain? (Shapiro, 1993)	Visual analogue scales; in-depth interviews
Do adults with chronic disease manifest a different pattern of health behavior than adults without diagnosed disease? (Laffrey, 1990)	Structured questionnaire and scales; semistructured interviews

structured scales were administered, including the CES-D Scale, the Self-Transcendence Scale (STS) that the author herself developed, and the Langner Scale of Mental Health Symptomatology (MHS). Additionally, because the construct of self-transcendence had not previously been widely studied, Reed used a semistructured interview designed to elicit the respondents' own descriptions of self-transcendence perspectives and behaviors that promoted their sense of well-being. The questions addressed the respondents' perspectives about their past, present, and future, and about the bodily changes they were experiencing. The questions also probed the respondents' tendency and ability to focus on things beyond themselves.

Reed used a highly systematic, iterative process to analyze the qualitative data. A conceptually clustered matrix was constructed to answer questions about patterns of variables across respondents. Cases were listed in the matrix by rows; the columns were arranged to bring together conceptually similar clusters of data. This analysis revealed four conceptual clusters that the researcher labeled Generativity, Introjectivity, Temporal Integration, and Body-Transcendence. Table 23-2 presents Reed's clusters and categories for the qualitative data.

The relationship between self-transcendence and depression was examined by juxtaposing the qualitatively generated self-transcendence patterns and quantitative depression scores for each respondent. Using correlational procedures, Reed found a relationship between self-transcendence and positive mental health among the very elderly.

Table 23-2.   *Reed's Clusters and Categories of Self-Transcendence*

CLUSTER, CATEGORIES	SAMPLE RESPONSES
I. Generativity	
(1)* Helping others	Visit the sick; volunteer work; teaching; church work
(1) Family involvement	Visiting siblings, helping children
II. Introjectivity	
(1) Interiority	Hobbies; travel; housework
(1) Lifelong learning	Reading; taking formal courses; spiritual or self-reflection
III. Temporal Integration	
Past	
(2) Active acceptance	Sense of pride in past; feelings of joy about past
(1) Passive acceptance	The past is gone; I have no regrets
(0) Negative acceptance	It saddens me; I regret it
Present	
(2) Active positive	I make the best of it; I am happy; one must change to grow
(1) Passive positive	Take one day at a time; you have to roll with the punches
(0) Negative	I am existing, not living; it is worrisome; discouraging
Future	
(2) Active anticipation	I look forward to it; I am at peace; I have hope
(1) Passive anticipation	Que sera sera; I don't think about it
(0) Negative anticipation	I worry about my health then; I have fears about it
IV. Body Transcendence	
(2) Flexibility	Learn how to live with it; have to accept it; don't dwell on it
(1) Maybe or unsure	Never thought about it; I think I'm able to accept the changes
(0) Negative	I get disgusted; I feel trapped by my body; I hate my body

*Indicates weighting used to code the score for each cluster.

Reed, P. G. (1991). Self-transcendance and mental health in oldest-old adults. *Nursing Research, 40,* 5–11. (Reprinted with permission)

❖ SUMMARY

The judicious blending of qualitative and quantitative data collection and analysis in a single project offers many advantages. The most obvious advantage is that the two methods have complementary strengths and weaknesses and offer the possibility of "mutually supplying each other's lack." Second, an integrated approach can lead to theoretical and substantive insights into the multidimensional nature of reality that might otherwise be unattainable. Third, integration can provide feedback loops that augment the incremental gains in knowledge that a single-method study could achieve. Fourth, the potential for confirmation of the study hypotheses through multiple and complementary types of data can strengthen the researcher's confidence in the validity of the findings. Fifth, when the multiple methods yield inconsistent findings, a careful scrutiny of the discrepancies could push the line of inquiry further than might otherwise have been possible.

The integration of qualitative and quantitative data can be used in many applications. In nursing, one of the most frequent uses of multimethod research has been in the area of instrument development. Qualitative data are also used in some studies to illustrate the meaning of quantified descriptions or relationships. Integrated analyses are also used in efforts to interpret and give shape to relationships and causal processes. Finally, the most ambitious application of an integrated approach is in the area of theory development.

Researchers can implement an integrated approach in a variety of ways, but three strategies are especially likely to be common. The first is to embed qualitative methods (such as in-depth interviews or unstructured observations) within a survey. The second is to add structured data collection (such as a survey or a systematic analysis of records data) into field work. The third is to collect both types of data within the context of an experimental or quasi-experimental design. In some studies, the simultaneous collection and analysis of qualitative and quantitative data may address the objectives of integration, but in many studies, a multistage approach is likely to yield more insights.

Despite the advantages of blending both types of data in a single study, there are several obstacles to doing so. These obstacles include epistemological biases, high costs, inadequate researcher training, and publication biases. However, these obstacles are not insurmountable; the potential contribution that integration would afford nursing science makes the effort to surmount them a worthwhile investment.

❖ STUDY SUGGESTIONS

Chapter 23 of the accompanying *Study Guide for Nursing Research: Principles and Methods, 5th ed.*, offers various exercises and study suggestions for reinforcing the concepts presented in this chapter. Additionally, the following study questions can be addressed:

1. Suppose you were interested in studying the psychological consequences of a miscarriage. Suggest ways in which qualitative and quantitative data could be gathered for such a study.
2. Read an article in a recent issue of a nursing research journal in which the researcher collected only quantitative data. Suggest some possibilities for how qualitative data might have enhanced the validity or interpretability of the findings.

3. Read one of the studies cited under Substantive References at the end of this chapter. To what extent were the qualitative and quantitative analyses integrated? Describe how the absence of either the quantitative or qualitative portions of the study might have affected the study quality and the study conclusions.

❖ SUGGESTED READINGS

METHODOLOGICAL REFERENCES

Brewer, J., & Hunter, A. (1989). *Multimethod research: A synthesis of styles.* Newbury Park, CA: Sage.

Bryman, A. (1988). *Quantity and quality in social research.* London: Unwin Hyman.

Carey, J. W. (1993). Linking qualitative and quantitative methods: Integrating cultural factors into public health. *Qualitative Health Research, 3,* 298–318.

Chesla, C. A. (1992). When qualitative and quantitative findings do not converge. *Western Journal of Nursing Research, 14,* 681–685.

Damrosch, S. P., & Strasser, J. A. (1988). A survey of doctorally prepared academic nurses on qualitative and quantitative research issues. *Nursing Research, 37,* 176–180.

Denzin, N. K. (1989). *The research act* (3rd ed.). Englewood Cliffs, NJ: Prentice-Hall.

Duffy, M. (1987). Methodological triangulation: A vehicle for merging quantitative and qualitative research methods. *Image, 19,* 130–133.

Haase, J. E., & Myers, S. T. (1988) Reconciling paradigm assumptions of qualitative and quantitative research. *Western Journal of Nursing Research, 10,* 128–137.

Jicks, T. D. (1979). Mixing qualitative and quantitative methods: Triangulation in action. *Administrative Science Quarterly, 24,* 602–611.

Mitchell, E. S. (1986). Multiple triangulation: A methodology for nursing science. *Advances in Nursing Science, 8,* 18–26.

Morse, J. M. (1991). Approaches to qualitative-quantitative methodological triangulation. *Nursing Research, 40,* 120–122.

Murphy, S. A. (1989). Multiple triangulation: Applications in a program of nursing research. *Nursing Research, 38,* 294–298.

Myers, S. T., & Haase, J. E. (1989). Guidelines for integration of quantitative and qualitative approaches. *Nursing Research, 38,* 299–301.

Seiber, S. D. (1973). Integrating field work and survey methods. *American Journal of Sociology, 78,* 1335–1359.

Tilden, V. P., Nelson, C. A., & May, B. A. (1990). Use of qualitative methods to enhance content validity. *Nursing Research, 39,* 172–175.

Tripp-Reimer, T. (1985). Combining qualitative and quantitative methodologies. In M. Leininger (Ed.), *Qualitative research methods in nursing.* New York: Grune & Stratton.

SUBSTANTIVE REFERENCES

Bargagliotti, L. A., & Trygstad, L. N. (1987). Differences in stress and coping findings: A reflection of social realities or methodologies. *Nursing Research, 36,* 170–173.

Dreher, M. C., & Hayes, J. S. (1993). Triangulation in cross-cultural research of child development in Jamaica. *Western Journal of Nursing Research, 15,* 216–229.

Grau, L., & Wellin, E. (1992). The organizational cultures of nursing homes: Influences on responses to external regulatory controls. *Qualitative Health Research, 2,* 42–60.

Gulick, E. E. (1991). Reliability and validity of the Work Assessment Scale for persons with multiple sclerosis. *Nursing Research, 40,* 107–112.

Hall, J. M., Stevens, P. E., & Meleis, A. I. (1992). Developing the construct of role integration: A narrative analysis of women clerical workers' daily lives. *Research in Nursing and Health, 15,* 447-457.

Hinds, P. S. (1989). Method triangulation to index change in clinical phenomena. *Western Journal of Nursing Research, 11,* 440–447.

Hough, E. E., Lewis, F. M., & Woods, N. F. (1991). Family response to mother's chronic illness: Case studies of well- and poorly-adjusted families. *Western Journal of Nursing Research, 13,* 568–596.

Laffrey, S. C. (1990). An exploration of adult health behaviors. *Western Journal of Nursing Research, 12,* 434–447.

Lee, H., Coenen, A., & Heim, K. (1994). Island living: The experience of loneliness in a psychiatric hospital. *Applied Nursing Research, 7,* 7–13.

Lewis, F. M., Woods, N. F., Hough, E. E., & Bensley, L. (1989). The family's functioning with chronic illness in the mother. *Social Science and Medicine, 29,* 1261–1269.

Lipson, J. G. (1992). The health and adjustment of Iranian immigrants. *Western Journal of Nursing Research, 14,* 10–24.

Matthews, M. K. (1993). Experiences of primiparous breast-feeding mothers in the first days following birth. *Clinical Nursing Research, 2,* 309–326.

Meleis, A. I., Norbeck, J. S., Laffrey, S. (1989). Role integration and health among female clerical workers. *Research in Nursing and Health, 12,* 355–364.

Murphy, S. A. (1986). Perceptions of stress, coping, and recovery one and three years after a natural disaster. *Mental Health Nursing, 8,* 63–77.

Murphy, S. A. (1987). Self-efficacy and social support: Mediators of stress on mental health following a natural disaster. *Western Journal of Nursing Research, 9,* 58–73.

Murphy, S. A. (1989). An explanatory model of recovery from disaster loss. *Research in Nursing and Health, 12,* 67–76.

Nyamathi, A. M., & Flaskerud, J. (1992). A Community-based Inventory of Current Concerns of impoverished homeless and drug-addicted minority women. *Research in Nursing and Health, 15,* 121–129.

Oberle, K., Allen, M., & Lynkowski, P. (1993). Submucous resection: Is it a simple procedure? *Clinical Nursing Research, 2,* 54–66.

Polit, D. F., Morton, T., & White, C. M. (1989). Sex, contraception, and pregnancy among children in foster care. *Family Planning Perspectives, 21,* 203–206.

Polit, D. F., White, C. M., & Morton, T. (1990). Child sexual abuse and premarital intercourse among high-risk adolescents. *Journal of Adolescent Health Care, 11,* 231–234.

Quint, J. C., Fink, B. L., & Rowser, S. L. (1991). *New Chance: Implementing a comprehensive program for disadvantaged young mothers and their children.* New York, NY: Manpower Demonstration Research Corporation.

Quint, J. C., & Musick, S. J. (1994). *Lives of promise, lives of pain: Young mothers after New Chance.* New York, NY: Manpower Demonstration Research Corporation.

Quint, J. C., Polit, D. F., Bos, H., & Cave, G. (1994). *New Chance: Interim findings on a comprehensive program for disadvantaged young mothers and their children.* New York, NY: Manpower Demonstration Research Corp.

Reed, P. G. (1991). Self-transcendence and mental health in oldest-old adults. *Nursing Research, 40,* 5–11.

Salazar, M. K., & Carter, W. B. (1993). Evaluation of breast self-examination beliefs using a decision model. *Western Journal of Nursing Research, 15,* 403–418.

Shapiro, C. R. (1993). Nurses' judgments of pain in term and preterm newborns. *Journal of Obstetric, Gynecologic, and Neonatal Nursing, 22,* 41–47.

Part VI

COMMUNICATION IN THE RESEARCH PROCESS

Chapter 24

Writing a research report

No scientific project is ever complete until a research report has been prepared. The most brilliant piece of work is of little value to the scientific community unless that work is known. The task of preparing a research report may appear to be anticlimactic: after all, the researcher has satisfied his or her curiosity. Nevertheless, the reporting of results adds to knowledge on some issue and is a scientist's responsibility. It is also to the researcher's advantage to have research findings known by others because proper credit should be given to the work that has been completed. This chapter offers general guidelines for helping researchers to communicate their research results.

❖ THE RESEARCH REPORT: CONTENT

Research reports are prepared for different audiences and for different purposes. A thesis or dissertation not only communicates the research strategy and results but also serves as documentation of the student's thoroughness and ability to perform scholarly empirical work. Theses and dissertations, therefore, are rather lengthy documents. Journal articles, on the other hand,

are typically short because they must compete with other reports for limited journal space and because they will be read by busy professionals. Oral reports and presentations at professional conferences are another mechanism for disseminating research results; they offer the possibility of immediate two-way communications and are therefore highly useful.

Despite differences among various types of research reports, their general form and content are similar. The major distinction lies in the amount of detail reported and the emphasis given to different parts. In this section, we expand on the information presented in Chapter 4 by reviewing in greater depth the type of material that is covered in four of the major sections of a research report: introduction, methods, results, and discussion. The distinctions among the various kinds of reports are described later in the chapter.

The Introduction

The purpose of the introductory section of a research report is to acquaint readers with the research problem, the significance of the problem for nursing and for a field of knowledge, and the context within which the problem was developed. The introduction sets the stage for a description of the study through the inclusion of a brief literature review; description of the conceptual framework; presentation of the problem statement, hypotheses, and any underlying assumptions; and discussion of the rationale for studying the problem.

Sometimes reports describe only the general purpose of an investigation. However, a precise and unambiguous problem statement is of immense value in communicating to the reader the major objectives of the study. If formal hypotheses have been developed, then they should also be identified in the introduction. It is often useful to number research questions or hypotheses so that they can be more readily referenced in reporting the results.

The researcher should explain enough of the background of the study to make clear the reasons that the problem was considered worth pursuing. The justification of a nursing research problem should ideally include both the practical and theoretical significance of the study. This ideal is not always feasible. Not all studies have a direct bearing on theoretical issues, nor should they all necessarily be expected to have such a bearing in a practicing profession such as nursing. With the current state of knowledge, no one should feel apologetic if a study can solve a practical problem but is not linked to a theory. Of course, studies that are framed within a theoretical context are most likely to make enduring contributions to knowledge about nursing and the nursing process. The introduction should make explicit such theoretical rationales when they exist. In most cases, the theoretical framework should be sufficiently explained that a reader who may be unfamiliar with the particular framework can nevertheless understand its main thrust and its link to the research problem.

The statement of the problem should also be accompanied by a summary of related research so that the research may be seen in an appropriate context. The review of the literature helps to clarify the theoretical and practical foundations of the research problem. Chapter 4 describes in greater detail the write-up of the literature review section.

Finally, the introduction should incorporate definitions of the concepts under investigation. Sometimes complete operational definitions are reserved for the methods section, but a reader should have a fairly good idea early in the report what the researcher had in mind with regard to such terms as "grief," "stress," "therapeutic touch," and so forth if they are the key concepts under study.

In many research reports, the introductory materials are not explicitly grouped under a heading labeled Introduction. In fact, research reports in journals typically begin without any header. Some introductory sections have headings or subheadings dedicated to specific aspects of the study's background, such as Literature Review, Conceptual Framework, or Hypotheses. In general, however, all the material before the methods section is considered to be the introduction to the report.

In summary, the introduction should prepare readers for the description of what was done and what was discovered. The introduction should answer the questions, What did the researcher want to know? Why did he or she want to know it? and What is the likely theoretical and practical significance of such a study?

The Methods Section

Consumers of a research report need to understand what the researcher did to address the problem identified in the introduction. The methods section should have as its goal a description of what was done to collect and analyze the data in sufficient detail that another researcher could replicate the study if desired. In theses and final reports to funding agencies, this goal should almost always be satisfied. In journal articles, however, it is often necessary to condense the methods section. For example, it is typically impossible to include a complete questionnaire, interview schedule, or observation schedule. Nevertheless, the degree of detail should be sufficiently adequate to permit a

reader to evaluate the manner in which the research problem was solved.

The methods section is often subdivided into several parts. The reader needs to know, first of all, who the subjects participating in the study were. The description of the subjects normally includes the specification of the population from which the sample was drawn and the setting for the research. The method of sample selection, the rationale for the sampling design, and the sample size should be clearly delineated so that the reader can understand the strengths and limitations of the sampling plan. It is also advisable to describe the basic characteristics of the subjects, such as their age, gender, and other relevant attributes. It is also helpful to indicate, if possible, the degree to which these characteristics are representative of the population. For instance, if it is known that a sample of nurses tends to underrepresent those with graduate degrees, then this fact should be pointed out.

The design of the study also needs to be described. The design is often given more detailed coverage in an experimental project than in a nonexperimental one. In an experiment, the researcher should indicate what variables were manipulated, how subjects were assigned to groups, the nature of the experimental intervention, and the specific design adopted. In longitudinal studies, the report should indicate the amount of time elapsed between waves of data collection. Regardless of study design, the report should offer a rationale for its use. Also, in quantitative studies, it is important to identify what steps were taken to control the research situation in general and extraneous variables in particular.

A description of the methods used to collect the data is a critical component of the methods section. In rare cases, this description may be accomplished in three or four sentences, such as when a standard physiologic measure has been utilized. More often, a detailed explanation of the instruments or procedures and a rationale for their use are required to communicate to the reader the manner in which the data were gathered and how the variables were operationalized. When it is not feasible to include the actual research instrument within the report, its form and content should be outlined in as much detail as possible. If the measuring devices were constructed specifically for the research project, then the report should describe how they were developed, the methods used for pretesting, revisions made as a result of pretesting, scoring procedures, and guidelines for interpretation. Any information relating to data quality and procedures used to evaluate data quality should also be mentioned. Such information is particularly important in a qualitative study because so much of the analysis depends on the researcher's interpretation of the data.

A procedures section provides information about what steps were followed in actually collecting the data. In an experiment, how much time elapsed between the intervention and the measurement of the dependent variable? In an interview study, where were the interviews conducted, who conducted them, and how long did the average interview last? In an observational study, what was the role of the observer in relationship to the subjects? When questionnaires are used, how were they delivered to respondents, were follow-up procedures used to increase the response rate, and what was the response rate? Any unforeseen events occurring during the collection of data that could affect the findings should be described and assessed. Those reading a report must be in a position to evaluate the quality of the data obtained, and a description of research procedures assists in this evaluation.

A delineation of the analytic procedures is sometimes incorporated into the methods section and sometimes put with the results of the analyses. In qualitative studies, in which there is less standardization than is true in analyzing quantitative data, analytic procedures are often described in some detail. In quantitative studies, it is usually sufficient to identify the statistical procedures used. It is unnecessary to give computational formulas or even references for commonly used statistics. For unusual procedures, or unusual applications of a common procedure, a technical reference justifying the approach should be noted.

Table 24-1 illustrates the content covered in the methods section of quantitative research reports, using excerpts from several studies published in nursing research journals. Table 24-2 presents analogous information for qualitative studies.

The Results Section

The results section summarizes the results of the analyses. In qualitative studies, the researcher presents a summary of the thematic analysis and the integration of the narrative materials, often including direct quotes to illustrate important points. Due to space constraints in journals, quotes cannot be extensive, and great care must be exercised in selecting the best possible exemplars. Figures and diagrams are often extremely useful in qualitative studies in summarizing an overall conceptualization of the phenomena under study.

In quantitative studies, if both descriptive and inferential statistics have been used, then the descriptive statistics ordinarily come first. If both quantitative and qualitative analysis has been performed, the qualitative analyses are often placed later because of their ability to explain the meaning of statistical analyses. On the other hand, in some cases, quantitative results may serve a useful summation or confirmatory function and may be more meaningful after a presentation of qualitative results.

The researcher must be careful to report all results as accurately and completely as possible, whether or not the hypotheses were supported. If there are too many analyses for inclusion in the report, then the criterion used to select analyses should be their relevance to the overall objectives of the study.

When the results of several statistical analyses are to be presented, it is frequently useful to summarize the findings in a *table*. Good tables, with precise headings and titles, are an important way to economize on space and to avoid dull, repetitious statements. Box 24-1 presents some suggestions regarding the construction of effective tables. *Figures* may also be used to summarize results. Figures that display the results in graphic form are used less as an economy than as a means of dramatizing important findings and relationships. Figures are especially helpful for displaying information for some phenomenon over time.

When the results of statistical tests are reported, three pieces of information are normally included: the value of the calculated statistic, the number of degrees of freedom, and the significance level. For instance, it might be stated, "A chi-square test revealed that patients who were exposed to the experimental intervention were significantly less likely to develop decubitus ulcers than patients in a control group ($\chi^2 = 8.23$, $df = 1$, $p < .01$)."

Although we will discuss style in a later section, it is difficult to avoid the mention of style here. The write-up of statistical results is often a difficult task for beginning researchers because they are unsure both about what should be said and about the style in which to say it. A few suggestions may prove helpful. By now, it should be clear that research evidence does not constitute proof of anything, but the point bears repeating here. The research report should never claim that the data proved, verified, confirmed, or demonstrated that the hypotheses were correct or incorrect. Hypotheses are supported or unsupported, accepted or rejected. It may seem a trivial point, but the presentation of results should be written in the past tense. For example, it is inappropriate to say, "Nurses who receive special training perform triage functions significantly better than those without training." In this sentence, "receive" and "perform" should be changed to "received" and "performed." The present tense implies that the results apply to all nurses, when in fact the statement pertains only to a particular sample whose behavior was observed in the past.

To further acquaint readers with the write-up of research results, Table 24-3 presents excerpts from the results sections of several quan-

Table 24-1.   *Excerpts From Methods Sections: Quantitative Nursing Research Reports*

METHODOLOGICAL ASPECT	EXCERPT
Research design	All patients entered an initial 4-week control period during which they learned to perform the physical tests used. . . . Testing was conducted at weekly intervals and data from the fourth measurement session were used for baseline data. At the end of the control period, patients were randomly assigned to either the treatment or control group. Data collectors were blinded to group assignment. (Kim, Larson, Covey, Vitalo, Alex, & Patel, 1993, p. 358)
Sampling plan	The sample consisted of 405 aspirates from small-bore nasogastric tubes and 389 aspirates from nasointestinal tubes. These samples were obtained from 605 subjects, ranging in age from 18 to 94 years. Over a 3½ year period, subjects were recruited from six acute care hospitals during daily rounds or were referred to the researchers by staff nurses and physicians. (Metheny, Reed, Wiersma, McSweeney, Wehrle, & Clark, 1993, p. 326)
Measurements	Blood pressure was determined every 3 min using a 1846 SX Dinamap automatic sphygmomanometer according to standard procedures. The Dinamap was calibrated with a mercury sphygmomanometer prior to use with each subject. Blood pressure and time of day were printed immediately after the cuff deflated. (Baker, Garvin, Kennedy, & Polivka, 1993, p. 417)
Data collection procedures	Physiologic and behavioral data were collected for each neonate before, during, and after a routine morning heel stick. The heel-stick procedure was subdivided into five phases, including baseline (60 seconds), heel warming (60 seconds), heel stick (15 seconds), heel squeezing (1–5 minutes), and return to baseline (60 seconds or until physiologic parameters returned to baseline values). (Stevens, Johnston, & Horton, 1993, p. 533)
Data quality	Content validity was established by a panel of experts that included two professors of maternal-child nursing, a certified nurse midwife, a clinical psychologist and a physician. . . . Construct validity was established by conducting a principal components factor analysis with oblique rotation. . . . Stability was determined to be substantial (Pearson's $r = .94$) for the 3 items of interest using a 2-week retest. Internal consistency also was determined to be substantial (alpha $= .95$) for the three items of interest. (Troy, 1993, p. 162)
Data analysis	Repeated measures ANOVAs were used to test for groups (low symptoms, high symptoms) by menstrual cycle phase (premenstrual, postmenstrual) interaction, for hassles scores and for uplift scores. Following this analysis, post hoc comparisons using t tests with Bonferroni corrections were carried out. (Brown & Lewis, 1993, p. 426)

Table 24-2.   *Excerpts From Methods Sections: Qualitative Nursing Research Reports*

METHODOLOGICAL ASPECT	EXCERPT
Research design	A combination of cross-sectional and longitudinal designs was employed. Both primiparous and multiparous mothers participated in the study and each participated three times over the early infant period. Data collection was scheduled at 6 weeks, 10 weeks, and 16 weeks postpartum. (Drummond, McBride, & Wiebe, 1993, p. 397)
Sampling plan	The sample was accessed through Compassionate Friends, an international support group of parents and children who have experienced the death of a child or sibling, respectively. . . . Criteria for inclusion in the sample were that the bereaved adolescents: (a) were between the ages of 13 and 18 at the time of the study; (b) were not engaged in professional mental health counseling; and (c) had a sibling die within the 5-year period prior to data collection. (Hogan & DeSantis, 1994, p. 134)
Data collection method	Interviews were semistructured, and we asked each informant to describe his experience with breastfeeding from the time his wife became pregnant until after weaning. Initially, we used open-ended questions such as "Tell me about your experience as the father of the breastfed infant." The issues and concerns raised in early interviews directed the course of subsequent interviews (Gamble & Morse, 1993, p. 359)
Data collection procedures	Participants were contacted by telephone to arrange interviews at a convenient time. Informed consent of participants was obtained before the implementation of the study procedure. The interviews were conducted in the participants' place of residence. Only the investigator and the participant were present during the actual interview. (Herth, 1993, p. 147)
Data quality	Investigator triangulation, the use of multiple interviewers and analysts, removed the potential bias of a single-investigator study and brought multiple perspectives to data gathering and analysis. Data triangulation, gathering data from several sources, was used as a system of checks and balances to obtain additional viewpoints when discrepancies appeared in the data. . . . Member checks, where the analysis is given to participants for correction and verification, was used as an interviewing strategy and as an opportunity to refine the final analysis. (Patterson, Douglas, Patterson, & Bradle, 1992, p. 369)
Data analysis	Transcriptions of interviews were analyzed using constant comparative analysis. . . . This yielded provisional hypotheses, which were tested through subsequent data collection and by reinspection of data in hand. New subjects were recruited until no new concepts were found in the data. (Bailey & Kahn, 1993, p. 59)

BOX 24-1   GUIDELINES FOR THE PREPARATION OF TABLES

- A table makes it possible to compare and comprehend patterns and relationships among data. Most quantitative studies benefit from the inclusion of one or more tables, but tables should be reserved for important substantive information that is too cumbersome to report in the text. Avoid very short tables, such as a table with two columns and two rows; it is more efficient to present such information in the text.
- Tables are effective only when the data are arranged in such a way that the patterns are obvious at a glance. Care needs to be taken in organizing the information in an intelligible way.
- If there is a choice between what to put on the horizontal and vertical dimensions of the table, keep in mind that it is easier for readers to compare numbers down a column than across a row.
- Every column of data should have a heading. Table headings should establish the logic of the table structure. The headings should be succinct but clear.
- Numerical values should be expressed in the number of decimal places justified by the precision of measurement. However, it is often preferable to report numbers in tables to a maximum of one decimal place (except correlation coefficients); rounded numbers are often easier to absorb and compare than more precise values. The number of decimal places should be the same across entries in the table.
- Probability values should be clearly indicated, as appropriate, either by indicating the actual p values or by using asterisks and a probability level note. When more than one probability level is indicated in the table, use one asterisk for the least stringent level, two for the next level, and so on (e.g., $*p < .05$, $**p < .01$). It is not necessary to use the same probability levels and number of asterisks from one table to the next.
- Every table should be comprehensible without reference to the text. All abbreviations (except commonly used ones such as N or SD) and special symbols should be explained in notes to the table.
- When applicable, the units of measurement for the numbers in the table should always be indicated (e.g., pounds, dollars, beats per minute, milligrams, etc.).
- Each table should be referred to in the text (e.g., "As shown in Table 2, patients who. . ."). Thus, every table should be numbered.
- Every table should have a clear, but brief, explanatory title.

titative studies published in nursing journals. Excerpts from the results sections of qualitative and integrated qualitative and quantitative studies are presented in Table 24-4.

The Discussion Section

A bare report of the findings is never sufficient to convey their full implications. The meaning that a researcher gives to the results plays a rightful and important role in the report. The discussion section is typically devoted to a consideration of the study's limitations, the interpretation of the results, and recommendations that incorporate the study's implications.

In qualitative studies, the findings and the interpretation are typically presented together in the results section because the task of integrating qualitative materials is necessarily interpretive. In quantitative studies, however, the interpretation is reserved for the discussion.

In quantitative studies, the interpretation of the results involves the translation of statistical findings into practical and conceptual meaning. The interpretative process is a global one, encompassing the investigator's knowledge of the results, the methods, the sample characteristics, related research findings, clinical dimensions, and theoretical issues. The researcher should justify his or her interpretations, explicitly stating why alternative explanations have been ruled out. If the findings conflict with those of earlier research investigations, then tentative explanations should be offered. A discussion of the generalizability of the study findings and an analysis of their importance should also be included.

Table 24-3.   *Excerpts From Results Sections: Quantitative Nursing Research Reports*

TYPE OF ANALYSES	EXCERPT
Descriptive statistics	The majority of patients (72.3%) had an identified caregiver; about one-third (31.7%) received services from community agencies other than the home care agency. . . . Considerable variation existed in the type and amount of coordination the patients received. Total coordination ranged from 0 to 97 nurse-patient encounters (M = 10.16, SD = 10.95). (Cloonan & Belyea, 1993, p. 746)
t-Tests	Women without spouses perceived they had obtained significantly less tangible support (M = 2.83, SD = .98) than women with spouses (M = 3.33, SD = .88, $t(78) = 2.12$, $p < .05$. These two groups of women did not vary on their perception of emotional support. (Friedman, 1993, p. 409)
Pearson's *r*	Educational level was significantly related to attitude towards caring for HIV positive patients ($r = .30$, $p = .04$), indicating that nurses with higher levels of education had more positive attitudes. A significant negative relationship was found between number of children and intentions to care for HIV positive patients ($r = -.32$, $p = .02$), indicating that those with several children were less likely to care for these patients. (Laschinger & Goldenberg, 1993, p. 447)
ANOVA	Analysis of variance was used to determine if total scores on the revised LaMonica-Obserst Patient Satisfaction Scale (LOPSS) differed by client group. The two-way ANOVA contained two independent variables: study with three levels (Cesarean section, diabetic, and hysterectomy) and Group with two levels (early and routine discharge). The early discharge group scored significantly higher ($F = 44.34$, $p = .001$) on the revised LOPSS (M = 125.1, SD = 13.4) than the routine discharge group (M = 112.6, SD = 18.3). (Munro, Jacobsen, & Brooten, 1994, p. 124)
Chi-square	Nausea was not significantly more prevalent in the morning hours compared to other times during the waking hours of 7 a.m. to 10 p.m. ($\chi^2 = 1.588$, df = 3, p = .662). There was, however, a significant difference in the frequency of nausea between day (7 a.m.–10 p.m.) and night (11 p.m.–6 am.) hours, with fewer occurrences of nausea during the night ($\chi^2 = 428.004$, df = 5, $p < .001$). (DiIorio, van Lier, & Manteuffel, 1992, p. 132)
Multiple regression	A regression using the six personal variables showed a significant relationship with Agitated Psychomotor Behaviors, $F(6, 253) = 6.90$; $p = .0001$. Addition of the two variables for physical environment in the model did not significantly increase explanatory power, $F(2, 251) = 1.58$; $p = .21$, nor did the addition of the five psychosocial milieu variables, $F(5, 248) = 1.89$; $p = .10$. The addition of one organizational variable, staff mix, did however significantly increase the amount of variance explained, $F(1, 252) = 10.79$; $p = .0012$. (Kolanowski, Hurwitz, Taylor, Evans, & Strumpf, 1994, p. 77)

Table 24-4. *Excerpts From Results Sections: Qualitative and Integrated Nursing Research Reports*

TYPE OF ANALYSES	EXCERPT
Qualitative	A diagnosis of genital herpes eroded self-esteem, raised suspicions of infidelity in a partner, lowered confidence in establishing close relationships, and threatened these young adults' sense of self. Resisting loss is the strategy used to withstand the interpretation or meaning of the disease in their lives. Acknowledging the loss occurred by comparing past and present selves. The theme of a past "body beautiful" and how herpes affected it persisted throughout the interviews. (Swanson & Chenitz, 1993, p. 281)
Integrated	[In the survey], the lack of a doctor's recommendation was the single most frequently given reason for never having had a mammogram, but one in three responses concerned knowledge barriers. . . . The focus group findings echoed the survey findings, adding a few dimensions and providing more specific information on other dimensions. As in the survey, lack of provider recommendation was the single most frequently mentioned reason for not getting breast cancer screening. It was not that providers were telling women not to get mammograms but that preventive care took a back seat to chronic illnesses, such as diabetes. (Saint-Germain, Bassford, & Montano, 1993, p. 360)
Qualitative	The study participants were clear that when they first began to manage life with a chronic condition the story was not "Our life is normal, we just have a few problems." Instead, the informants reported that life was problem saturated— there was little life beyond the problem. The story at that time was characterized by despair; however, at some point, it began to shift. A problem existed, but there was clearly life beyond the problem . (Robinson, 1993, p. 10)

Although the readers should be told enough about the methods of the study to identify its major weaknesses, report writers should point out the limitations themselves. The researcher is in the best position to detect and assess the impact of sampling deficiencies, design constraints, data quality problems, and so forth, and it is a professional responsibility to alert the reader to these difficulties. Moreover, if the writer shows that he or she is aware of the study's limitations, then the reader will know that these limitations were not ignored in the development of the interpretation.

The implications derived from a study are often speculative and, therefore, should be couched in tentative terms. For instance, the kind of language appropriate for a discussion of the interpretation is illustrated by the following sentence: "The results suggest that it may be possible to improve nurse–physician interaction by modifying the medical student's stereotype of the nurse as the physician's 'handmaiden'." The interpretation is, in essence, a hypothesis and as such can presumably be tested in another research project. The discussion section, therefore, should include recommendations for studies that would help to test this hypothesis as well as suggestions for other research to answer questions raised by the findings.

Other Aspects of the Report

The materials covered in the four major sections are found in some form in virtually all research reports, although the organization might differ slightly. In addition to these major divisions, some other aspects of the report deserve mention.

Every research report should have a title. The phrases "Research Report" or "Report of a Nursing Research Investigation" are inadequate. The title should indicate to prospective readers the nature of the study. Insofar as possible, the dependent and independent variables (or central phenomenon under study) should be named in the title. It is also desirable to indicate the study population. However, the title should be brief (no more than about 15 words), so the writer must balance clarity with brevity. Some examples of titles include the following:

The Effect of Advance Information on Pain Perception in Hospitalized Children
Attitudes Toward Preventive Health Care in the Urban Working Class
Educational Preparation: Its Effects on Role Conflict Among Nurses

If the title gets too unwieldy, its length can often be reduced by omitting unnecessary terms such as "A Study of . . ." or "An Investigation To Examine the Effects of . . ." and so forth. The title should communicate clearly and concisely the phenomena that were researched.

Research reports often include an abstract or a summary. *Abstracts* are brief descriptions of the problem, methods, and findings of the study, written so that a reader can assess whether the entire report should be read. Sometimes a report concludes with a brief summary, and the summary, in such cases, usually substitutes for the abstract. Abstracts and summaries are typically only 100 to 200 words in length. Finally, each report concludes with a list of cited references so that the reader can locate other relevant materials.

❖ THE STYLE OF A RESEARCH REPORT

Research reports are generally written in a distinctive style. Some stylistic guidelines were discussed previously in this chapter and in Chapter 4, but additional points are elaborated on in this section.

A scientific report is not an essay but rather a factual account of how and why a problem was studied and what results were obtained. The report should generally not include overtly subjective statements, emotionally laden statements, or exaggerations. When opinions are stated, they should be clearly identified as such, with proper attribution if the opinion was expressed by another writer. In keeping with the goal of objective reporting, personal pronouns such as "I," "my," and "we" are often avoided because the passive voice and impersonal pronouns do a better job of conveying impartiality. However, some journals are beginning to break with this tradition and are encouraging a greater balance between active and passive voice and first-person and third-person narration. If a direct presentation can be made without sacrificing objectivity, a more readable and lively product usually will result.

It is not easy to write simply and clearly, but these are important goals of scientific writing. The use of pretentious words or technical jargon does little to enhance the communicative value of the report, although colloquialisms should be avoided. Avoiding jargon and highly technical terms is especially important in communicating research findings to practicing nurses. Also, complex sentence constructions are not necessarily the best way to convey ideas. The style should be concise and straightforward. If writers can add elegance to their reports without interfering with clarity and accuracy, so much the better, but the product is not expected to be a literary achievement. Needless to say, this does not imply that grammatical and spelling accuracy should be sacrificed. The research report should reflect scholarship, not pedantry.

With regard to references and specific technical aspects of the manuscript, various styles have been developed. The writer may be able to select a style, but often such considerations are imposed by journal editors and university regulations. Specialized manuals such as those of the University of Chicago Press (1993), the American Psychological Association (1983), and the American Medical Association (1989) are widely used. Most nursing research journals (e.g., *Nursing Research, Research in Nursing and Health, Western Journal of Nursing Research, Clinical Nursing Research,* and *Applied Nursing Research*) use the reference style recommended by the American Psychological Association, which is the reference style used in this book.

A common flaw in the reports of beginning researchers is inadequate organization. The overall structure is fairly standard and, therefore, should pose no difficulties, but the organization within sections and subsections needs careful attention. Sequences should be in an orderly progression with appropriate transition. Themes or ideas should not be introduced abruptly nor abandoned suddenly. Continuity and logical thematic development are critical to good communication.

❖ TYPES OF RESEARCH REPORTS

Although the general form and structure of a research report are fairly consistent across different types of reports, certain requirements vary. This section describes the content, structure, and features of three major kinds of research reports: theses and dissertations, journal articles, and papers for professional meetings. Reports for class projects are excluded—not because they are unimportant but rather because they so closely resemble theses on a smaller scale. Final reports to agencies that have sponsored research are also not described. Most funding agencies issue guidelines for their reports, and these guidelines can be secured from project officers. In most cases, reports to funding agencies require nearly as much detail and documentation as dissertations.

Theses and Dissertations

Most doctoral degrees are granted on the successful completion of an empirical research project. Empirical theses are sometimes required of master's degree candidates as well. Theses and dissertations typically document completely the steps performed in carrying out the research investigation. Faculty members overseeing the project must be able to judge whether the student has understood the research problem both substantively and methodologically. The length of most doctoral dissertations is between 150 and 250 typed or printed double-spaced pages.

Most universities have a preferred format for their dissertations, but the following format is fairly typical:

Preliminary Pages
    Title Page
    Acknowledgment Page
    Table of Contents
    List of Tables
    List of Figures
Main Body
    Chapter I. Introduction
    Chapter II. Review of the Literature
    Chapter III. Methods
    Chapter IV. Results
    Chapter V. Discussion and Summary
Supplementary Pages
    Bibliography
    Appendix

The preliminary pages for a dissertation are much the same as those for a scholarly book. The title page indicates the title of the study, the author's name, the degree requirement being fulfilled, the name of the university awarding the degree, the date of submission of the report, and the signatures of the dissertation committee members. The acknowledgment page gives the writer the opportunity to express appreciation to those who contributed to the completion of the project. The table of contents outlines the major sections and subsections of the report, indicating on which page the reader will find those sections of interest. The lists of tables and figures identify by number, title, and page the tables and figures that appear in the text.

The main body of a dissertation incorporates those sections that were described earlier. The literature review often is so extensive for doctoral dissertations that a separate chapter may be devoted to it. When a short review is sufficient, the first two chapters may be combined. In some cases, a separate chapter may also be required to elaborate the study's conceptual framework.

The supplementary pages include a bibliography or list of references used to prepare the report, and one or more appendixes. An appendix contains information and materials relevant to the study that are either too lengthy or too unimportant to be incorporated into the body of the report. Data collection instruments, listings of special computer programs, detailed scoring instructions, cover letters, permission letters, listings of the raw data, codebooks, category schemes, and peripheral statistical tables are examples of the kinds of materials included in the appendix. Some universities also require the inclusion of a brief *curriculum vitae,* or autobiography, of the author.

Journal Articles

Progress in nursing research depends on researchers' efforts to share their work with others. Dissertations and final reports to funders are rarely read by more than a handful of individuals. They are too lengthy and too inaccessible for widespread use. Publication in a professional journal ensures broadest possible circulation of scientific findings. From a personal point of view, it is exciting and professionally advantageous to have one or more publications.

A journal article generally follows the same form as that for the main body of a thesis, but articles are much shorter. The purpose of an article is not to demonstrate research competence but rather to communicate the contribution that the study makes to knowledge. Because readers are particularly interested in the findings of a research project, a relatively large proportion of the journal report normally is devoted to the results and discussion sections. For

the sake of economy of journal space, the typical research article is only about 10 to 25 typewritten double-spaced pages.

Several nursing journals accept research articles for publication. *Nursing Research,* which is published six times annually, is a major communication outlet for research in the field of nursing and has been published for four decades. Other nursing journals that focus primarily on empirical studies are *Advances in Nursing Science, Applied Nursing Research, Clinical Nursing Research, Qualitative Health Research, Research in Nursing and Health,* and the *Western Journal of Nursing Research.* Nursing journals that are not devoted exclusively or even primarily to research but do accept research reports for publication include the *American Journal of Nursing; Heart and Lung; Image; Nursing Forum; Journal of Advanced Nursing; Journal of Obstetric, Gynecologic, and Neonatal Nursing; Oncology Nursing Forum; Psychiatric Nursing Forum; Public Health Nursing;* and the *Journal of Gerontological Nursing.* Many journals that do not directly focus on nursing also publish articles by nurse authors, such as *The American Journal of Public Health, Journal of School Health, Journal of Adolescent Health,* and numerous others.

The prospective author should check through recent issues of journals under consideration for guidance concerning the journals' stylistic requirements and content coverage. Many publications make an explicit statement concerning the type of manuscripts they are seeking. Swanson, McCloskey, and Bodensteiner (1991) prepared a valuable report on publishing opportunities for nurses in journals. This article includes information on the circulation of the journal, number of copies of a manuscript required for submission, typical article word length, time needed to arrive at an editorial decision, and acceptance rate for 92 U.S. journals in nursing and related health fields.

When the manuscript is finally prepared for journal submission, the required number of copies should be sent to the editor with a brief cover letter indicating the mailing address of at least one author.* Generally, the receipt of the manuscript is acknowledged immediately, but the final decision concerning the paper's acceptance or rejection may require several months.

Many journals have a policy of independent, anonymous (sometimes referred to as *blind*) *peer reviews* by two or more knowledgeable people. By anonymous, we mean that the reviewers do not know the identity of the authors of the article, and the authors do not learn the identity of the reviewers. Journals that have such a policy are sometimes described as *refereed journals* and are generally more prestigious than nonrefereed journals.

Accepted manuscripts almost invariably are revised somewhat, either by the authors at the editor's request or by the editorial staff of the journal. If the manuscript is not accepted, authors are usually sent copies of the reviewers' comments or a summary of the reasons for its rejection. This information can be used to revise a manuscript before submitting it to another journal.

Presentations at Professional Conferences

Numerous professional organizations sponsor annual national meetings at which research activities are presented, either through the reading of a research report or through visual display in a poster session. The American Nurses' Association is an example of an organization that holds meetings where nurses have an opportunity to share their knowledge with others interested in their research topic. Many local chapters of Sigma Theta Tau devote one or more of their annual activities to research reports. Examples of regional organizations that sponsor research conferences are the Western Society for Research in Nursing, the Southern Council on Collegiate Education for Nursing,

the Eastern Nursing Research Society of MARNA/NEON, and the Midwest Nursing Research Society. Other nursing organizations such as the Society for Research in Nursing Education, the American Association of Critical Care Nurses, the American Association of Neurosurgical Nurses, the Congress of Nursing in Child Health, and many others sponsor research conferences.

Presentation of research results at a conference has at least two advantages over journal publication. First, there is generally less time elapsed between the completion of a research project and its communication to others when a presentation is made at a meeting. Second, there is an opportunity for dialogue between the researcher and the audience at a professional conference. The listeners can request clarification on certain points and can suggest interesting modifications to the research paradigm. For this reason, a professional conference is a particularly good forum for presenting results to a clinical audience. At professional conferences, researchers also can take advantage of meeting and talking with others who are working on the same or similar problems in different parts of the country.

The mechanism for submitting a presentation to a conference is somewhat simpler than in the case of journal submission. The association sponsoring the conference ordinarily publishes a *Call for Papers* in its newsletter or journal about 6 to 9 months before the meeting date. The notice indicates requirements and deadlines for submitting a paper. The journal *Nursing Research* publishes a Call for Papers section as one of its regular departments, and most universities and major health care agencies also receive and post Call for Papers notices. Usually, an abstract of 500 to 1000 words is submitted rather than a full paper. If the submission is accepted, the researcher is committed to appear at the conference to make a presentation.

Papers of empirical work presented at professional meetings follow much the same format as a journal article. The report is typically condensed because the time allotted for presen-

* By convention, the ordering of authors' names on a research report usually is alphabetic if authors have contributed equally, or in order of the importance of their contribution if otherwise. See Waltz, Nelson, & Chambers (1985) and Hanson (1988) for a discussion of author credits.

tation usually ranges from 10 to 20 minutes. Therefore, only the most important aspects of the study can be included in the paper. A handy rule of thumb is that a page of double-spaced text requires 2½ to 3 minutes to read aloud. Presentations are usually more effective, however, if they are informal summaries of research than if they are read verbatim from a written text.

Researchers sometimes elect to present their findings in a *poster session*. In such a session, several researchers simultaneously present visual displays summarizing the highlights of the study, and conference attendees circulate around the room perusing these displays. In this fashion, those interested in a particular topic can devote considerable time to discussing the study with the researcher and avoid those posters dealing with topics of lesser personal interest. Poster sessions are thus efficient and encourage one-on-one discussions. Several nurse researchers have prepared useful tips for poster sessions (e.g., Lippman & Ponton, 1989; McDaniel, Bach, & Poole, 1993; Ryan, 1989).

❖ TIPS FOR WRITING RESEARCH REPORTS

If you are beginning to write a research report for the first time, the following suggestions may help you to get started:

- Do not begin to write until you have carefully examined a high-quality research report that you can use as a model. If you are writing a manuscript for submission to a journal, select as a model a journal article on a topic similar to your own. If you are preparing a dissertation, you are less likely to be able to find a model on a similar topic—but it is more important to find a dissertation that is considered to be of exceptional quality. Your adviser may be able to suggest a good example.
- If you are reporting quantitative findings, do not repeat all statistical information in both the text and in tables. Tables should be used to display information that would be monot-

onous to present in the text—and to display it in such a way that the numbers and patterns among the numbers are more comprehensible. The text can then be used to highlight the major thrust of the tables.

- It is usually best to limit the number of tables in a manuscript for journal submission to 4 or 5 tables because tables are complicated and expensive to typeset. Tables (and figures) should be numbered for easy reference. If you use tables, be sure that you reference each one in the text.
- It is often useful to study carefully tables presented in research journals to acquaint yourself with the format and content normally considered appropriate for reporting the kinds of analysis other researchers have undertaken. Because some people do not like to read tables, it is best to keep them as simple as possible. A cluttered table with hundreds of numbers in it is daunting to even a seasoned researcher—and even more so to a clinical nurse who is reading research to keep up with a field. It is usually unnecessary to report numbers beyond one decimal point (e.g., 10.2 rather than 10.18), and in some cases it might be better to round to the nearest whole number. Every table should have a concise but clearly explanatory title. Care should also be taken to use column headings that are clearly labeled and comprehensible.
- First drafts of research reports are almost never perfect. The assistance of a colleague or an adviser can be invaluable in improving the quality of a scientific paper. Objective criticism can often be achieved by simply putting the report aside for a few days and then rereading it with a fresh outlook. As a final check, you might want to subject your own manuscript to an evaluation according to the guidelines presented in Chapter 25.
- If you are hoping to publish your report in a journal, do not be too disheartened by a rejection. A rejection by one journal should not discourage you from sending the manuscript to another journal. The competition for jour-

nal space is keen, and a rejection does not necessarily mean that a study is unworthy of publication. Although it is considered unethical to submit an article to two journals simultaneously, manuscripts may need to be reviewed by several journals before final acceptance.

❖ SUMMARY

A research project is not complete until the results have been communicated in the form of a report. Despite some differences in the length, purposes, and audience of different types of research reports, the general form and content are similar. In general, the four major sections of a research report are the introduction, methods, results, and discussion.

The purpose of the introduction is to acquaint the reader with the research problem. This section includes the problem statement, the research hypothesis, a justification of the importance or value of the research, a summary of relevant related literature, the identification of a theoretical framework, and definitions of the concepts being studied. The methods section acquaints the reader with what the researcher did to solve the research problem. This section normally includes a description of the subjects, how they were selected, the instruments and procedures used to collect the data, and the techniques used to analyze the data. In the results section, the findings obtained from the analyses are summarized. Finally, the discussion section of a research report presents the researcher's interpretation of the results, a consideration of the study's limitations, and recommendations for future research and for utilization of the findings.

Scientific communications should be written as simply and clearly as possible. Emotionally laden statements and overtly subjective statements should be excluded from research reports. Various reference manuals exist to assist the researcher in selecting a consistent and acceptable style for noting references and han-

dling other technical aspects of report writing. The style should be congruent with that of the university or journal to which the report is submitted.

The major types of research reports are theses and dissertations, reports to funding agencies, journal articles, and presentations at professional meetings. When space or time are at a premium—as in the case of journal articles and conference papers—detail should be kept to a minimum. In other types of reports, however, extensive documentation may be required.

❖ STUDY SUGGESTIONS

Chapter 24 of the accompanying *Study Guide for Nursing Research: Principles and Methods, 5th ed.*, offers various exercises and study suggestions for reinforcing the concepts presented in this chapter. Additionally, the following questions can be addressed:

1. Write an abstract for an article appearing in a 1992 or 1993 issue of the *Western Journal of Nursing Research*. Compare your abstract with that written by a classmate.
2. What are the similarities and differences of research reports that are written for journal publication and for presentation at a professional meeting?
3. Read a research report. Now write a two- to three-page summary of the report that communicates the major points of the report to a clinical audience with minimal research skills.

❖ SUGGESTED READINGS

METHODOLOGICAL/STYLISTIC REFERENCES

Aaronson, L. S. (1994). Milking data or meeting commitments: How many papers from one study? *Nursing Research, 43,* 60–62.

American Medical Association. (1989). *American Medical Association manual of style* (8th ed.). Baltimore: Williams & Wilkins.

American Psychological Association. (1983). *Publication manual of the American Psychological Association* (3rd ed.). Washington, DC: Author.

Burns, N. (1989). Standards for qualitative research. *Nursing Science Quarterly, 2,* 44–52.

Ehrenberg, A. S. C. (1977). Rudiments of numeracy. *Journal of the Royal Statistical Society, 140* (part 3), 277–297.

Fuller, E. O. (1983). Preparing an abstract of a nursing study. *Nursing Research, 32,* 316–317.

Gay, J. T., & Edgil, A. E. (1989). When your manuscript is rejected. *Nursing and Health Care, 10,* 459–461.

Hanson, S. M. H. (1988). Collaborative research and authorship credit: Beginning guidelines. *Nursing Research, 37,* 49–52.

Hayes, P. (1992). "De-jargonizing" research communication. *Clinical Nursing Research, 1,* 219–220.

Huth, E. J. (1990). *How to write and publish papers in the medical sciences.* (2nd ed.). Philadelphia: Institute for Scientific Information.

Jackle, M. (1989). Presenting research to nurses in clinical practice. *Applied Nursing Research, 2,* 191–193.

Johnson, S. H. (1982). Selecting a journal. *Nursing and Health Care, 3,* 258–263.

Juhl, N., & Norman, V. L. (1989). Writing an effective abstract. *Applied Nursing Research, 2,* 189–191.

Knafl, K. A., & Howard, M. T. (1984). Interpreting and reporting qualitative research. *Research in Nursing and Health, 7,* 17–24.

Kolin, P. C., & Kolin, J. L. (1980). *Professional writing for nurses in education, practice, and research.* St. Louis: C. V. Mosby.

Lippman, D. T., & Ponton, K. S. (1989). Designing a research poster with impact. *Western Journal of Nursing Research, 11,* 477–485.

Markman, R. H., & Waddell, M. J. (1989). *Ten steps in writing the research paper* (4th ed.). Woodbury, NY: Barron's Educational Series.

McDaniel, R. W., Bach, C. A., & Poole, M. J. (1993). Poster update: Getting their attention. *Nursing Research, 42,* 302–304.

McKinney, V., & Burns, N. (1993). The effective presentation of graphs. *Nursing Research, 42,* 250–252.

Mirin, S. K. (1981). *The nurse's guide to writing for publication.* Wakefield, MA: Nursing Resources.

Ryan, N. M. (1989). Developing and presenting a research poster. *Applied Nursing Research, 2,* 52–55.

Selby, M., Tornquist, E., & Finerty, E. (1989). How to present your research. *Nursing Outlook, 37,* 172–175.

Strunk, W., Jr., & White, E. B. (1979). *The elements of style* (3rd ed.). New York: Macmillan.

Swanson, E., & McCloskey, J. (1982). The manuscript review process of nursing journals. *Image, 14,* 72–76.

Swanson, E., McCloskey, J., & Bodensteiner, A. (1991). Publishing opportunities for nurses: A comparison of 92 U.S. journals. *Image, 23,* 33–38.

Tornquist, E. M. (1986). *From proposal to publication: An informal guide to writing about nursing research.* Menlo Park, CA: Addison-Wesley.

Tornquist, E. M., Funk, S. G., & Champagne, M. T. (1989). Writing research reports for clinical audiences. *Western Journal of Nursing Research, 11,* 576–582.

University of Chicago Press. (1993). *The Chicago manual of style* (15th ed.). Chicago: Author.

Van Till, W. (1985). *Writing for professional publication* (2nd ed.). Boston: Allyn & Bacon.

Waltz, C. F., Nelson, B., & Chambers, S. B. (1985). Assigning publication credits. *Nursing Outlook, 33,* 233–238.

SUBSTANTIVE REFERENCES

Baker, C. F., Garvin, B. J., Kennedy, C. W., & Polivka, B. J. (1993). The effect of environmental sound and communication on CCU patients' heart rate and blood pressure. *Research in Nursing and Health, 16,* 415–421.

Bailey, B. J., & Kahn, A. (1993). Apportioning illness management authority: How diabetic individuals evaluate and respond to spousal help. *Qualitative Health Research, 3,* 55–73.

Brown, M. A., & Lewis, L. L. (1993). Cycle-phase changes in perceived stress in women with varying levels of premenstrual symptomatology. *Research in Nursing and Health, 16,* 423–429.

Cloonan, P. A., & Belyea, M. J. (1993). Limits of using patient characteristics in predicting home health care coordination. *Western Journal of Nursing Research, 15,* 742–751.

DiIorio, C., van Lier, D., & Manteuffel, B. (1992). Patterns of nausea during first trimester of pregnancy. *Clinical Nursing Research, 1,* 127–140.

Drummond, J. E., McBride, M. L., & Wiebe, C. F.

(1993). The development of mothers' understanding of infant crying. *Clinical Nursing Research, 2,* 396–410.

Friedman, M. M. (1993). Social support sources and psychological well-being in older women with heart disease. *Research in Nursing and Health, 16,* 405–413.

Gamble, D., & Morse, J. M. (1993). Fathers of breastfed infants: Postponing and types of involvement. *Journal of Gynecologic, Obstetric, and Neonatal Nursing, 22,* 358–365.

Herth, K. A. (1993). Humor and the older adult. *Applied Nursing Research, 6,* 146–153.

Hogan, N. S., & DeSantis, L. (1994). Things that help and hinder adolescent sibling bereavement. *Western Journal of Nursing Research, 16,* 132–145.

Kim, M. J., Larson, J. L., Covey, M. K., Vitalo, C. A., Alex, C. G., & Patel, M. (1993). Inspiratory muscle training in patients with chronic obstructive pulmonary disease. *Nursing Research, 42,* 356–362.

Kolanowski, A., Hurwitz, S., Taylor, L. A., Evans, L., & Strumpf, N. (1994). Contextual factors associated with disturbing behaviors in institutionalized elders. *Nursing Research, 43,* 73–79.

Laschinger, H. K. S., & Goldenberg, D. (1993). Attitudes of practicing nurses as predictors of intended care behavior with persons who are HIV positive. *Research in Nursing and Health, 16,* 441–450.

Metheny, N., Reed, L., Wiersma, L., McSweeney, M., Wehrle, M., & Clark, J. (1993). Effectiveness of pH measurements in predicting feeding tube placement: An update. *Nursing Research, 42,* 324–331.

Munro, B. H., Jacobsen, B. S., & Brooten, D. A. (1994). Re-examination of the psychometric characteristics of the LaMonica-Oberst Patient Satisfaction Scale. *Research in Nursing and Health, 17,* 119–125.

Patterson, E. T., Douglas, A. B., Patterson, P. M., & Bradle, J. B. (1992). Symptoms of preterm labor and self-diagnostic confusion. *Nursing Research, 41,* 367–372.

Robinson, C. A. (1993). Managing life with a chronic condition: The story of normalization. *Qualitative Health Research, 3,* 6–28.

Saint-Germain, M. A., Bassford, T. L., & Montano, G. (1993). Surveys and focus groups in health research with older Hispanic women. *Qualitative Health Research, 3,* 341–367.

Stevens, B. J., Johnston, C. C., & Horton, L. (1993). Multidimensional pain assessment in premature neonates. *Journal of Gynecologic, Obstetric, and Neonatal Nursing, 22,* 531–541.

Swanson, J. M., & Chenitz, W. C. (1993). Regaining a valued self: The process of adaptation to living with genital herpes. *Qualitative Health Research, 3,* 270–297.

Troy, N. W. (1993). Early contact and maternal attachment among women using public health care facilities. *Applied Nursing Research, 6,* 161–166.

Chapter 25

EVALUATING RESEARCH REPORTS

Research in a practicing profession such as nursing contributes not only scholarly knowledge but also information concerning how that practice can be improved. Nursing research, then, has relevance for all nurses, not just the minority of nurses who actually engage in research projects. As professionals, nurses should possess skills to evaluate reports of research in their field. We hope that this text has provided a foundation for the development of such skills. In this chapter, more specific guidelines for the critical and intelligent review of research are presented.

❖ THE RESEARCH CRITIQUE

If nursing practice is to be based on a solid foundation of scientific knowledge, then the worth of studies appearing in the nursing literature must be critically appraised. Sometimes consumers have the mistaken belief that if a research report was accepted for publication, then it must be a good study. Unfortunately, this is not the case. Indeed, *most* research has limitations and weaknesses, and for this reason, no

single study can provide unchallengeable answers to research inquiries. Nevertheless, the scientific method continues to provide us with the best possible means of answering certain questions. Knowledge is accumulated not by an individual researcher conducting a single, isolated study but rather through the conduct—and the evaluation—of several studies addressing the same or similar research questions. Thus, consumers who can thoughtfully critique research reports also have a role to play in the advancement of scientific knowledge.

Critiquing Research Decisions

Although no single study is infallible, there is a tremendous range in the quality of studies—from nearly worthless to exemplary. The quality of the research is closely tied to the kinds of decisions the researcher makes in conceptualizing, designing, and executing the study and in interpreting and communicating the study results. Each study tends to have its own peculiar flaws because each researcher, in addressing the same or a similar research question, makes somewhat different decisions about how the study should be done. It is not uncommon for researchers who have made different research decisions to arrive at different answers to the same research question. It is precisely for this reason that consumers of research must be knowledgeable about the research process. As a consumer, you must be able to evaluate the decisions that investigators made so that you can determine how much faith should be put in their conclusions. The consumer must ask, What other approaches could have been used to study this research problem? and If another approach had been used, would the results have been more reliable, believable, or replicable? In other words, the consumer must evaluate the impact of the researcher's decisions on the study's ability to reveal the truth.

Much of this book has been designed to acquaint consumers with a range of methodological options for the conduct of research—options on how to develop a research design, collect and analyze data, select a study sample, operationalize variables, and so on. We hope that an acquaintance with these options has provided you with the tools to challenge a researcher's decisions and to suggest alternative methods.

Purpose of a Research Critique

Research reports are evaluated for a variety of purposes. Students are often asked to prepare a critique to demonstrate their mastery of methodological and analytic skills. Seasoned researchers are sometimes asked to write critiques of manuscripts to help journal editors make publication decisions or to accompany the report as published commentaries.* Journal clubs in clinical or other settings may meet periodically to critique and discuss research studies. For all these purposes, the goal is generally to develop a balanced evaluation of the study's contribution to knowledge.

A research critique is not just a review or summary of a study; rather, it is a careful, critical appraisal of the strengths and limitations of a piece of research. A written critique should serve as a guide to researchers and practitioners. The critique also should inform the research community of the ways in which the study results may have been compromised, and it should alert them to how to better go about addressing the research question. The critique should thus help to advance a particular area of knowledge. When the audience is clinical nurses, the critique should help those who are practicing nursing to decide how the findings from the study can best be incorporated into their practice, if at all.

The function of critical evaluations of scientific work is not to hunt for and expose mistakes. A good critique objectively and critically identifies adequacies and inadequacies, virtues as well as faults. Sometimes the need for such balance is obscured by the terms *critique* and *critical appraisal,* which connote unfavorable observations. The merits of a study are as important as its limitations in coming to conclusions about the worth of its findings. Therefore, the research critique should reflect a thoughtful, objective, and balanced consideration of the study's validity and significance. If the critique is not balanced, then it will be of little utility to the researcher who conducted the study because it might engender defensiveness, and the practitioner may erroneously get the impression that the study has no merit at all.

Box 25-1 summarizes general guidelines to consider in preparing a written research critique. In the section that follows, we present some specific guidelines for evaluating various aspects of a research report.

❖ ELEMENTS OF A RESEARCH CRITIQUE

Each research report has several important dimensions that should be considered in a critical evaluation of the study's worth. In this section,

---

* The *Western Journal of Nursing Research,* for example, usually publishes a research report followed by one or two commentaries that include appraisals of the report.

BOX 25-1   GUIDELINES FOR THE CONDUCT OF A WRITTEN RESEARCH CRITIQUE

1. Be sure to comment on the study's strengths as well as its weaknesses. The critique should be a balanced consideration of the worth of the research. Each research report has at least *some* positive features—be sure to find them and note them.
2. Give specific examples of the study's weaknesses and strengths. Avoid vague generalities of praise and fault finding.
3. Try to justify your criticisms. Offer a rationale for how a different approach would have solved a problem that the researcher failed to address.
4. Be as objective as possible. Try to avoid being overly critical of a study because you are not particularly interested in the topic or because you have a bias against a certain research approach (e.g., qualitative vs. quantitative).
5. Without sacrificing objectivity, be sensitive in handling negative comments. Try to put yourself in the shoes of the researcher receiving the critical appraisal. Try not to be condescending or sarcastic.
6. Suggest alternatives that the researcher (or future researchers) might want to consider. Do not just identify the problems in the research study—offer some recommended solutions, making sure that the recommendations are practical ones.
7. Evaluate all aspects of the study—its substantive, methodological, interpretive, ethical, and presentational dimensions.

we review the substantive and theoretical, methodological, interpretive, ethical, and presentational and stylistic dimensions of a study.

Substantive and Theoretical Dimensions

The reviewer needs to determine whether the study was an important one in terms of the significance of the problem studied, the soundness of the conceptualizations, and the creativity and appropriateness of the theoretical framework. The research problem is one that should have obvious relevance to some aspect of the nursing profession. It is not enough that a problem be interesting if it offers no possibility of contributing to nursing knowledge or improving nursing practice. Even before the reader learns *how* a study was conducted, there should be an evaluation of whether the study should have been conducted in the first place.

The reader's own disciplinary orientation should not intrude in an objective evaluation of the study's significance. A clinical nurse might not be intrigued by a study focusing on the determinants of nursing turnover, but a nursing administrator trying to improve staffing decisions might find such a study highly useful. Similarly, a psychiatric nurse might find little value in a study of the sleep–wake patterns of low-birthweight infants, but nurses in neonatal intensive care units might not agree. It is important, then, not to adopt a myopic view of the study's importance and relevance to nursing.

Many problems that are relevant to nursing are still not necessarily substantively worthwhile. The reviewer must ask a question such as, Given what we know about this topic, is this research the right next step? Knowledge tends to be incremental. Researchers must consider how to advance knowledge on a topic in the most beneficial way. They should avoid unnecessary replications of a study once a body of research clearly points to an answer, but they should also not leap several steps ahead when there is an insecure foundation. Sometimes replication is exactly what is needed to enhance the believability or generalizability of earlier findings.

A final issue to consider is whether the researcher has appropriately placed the research problem into some larger theoretical context. As we stressed in Chapter 5, a researcher does little to enhance the value of the study if the connection between the research problem and a conceptual framework is artificial and contrived. However, a specific research problem that is genuinely framed as a part of some larger intellectual problem can generally go much farther in advancing knowledge than a problem that ignores its theoretical underpinnings.

The substantive and theoretical dimensions of a study are normally communicated to readers in the introduction to a report. The manner in which the introductory materials are presented is vital to the proper understanding and appreciation of what the researcher has accomplished. Specific guidelines for critiquing the introduction of a research report are presented in Boxes 25-2 through 25-4.* Box 25-2 provides guidelines for critiquing the researcher's statement of the problem and the hypotheses. Boxes 25-3 and 25-4 suggest considerations relevant to a critique of the literature review and conceptual framework, respectively.

Methodological Dimensions

Once a research problem has been identified, the researcher must make a number of important decisions regarding how to go about answering the research questions or testing the research hypotheses. It is the consumer's job to evaluate the consequences of those decisions. In fact, the heart of the research critique lies in the analysis of the methodological decisions adopted in addressing the research question. Although the researcher makes hundreds of methodologically relevant decisions in conducting a study, the four major decisions on which the consumer should focus critical attention are as follows:

Decision 1. What design should be used that will yield the most meaningful, unambiguous, and valid results about either the relationship between the independent and dependent variable or the nature of the phenomena under study?

---

* The questions included in the boxes in this chapter are not exhaustive. Many additional questions will need to be raised in dealing with a particular piece of research. Moreover, the boxes include many questions that do not apply to every piece of research. The questions are intended to represent a useful point of departure in undertaking a critique.

BOX 25-2   GUIDELINES FOR CRITIQUING PROBLEM STATEMENTS AND HYPOTHESES

1. Does the research report clearly present the research problem? Was the problem statement introduced promptly? Was it placed in a logical and easy-to-find location?
2. Does the problem have significance to the nursing profession, and does the researcher describe what that significance is?
3. Does the problem seem sensible and justifiable? Does it flow from prior scientific information, experience in the topic area, or a theory? In the context of current knowledge on the topic, is the problem the right one to address?
4. Has the researcher appropriately delimited the scope of the problem, or is the problem too big or complex for a single investigation?
5. Does the problem statement clearly identify the research variables and the nature of the population being studied? Are the research variables adequately defined? Is the problem statement clearly and concisely articulated?
6. Does the research report contain formally stated hypotheses? If not, is their absence justifiable? Are the hypotheses directly and logically tied to the research problem?
7. Do the hypotheses flow logically from the theoretical framework or from prior research? If not, is adequate justification offered for the researcher's predictions?
8. Can the hypotheses be tested in such a way that it is clear whether the hypotheses are supported?
9. Are the hypotheses properly worded? Does each hypothesis express a predicted relationship between two or more variables? Are they worded clearly and objectively and written as a stated prediction?
10. Are the hypotheses stated as research hypotheses rather than as null hypotheses? Are the hypotheses directional? If not, is there a rationale for the nondirectional hypotheses?

BOX 25-3   GUIDELINES FOR CRITIQUING RESEARCH LITERATURE REVIEWS

1. Does the review seem thorough? Does it appear that the review includes all or most of the major studies that have been conducted on the topic of interest? Does the review include recent literature?
2. Is there an overdependence on secondary sources when primary sources could have been obtained?
3. Is there an overreliance on opinion articles and an underemphasis on research studies?
4. Does the content of the review relate directly to the research problem, or is it only peripherally related?
5. Is the review merely a summary of past work, or does it critically appraise and compare the contributions of key studies? Does it discuss weaknesses in existing studies and identify important gaps in the literature?
6. Is the review paraphrased adequately, or is it a string of quotations from the original sources?
7. Does the review use appropriate language, suggesting the tentativeness of prior findings? Is the review objective?
8. Is the review well organized? Is the development of ideas clear? Does the organization lay the foundation for undertaking the new study?
9. Does the review conclude with a brief synopsis of the state-of-the-art of the literature on the topic?

BOX 25-4   GUIDELINES FOR CRITIQUING THEORETICAL AND CONCEPTUAL FRAMEWORKS

1. Does the research report describe a theoretical or conceptual framework for the study? If not, does the absence of a theoretical framework detract from the usefulness or significance of the research?
2. Does the report adequately describe the major features of the theory so that readers can understand the conceptual basis of the study?
3. Is the theory appropriate to the research problem? Would a different theoretical framework have been more appropriate?
4. Is the theoretical framework based on a conceptual model of nursing, or is it borrowed from another discipline? Is there adequate justification for the researcher's decision about the type of framework used?
5. Do the research problem and hypothesis flow naturally from the theoretical framework, or does the link between the problem and theory seem contrived?
6. Are the deductions from the theory or conceptual framework logical?
7. Are all the concepts adequately defined in a way that is consistent with the theory?

Decision 4.   What analyses will provide the most appropriate and meaningful tests of the research hypotheses or answers to the research questions?

Because of practical constraints, research studies almost always involve making some compromises between what is ideal and what is feasible. For example, the researcher might ideally like to work with a sample of 1000 subjects, but because of limited resources, he or she might have to be content with a sample of 200 subjects. The person doing a research critique cannot realistically demand that researchers attain these methodological ideals but must be prepared to evaluate how much damage has been done by failure to achieve them.

After the reader evaluates the types of decisions that the researcher made, a further step

Decision 2.   Who should be the subjects of the study? What are the characteristics of the population to which the findings should be generalized? How large should be the sample of subjects be, where should they be recruited from, and what sampling approach should be used to select the sample?

Decision 3.   How should the research data be gathered? How can the validity and trustworthiness of the data be maximized?

is necessary. The reviewer must assess how well the research plan was actually executed. A well-conceived research plan may go awry because of time pressures, financial constraints, personnel changes, researcher inexperience, administrative problems, and so on. Therefore, the methodological aspects of a study must be critiqued not only as they were conceived but also as they were put into operation.

Various boxes are presented to guide the reader in performing a critical analysis of the research methods, which are generally described in the methods section of a research report. Box 25-5 presents guidelines for critiquing the overall research design. The sampling strategy and the researcher's selection of a target population can be evaluated using the questions included in Box 25-6.

Five separate boxes are included here to assist with a critique of the researcher's data collection plan. Explicit guidelines are provided for evaluating self-report approaches (Box 25-7); observational methods (Box 25-8); and biophysiologic measures (Box 25-9). Criteria are not provided for evaluating infrequently used data collection techniques, such as Q sorts and records. However, in addition to questions adapted from Boxes 25-7 through 25-9, other methods can be evaluated by considering one overarching question: Did the researcher's method of measurement and data collection yield the best possible measure of the key research variables? Box 25-10 provides suggestions for critiquing the actual procedures used to collect the data. Box 25-11 suggests some guidelines for evaluating the overall quality of the data.

BOX 25-5   GUIDELINES FOR CRITIQUING RESEARCH DESIGNS

1. Given the nature of the research question, what type of design is most appropriate? How much flexibility does the research question call for, and how much structure is needed?
2. Does the design involve an experimental intervention? Was the full nature of any intervention described in detail?
3. If there is an intervention, was a true experimental, quasi-experimental, or preexperimental design used? Should a more rigorous design have been used?
4. If the design is nonexperimental, what is the reason that the researcher decided not to manipulate the independent variable? Was this decision appropriate?
5. What types of comparisons are specified in the research design (e.g., before–after, the use of one or more comparison group)? Are these comparisons the most appropriate ones?
6. If the research design does not call for any comparisons, what difficulties, if any, does this pose for understanding what the results mean?
7. How many times were data collected or observations recorded? Is this number appropriate, given the research questions?
8. What procedures, if any, did the researcher use to control external (situational) factors? Were these procedures appropriate and adequate?
9. What procedures, if any, did the researcher use to control extraneous subject characteristics? Were these procedures appropriate and adequate?
10. To what extent did the design affect the internal validity of the study? What alternative explanations must be considered, given the design that was used?
11. To what extent did the design enhance the external validity of the study? Can the design be criticized for its artificiality, or praised for its realism?
12. Does the research design enable the researcher to draw causal inferences about the relationships among research variables?
13. What are the major limitations of the design used? Are these limitations acknowledged by the researcher?

BOX 25-6   GUIDELINES FOR CRITIQUING SAMPLING PLANS

1. Is the target or accessible population identified and described? Are the eligibility criteria clearly specified?
2. Given the research problem and limitations on resources, is the target population appropriately designated? Would a more limited population specification have controlled for important sources of extraneous variation not covered by the research design?
3. Are the sample selection procedures clearly described? Does the report make clear whether probability or nonprobability sampling was used?
4. How were subjects recruited into the sample? Does the method suggest potential biases?
5. Is the sampling plan one that is likely to have produced a representative sample?
6. If the sampling plan is relatively weak (such as in the case of a convenience sample), are potential sample biases identified? If the sampling plan is relatively weak, is it justified on the basis of the nature of the problem?
7. Did some factor other than the sampling plan itself (such as a low rate of response) affect the representativeness of the sample?
8. Are the size and key characteristics of the sample described?
9. Is the sample sufficiently large? Was the sample size justified on the basis of a power analysis?
10. To whom can the study results reasonably be generalized?

The researcher's analytic plan is the final methodological area that requires a critical analysis. The analytic strategy is sometimes presented in the methods section of a research report but is usually more fully explicated in the results section, where the actual findings are reported. Box 25-12 lists a number of guiding questions of relevance for evaluating quantitative analyses, and Box 25-13 identifies questions for qualitative analyses. When a study has used both qualitative and quantitative analyses, questions from both boxes are likely to be applicable. In addition, the reader should ask: Were the qualitative and quantitative analyses meaningfully integrated, and did they complement each other in appropriate ways?

Interpretive Dimensions

Research reports almost always conclude with a Discussion, Conclusions, or Implications section. It is in this final section that the researcher attempts to make sense of the analyses, to understand what the findings mean in relation to the research hypotheses, to consider whether the findings support or fail to support a theoretical framework, and to discuss what the findings might mean for the nursing profession. Inevitably, the discussion section is more subjective than other sections of the report. This subjectivity is not necessarily detrimental because great insights spring from researchers' personal experience, knowledge, and creative capacities—not from the data themselves. However, subjectivity can sometimes block insights if researchers read into the data only what they want to see.

The task of the reviewer is generally to contrast his or her own interpretation with that of the researcher and to challenge conclusions that do not appear to be warranted by the empirical results. If the reviewer's objective reading of the research methods and study findings leads to an interpretation that is notably different from that endorsed by the researcher, then the interpretive dimension of the study may well be faulty. Box 25-14 presents questions to assist readers in assessing the researcher's conclusions.

Ethical Dimensions

The person performing a research critique should consider whether there is any evidence that the rights of human subjects were violated

BOX 25-7   GUIDELINES FOR CRITIQUING SELF-REPORTS

Interviews/Questionnaires

1. Does the research question lend itself to a self-report approach? Would an alternative method have been more appropriate?
2. Is the degree of structure of the researcher's approach consistent with the nature of the research question?
3. Do the questions posed to respondents adequately cover the complexities of the problem under investigation?
4. Did the researcher use the best possible mode for the collection of self-report data (i.e., personal interview, telephone interview, self-administered questionnaire), given the nature of the research question and the characteristics of the respondents? Would an alternative mode have improved the quality of data collected?
5. Was there an appropriate balance of open-ended and closed-ended questions?
6. [If an instrument is included for review] Are the questions clearly worded? Do the questions tend to bias responses in a certain direction? Do response options to closed-ended questions adequately cover the alternatives? Is the ordering of questions appropriate? Are the questions sensitively worded to minimize psychological distress?
7. Was there an appropriate number of questions? Was the instrument too long? Too brief?
8. Was the instrument adequately pretested?
9. Was the response rate adequately high? Did the researcher take steps to produce a high response rate? Does the researcher discuss the nature and extent of biases (if any) resulting from nonresponse?

Scales

10. If a scale was used, is its relevance to the objectives of the study clearly explained? Does it, in fact, adequately capture the construct of interest?
11. If a new scale was developed, is there adequate justification for failure to use an existing one? Was the new scale pretested and refined?
12. Is the rationale for selecting one scaling procedure as opposed to another (e.g., Likert vs. semantic differential) explained? Is the rationale convincing?
13. Is the scale sufficiently long?
14. Are procedures for eliminating or minimizing response-set biases described, and are they appropriate? For example, are negative and positive items counterbalanced?

---

during the course of the investigation. If there are any potential ethical problems, then the reviewer must consider the impact of those problems on the scientific merit of the study on the one hand and on subjects' well-being on the other. Guidelines for evaluating the ethical dimensions of a research report are presented in Box 25-15.

There are two main types of ethical transgressions in research studies. The first class consists of inadvertent actions or activities that the researcher did not interpret as creating an ethical dilemma. For example, in a study that examined married couples' experiences with sexually transmitted diseases, the researcher might inadvertently have scheduled the interview at a time when privacy for the members of the couple could not be ensured.

In other cases, the researcher may have been aware of having committed some violation of ethical principles, but made a conscious decision that the violation was relatively minor in relation to the knowledge that could be gained by doing the study in a certain way. For example, the researcher may have decided not to obtain informed consent from the parents of minor children attending a family planning clinic because to require such consent would probably

BOX 25-8 GUIDELINES FOR CRITIQUING OBSERVATIONAL METHODS

1. Does the research question lend itself to an observational approach? Would an alternative method have been more appropriate?
2. Is the degree of structure of the observational method consistent with the nature of the research question?
3. To what degree were the observers concealed during data collection? What effect might their presence have had on the behaviors and events they were observing?
4. What was the unit of analysis in the study? How much inference was required on the part of the observers, and to what extent did this lead to a potential for bias?
5. Where did the observations actually take place? To what extent did the setting influence the "naturalness" of the behaviors being observed?
6. How were data actually recorded (e.g., on field notes or checklists)? Did the recording procedure appear appropriate?
7. What steps were taken to minimize observer biases? For example, how were observers trained? How detailed were the explanations of the behaviors to be recorded?
8. If a category scheme was developed, was it exhaustive? Was the scheme overly demanding of observers, leading to the potential for inaccurate data? If the scheme was not exhaustive, did the omission of large realms of subject behavior lead to an inadequate context for understanding the behaviors of interest? Do the categories included in the instrument adequately cover the relevant behaviors?
9. What was the plan by which events or behaviors were sampled for observation? Did this plan appear to yield a representative sample of relevent behaviors?

BOX 25-9 GUIDELINES FOR CRITIQUING BIOPHYSIOLOGIC MEASURES

1. Does the research question lend itself to a biophysiologic approach? Would an alternative method have been more appropriate?
2. Was the proper instrumentation used to obtain the biophysiologic measurements? Would an alternative instrument or method have been more appropriate? Did the researcher present a rationale for the use of the particular method, and was that rationale convincing?
3. Were the procedures for data collection adequately described? Did the procedures appear to be appropriate?
4. Does the report suggest that care was taken to obtain accurate data? For example, did the researcher's activities permit accurate recording if an instrument system without recording equipment was used?
5. Does the researcher appear to have the skills necessary for proper interpretation of the biophysiologic measurements?

6, the reviewer must evaluate the decision itself *and* the researcher's rationale.

The reviewer who comments on the ethical aspects of a study based on a report of completed research is obviously too late to prevent an ethical transgression from occurring. Nevertheless, the critique can bring the ethical problems to the attention of those who may be replicating the research.

Presentational and Stylistic Dimensions

Although the worth of the study itself is primarily reflected in the dimensions we have reviewed thus far, the manner in which the information is communicated in the research report is also fair game in a comprehensive critical appraisal. Box 25-16 summarizes the major points that should be considered in evaluating the presentation of a research report.

have dramatically reduced the number of minors willing to participate in the research and would have lead to a biased sample of clinic users; it could also have violated the minors' right to confidential treatment at the clinic. When the researcher knowingly elects not to follow the ethical principles outlined in Chapter

BOX 25-10   GUIDELINES FOR CRITIQUING DATA COLLECTION PROCEDURES

1. Who collected the research data? Were the data collectors appropriate, or is there something about them (e.g., their professional role, their prior relationship with subjects) that could undermine the collection of unbiased, high-quality data?
2. How were the data collectors trained? Were steps taken to improve their ability to elicit or produce high-quality data? Were steps taken to evaluate their performance?
3. Where and under what circumstances were the data gathered? Were others present during the data collection? Could the presence of others have created any distortions?
4. To what risks did the subjects expose themselves in providing the research data (e.g., admitting to criminal behavior or putting themselves in a bad light)? How might these risks have introduced biases? What, if anything, did the researcher do to minimize such biases?
5. Did the collection of data place any undue burdens (in terms of time or stress) on subjects? How might this have affected data quality?

BOX 25-11   GUIDELINES FOR EVALUATING DATA QUALITY

1. Does there appear to be a strong congruence between the research variables as conceptualized (i.e., as discussed in the introduction) and as operationalized (i.e., as discussed in the methods section)?

Quantitative Data

2. If operational definitions (or scoring procedures) are specified, do they clearly indicate the rules of measurement? Do the rules seem reasonable?
3. Does the report provide any evidence of the reliability of the data? Does the evidence come from the research sample itself, or is it based on other studies? If the latter, is it reasonable to believe that data quality would be the same for the research sample as for the reliability sample?
4. If there is evidence of reliability, which estimation method was used? Was this method appropriate? Should an alternative or additional method of reliability appraisal have been used? Is the reliability adequate?
5. If the report does not provide evidence of the reliability of the measures, are there any indications of efforts the researcher made to minimize errors of measurement?
6. Does the report offer any evidence of the validity of the measures? Does the evidence come from the research sample itself, or is it based on other studies? If the latter, is it reasonable to believe that data quality would be the same for the research sample as for the validation sample?
7. If there is evidence of validity, which validity approach was used? Was this approach appropriate? Should an alternative or additional method of validation have been used? Does the validity of the instrument appear to be adequate?
8. Were the research hypotheses supported? If not, might data quality play a role in the failure of the hypotheses to be confirmed?

Qualitative Data

9. Does the research report discuss efforts the researcher made to enhance or evaluate the trustworthiness of the data? If so, is the documentation sufficiently detailed and clear? If not, is there other information that allows readers to conclude that the data are believable?
10. Which techniques (if any) did the researcher use to enhance and appraise data quality? Was any type of triangulation used? Were there member checks? Was there an external audit of the data? How adequate were the procedures? What techniques could have been used profitably to improve data quality?
11. Given the procedures that were used to enhance data quality, what can you conclude about the credibility, transferability, dependability, and confirmability of the data? Given this assessment, how much faith can be placed in the results of the study?

BOX 25-12   GUIDELINES FOR CRITIQUING QUANTITATIVE ANALYSES

1. Do the research data lend themselves to quantitative analysis? Would a qualitative approach to data analysis have been more appropriate?
2. Does the report include any descriptive statistics? Do these statistics sufficiently describe the major characteristics of the researcher's data set?
3. Were indices of both central tendency and variability provided in the report? If not, how does the absence of this information affect the reader's understanding of the research variables?
4. Were the correct descriptive statistics used (e.g., was a median used when a mean would have been more appropriate)?
5. Does the report include any inferential statistics? Was a statistical test performed for each of the hypotheses or research questions? If inferential statistics were not used, should they have been?
6. Was the selected statistical test appropriate, given the level of measurement of the variables?
7. Was a parametric test used? Does it appear that the assumptions for the use of parametric tests were met? If a nonparametric test was used, should a more powerful parametric procedure have been used instead?
8. Were any multivariate procedures used? If so, does it appear that the researcher chose the appropriate test? If multivariate procedures were not used, should they have been? Would the use of a multivariate procedure have improved the researcher's ability to draw conclusions about the relationship between the dependent and independent variables?
9. In general, does the research report provide a rationale for the researcher's decision to use certain statistical tests but not others? Does the report contain sufficient information for the reader to judge whether appropriate statistics were used?
10. Was there an appropriate amount of statistical information reported? Are the findings clearly and logically organized?
11. Were the results of any statistical tests significant? What do the tests tell the reader about the plausibility of the research hypotheses?
12. Were tables used judiciously to summarize large masses of statistical information? Are the tables clearly presented, with good titles and carefully labeled column headings? Is the information presented in the text consistent with the information presented in the tables? Is the information totally redundant?
13. Could the study have been strengthened by the inclusion of some qualitative data?

An important consideration is whether the research report has provided sufficient information for a thoughtful critique of the other dimensions. For example, if the report does not describe how the sample was selected, then the reviewer cannot comment on the adequacy of the sampling plan, but he or she can criticize the researcher's failure to include information on sampling. When vital pieces of information are missing, the researcher leaves the reader little choice but to assume the worst because this would lead to the most cautious interpretation of the results.

The writing in a research report, as in any published document, should be clear, grammatically correct, concise, and well-organized. Un-necessary jargon should be kept to a minimum, although colloquialisms should also be avoided. The reader should try to observe whether the researcher's view intruded too much in the report, especially in the reporting of the results.

❖ CONCLUSION

In concluding this chapter, several points about the research critique should be made. It should be apparent to those who have glanced through the questions in the boxes in this chapter that it will not always be possible to answer the questions satisfactorily on the basis of the research report. This is especially true for journal articles

BOX 25-13   GUIDELINES FOR CRITIQUING QUALITATIVE ANALYSES

1. Are the data best analyzed qualitatively, or would a quantitative approach have been more appropriate?
2. Is the research tradition within which the study was undertaken identified (e.g., ethnographic, phenomenological)? Do the methods of data collection and analysis appear to be congruent with this tradition?
3. What sources of data were used to yield the qualitative materials (e.g., unstructured interview, observation)? Are these sources sufficient to provide a broad array of information and to capture the full range of likely variation regarding the phenomenon under investigation?
4. Are the coding categories used to organize the data described? Are examples of data fitting each category presented? Does the report describe the rules used to place data into the categories? Do the categories seem to be logical and complete? Does there seem to be unnecessary overlap or redundancy in the categories?
5. Is the reasoning process through which the thematic analysis occurred clearly described? What were the major themes that emerged? If excerpts from the narrative materials are provided, do these themes appear to capture the meaning of the narratives (i.e., did the researcher adequately interpret and conceptualize the themes)?
6. Is the analysis parsimonious? That is, could two or more themes have been collapsed into some broader and perhaps more useful conceptualization of the issues?
7. What efforts did the researcher make to validate the findings? Were quasi-statistical procedures used? Did two or more researchers indpendently code and analyze the data? Did the researcher specifically mention a search for contrary occurrences? What evidence does the report provide that the researcher's analysis is accurate, objective, and replicable?
8. Was the grounded theory approach used? If so, does it appear to have been used appropriately? Did data collection continue until saturation occurred? Were data collection and analysis undertaken concurrently?
9. Were the data displayed in a manner that allows the reader to verify the researcher's theoretical conclusions? Was a conceptual map or framework displayed to communicate important processes?
10. Was the context of the phenomenon under investigation adequately described? Does the report give the reader a clear picture of the social world of those people under study?
11. Does the theoretical schema yield a meaningful picture of the phenomenon under study? Are the relationships among the concepts clearly expressed? Do these relationships seem logical, and do they accurately reflect the data? Is the resulting theory trivial and obvious?
12. Could the study have been strengthened by the inclusion of some quantitative data?

in which the need for economy often translates into a severe abridgement of methodological descriptions. Furthermore, there are many questions listed that may have little or no relevance for a particular study. The inclusion of a question in the list does not necessarily imply that all reports should have all the components mentioned. The questions are meant to suggest aspects of a study that often are deserving of consideration; they are not meant to lay traps for identifying omitted and perhaps unnecessary details.

It must be admitted that the answers to many questions will call on the reader's judgment as much as, or even more than, his or her knowledge. An evaluation of whether the most appropriate data collection procedure was used for the research problem necessarily involves a degree of subjectiveness. Issues concerning the appropriateness of various strategies and techniques are topics about which even experts disagree. One should strive to be as objective as possible and to indicate one's reasoning for the judgments made.

BOX 25-14   GUIDELINES FOR CRITIQUING THE INTERPRETIVE DIMENSIONS OF A RESEARCH REPORT

Interpretation of the Findings

1. Are all the important results discussed? Are the interpretations consistent with the results?
2. Is each result interpreted in terms of the original hypothesis to which it relates and to the conceptual framework? Is each result interpreted in light of findings from similar research studies?
3. Are alternative explanations for the findings mentioned, and is the rationale for their rejection discussed?
4. Do the interpretations give due consideration to the limitations of the research methods?
5. Are any unwarranted interpretations of causality made?
6. Is there evidence of bias in the interpretations?
7. Does the interpretation distinguish between practical and statistical significance?

Implications

8. Are implications of the study ignored, although a basis for them is apparent?
9. Are the implications of the study discussed in terms of the retention, modification, or rejection of a theory or conceptual framework?
10. Are the implications of the findings for nursing practice described?
11. Are the discussed implications appropriate, given the study's limitations?
12. Are generalizations made that are not warranted on the basis of the sample used?

Recommendations

13. Are recommendations made concerning how the study's methods could be improved? Are recommendations for future research investigations made?
14. Are recommendations for specific nursing actions made on the basis of the implications?
15. Are the recommendations thorough, consistent with the findings, and consistent with related research results?

BOX 25-15   GUIDELINES FOR CRITIQUING THE ETHICAL ASPECTS OF A STUDY

1. Were the subjects unnecessarily subjected to any physical harm or psychological distress or discomfort?
2. Did the researchers take appropriate steps to remove or prevent harm?
3. Did the benefits that accrued from the research outweigh any potential risks or actual discomfort to the subjects?
4. Was information gathered from study participants by personnel with appropriate qualifications?
5. Were the subjects told about any real or potential risks that might result from participation in the study? Were the purposes and procedures of the study fully described in advance?
6. Was any type of coercion or undue influence used in recruiting subjects for the study? Were vulnerable subjects used?
7. Did all the subjects know they were subjects in a study? Did they have an opportunity to decline participation? Were subjects deceived in any way?
8. Was informed consent obtained from all subjects or their representatives? If not, was there a valid and justifiable reason for not doing so?
9. Were appropriate steps taken to safeguard the privacy of the research subjects?
10. Was the research study approved and monitored by an Institutional Review Board or other similar committee on ethics?

❖ SUMMARY

Evaluating research reports involves critically appraising both the merits and the limitations of the published report. A systematic assessment of the various aspects of a research report is essential in judging the utility and value of a study. This chapter offers suggestions for assessing the substantive, methodological, interpretive, ethical, and stylistic aspects of a written research report.

BOX 25-16 GUIDELINES FOR CRITIQUING THE PRESENTATION OF A RESEARCH REPORT

1. Does the report include a sufficient amount of detail to permit a thorough critique of the study's purpose, conceptual framework, design and methods, handling of critical ethical issues, and interpretation?
2. Is the report well written? Are pretentious words or jargon used when simpler wording would have been possible? Are the grammar and spelling correct?
3. Is the report well-organized, or is the presentation confusing? Is there an orderly, logical presentation of ideas? Are transitions smooth, and is the report characterized by continuity of thought and expression?
4. Is the report sufficiently concise, or does the author include a lot of irrelevant details?
5. Is the report written in an objective style, or are the author's biases and viewpoints overly intrusive? Are attributions made for any opinions presented in the report?
6. Is the report written using tentative language as befits the nature of scientific inquiry, or does the author talk about what the study did or did not "prove"?
7. Is sexist language avoided?
8. Does the title of the report adequately capture the variables and population under investigation?
9. Does the report have a summary or abstract? Does the abstract adequately summarize the research problem, the study methods, and important findings?
10. Does the author include a reference for every citation made in the text, so that readers can refer to earlier work on the topic?

❖ STUDY SUGGESTIONS

Chapter 25 of the accompanying *Study Guide for Nursing Research: Principles and Methods, 5th ed.*, offers various exercises and study suggestions for reinforcing the concepts presented in this chapter. Additionally, the following study questions can be addressed:

1. Read the article, "Nipple feeding premature infants in the neonatal intensive-care unit: Factors and decisions" by M. D. Kinner and P. Beachy (1994), *Journal of Obstetric, Gynecologic, and Neonatal Nursing, 23*, 105–112. What limitations of the research methods did the authors identify? Do these limitations alter your acceptance of the findings?
2. Read an article from any issue of *Nursing Research* or any other nursing research journal and systematically assess the article according to the questions contained in this chapter. What are the merits and limitations of the report?
3. Review the research critique presented in Polit and Hungler (1993), pages 388–402.

❖ SUGGESTED READINGS

Aamodt, A. M. (1983). Problems in doing nursing research: Developing criteria for evaluating qualitative research. *Western Journal of Nursing Research, 5,* 398–402.

Becker, P. H. (1993). Common pitfalls in published grounded theory research. *Qualitative Health Research, 3,* 254–260.

Burns, N. (1989). Standards for qualitative research. *Nursing Science Quarterly, 2,* 44–52.

Field, W. E. (1983). Clinical nursing research: A proposal of standards. *Nursing Leadership, 6,* 117–120.

Gehlbach, S. H. (1992). *Interpreting the medical literature.* (3rd ed.). Lexington, MA: The Collamore Press.

Horsley, J., & Crane, J. (1982). *Using research to improve nursing practice: A guide.* New York: Grune & Stratton.

LoBiondo-Wood, G., & Haber, J. (1994). *Nursing research: Methods, critical appraisal, and utilization.* (3rd ed.). St. Louis: C. V. Mosby.

Morse, J. M. (1991). Evaluating qualitative research. *Qualitative Health Research, 1,* 283–286.

Parse, R., Coyne, A., & Smith, M. (1985). *Nursing research: Qualitative methods.* (Chapter 11). Bowie, MD: Brady Communications.

Polit, D. F., & Hungler, B. P. (1993). *Essentials of nursing research: Methods, appraisal, and utilization* (3rd ed.). Philadelphia: J. B. Lippincott.

Ryan-Wenger, N. M. (1992). Guidelines for critique of a research report. *Heart and Lung, 21,* 394–401.

Topham, D. L., & DeSilva, P. (1988). Evaluating congruency between steps in the research process: A critique guide for use in clinical nursing practice. *Clinical Nurse Specialist, 2,* 97–102.

Chapter 26

UTILIZATION OF NURSING RESEARCH

Nurse researchers are usually not interested in pursuing knowledge simply for the sake of knowledge itself. In a practicing profession such as nursing, researchers generally want to have their findings incorporated into nursing protocols and into diagnostic decision making. In fact, it might be argued that the ultimate worth of a nursing research study is demonstrated by the extent to which its findings are eventually used to improve the delivery of nursing services.

Over the past two decades, a number of changes in nursing education and in nursing research have been prompted by the desire to develop a better knowledge base for the practice of nursing. In education, most schools of nursing changed their curricula to include courses on nursing research. Now, almost all baccalaureate and graduate nursing programs offer courses to instill some degree of research competence in their students. In the research arena, as indicated in Chapter 1, there has been a dramatic shift toward a focus on clinical nursing problems. These two changes alone, however, have not in and of themselves been enough to effect widespread modifications to the delivery

of nursing care on the basis of scientific research. There appears to have been an unwarranted assumption that the production of clinically relevant studies would lead automatically to improved nursing practice—if only there were an audience of practicing nurses who were competent in critically evaluating these studies. Research utilization, as the nursing community has increasingly begun to recognize, is a complex and nonlinear phenomenon. In this chapter, we discuss various aspects of the utilization of nursing research.

❖ WHAT IS RESEARCH UTILIZATION?

Broadly speaking, *research utilization* refers to the use of some aspect of a scientific investigation in an application unrelated to the original research. Current conceptions of research utilization recognize a continuum in terms of the specificity or diffuseness of the use to which knowledge is put. At one end of the continuum are discrete, clearly identifiable attempts to base some specific action on the results of research

Polit DF, Hungler BP: NURSING RESEARCH: PRINCIPLES AND METHODS, 5th ed. © 1995 J. B. Lippincott Company.

findings. For example, a series of studies in the 1960s and 1970s demonstrated that the optimal placement time for accurate oral temperature determination is 9 minutes (e.g., Nichols & Verhonick, 1968). When nurses specifically altered their behavior from shorter placement times to the empirically based recommendation of 9 minutes, this constituted an instance of research utilization at this end of the continuum. Research utilization is sometimes defined in terms of such direct, specific impacts. For example, Horsley and her colleagues (1983), who were involved in a major project on the utilization of research in nursing, defined research utilization as a "process directed toward transfer of specific research-based knowledge into practice through the systematic use of a series of activities" (pp. 100–101). This type of utilization has been referred to as *instrumental utilization* (Caplan & Rich, 1975).

However, there is growing recognition that research can be utilized in a more diffuse manner—in a way that promotes cumulative awareness, understanding, or enlightenment. Caplan and Rich (1975) refer to this end of the utilization continuum as *conceptual utilization.* Thus, a practicing nurse may read a research report in which the investigators report that nonnutritive sucking among preterm infants in a neonatal intensive care unit had a beneficial effect on the number of days to the infant's first bottle feeding and on the number of days of hospitalization. The nurse may be reluctant to alter his or her own behavior or suggest an intervention based on the results of a single study. However, the nurse's reading of the research report may make the nurse more observant in his or her own work with preterm infants and may lead the nurse to collect informal data regarding the benefits of nonnutritive sucking in the nurse's own setting. Conceptual utilization, then, refers to situations in which users are influenced in their thinking about an issue based on their knowledge of one or more studies but do not put this knowledge to any specific, documentable use.

The middle ground of this continuum involves the partial impact of research findings on nursing activities. Here, nursing actions or decisions are based to some extent on research findings, but other factors such as first-hand experience, tradition, and situational constraints are also considered. This middle ground is frequently the result of a slow evolutionary process that does not reflect a conscious decision to use an innovative procedure but rather reflects what Weiss (1980) termed knowledge creep and decision accretion. *Knowledge creep* refers to an evolving "percolation" of research ideas and findings. *Decision accretion* refers to the manner in which momentum for a decision builds over time based on accumulated information gained through readings, informal discussions, meetings, and so on.

Research utilization at all points along this continuum appears to be an appropriate goal for nurses.

❖ RESEARCH UTILIZATION IN NURSING

Numerous commentators have noted that progress in utilizing the results of nursing research studies has proceeded slowly—too slowly for many who are anxious to establish a scientific base for nursing actions. In this section, we consider the possibilities for research utilization and evidence on the extent to which utilization has occurred.

Incorporating Research Into Practice: The Potential

The nursing process is complex and requires nurses to engage in many decision-making activities. In the course of delivering patient care, nurses collect relevant information, make assessments and diagnoses, develop plans for appropriate nursing actions, initiate interventions, and evaluate the effects of these interventions. These activities correspond to the five phases of nursing outlined in the *Standards for*

Practice established by the American Nurses' Association Congress for Practice (1973). Within each of these phases, the findings from research can assist nurses in making more informed decisions and in taking actions that have a solid, scientifically based rationale. Thus, research conducted by nurses can potentially play a pivotal role in improving the quality of nursing care, the efficiency with which it is delivered, and the process by which the care is delivered.

ASSESSMENT PHASE

Nurses collect information to assess patient needs from a variety of sources. The information may come from interviews with clients, family members, other nurses, and other types of health professionals as well as from records, charts, and nurses' observations. Each source contributes its unique part to the total assessment. Research can focus on how best to collect the information, what types of information need to be collected, how to integrate various pieces of assessment data, and how to improve the accuracy of gathering information. Research can also help nurses select alternative methods or forms for particular types of clients, settings, and situations. Through research, nurses can determine the extent to which the forms produce comparable information.

DIAGNOSIS PHASE

Based on an analysis of the information collected in the assessment phase of the nursing process, nurses are expected to develop nursing diagnoses. Research can play an important role in helping nurses make more accurate nursing diagnoses by validating the etiology of each diagnosis against the recorded assessment information. In addition, nursing research can help to determine the frequency of occurrence for each defining characteristic or cue associated with each diagnosis. The documentation can be helpful to the nursing profession, which has only recently begun the task of building up its taxonomy of diagnoses. Continued efforts in this area hold promise for the clustering of nursing diagnostic groups and for the refinement of accepted nursing diagnoses.

PLANNING PHASE

The planning phase of the nursing process involves decisions concerning *what* nursing actions or interventions are needed; *when* the nursing actions are most appropriately instituted for each nursing diagnosis; *whom* the recipients of the nursing interventions should be; and under *what* conditions the interventions are to be implemented. Research findings can fruitfully be used by nurses in planning care by indicating the nursing interventions that are especially effective for particular cultural groups, settings, types of problems, and client characteristics. Research can also help nurses to evaluate the holism of the plan of care and to make more informed decisions about whether the established goals are realistic in a given situation.

INTERVENTION PHASE

Ideally, professionally accountable nurses would base as many of their nursing interventions as possible on research findings. Consider, for example, the many decisions made by nurses working the night shift in a nursing home. At what point do they decide that the nursing interventions are no longer producing the desired results for a resident in the process of dying? When is it time to notify the family or physician? What alterations in nursing interventions are available that facilitate, with as much ease as is possible, the transition from a state of life to a state of death? What approach might be used with families? What response might be expected from other residents of the home, and how might their stresses be appropriately alleviated? The systematic documentation of nursing interventions that have been found to be helpful may benefit other nurses facing the same kinds of situations.

EVALUATION PHASE

The last stage of the nursing process involves the evaluation of the degree to which the behavioral outcomes or goals developed at the planning stage have been met. Research can help document success or failure in achieving the various outcomes. When success occurs with relative frequency, it may offer other nurses the opportunity to implement the plan in other comparable situations with a fair degree of confidence. When the plan has been unsuccessful, nurses are redirected to examine the accuracy of the assessment, the nursing diagnoses, the plan, and the nursing interventions. Such information, collected systematically, may aid other nurses in avoiding the same dilemmas and should lead to improvements in nursing care.

Incorporating Research Into Practice: The Record

As suggested previously, there is ample potential for utilizing research throughout the various phases of the nursing process. Currently, however, there is considerable concern that nurses have thus far failed to realize this potential for using research findings as a basis for making decisions and for developing nursing interventions. This concern is based on some evidence suggesting that nurses are not always aware of research results and do not effectively incorporate these results into their practice.

One of the first pieces of evidence about the gap between research and practice was a study by Ketefian (1975), who reported on the oral temperature determination practices of 87 registered nurses. Ketefian's study was designed to learn what "happens to research findings relative to nursing practice after five or ten years of dissemination in the nursing literature" (p. 90). The results of a series of investigations in the late 1960s had clearly demonstrated that the optimal placement time for oral temperature determination using glass thermometers is 9 minutes. In Ketefian's study, only one out of 87 nurses reported the correct placement time, suggesting

that these practicing nurses were unaware of or ignored the research findings about optimal placement time.

In another study investigating research utilization, Kirchhoff (1982) investigated the discontinuance of coronary precautions in a nationwide sample of 524 intensive care nurses. Several published studies had failed to demonstrate that the practices of restricting ice water and rectal temperature measurement were necessary, yet Kirchhoff's results indicated that these coronary precautions were still widely practiced. Only 24% of the nurses had discontinued ice water restrictions, and only 35% had discontinued rectal temperature restrictions.

More recently, Coyle and Sokop (1990) investigated practicing nurses' adoption of 14 nursing innovations that had been reported in the nursing literature, replicating a study by Brett (1987). Brett used the utilization criteria suggested by Haller and colleagues (1979) in selecting 14 studies. These criteria included scientific merit, significance and usefulness of the research findings to the practice setting, and the suitability of the finding for application to practice. A sample of 113 nurses practicing in 10 hospitals (randomly selected from the medium-sized hospitals in North Carolina) completed questionnaires that measured the nurses' awareness and use of the study findings. The results indicated much variation across the 14 studies. For example, from 34% to 94% of the nurses reported awareness of the various innovations. Coyle and Sokop used Brett's original scheme to categorize each study according to its stage of adoption: awareness (indicating knowledge of the innovation); persuasion (indicating the nurses' belief that nurses should use the innovation in practice); occasional use in practice; and regular use in practice. Only one of the 14 studies was at the regular-use stage of adoption. Six of the studies were in the persuasion stage, indicating that the nurses knew of the innovation and thought it *should* be incorporated into nursing practice but were not basing their own nursing decisions on it. Table 26-1 describes 4 of the 14 nursing innovations, one for each of the

Table 26–1.   *Extent of Adoption of Four Nursing Practices**

STAGE	NURSING INNOVATION	AWARE (%)	PERSUADED (%)	USE SOMETIMES (%)	USE ALWAYS (%)
Awareness	Elimination of lactose from the formulas of tube-feeding diets for adult patients minimizes diarrhea, distention, flatulence, and fullness and reduces patient rejection of feedings (Horsley, Crane, & Haller, 1981)	38	36	13	19
Persuasion	Accurate monitoring of oral temperatures can be achieved on patients receiving oxygen therapy by using an electronic thermometer placed in the sublingual pocket (Lim-Levy, 1982)	68	55	35	29
Occasional use	A formally planned and structured preoperative education program preceding elective surgery results in improved patient outcomes (King & Tarsitano, 1982)	83	81	48	23
Regular use	A closed sterile system of urinary drainage is effective in maintaining the sterility of urine in patients who are catheterized for less than 2 weeks; continuity of the closed drainage system should be maintained during irrigations, sampling procedures, and patient transport (Horsley,Crane, Haller, & Bingle, 1981)	94	91	84	6

* Based on findings reported in Coyle, L. A., & Sokop, A. G. (1990). Innovation adoption behavior among nurses. *Nursing Research, 39,* 176–180. The sample consisted of 113 practicing nurses.

four stages of adoption, according to Coyle and Sokop's results. The results of this study (and the results of Brett's earlier study) are more encouraging than the studies by Ketefian and Kirchhoff in that they suggest that, on average, the practicing nurses were aware of many innovations based on research results, were persuaded that the innovations should be used, and were beginning to use them on occasion. Of course, it is possible that the respondents overstated their awareness and use of nursing innovations.

It is clear that a gap exists between knowledge production and knowledge utilization in nursing and in other disciplines. Some gap is inevitable and, given the imperfection of scientific research as a means of knowing, even desirable. Moreover, it seems likely that the gap as identified in studies such as those described previously is somewhat overstated for three reasons. First, utilization studies do not always consider technological changes that might make the knowledge irrelevant. Thus, as Downs (1979) pointed out, electronic thermometers that rapidly replaced glass thermometers in the mid-1970s made the placement-time findings obsolete and could account for Ketefian's results. Second, an important factor in research utilization is a cost/benefit assessment, as we describe later in this chapter. The subjects in Kirchhoff's study may have continued using coronary care precautions because the risk of problems that might arise by eliminating them (e.g., if the study results were incorrect) outweighed the benefits (e.g., more efficient use of staff time) that could accrue. Third, utilization studies have focused primarily on utilization at one end of the utilization continuum—the end we refer to as *instrumental utilization*. That is, utilization studies have been interested primarily in the extent to which specific types of information are used in specific nursing situations. The studies by Brett (1987) and Coyle and Sokop (1990), which found that about half of the innovations were in the persuasion stage, supported the notion of a great middle ground when it comes to research utilization. No study has investigated conceptual utilization, but we suspect that, with the growing emphasis on nursing research in nursing curricula, there is a much higher level of conceptual utilization throughout the nursing community today than there was 10 years ago. Nurses are becoming enlightened with regard to the value of research and enlightened by a growing body of research that is challenging traditional ways of practicing nursing.

Efforts To Improve Utilization

The need to reduce the gap between nursing research and nursing practice has been the topic of much discussion, but there have been relatively few formal efforts to achieve that goal. In this section, we briefly describe the most prominent of these efforts.

THE WICHE PROJECT

One of the earliest research utilization projects was the Western Interstate Commission for Higher Education (WICHE) Regional Program for Nursing Research Development. The project, a 6-year effort funded by the Division of Nursing of the U.S. Department of Health, Education, and Welfare, had as its original goal investigating the feasibility of increasing nursing research activities through regional collaborative activities. According to the final report (Krueger, Nelson, & Wolanin, 1978), the three major project activities were 1) collaborative, nontargeted research (bringing together nurses from educational and practice settings to design studies based on mutually identified nursing problems); 2) collaborative, targeted research (multiple studies in different settings all designed to investigate the concept of quality of care); and 3) research utilization. The project team visualized research utilization as part of a five-phase resource linkage model. In this model, nurses were conceived as organizational change agents who could provide a link between research and practice. Through a support system (e.g., through workshops, conferences, and consultations), participant nurses were to utilize research results to solve problems identified as occurring in practice.

Nurses who participated in the WICHE project were given the opportunity to identify problems that needed research-based solutions and were then provided with opportunities to develop skills in reading and evaluating research for use in practice. They also developed detailed plans for introducing research innovations into their clinical practice settings. The final report indicated that the project was successful in increasing research utilization, but it also identified a stumbling block. The problem that posed the greatest difficulty was finding scientifically sound, reliable nursing studies with clearly identified implications for nursing care.

THE NCAST PROJECT

The Nursing Child Assessment Satellite Training (NCAST) Project was a 2-year research dissemination project, also funded by the Division of Nursing. The primary objectives of the project were to determine whether satellite communication technology is an efficient means of disseminating nursing research and whether an interactive communication facility would promote effective application of new health care assessment techniques (Barnard & Hoehn, 1978). The results of the study supported the use of satellite communication for research dissemination. In terms of research utilization, the project directors proposed a model with four components: 1) recruitment (i.e., the identification and recruitment of an appropriate practitioner audience); 2) translation (i.e., the transformation of research results into a format and idiom that can easily be understood by nurse practitioners); 3) dissemination (i.e., the communication of research findings in an effective and efficient manner); and 4) evaluation (i.e., the determination of the impact of the other three processes).

THE CURN PROJECT

The best-known nursing research utilization project is the Conduct and Utilization of Research in Nursing (CURN) Project, a 5-year development project awarded to the Michigan Nurses' Association by the Division of Nursing. The major objective of the CURN project was to increase the use of research findings in the daily practice of RNs by disseminating current research findings, facilitating organizational changes needed for the implementation of innovations, and encouraging the conduct of collaborative research that has relevance to nursing practice.

One of the activities of the CURN project was to stimulate the conduct of research in clinical settings. The project resulted in a set of nine volumes on various clinical problems. The titles of these volumes (e.g., *Pain, Preventing Decubitus Ulcers, Structured Preoperative Teaching,* and *Reducing Diarrhea in Tube-Fed Patients*) indicate that a wide range of clinical issues were studied.

The CURN project also focused on helping nurses to utilize research findings in their practice. The CURN project staff saw research utilization as primarily an organizational process (Horsley, Crane, & Bingle, 1978). According to their view, the commitment of organizations that employ practicing nurses to the research utilization process is essential for research to have any impact on nursing practice. They conceptualized the six phases of the research utilization process as follows (Horsley, Crane, Crabtree, & Wood, 1983):

1. Identification of practice problems that need solving and assessment of valid research bases to use in nursing practice
2. Evaluation of the relevance of the research-based knowledge as it applies to the identified clinical problem, the organization's values, current policies, and potential costs and benefits
3. Design of a nursing practice innovation that addresses the clinical problem but does not exceed the scientific limitations of the research base
4. Clinical trial and evaluation of the innovation in the practice setting
5. Decision making to adopt, revise, or reject the innovation
6. Development of strategies to extend the innovation to other appropriate settings

The CURN project team concluded that research utilization by practicing nurses is feasible, but only if the research is relevant to practice and if the results are broadly disseminated.

❖ BARRIERS TO UTILIZING NURSING RESEARCH

Typically, several years elapse between the time a researcher conceptualizes and designs a study and the time the results are reported in the research literature. Many more years may elapse between the time the results are reported and the time practicing nurses learn about the results and attempt to incorporate them into practice. Thus, it is not unusual for there to be an interim of a decade or so between the posing of a research problem and the implementation of a solution—if, in fact, there is *ever* an effort to implement. In the next section of this chapter, we discuss some strategies for bridging the gap between nursing research and nursing practice. First, however, we review some of the barriers to research utilization in nursing. These barriers can be broadly grouped into four categories relating to characteristics of the source of the barrier: 1) the research itself, 2) practicing nurses, 3) organizational settings, and 4) the nursing profession.

Research Characteristics

Because nursing research is a relatively new area of inquiry, state-of-the-art research knowledge on any given problem is often at a relatively rudimentary level. Studies reported in the literature often do not warrant the incorporation of their findings into practice. Flaws in research design, sample selection, data collection instruments, or data analysis often raise questions about the soundness or generalizability of the study findings. Thus, a major impediment to research utilization by practicing nurses is that, for many problems, an extensive base of valid, reliable, and generalizable study results has not yet been developed.

As we have repeatedly stressed throughout this book, most scientific studies have flaws of one type or another. The study may be flawed conceptually or methodologically, and the flaws may be minor or major. There are few, if any, perfect studies. If one were to wait for the perfect study before basing clinical decisions and interventions on research findings, however, one would have a very long wait indeed. It is precisely because of the limits of the scientific approach that replication becomes essential. When repeated testing of a hypothesis in different settings and with different types of subjects yield similar results, then there can be greater confidence that the truth has been discovered.

Isolated studies can almost never provide an adequate basis for making changes in nursing practice. Therefore, another constraint to research utilization is the dearth of reported replications of studies.

Nurses' Characteristics

Practicing nurses as individuals have characteristics that impede the incorporation of research findings into nursing care. Perhaps the most obvious is the educational preparation of nurses. Most practicing nurses—graduates of diploma or associate degree programs—have not received any formal instruction in research. They may therefore lack the skills to judge the merits of scientific projects. Furthermore, because research played a limited role in their training, these nurses may not have developed positive attitudes toward research and may not be aware of the beneficial role it can play in the delivery of nursing care. Champion and Leach (1989) found that nurses' attitudes toward research were strong predictors of the utilization of research findings. Courses on research methodology are now typically offered in baccalaureate nursing programs, but there is generally insufficient attention paid to research utilization. The ability to critique a research report is a necessary, but not sufficient, condition for effectively incorporating research results into daily decision making.

Another characteristic is one that is common to most humans. People are generally resistant to change. Change requires effort, retraining, and restructuring one's work habits. Change may also be perceived as threatening; for example, proposed changes may be perceived as potentially affecting one's job security. Thus, there is likely to be some opposition to introducing innovations in the practice setting.

Organizational Characteristics

Some of the impediments to research utilization, as the CURN project staff so astutely noted, stem from the organizations that train and employ practicing nurses. Organizations, perhaps to an even greater degree than individuals, resist change, unless there is a strong organizational perception that there is something fundamentally wrong with the status quo. In many settings, the organizational climate is simply not conducive to research utilization. To challenge tradition and accepted practices, a spirit of intellectual curiosity and openness must prevail.

In many practice settings, administrators have established protocols and procedures to reward expertise and competence in nursing practice. However, few practice settings have established a system to reward nurses for critiquing nursing studies, for utilizing research in practice, or for discussing research findings appropriate to clients. Thus, organizations have failed to motivate or reward nurses to seek ways to implement appropriate findings into their practice. Research review and utilization are often considered appropriate activities only when time is available, but available time is generally limited. In a recent national survey of nearly 1000 clinical nurses, one of the greatest reported barriers to research utilization was "insufficient time on the job to implement new ideas," which was reported as a moderate or great barrier by about 75% of the sample (Funk, Champagne, Wiese, & Tornquist, 1991).

Finally, organizations may be reluctant to expend the necessary resources for attempting utilization projects or for implementing changes to organizational policy. Resources may be required for the use of outside consultants, for staff release time, for administrative review, for evaluating the effects of an innovation, and so on. With the push toward cost containment in health care settings, resource constraints may therefore pose a barrier to research utilization.

Overall, in the national survey of perceived barriers, those stemming from the organizational setting were viewed by clinical nurses as posing the greatest obstacles to research utilization (Funk et al., 1991).

Characteristics of the Nursing Profession

Some of the impediments that contribute to the gap between research and practice are more global than those discussed previously and can be described as reflecting the state of the nursing profession or, even more broadly, the state of American society.

One of the difficulties is that it has sometimes been difficult to encourage clinicians and researchers to interact and collaborate. They are generally in different settings, have many different professional concerns, interact with different networks of nurses, and operate according to different philosophical systems. Relatively few systematic attempts have been made to form collaborative arrangements, and to date, even fewer of these arrangements have been institutionalized as formal, permanent entities. Moreover, attempts to develop such collaboration will not necessarily be welcomed by either group. As Phillips (1986) observed, there is often a deep-seated lack of trust between nurse researchers and nurse clinicians.

A related issue is that communication between practitioners and researchers is problematic. Most practicing nurses do not read nursing research journals, nor do they usually attend professional conferences where research results are reported. Many nurses involved in the direct delivery of care are too overwhelmed by the jargon, the statistical symbols, and the wealth of quantitative information contained in research reports to understand fully such reports even when they do read them. Furthermore, nurse researchers may too infrequently attend to the needs of clinical nurses as identified in specialty journals. For research utilization to happen, there must be two-way communication between the practicing nurse and the nurse researcher. The recent emergence of two journals—*Applied Nursing Research* and *Clinical Nursing Research*—represents an important step in this direction.

Phillips (1986) also noted two other noteworthy barriers to bridging the research–practice gap. One is the shortage of appropriate role models. Phillips commented that, "even if a nurse wants to assume the role of nursing research consumer, there are few colleagues available to give support for the endeavor and fewer still available to emulate" (p. 8). The other barrier is the historical "baggage" that has defined nursing in such a way that practicing nurses may not typically perceive themselves as independent professionals capable of recommending changes based on nursing research results. If practicing nurses believe that their role is to await direction from the medical community, and if they believe they have no power to be self-directed, then they will have difficulty in initiating innovations based on nursing research results. In the previously mentioned national survey, the barrier perceived by the largest percentage of nurses was the nurse's feeling that he or she did not have "enough authority to change patient care procedures" (Funk, et al., 1991).

❖ TIPS FOR IMPROVING RESEARCH UTILIZATION

Where does the responsibility for bridging the gap between research and practice lie? Should individual practicing nurses pursue appropriate nursing innovations? Should organizations and their administrative staff take the lead? Or should the direction come from researchers themselves? In our view, the entire nursing community must be involved in the process of putting research into practice. In this section, we discuss some research utilization strategies that various segments of the nursing community can adopt.

Strategies for Researchers

A great deal of the responsibility for research utilization rests in the hands of researchers. There is little point in pursuing scientific investigations if the results do not get used, so it behooves researchers to take steps to en-

sure that utilization can occur. Some suggestions for strategies that researchers could implement to foster better adoption of their research results are as follows:

- *Do high-quality research.* A major impediment to utilizing nursing research results, as indicated in the previous section, is that there is often an inadequate scientific basis for introducing innovations or for making changes. The quality of nursing studies has improved dramatically in the past two decades, but much progress remains to be made. The inadequacy of sampling plans remains one of the greatest weaknesses of nursing studies. If a study is based on an unrepresentative sample of 50 subjects, then utilization efforts based on the study findings are likely to be inappropriate.

- *Replicate.* As noted earlier, utilization of research results can almost never be justified on the basis of a single isolated study, so researchers must make a real commitment to replicating studies. It is also important to publish the results of replications even if—in fact, especially if—the results are exactly the same as those obtained in an earlier investigation. The journal *Clinical Nursing Research* has explicitly noted its intent to publish the results of replication studies (Hayes, 1993).

- *Collaborate with practitioners.* Academic researchers will never succeed in having much of an impact on nursing practice unless they become better attuned to the needs of practicing nurses and the clients they serve, the problems that practicing nurses face in delivering nursing care, and the constraints that operate in practice settings. Practicing nurses will be more willing to change their behaviors and modes of delivering care if they perceive that researchers are addressing issues of concern and importance to them. Researchers should seek opportunities to exchange ideas for research problems with nurse clinicians. They also need to involve clinicians in the actual conduct of research and in the interpretation of study results.

- *Disseminate aggressively.* If a researcher fails to communicate the results of a completed study to other nurses, it is obvious that the results will never be utilized by practicing nurses. Even studies with a variety of methodological shortcomings can make a contribution, if only to illuminate the researcher's conceptualization of a practice problem or to suggest how the research question might be better addressed in some subsequent study. It is the researcher's *responsibility* to find some means of communicating research results. Researchers should submit their manuscripts to at least two or three journals before abandoning hope of getting their reports published.

- *Disseminate broadly.* A researcher's responsibility for dissemination does not end at the point at which an article has been accepted for publication. Most nurses read only one or two professional journals, so a researcher who is truly committed to having his or her results known by the nursing community often publishes study results in several journals. It is unethical to submit *exactly* the same manuscript to two different journals, but a study generally yields more information than can be concisely reported in a single journal anyway. It is especially important from a utilization standpoint for researchers to report their results in specialty journals, which are more likely to be read by practicing nurses than the nursing research journals. Researchers should also take steps to disseminate study findings at conferences, colloquia, and workshops that are known to be attended by nurse clinicians. Collaboration with practicing nurses should prove useful in developing effective dissemination plans.

- *Communicate clearly.* It is not always possible to present the results of a research project in a way that is readily comprehensible to all nonresearchers. However, researchers need to be encouraged to avoid unnecessary jar-

gon whenever possible, to define any terms that are technically difficult, to construct tables carefully so that a nonresearcher can get a sense of the findings, and to compose the abstract of the report so that virtually any intelligent reader can understand the research problem, the general approach, and the most salient findings. A general aim should be to write research reports that are user-friendly.

- *Suggest clinical implications.* In the introduction to a research report, the researcher should explain the potential clinical significance of the study. In the discussion section, the researcher should suggest how the results of their research can be utilized by practicing nurses: How would a staff nurse currently working in the area apply the findings? The researcher should be careful to discuss study limitations and to make some assessment of the generalizability of the study findings. If an implications section with suggestions for clinical practice became a standard feature of research reports, then the burden of utilization would be much lighter for the nurse clinician.

Strategies for Scholars and Educators

Some overlap exists between the categories of nurse researcher and nurse academician, but the overlap is imperfect because not all educators are researchers and not all researchers are in academia. Several of the following suggested strategies could, however, be undertaken by nonacademic researchers as well as by educators.

- *Incorporate research findings into the curriculum.* Research findings should be integrated throughout the curriculum. Whenever possible, faculty should document the efficacy of a specific procedure or technique by referring to a relevant study. When there is no relevant research, the instructor can note the absence of empirical evidence supporting the technique—this could help to stimulate the students' interest in a research-based verification.

• *Encourage research and research utilization.* Either by acting as role models to students (e.g., by discussing their own research) or by clearly demonstrating positive attitudes toward research and its use in nursing, instructors can help to foster a spirit of inquiry and openness that is a precondition to effective utilization of research. Instructors of research methods can also encourage students to become better consumers of nursing research, to do their own research, or to develop a plan for a utilization project.

• *Prepare integrative reviews.* There is a desperate need for high-quality critical reviews of research on specific research topics. If a research question has been studied by several different researchers—in other words, if there have been several replications of a study—then the question may be ripe for a review that will summarize the state of knowledge. Such reviews can play an invaluable role for practicing nurses, who generally do not have the time to do extensive literature reviews and who may have some difficulty in critically evaluating individual studies. When an integrative review takes the form of a meta-analysis—which involves the use of statistical procedures to integrate the findings—the researcher should take pains to translate the results into clinical terms. Integrative reviews should ideally conclude with some strong statements about the implications of the body of research for nursing practice.

• *Place demands on researchers.* Faculty (especially if they have done research themselves) are often asked to be anonymous reviewers of research proposals and reports. Funding sources that offer financial support for the conduct of nursing research generally rely on a panel of experts to help them review research proposals before awarding any grants. Peer reviewers of such proposals should demand that researchers demonstrate the proposed study's potential for practical

utility. Moreover, peer reviewers can demand that the researchers include a specific plan for dissemination or utilization. Reviewers of journal articles of completed research should also criticize reports that have failed to include a discussion of the study's implications for practice.

Strategies for Practicing Nurses and Nursing Students

Practicing nurses cannot by themselves launch institution-wide utilization projects, but their behaviors and attitudes are nevertheless critical to the success of any efforts to base nursing interventions and nursing diagnoses on research findings. Furthermore, individual nurses can engage in and benefit from conceptual utilization. Therefore, every nurse has an important role to play in utilizing nursing research.

• *Read widely and critically.* Professionally accountable nurses continue their nursing education on an ongoing basis by keeping abreast of important developments in their field. All nurses should regularly read journals relating to their specialty, including the research reports in them. Research reports should be critically appraised, according to guidelines such as those suggested in Chapter 25. It is especially important for nurse clinicians to read critical reviews of research that integrate numerous studies on a problem. Brett's (1987) study confirms the importance of reading. Her findings revealed that nurses who spent more time each week reading professional journals were more likely to adopt a research-based innovation than nurses who read infrequently.

• *Attend professional conferences.* Many nursing conferences include presentations of studies that have clinical relevance. It is often more rewarding to attend research presentations at a conference than to read a research report because the lag time between the conduct of a study and a conference presentation is generally less than the lag time for publication. Thus, conference attendees usually hear of an innovation much sooner than those who wait to read about it in a journal. Furthermore, those attending a conference get an opportunity to meet the researcher and to ask questions about practice implications. Brett's (1987) utilization study revealed a positive relationship between nurses' conference attendance and the degree to which they adopt research-based innovations. Nurses should ask their supervisors about the possibility of obtaining stipends to defray the cost of attending such conferences.

- *Learn to expect evidence that a procedure is effective.* Every time nurses or nursing students are told about a standard nursing procedure, they have a right to ask: Why? Nurses need to develop expectations that the decisions they make in their clinical practice are based on sound rationales. It is not inappropriate for the nursing student or practitioner to challenge the principles and procedures that are currently in use, although tact is advisable so that defensiveness is not engendered by such challenges.

- *Seek environments that support research utilization.* Organizations differ in their openness to research utilization, so nurses interested in basing their practice on research have some control through their employment decisions. If organizations perceive that nurses are basing their employment decisions on such factors as the organizational climate in relationship to research, there will be some pressure to support research utilization.

- *Become involved in a journal club.* Many organizations that employ nurses sponsor journal clubs that meet regularly to review research articles that have potential relevance to practice. Generally, members take turns reviewing and critically appraising a study and presenting the critique to the club's members. If there is no such club in existence, it might be possible to work with the organization to initiate one. Although the bulk of the responsibility for disseminat-

ing research results lies with the researcher, this is a responsibility that can be shared by practitioners.

- *Collaborate with a nurse researcher.* Collaboration, which we previously mentioned as a strategy for nurse researchers, is a two-way street. Practicing nurses who have identified a clinical problem in need of a solution and who lack methodological skills for the conduct of a study should consider initiating a collaborative relationship with a local nurse researcher. Collaboration with a nurse researcher could also be a useful approach for formal, institutional utilization projects.

- *Pursue and participate in institutional utilization projects.* Sometimes ideas for utilization projects come from staff nurses. Although large-scale utilization projects require organizational and administrative support, individual nurses or groups of nurses can propose such a project to the nursing department. For example, an idea for such a project may emerge in the context of a journal club. If the idea for a research utilization effort originates from within the administration, then individual nurses are still likely to play an important role in carrying out the project. Indeed, a utilization project can easily be undermined by reluctant or uncooperative staff. Although change is not always easy, it is in the interest of the profession to have practicing nurses who are open-minded about the possibility that a new technique or procedure can improve the quality of care that nurses provide.

- *Pursue appropriate personal utilization projects.* Not all findings from research studies are ones that require organizational commitment or policy directives. For example, a study might reveal that the health beliefs of an immigrant group are different from those of the predominant cultural group, and this may lead a nurse to ask several additional questions informally of clients of that immigrant group during assessment. If the nurse discovers that important and relevant information is gleaned from these additional questions, it may then be appropriate to recommend to the administration a more formal utilization project, which might involve changes to the standard assessment protocols. Of course, not all research findings are amenable to such informal personal utilization projects. If the results of a study or series of studies suggest an action or decision that is contrary to organizational policy or that has *any* potential risk for the clients, then nurses should not pursue such projects without supervisory approval. Some criteria for research utilization are discussed in the next section of this chapter.

Strategies for Administrators

According to several models of research utilization, the organizations that employ nurses play a fundamental role in supporting or undermining the nursing profession's efforts to develop a scientific base of practice. In the national survey, respondents viewed "enhancing administrative support and encouragement" as the single most effective means of facilitating research utilization (Funk, et al., 1991). In a more recent survey of over 1000 practicing nurses, Rizzuto and her colleagues (1994) found that nurses value research and want more time for research-related activities. Although the readers of this book are not likely to include a large audience of nursing or hospital administrators, the following suggested strategies are included primarily to alert practicing nurses to the kinds of issues facing these groups:

- *Foster a climate of intellectual curiosity.* If there is a great deal of administrative rigidity and opposition to change, then the staff's interest in research utilization is unlikely to become ignited. The administrator can take steps to encourage reading and critical thinking about the challenges facing practicing nurses. Open communication is an important ingredient in persuading staff nurses that their experiences and problems are important and that the administration is willing to consider innovative solutions.

- *Offer emotional or moral support.* If nurse administrators are unsupportive of research utilization, then there is little chance that any utilization efforts will get off the ground. Administrators need to make their support visible by informing staff and prospective staff on an individual basis, by establishing research utilization committees, by helping to develop research journal clubs, and so on. Administrators can perhaps offer the greatest degree of personal support by being a role model for the staff nurses. They can accomplish this by, for example, engaging in their own program of research, by actively participating themselves in the research journal clubs, and by playing a role in any utilization projects.

- *Offer financial or resource support for utilization.* Utilization projects often require some resources, although resource demands may not be great. Resources may be required for release time for nurses engaged in utilization projects, for outside consultation, for supplies and computer time, for registration at conferences, and so on. If the administration expects nurses to engage in research utilization activities on their own time and at their own expense, then the not-so-subtle message is that research utilization is unimportant to those running the organization.

- *Reward efforts for utilization.* When administrators evaluate nursing performance, they use a number of different criteria. Although research utilization should not be a primary criterion for evaluating a nurse's performance, its inclusion as one of several important criteria is likely to have a large impact on nurses' behaviors.

❖ THE UTILIZATION PROCESS AND CRITERIA FOR UTILIZATION

In this section, we discuss how a research utilization project can be planned and executed. Although the processes described here are ones that most likely will apply to an organization or a group of nurses working together, many of the steps in the processes are important ones for individual nurses to consider as they attempt to base their clinical decisions on scientific findings.

Approaches to Research Utilization

Nurses interested in utilizing research findings in their nursing practice generally set about the task in one of two ways. One approach to utilization, shown schematically as path A in Figure 26-1, begins with the identification of a clinical problem that needs solution. This problem identification approach, which corresponds to the first step in the six-phase process described by the CURN project team, is likely to have considerable internal staff support if the selected problem is one that numerous nurses in the practice setting have encountered. This approach to utilization is likely to be high on clinical relevance because a specific clinical situation generated the interest in resolving the problem in the first place.

The next step is a search for relevant literature to determine whether nurse researchers have addressed the problem through scientific research. If there is no research base related to the identified problem, then there are two choices: 1) to abandon the original problem and select an alternative one; or 2) to consider initiating an original research project on the topic (i.e., to initiate steps to *create* a knowledge base). This decision is likely to depend on the research skills of the staff and on the availability of research consultants.

Next, the knowledge base must be assessed. If the knowledge base is sound (according to criteria to be described later), then the subsequent step is to conduct an *implementation assessment*. If, however, the existing knowledge base inspires little confidence that the research could effectively be utilized by nurses, then there remain the two previously suggested alternatives: 1) to "go back to the drawing board" and select a new problem or 2) to investigate the possibility of doing original research to improve the knowledge base.

The implementation assessment involves three primary aspects: 1) an assessment of the transferability of the research findings; 2) an analysis of the cost/benefit ratio; and 3) an evaluation of the feasibility of implementing the innovation. These criteria will be elaborated in the next section. If all the implementation criteria are met, the team can then proceed to design the protocols for the innovation and its clinical evaluation, test the innovation in the practice setting, evaluate its effectiveness and costs, and then decide whether the new practice should be institutionalized. A final optional step, but one that is highly advisable, is the dissemination of the results of the utilization project so that other practicing nurses can benefit. If the implementation analysis suggests that there might be problems in testing the innovation within that particular practice setting, then the team can either identify a new problem and begin the process anew or consider adopting a plan to improve the implementation potential (e.g., seeking external resources if cost considerations were the inhibiting factor).

The second major approach to conducting a utilization project, shown schematically as path B in Figure 26-1, has many of the same components as the first approach. The major difference, however, is the starting point. Here, the process starts with the research literature. This could occur if, for example, a utilization project emerged as a result of discussions within a journal club. In this approach, the team would proceed through most of the same steps as outlined previously, except that a preliminary assessment would need to be made of the clinical relevance of the research findings. If it is determined that the research base is not clinically relevant, then the next step involves further reading and reviewing of the research literature.

Both these approaches involve several types of assessments, the results of which affect the appropriateness of proceeding with the utilization project. Criteria for making these assessments are presented next.

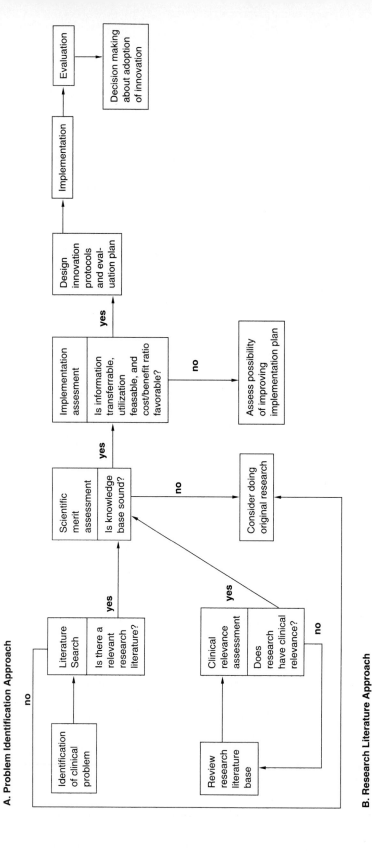

A. Problem Identification Approach

B. Research Literature Approach

Figure 26-1. *Two models of research utilization*

Utilization Criteria

As the model shown in Figure 26-1 suggests, there are three broad classes of criteria that are important in undertaking a utilization project: clinical relevance, scientific merit, and implementation potential. Boxes 26-1 and 26-2 present some assessment questions for these categories, each of which is elaborated on here.

CLINICAL RELEVANCE

Of critical importance is whether the problem and its solution have a high degree of clinical relevance. The central issue here is whether a problem of significance to nurses will be solved by making some change or introducing a new intervention. There is little point in undertaking a utilization project if the nursing profession or the clients it serves cannot benefit from the effort. If, under the best of circumstances, there is little potential for solving a nursing problem or helping nurses to make important clinical decisions, then the project probably should not be undertaken.

The five questions relating to clinical relevance, shown in Box 26-1, can be applied to a research report or set of related reports and can generally be answered based on a reading of the introduction to the reports. According to Tanner (1987), from whom these questions were adapted, if the answer is yes to any one of the five questions, then the next step in the process can be pursued because the innovation has the potential for being useful in practice. If, however, the answers to all the questions are negative, then the prospect of clinical relevance is small, and there is probably little point in pursuing the problem area any further.

SCIENTIFIC MERIT

We have discussed the criteria for scientific merit throughout this book, and in Chapter 25, we presented guidelines for assessing whether the findings and conclusions of a study are accurate, believable, and generalizable. When it comes to utilization, however, some additional concerns must be kept in mind. First and foremost is the issue of replication, the repeating of a study in a new setting, with a new sample of subjects. It is unwise to base an entire utilization project on a single study that has not been replicated, even if the study is extremely rigorous. Ideally, there would be several replications—each providing similar evidence of the effectiveness of the innovation being considered. At least one and ideally more of the studies should have

---

BOX 26–1   CRITERIA FOR EVALUATING THE CLINICAL RELEVANCE OF A BODY OF RESEARCH

1. Does the research have the potential to help solve a problem that is currently being faced by practitioners?
2. Does the research have the potential to help with clinical decision making with respect to (a) making appropriate observations, (b) identifying client risks or complications, or (c) selecting an appropriate intervention?
3. Are clinically relevant theoretical propositions tested by the research?
4. If the research involves an intervention, does the intervention have potential for implementation in clinical practice? Do nurses have control over the implementation of such interventions?
5. Can the measures used in the study be used in clinical practice?

Adapted from Tanner, C. A. (1987). Evaluating research for use in practice: Guidelines for the clinician. *Heart and Lung, 16*, 424–430.

been conducted in a clinical setting, with real clients.

Replications are seldom exact duplications of an earlier study; usually, a replication involves making some changes to some aspects of the research methods, such as the data collection instruments, the sampling plan, and so on. It is not essential that the replications be identical to provide a useful basis for pursuing a utilization project. Rather, it is more important that the *problem* being addressed is the same and that the innovations being tested are conceptually similar to each other. For example, several nurse researchers have investigated the use of therapeutic touch as a means of reducing stress and enhancing the psychological well-being of patients. Although these studies have all operationalized therapeutic touch in somewhat different ways and have examined somewhat different outcomes, it would be reasonable for a utilization project to consider the whole body of research on therapeutic touch.

IMPLEMENTATION POTENTIAL

Even when it has been determined that a problem has clinical significance and when there is a sound knowledge base relating to that clinical problem, it is not necessarily true that a utilization project can be planned and implemented. A number of other issues must be considered, which we have grouped under three headings: the transferability of the knowledge, the feasibility of implementation, and the cost/benefit ratio of the innovation. Box 26-2 presents some assessment questions for these categories.

TRANSFERABILITY. The main issue in the transferability question is whether it makes good sense to attempt the selected innovation in the new practice setting. If there is some aspect of the practice setting that is fundamentally incongruent with the innovation—in terms of its philosophy, the type of clients it serves, its personnel, or its financial or administrative

structure—then it makes little sense to try to transfer the innovation, even if a clinically significant innovation has been shown to be effective in various research contexts.

FEASIBILITY. The feasibility questions address a number of practical concerns about the availability of resources, the availability of staff, the organizational climate, the need for and availability of external assistance, and the potential for clinical evaluation. An important issue here is whether nurses will have control over the innovation (often this means having the ability to manipulate the independent variable). When nurses do not have full control over the new procedure being introduced, it is important to recognize the interdependent nature of the utilization project and to proceed as early as possible to establish the necessary cooperative arrangements.

COST/BENEFIT RATIO. A critical part of any decision to proceed with a utilization project is a careful assessment of the costs and benefits of the innovation. The *cost/benefit assessment* should encompass likely costs and benefits to various groups, including clients, staff, the organization as a whole, and even the nursing profession as a whole. Clearly, the most important factor is the client. If the degree of risk in introducing a new procedure is high, then the potential benefits must be great. Moreover, if there are risks to client well-being, it is essential that the knowledge base be sound. That is, an innovation that involves client risks should only be implemented when there is a solid body of evidence from several methodologically rigorous studies that the new practice is effective. A cost/benefit assessment should consider the reverse side of the coin as well: the costs and benefits of *not* implementing the innovation. It is sometimes easy to forget that the status quo bears its own risks and that failure to change—especially when such change is based on a firm knowledge base—is costly to clients, to organizations, and to the entire nursing community.

BOX 26–2   CRITERIA FOR EVALUATING THE IMPLEMENTATION POTENTIAL OF AN INNOVATION UNDER SCRUTINY

Transferability of the Findings

1. Will the innovation "fit" in the proposed setting?
2. How similar are the target population in the research and that in the new setting?
3. Is the philosophy of care underlying the innovation fundamentally different from the philosophy prevailing in the practice setting? How entrenched is the prevailing philosophy?
4. Is there a sufficiently large number of clients in the practice setting who could benefit from the innovation?
5. Will the innovation take too long to implement and evaluate?

Feasibility

6. Will nurses have the freedom to carry out the innovation? Will they have the freedom to terminate the innovation if it is considered undesirable?
7. Will the implementation of the innovation interfere inordinately with current staff functions?
8. Does the administration support the innovation? Is the organizational climate conducive to research utilization?
9. Is there a fair degree of consensus among the staff and among the administrators that the innovation could be beneficial and should be tested? Are there major pockets of resistance or uncooperativeness that could undermine efforts to implement and evaluate the innovation?
10. To what extent will the implementation of the innovation cause friction within the organization? Does the utilization project have the support and cooperation of departments outside the nursing department?
11. Are the skills needed to carry out the utilization project (both the implementation and the clinical evaluation) available within the nursing staff? If not, how difficult will it be to collaborate with or to secure the assistance of others with the necessary skills?
12. Does the organization have the equipment and facilities necessary for the innovation? If not, is there a way to obtain the needed resources?
13. If nursing staff need to be released from other practice activities to learn about and implement the innovation, what is the likelihood that this will happen?
14. Are appropriate measuring tools available for a clinical evaluation of the innovation?

Cost/Benefit Ratio of the Innovation

15. What are the risks to which clients would be exposed during the implementation of the innovation?
16. What are the potential benefits that could result from the implementation of the innovation?
17. What are the risks of maintaining current practices (i.e., the risks of *not* trying the innovation)?
18. What are the material costs of implementing the innovation? What are the costs in the short-term during utilization, and what are the costs in the long run, if the change is to be institutionalized?
19. What are the material costs of *not* implementing the innovation (i.e., could the new procedure result in some efficiencies that could lower the cost of providing service)?
20. What are the potential nonmaterial costs of implementing the innovation to the organization (e.g., lower staff morale, staff turnover, absenteeism)?
21. What are the potential nonmaterial benefits of implementing the innovation (e.g., improved staff morale, improved staff recruitment)?

❖ RESEARCH EXAMPLES

Many utilization projects undoubtedly are being undertaken by nurses in practice settings. Regrettably, relatively few of these efforts are documented in the nursing literature. One such project, described below, illustrates the potential of such projects to result in improved nursing care.

> Kilpack, Boehm, Smith, and Mudge (1991) undertook a utilization project that focused on efforts to decrease patient falls in their hospital, the Dartmouth-Hitchcock Medical Center. The project began when the hospital's Nursing Quality Assurance Committee noted an increase in patient falls and established a study group to address the problem.
>
> The group began by undertaking a thorough review of the literature to identify nursing interventions that have been documented as being effective in reducing patient falls. After the review, a fall prevention program was implemented in the two units that had especially high rates of in-patient falls. The special program was designed to prevent repeat falls among those who had a fall identified by an incident report.
>
> During the 1-year study period, incident reports were screened, and for each patient who had experienced a fall, the staff nurse caring for the patient completed a form that listed the research-based interventions that previously had been identified in the literature review. The nurse was asked to select those interventions that he or she thought should be incorporated into the plan of care. With this information, the clinical nurse specialist developed a written plan of care using the nursing diagnosis of potential for injury. The staff nurse was asked to implement the plan, and adherence to the plan was monitored. Care plans were adjusted as needed when there was a recurrence of a fall.
>
> The researchers gathered data on falls during the study period and documented their incidence and nature; they also documented the interventions that were utilized. They found that the patient fall rate on the two targeted units decreased (relative to the previous year), while the overall rate in the hospital increased. As a result of the project, six major clinical practice recommendations were made to the institution, and all six were implemented.

❖ SUMMARY

In nursing, *research utilization* refers to the use of some aspect of a scientific investigation in a clinical application unrelated to the original research. Research utilization can best be characterized on a continuum, with direct utilization of some specific innovation (*instrumental utilization*) at one end and more diffuse situations in which users are influenced in their thinking about an issue based on some research (*conceptual utilization*) at the other end.

There is tremendous potential for research utilization at all points along this continuum throughout the nursing process. To date, however, there is little evidence that utilization has occurred—at least not with respect to instrumental utilization. It seems likely, though, that more diffuse forms of utilization have occurred as nurses have increased their research productivity and their awareness of the need for research.

Several major utilization projects have been implemented, the most noteworthy being the WICHE, NCAST, and CURN projects. These utilization projects demonstrated that it is possible to increase research utilization, but they also shed light on some of the barriers to utilization. These barriers include such factors as an inadequate scientific base, nursing staff with little training in research and utilization, resistance to change among nurses and institutions that employ them, unfavorable organizational climates, resource constraints, limited collaboration among practitioners and researchers, poorly developed communication channels among these two groups, and the shortage of appropriate role models.

Responsibility for research utilization should be borne by the entire nursing community. Researchers, educators, members of peer review panels, practicing nurses, nursing students, and nurse administrators can adopt a number of strategies to improve the extent to which research findings form the basis for nursing practice.

In planning a major utilization project, practicing nurses can begin with the identification of an important clinical problem and then proceed to identify and critique the knowledge base and perform an assessment of the implementation potential of the innovation. Under favorable conditions, the nurses can then plan the innovation protocols, implement and evaluate the innovation, and make a rational decision regarding the adoption of the innovation based on the evaluation. Alternatively, nurses can begin with the knowledge base and then perform an evaluation of the clinical relevance of a research area before proceeding through the other steps of the utilization process. In either case, there are three major categories of *utilization criteria* that must be considered before proceeding with a utilization plan: clinical relevance, scientific merit, and implementation potential. The implementation potential category includes the dimensions of transferability of knowledge, feasibility of utilization in the particular setting, and the cost/benefit ratio of the innovation.

❖ *STUDY SUGGESTIONS*

Chapter 26 of the accompanying *Study Guide for Nursing Research: Principles and Methods, 5th ed.*, offers various exercises and study suggestions for reinforcing the concepts taught in this chapter. Additionally, the following study questions can be addressed:

1. Find an article in a recent issue of a nursing research journal that does not discuss the implications of the study for nursing practice. Evaluate the study's relevance to nursing practice and, if appropriate, write one to two paragraphs summarizing the implications.
2. Consider your personal situation. What are the barriers that might inhibit your use of research findings? What steps might be taken to address those barriers?

❖ *SUGGESTED READINGS*

METHODOLOGICAL REFERENCES

American Nurses' Association Congress for Practice. (1973). *Standards for practice.* Kansas City, MO: Author.

Barnard, K. E., & Hoehn, R. E. (1978). *Nursing child assessment satellite training: Final report.* Hyattsville, MD: Department of Health, Education, and Welfare, Division of Nursing.

Brodish, M. S., Tranbarger, R. E., & Chamings, P. A. (1987). Clinical nursing research: A model for collaboration. *Journal of Nursing Administration, 17,* 6, 32.

Caplan, N., & Rich, R. F. (1975). *The use of social science knowledge in policy decisions at the national level.* Ann Arbor, MI: Institute for Social Research, University of Michigan.

Downs, F. S. (1979). Clinical and theoretical research. In F. S. Downs & J. W. Fleming (Eds.), *Issues in nursing research.* New York: Appleton-Century-Crofts.

Funk, S. G., Champagne, M. T., Wiese, R. A., & Tornquist, E. M. (1991). Barriers to using research findings in practice: The clinician's perspective. *Applied Nursing Research, 4,* 90–95.

Funk, S. G., Tornquist, E. M., & Champagne, M. T. (1989a). A model for improving the dissemination of nursing research. *Western Journal of Nursing Research, 11,* 361–367.

Funk, S. G., Tornquist, E.M., & Champagne, M. T. (1989b). Application and evaluation of the dissemination model. *Western Journal of Nursing Research, 11,* 485–491.

Gennaro, S. (1994). Research utilization: An overview. *Journal of Obstetric, Gynecologic, and Neonatal Nursing, 23,* 313–319.

Green, S., & Houston, S. (1993). Promoting research activities: Institutional strategies. *Applied Nursing Research, 6,* 97–98.

Haller, D., Reynolds, M., & Horsley, J. (1979). Developing research-based innovation protocols: Process, criteria, and issues. *Research in Nursing and Health, 2,* 45–51.

Hayes, P. (1993). Replicative studies. *Clinical Nursing Research, 2,* 243–244.

Horsley, J. A., Crane, J., & Bingle, J. D. (1978). Research utilization as an organizational process. *Journal of Nursing Administration, 8,* 4–6.

Horsley, J., Crane, J., Crabtree, M., & Wood, D. (1983). *Using research to improve nursing practice: A guide.* New York: Grune & Stratton.

Jackel, M. (1989). Presenting research to nurses in clinical practice. *Applied Nursing Research, 2,* 191–193.

Janken, J. K., Rudisill, P., & Benfield, L. (1992). Product evaluation as a research utilization strategy. *Applied Nursing Research, 5,* 188–194.

Keefe, M. R., Pepper, G., & Stoner, M. (1988). Toward research-based nursing practice: The Denver collaborative research network. *Applied Nursing Research, 1,* 109–115.

Krueger, J. C., Nelson, A. H., & Wolanin, M. O. (1978). *Nursing research: Development, collaboration, and utilization.* Germantown, MD: Aspen Systems.

Lambert, C. E., & Lambert, V. A. (1988). Clinical nursing research: Its meaning to the practicing nurse. *Applied Nursing Research, 1,* 54–57.

Larson, E. (1989). Using the CURN project to teach research utilization in a baccalaureate program. *Western Journal of Nursing Research, 11,* 593–599.

Maurin, J. T. (1990). Research utilization in the social-political arena. *Applied Nursing Research, 3,* 48–51.

Phillips, L. R. F. (1986). *A clinician's guide to the critique and utilization of nursing research.* Norwalk, CT: Appleton-Century-Crofts.

Reynolds, M. A., & Haller, K. B. (1986). Using research in practice: A case for replication in nursing. *Western Journal of Nursing Research, 8,* 113–116.

Rizzuto, C., Bostrum, J., Suter, W. N., & Chenitz, W. C. (1994). Predictors of nurses' involvement in research activities. *Western Journal of Nursing Research, 16,* 193–204.

Stetler, C. B. (1985). Research utilization: Defining the concept. *Image, 17,* 40–44.

Tanner, C. A. (1987). Evaluating research for use in practice: Guidelines for the clinician. *Heart and Lung, 16,* 424–430.

Weiss, C. (1980). Knowledge creep and decision accretion. *Knowledge: Creation, Diffusion, Utilization, 1,* 381–404.

SUBSTANTIVE REFERENCES

Brett, J. L. L. (1987). Use of nursing practice research findings. *Nursing Research, 36,* 344–349.

Brett, J. L. L. (1989). Organizational integrative mechanisms and adoption of innovations by nurses. *Nursing Research, 38,* 105–110.

Champion, V. L., & Leach, A. (1989). Variables related to research utilization in nursing. *Journal of Advanced Nursing, 14,* 705–710.

Coyle, L. A., & Sokop, A. G. (1990). Innovation adoption behavior among nurses. *Nursing Research, 39,* 176–180.

Horsley, K., Crane, J., & Haller, J. (1981). *Reducing diarrhea in tube-fed patients (CURN Project).* New York: Grune & Stratton.

Horsley, K., Crane, J., Haller, J., & Bingle, J. (1981). *Closed urinary drainage system (CURN Project).* New York: Grune & Stratton.

Ketefian, S. (1975). Application of selected nursing research findings into nursing practice. *Nursing Research, 24,* 89–92.

Kilpack, V., Boehm, J., Smith, N., & Mudge, B. (1991). Using research-based interventions to decrease patient falls. *Applied Nursing Research, 4,* 50–56.

King, I., & Tarsitano, E. (1982). The effect of structured and unstructured preoperative teaching: A replication. *Nursing Research, 31,* 324–329.

Kirchhoff, K. T. (1982). A diffusion survey of coronary precautions. *Nursing Research, 31,* 196–201.

Lim-Levy, F. (1982). The effect of oxygen inhalation on oral temperature. *Nursing Research, 31,* 150–152.

Longman, A. J., Verran, J. A., Ayoub, J., Neff, J., & Noyes, A. (1990). Research utilization: An evaluation and critique of research related to oral temperature measurement. *Applied Nursing Research, 3,* 14–19.

Nichols, G. A., & Verhonick, P. J. (1968). Placement times for oral temperatures: A nursing study replication. *Nursing Research, 17,* 159–161.

Chapter 27

WRITING A RESEARCH PROPOSAL

This chapter brings us, in a sense, full circle: back to the beginning of a research project. A *research proposal* is a written document specifying what the investigator proposes to study and therefore is written before the project has commenced. Proposals serve to communicate the research problem, its significance, and planned procedures for solving the problem to some interested party.

Proposals are written for various reasons. A student enrolled in a research class is often expected to submit a brief plan to the professor before data collection actually begins. Most universities require a formal proposal and a proposal hearing for students about to engage in research for a thesis or dissertation. Funding agencies that sponsor research almost always award funds competitively and use proposals as a basis for their funding decisions.

Proposals prepared for different reasons vary in the amount of detail expected but, like research reports, often have similar content. In the next section, we provide some general information regarding the content and prepara-

tion of research proposals. In a subsequent section, we offer more specific guidelines for the preparation of a proposal for the National Institutes of Health (NIH), the federal agency that sponsors a great number of nursing studies.

❖ OVERVIEW OF PROPOSAL PREPARATION

Reviewers of research proposals, whether they are faculty, funding sponsors, or peer reviewers, want a clear idea of what the researcher plans to do, how and when various tasks are to be accomplished, and whether the researcher is capable of successfully following the proposed plan of action. Proposals are generally evaluated on a number of criteria, including the importance of the research question, its theoretical relevance, the adequacy of the research methods, the availability of appropriate personnel and facilities, and, if money is being requested, the reasonableness of the budget. General guidelines for preparing research proposals follow.

Proposal Content

A researcher preparing a proposal will almost always be given a set of instructions that indicate the format to be followed. Funding agencies often supply an application kit that includes forms to be completed and a specified format for organizing the contents of the proposal. Despite the fact that formats and the amount of detail required may vary widely, there is considerable similarity in the type of information that is expected in research proposals. The major components normally included in research proposals are described in the following sections.

ABSTRACT

Proposals often begin with a brief synopsis of the proposed research. The abstract helps to establish a frame of reference for the reviewers as they begin to read the proposal. The abstract should be brief (usually about 200 to 300 words in length) and should concisely state the study objectives and methods to be used.

STATEMENT OF THE PROBLEM

The problem that the intended research will address is ordinarily identified early in the proposal. The problem should be stated in such a way that its importance is apparent to the reviewer. On the other hand, the researcher should not promise more than can be produced. A broad and complex problem is unlikely to be solvable or manageable.

SIGNIFICANCE OF THE PROBLEM

The proposal needs to describe clearly how the proposed research will make a contribution to knowledge. The proposal should indicate the expected generalizability of the research, its contribution to theory, its potential for improving nursing practice and patient care, and possible applications or consequences of the knowledge to be gained.

BACKGROUND OF THE PROBLEM

A section of the proposal is often devoted to an exposition of how the intended research builds on what has already been done in an area. The background material should strengthen the author's arguments concerning the significance of the study, orient the reader to what is already known about the problem, and indicate how the proposed research will augment that knowledge; it should also serve as a demonstration of the researcher's command of current knowledge in a field.

OBJECTIVES

Specific, achievable objectives provide the reader with clear criteria against which the proposed research methods can be assessed. Objectives stated as research hypotheses or specific models to be tested are often preferred. Whenever the theoretical background of the study, existing knowledge, or the researcher's experience permit an explicit prediction of outcomes, these predictions should be included in the proposal. Avoid the use of null hypotheses, which create an amateurish impression. In exploratory or descriptive research, the formulation of hypotheses might not be feasible. Objectives, in such cases, may be most conveniently phrased as questions.

METHODS

The explanation of the research methods should be thorough enough that a reader will have no question about how the research objectives will be addressed. A thorough methods section includes a description of the sampling plan, research design, instrumentation, specific procedures, and analytic strategies, together with a discussion of the rationale for the methods, potential methodological problems, and intended strategies for handling such problems.

THE WORK PLAN

Researchers often describe in the proposal their plan for managing the flow of work on a research project. The researchers indicate in the *work plan* the sequence of tasks to be performed, the anticipated length of time required for their completion, and the personnel required for their accomplishment. The work plan indicates to the reader how realistic and thorough the researcher has been in designing the study.

PERSONNEL

In proposals addressed to funding agencies, the qualifications of key project personnel should be described. The research competencies of the project director and other team members are typically given major consideration in evaluating a proposal.

FACILITIES

The proposal should document the extent to which special facilities required by the project will be available. Access to physiologic instrumentation, libraries, data processing equipment, computers, special documents or records, and subjects should be described to reassure sponsors or advisers that the project will be able to proceed as planned. The willingness of the institution with which the researcher is affiliated to allocate space, equipment, services, or data should also be indicated.

BUDGET

The budget translates the project activities into monetary terms. It is a statement of how much money will be required to accomplish the various tasks. A well-conceived work plan greatly facilitates the preparation of the budget. If there are inordinate difficulties in detailing financial needs, there may be reason to suspect that the work plan is insufficiently developed.

General Tips on Proposal Preparation

Although it would be impossible to tell readers exactly what steps to follow to produce a successful proposal, we can offer some advice that might help to minimize the anxiety and frustration that often accompany the preparation of a proposal. Many of the tips we provide are especially relevant for researchers who are preparing a proposal for the purpose of securing funding for a research project.

1. REVIEW A SUCCESSFUL PROPOSAL

Although there is no substitute for actually doing one's own proposal as a learning experience, beginning proposal writers can often profit considerably by actually seeing the real thing. The information in this chapter is useful in providing some guidelines, but reviewing an actual successful proposal can do more to acquaint the novice with how all the pieces fit together than all the textbooks in the world.

Chances are some of your colleagues or advisors have written a proposal that has been accepted (either by a funding sponsor or by a dissertation committee), and many people are glad to share their successful efforts with others. Also, proposals funded by the federal government are generally in the public domain. That means that you can ask to see a copy of proposals that have obtained federal funding by writing to the sponsoring agency.

In recognition of the need of beginning researchers to become familiar with successful proposals, several journals (including *The Western Journal of Nursing Research* and *Research in Nursing and Health*) have published proposals in their entirety (with the exception of administrative information such as budgets), together with the critique of the proposal prepared by a panel of expert reviewers. For example, the first such published proposal was a grant application funded by the Division of Nursing entitled, "Couvade: Patterns, Predictors, and Nursing Management" (Clinton, 1985). A more recent example is a proposal for a study of comprehensive discharge planning for the elderly (Naylor, 1990). Another journal, *Grants Magazine,* also publishes successful proposals.

2. PAY ATTENTION TO REVIEWERS' CRITERIA

In most instances in which research funding is at stake, the funding agency will provide the researcher with information about the criteria that reviewers use in making funding decisions. In some cases, the criteria will simply consist of a list of questions that the reviewers must address in making a global assessment of the proposal's quality. In other cases, however, the agency will be able to specify exactly how many points will be assigned to different aspects of the proposal on the basis of specified criteria. As an example, the National Institute of Child Health and Human Development funded some research projects relating to fertility regulation using the following evaluation criteria:

Conceptualization of the problem. Ability of the researcher to conceptualize the problem, including the operationalizing and quantifying of measures, and the development of a theoretical or conceptual framework (0 to 30 points)
Project staff qualifications and availability. Adequacy of the relevant training and experience of the proposed staff (0 to 15 points) Appropriateness of allocation of personnel and time to accomplish objectives of the project (0 to 10 points)
Data sources and analysis. Demonstration of capability for identifying and obtaining access to pertinent and relevant sources of data and

adequacy of plans for data analysis (0 to 20 points)
Review and analysis of literature. Adequacy of the review and analysis of the literature in terms of scope and depth and extent to which research needs are delineated in theoretical, methodological, and analytic areas (0 to 15 points)
Facilities and equipment. Adequacy of computer facilities and other equipment that would be needed in the performance of the research (0 to 10 points)

In this example, a maximum of 100 points was awarded for each competing proposal. The proposals with the highest scores would ordinarily be most likely to obtain funding. Therefore, the researcher should pay particular attention to those aspects of the proposal that contribute most to an overall high score. In this example, it would have made little sense to put 85% of the proposal development effort into the literature review section, when a maximum of 15 points could be given for this part of the proposal.

Different agencies establish different criteria for different types of research projects. The wise researcher will learn what those criteria are and pay careful attention to them in the development of the proposal.

3. BE JUDICIOUS IN DEVELOPING A RESEARCH TEAM

For projects that are funded, reviewers often give considerable weight to the qualifications of the people who will conduct the research. In the example cited earlier, a full 25 of the 100 points were based on the expertise of the research personnel and their time allocations.

The person who is in the lead role on the project—often referred to as the principal investigator (PI)—should carefully scrutinize the qualifications of the research team. It is not enough to have a team of competent people. It is necessary to have the right mix of competence. A project team of three brilliant theorists without statistical skills in a project that proposes sophisticated multivariate techniques may have difficulty convincing reviewers that the project would be successful. Gaps and weaknesses can often be compensated for by the judicious use of consultants.

Another shortcoming of many project teams is that they often look as though there are too many managers. It is generally unwise to load up a project staff with five or more top-level professionals who are only able to contribute 5% to 10% of their time to the project. Such projects often run into management difficulties because no one person is ever really in control of the flow of work. Although collaborative efforts are to be commended, you should be able to *justify* the inclusion of every staff person and to identify the unique contribution that each will make to the successful completion of the project.

4. JUSTIFY AND DOCUMENT YOUR DECISIONS

Unsuccessful proposals often fail because they do not provide the reviewer with confidence that adequate thought and consideration have been given to a rationale for decisions. Almost every aspect of the proposal involves a decision—the problem selected, the population studied, the size of the sample, the data collection procedures to be used, the comparison group to be used, the extraneous variables to be controlled, the analytic procedures to be used, the personnel who will work on the project, and so on. These decisions should be made carefully, keeping in mind the costs and benefits of an alternative decision. When you are satisfied that you have made the right decision, you should be ready to defend your decision by sharing the rationale with the reviewers. In general, insufficient detail is more detrimental to the proposal than an overabundance of detail, although page constraints may make full detail impossible.

5. ARRANGE FOR A CRITIQUE OF THE PROPOSAL

Before formal submission of a proposal, a draft should be reviewed by at least one other person, preferably someone with relevant methodological and substantive strengths in the proposed area of research. (Ideally, if the proposal is being submitted for funding, then the reviewer will be someone who is knowledgeable about the funding source.) If a consultant has been proposed because of specialized expertise that you believe will strengthen the study; then it would be advantageous to have that consultant participate in the proposal development by reviewing the draft and making recommendations for its improvement.

❖ GRANT APPLICATIONS TO THE NATIONAL INSTITUTES OF HEALTH

The National Instiues of Health (NIH) funds a considerable number of nursing research studies through the National Institute of Nursing Research (NINR) and through other institutes and agencies within NIH. Applications for grant funding through NIH are made by completing Public Health Service Grant Application Form PHS 398, which is available through the research offices of most universities and hospitals. Copies of the application kit can also be obtained by writing to the following address:

Division of Research Grants
National Institutes of Health
Westwood Building Room 449
5333 Westbard Avenue
Bethesda, MD 20892

New grant applications are generally processed in three cycles annually. The schedule for submission and review of new grant applications is shown in Table 27-1. Proposals (grant applications) may be submitted on the proper forms at any time during the year. However, proposals received after one receipt date

Table 27-1. *Schedule for Processing General National Institutes of Health Grant Applications**

RECEIPT DATES	INITIAL (PEER) REVIEW DATES	NATIONAL ADVISORY COUNCIL REVIEW DATES	EARLIEST POSSIBLE START DATES
February 1	June/July	September/October	December 1
June 1	October/November	January/February	April 1
October 1	February/March	May/June	July 1

* Research applications relating to AIDS undergo an expedited review and award process. Receipt dates for R01 and R29 grant applications for AIDS-related research are January 2, May 1, and September 1 of each year.

will be held for another cycle. For example, if a proposal is received by NIH on February 2, it will be considered with the proposals received by June 1, not February 1.

The Review Process

Grant applications submitted to NIH are received by the Division of Research Grants (DRG), where they are reviewed for relevance to the overall mission of NIH. Acceptable applications are assigned to an appropriate Institute or Center. Figure 27-1 presents the NIH Institutes and Centers, as of September 1993. Most applications by nurse researchers are assigned to NINR, unless the content of the proposal is better suited to another Institute.

As the schedule in Table 27-1 indicates, NIH uses a dual review system for making decisions about its grant applications. The first level involves a panel of peer reviewers (not employed by NIH), who evaluate the grant application for its scientific merit. This panel (usually referred to as an *Initial Review Group* or *Study Section*) consists of about 15 to 20 scientists with backgrounds appropriate to the specific Study Section for which they have been selected. Appointments to the review panels are generally for 4-year terms and are staggered so that about one fourth of each panel is new each year. The second level of review is by a National Advisory Council, which includes both scientific and lay representatives. The National Advisory Council considers not only the scientific merit of an application but also the relevance of the proposed

study to the programs and priorities of the Center or Institute to which the application has been submitted as well as budgetary considerations.

The peer review panel members, after discussing the strengths and weaknesses of a given application, normally make one of three decisions: 1) to approve and score an application; 2) to not recommend an application for further consideration (NRFC);* or 3) to defer an application. Deferrals are relatively rare and usually involve an application that the review panel considers meritorious but missing some crucial information that would permit the panel to make a final determination. Most proposals are either approved or given an NRFC designation immediately. Review panels vary considerably from one Study Section to another in the proportion of applications that are approved. In part, this reflects the quality of the proposals themselves, but it also reflects the philosophy of different panels. Because only a relatively small percentage of proposals that are approved are actually funded, some panels decide to use the NRFC category for only a small minority of applications, reserving this classification for projects that are judged potentially to "set back science." In the NINR Study Section, over 90% of all grant applications typically are approved at each meeting.

All applications that are *approved* are privately assigned a priority rating by each member of the review panel. The ratings range from 1.0

* The NRFC category has replaced the category previously designated as disapprovals.

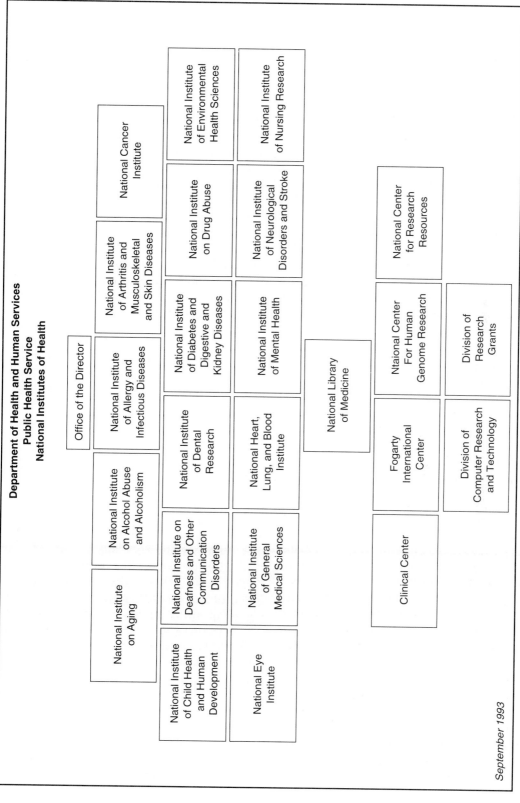

Figure 27-1. *National Institutes of Health Organizational Chart*

(the best possible score) to 5.0 (the least favorable score), in increments of 0.1. NIH has established the following guidelines for assigning priority scores:

Outstanding: 1.0–1.5
Excellent: 1.5–2.0
Very good: 2.0–2.5
Good: 2.5–3.5
Acceptable: 3.5–5.0

The individual ratings from different panel members are then combined, averaged, and multiplied by 100 to yield scores that range from 100 to 500, with 100 being the best possible score. Among all approved applications, only those with the best priority scores actually obtain funding. Cutoff scores for funding vary from agency to agency and year to year. It is often necessary to obtain a rating of 200 or better to become funded. Within NIH overall, fewer than 20% of all grant applications are actually funded.*

Applications for clinical research, defined as human biomedical and behavioral studies of the etiology, epidemiology, prevention (and preventive strategies), diagnosis, or treatment of diseases, disorders, or conditions, are also evaluated based on whether the proposed project appropriately includes women and minorities in the study population. The Study Section codes each application into one of five categories based on the adequacy of representation of women and minorities (coded separately) in the study population: 1) not clinical research; 2) representation not germane; 3) representation appropriate; 4) representation inappropriate, but justification adequate; and 5) representation inappropriate, justification inadequate. Awards cannot be granted to applications in the fifth category.

Each applicant, regardless of the decision of the Study Section, is sent a summary of the peer review panel's evaluation. These "pink sheets" (so called because they are printed on pink paper) summarize the reviewers' comments in six areas: 1) an overall description of the project; 2) a critique of the strengths and weaknesses of the methodological and conceptual aspects of the proposal; 3) an evaluation of the project team; 4) an evaluation of the facilities and resources; 5) an assessment of the reasonableness of the budget; and 6) a discussion of other considerations, with emphasis on the protection of the rights of human subjects or the welfare of animal subjects. The applicant is also advised of the panel's decision (approval, not recommended for further consideration, or deferral), and, if the proposal was approved, the priority score and percentile rank.

Unless an unfunded proposal is criticized in some fundamental way (e.g., the problem area was not judged to be significant, or the basic design was considered inappropriate), it is often worthwhile to resubmit an application, making revisions that reflect the concerns of the peer review panel. Unfunded proposals that receive encouraging priority scores (in the 200–300 range) are especially likely to fare well in a resubmission. When a proposal is resubmitted, the next review panel usually is given a copy of the original application and the pink sheet so that they can evaluate the degree to which the original criticisms have been addressed.

Types of National Institutes of Health Grants

The NIH awards different types of grants, and each has its own objectives and review criteria. Four types of grants that represent the bulk of awards are discussed next, but other types are also available.

The basic grant program is the *Research Project Grant* (R01). The objective of the R01 grant is to support discrete, specific research projects in areas reflecting the interests and competencies of a PI. The review criteria include 1) the significance and originality of the proposed research; 2) the appropriateness and adequacy of the proposed research methods; 3) the qualifications and experience of the PI and other staff; 4) the availability of needed resources; 5) the reasonableness of the proposed

---

* Within the NINR Study Section, the median priority score has typically been in the 250 to 270 range.

budget; and 6) the adequacy of proposed means for protecting human subjects or research animals.

There are also a limited number of *Small Grants* (R03) that provide funding for small-scale studies, pilot work, or feasibility studies in specific areas that are announced annually by NIH institutes. These grants award up to $35,000 of project funds (nonrenewable) for a project period of up to 2 years.

A special program (R15) has been established for researchers working in educational institutions that have not been major participants in NIH programs. These are the *Academic Research Enhancement Awards* (AREA), the objective of which is to stimulate research in institutions that provide baccalaureate training for many individuals who go on to do health-related research. AREA grants enable qualified researchers to obtain support for small-scale research projects. The review criteria for AREA grants are basically the same as for R01 grants.

Another special program has been established for new investigators. The *First Independent Research Support and Transition*, or FIRST (R29), program is designed to provide an initial period of support for newly independent researcher scientists. These grants are intended to provide an opportunity for new scientists to demonstrate creativity and productivity and to assist them in making the transition to other NIH grants. FIRST awards are made for a period of 5 years, and the total direct costs must not exceed $350,000. The review criteria are similar to those for R01 grants, but less emphasis is placed on the investigator's experience than on his or her potential for productive research. Letters of reference must accompany the proposal and are carefully evaluated.

Preparing a Grant Application for National Institutes of Health

As indicated earlier, proposals to NIH must be submitted according to procedures described in the Public Health Service application kit. Each kit specifies exactly how the grant application should be prepared and what forms are to be used for supplying critical pieces of information. It is important to follow these instructions precisely. In the sections that follow, we describe the various components of an application and provide some tips that should be helpful in completing certain sections.*

FRONT MATTER

The *front matter* of the grant application consists of various forms that help in the processing of the application or that provide administrative information about the conduct of the research. Proposal writers often fail to give this section the attention it merits because all the intellectual work is presented in the research plan section. However, we urge researchers to pay as much attention to detail in this first section as in the second. Each form included in Section 1 is briefly described to acquaint the reader with its contents.

- *Title page.* On the title page form, the researcher provides the title of the application (not to exceed 56 spaces), the name of the PI, the name of the PI's institutional affiliation, the amount of money requested, the proposed time period of the project, and other administrative information.
- *Abstract of research plan.* Page 2 is a form that asks for a listing of the key professional personnel who would work on the study and a half-page abstract of the investigator's aims and methods. The abstract *must* fit into the space allocated.
- *Table of contents.* Page 3 indicates on what pages various sections and subsections of the proposal are to be found.
- *Budget.* Pages 4 and 5 consist of budgetary forms. Page 4 asks for an itemization of all costs that would be incurred by the project during the first 12 months. Page 5 asks for a summary of the budget for the entire project

---

* The application kit for NIH grants changes periodically. Therefore, the instructions in a current version of Form PHS 398 should be carefully reviewed and followed in preparing a grant application rather than relying exclusively on information in this chapter.

period. For R01 grants, support can be requested for up to 5 years, but most projects are completed in 3 years or less. Beginning at the bottom of page 5 (and continuing for as many pages as necessary), the researcher must provide a narrative justification of all budgeted items. New researchers often make the mistake of submitting a budget justification that is insufficiently detailed. Remember that the reviewers need to be able to tell whether the budget is reasonable, and part of your job is to convince them that you would use funding judiciously. Normally, two or three single-spaced pages are needed to justify budgetary items.

Figure 27-2 presents a hypothetical page 4 (detail of first-year expenditures), and Figure 27-3 presents a hypothetical page 5 for a study that would require 2 years of support. The bottom of Figure 27-3 presents the first few paragraphs of a budget justification, showing the level of detail that is ordinarily considered appropriate. For most projects, personnel costs (wages and fringe benefits) represent the bulk of the requested funds, and personnel costs are generally represented as a percentage of a person's time (e.g., 20 hours per week would be designated as a 50% level of effort on the proposed project). Other costs include the cost for consultants, project-specific equipment, supplies, travel costs, patient care costs, costs associated with a subcontract or consortium arrangements, and other expenses. The final category might include such items as laboratory fees, subject stipends, transcriptions, computer time, and data entry expenses. Note that the NIH budget forms should indicate *direct costs* (specific project-related costs) only. *Indirect costs* (institutional *overhead*) are not shown on the budget forms. Beginning researchers are likely to need the assistance of a research administrator or an experienced, funded researcher in developing their first budget.

- *Biographic sketches.* Forms are provided to summarize salient aspects of the education and experience of key project personnel. The PI and any other proposed staff who are considered important contributors to the project's success must have their biographic sketches included. A maximum of two pages is permitted for each person.

- *Other support.* Key personnel must identify any sources of support they are now receiving or sources of support that they have pending on the form of other planned or submitted proposals. This form is designed to help reviewers determine whether important staff may be overcommitted and therefore be potentially unable to devote a sufficient amount of time to the proposed project.

- *Resources and environment.* On this form, the author must designate the availability of needed facilities and equipment, such as office space, computers, laboratories, medical apparatus, and so on.

RESEARCH PLAN SECTION

The main section of the NIH grant application is reserved for the investigator's research plan. This section consists of nine parts (though not all nine are relevant to every application). Parts 1 through 4 of the research plan, combined, must not exceed 25 single-spaced pages, including any figures, charts, or tables. If the proposal does not adhere to this page restriction, then the application will be returned without review. Within the overall 25-page limitation, the text can be distributed among Parts 1 through 4 in any manner the researcher considers appropriate, although guidelines are suggested.

1. *Specific aims.* The researcher must provide a succinct summary of the research problem and the specific objectives to be undertaken during the course of the project, including any hypotheses to be tested. The application guidelines suggest that Part 1 be restricted to a single page.

2. *Background and significance.* In Part 2, the researcher must convince the review

DD　　　　　　　Principal Investigator/Program Director *(Last, first, middle):*　Miller, Susan

DETAILED BUDGET FOR INITIAL BUDGET PERIOD **DIRECT COSTS ONLY**					FROM 12/1/95	THROUGH 11/30/96	
PERSONNEL *(Applicant organization only)*			%		DOLLAR AMOUNT REQUESTED *(omit cents)*		
NAME	ROLE ON PROJECT	TYPE APPT. *(months)*	EFFORT ON PROJ.	INST. BASE SALARY	SALARY REQUESTED	FRINGE BENEFITS	TOTALS
Susan Miller	Principal Investigator	12	25%	60,000	15,000	4,500	19,500
Stacie Mayette	Co-Invest.	12	25%	40,000	10,000	3,000	13,000
To Be Hired	Interviewr	9	100%	20,000	15,000	4,500	19,500
To Be Hired	Res. Asst.	12	20%	15,000	3,000	900	3,900
To Be Hired	Secretary	12	40%	16,000	6,400	1,920	8,320
	SUBTOTALS⟶				49,400	14,820	64,220

CONSULTANT COSTS
Michael Burns, statistical consultant　5 days @ $400/day
Michael Wilcox, programming consultant 20 days @ $200/day　　　　　　　6,000

EQUIPMENT *(Itemize)*

Modem

　　　　　　　　　　　　　　　　　　　　　　　　　　　　　　　500

SUPPLIES *(Itemize by category)*
Office supplies　　$75/month X 12
Photocopying　　　$50/month X 12
Postage　　　　　　$50/month X 12
Subject stipends　200 @ $15
Telephone　　　　　$1,000

　　　　　　　　　　　　　　　　　　　　　　　　　　　　　　　6,100

TRAVEL
1 professional conference ($1,000); interviewer travel ($750)
　　　　　　　　　　　　　　　　　　　　　　　　　　　　　　　1,750

PATIENT CARE COSTS　　INPATIENT
　　　　　　　　　　　OUTPATIENT

ALTERATIONS AND RENOVATIONS *(Itemize by category)*

OTHER EXPENSES *(Itemize by category)*
Computer time on mainframe
　　　　　　　　　　　　　　　　　　　　　　　　　　　　　　　1,000

SUBTOTAL DIRECT COSTS FOR INITIAL BUDGET PERIOD　　　　　　79,570

CONSORTIUM/CONTRACTUAL COSTS
　DIRECT COSTS　$　10,000　　　　　　　　　　TOTAL⟶
　INDIRECT COSTS　$　4,500　　　　　　　　　　　　　　　　　14,500

TOTAL DIRECT COSTS FOR INITIAL BUDGET PERIOD *(Item 7a, Face Page)* ⟶　$　94,070

PHS 398 (Rev. 9/91)　　　　　　　　(Form Page 4) Page _____
Number pages consecutively at the bottom throughout the application. Do *not* use suffixes such as 3a, 3b..　　　　DD

Figure 27-2.　*Example of first-year budget*

EE   Principal Investigator/Program Director *(Last, first, middle):*   Miller, Susan

BUDGET FOR ENTIRE PROPOSED PROJECT PERIOD
DIRECT COSTS ONLY

BUDGET CATEGORY TOTALS		INITIAL BUDGET PERIOD *(from page 4)*	ADDITIONAL YEARS OF SUPPORT REQUESTED			
			2nd	3rd	4th	5th
PERSONNEL: *Salary and fringe benefits* Applicant organization only		64,220	70,844			
CONSULTANT COSTS		6,000	8,000			
EQUIPMENT		500	0			
SUPPLIES		6,100	5,000			
TRAVEL		1,750	2,000			
PATIENT CARE COSTS	INPATIENT	0	0			
	OUTPATIENT	0	0			
ALTERATIONS AND RENOVATIONS		0	0			
OTHER EXPENSES		1,000	2,000			
SUBTOTAL DIRECT COSTS		79,570	87,844			
CONSORTIUM/ CONTRACTUAL COSTS		14,500	7,250			
TOTAL DIRECT COSTS		94,070	95,094			

TOTAL DIRECT COSTS FOR ENTIRE PROPOSED PROJECT PERIOD *(Item 8a)* ⟶ $ 189,164

JUSTIFICATION (Use continuation pages if necessary):
   From Budget for Initial Period: Describe the specific functions of the personnel, collaborators, and consultants and identify individuals with appointments that are less than full time for a specific period of the year, including VA appointments.

   For All Years: Explain and justify purchase of major equipment, unusual supplies requests, patient care costs, alterations and renovations, tuition remission, and donor/volunteer costs.

   From Budget for Entire Period: Identify with an asterisk (*) on this page and justify any significant increase or decrease in any category over the initial budget period. Describe any change in effort of personnel.

   For Competing Continuation Applications: Justify any significant increases or decreases in any category over the current level of support.

Personnel
   Miller, the PI, will be responsible for overall project management, instrument development, data quality control, data analysis and report preparation. She is budgeted for 25% effort in the first 18 months of the project. In the final 6 months, Miller will devote 50% of her time to the proposed project to perform the data analyses and prepare a final report. Mayette, the Co-Investigator, will devote 25% of her time to the project throughout the 2-year period. She will participate in the instrumentation, training of the interviewer, development of a coding scheme, analysis of the data, and report preparation.
   The interviewer will be hired in Month 4. She will work for 15 months at 100% effort and will be responsible for all data collection. A research assistant (RA) will be hired to assist with such tasks as library research, instrument pretests, and data coding. The RA will work at 20% level of effort in both years of the project. A secretary will be hired at 40% effort to perform secretarial and clerical functions.
   A 5% salary increase has been budgeted for all personnel in Year 2.

PHS 398 (Rev. 9/91)   (Form Page 5) Page _____   EE
Number pages consecutively at the bottom throughout the application. Do *not* use suffixes such as 3a, 3b.

Figure 27-3. *Example of overall summary budget*

panel that the proposed study idea is sound and has important clinical or theoretical relevance. In this section of the research plan, the researcher provides the context for the conduct of the study, usually through a brief analysis of existing knowledge on the topic and through a discussion of a conceptual framework. Within this context, the investigator must demonstrate the significance of, and need for, the proposed new project. Beginning researchers often have an especially difficult time with this section because only two to three pages are recommended. This is often a challenging task, especially if you have a firm grasp on the broad range of literature relating to your topic. However, we again urge researchers not to be tempted to exceed the three-page guideline. Space should be conserved for a full elaboration of the proposed research methods.

3. *Preliminary studies.* This section is reserved for a description of the project team's previous studies that are relevant to the new proposed investigation. Many novice researchers mistakenly believe that this section is designed for a literature review. If you make this mistake, it will indicate that you are a novice and unable to follow instructions. This section (although it is optional for new applications and is only required for continuation proposals) provides an opportunity to persuade the reviewers that you have the skills and background needed to do the research. Because the biographic sketch included in the front matter is limited to only two pages, the Preliminary Studies section provides a forum for the description of any relevant work you and other key staff have either completed or are in the process of doing. If the only relevant research you have completed is your dissertation, here is an opportunity to describe that research in full. If you have completed relevant research that has led to publications, you should reference them in this section and

include copies of them as appendixes. Other items that might be described in this section include previous uses of an instrument or an experimental procedure that will be used in the new study, relevant clinical or teaching experience, membership on task forces or in organizations that have provided you with a perspective on the research problem, or the results of a pilot study that involved the same research problem. The point is that this section allows you to demonstrate that the proposed work grew out of some ongoing commitment to, interest in, or experience with the topic. For new applications, no more than six to eight pages should be devoted to Part 3, and fewer pages are often sufficient.

4. *Research design and methods.* It is in Part 4 that you must describe the methods you will use to conduct the study. This section should be succinct but with sufficient detail to persuade reviewers that you have a sound rationale for your methodological decisions. Although there are no specific page limitations associated with this section of the application, keep in mind that you have up to 25 pages in total for Parts 1 through 4 combined.

The number of subsections in the methods section varies from one application to another. Each subsection should be labeled clearly to facilitate the review process. As is true in organizing any written material, it is often useful to begin with an outline. Here is an outline of the sections used in a successful grant application for a nonexperimental study of parenting behavior and family environments among low-income teenaged mothers:
- Overview of the Research Design
- Sampling Considerations
- Research Variables and Measuring Instruments
- Data Collection Procedures
- Data Analysis
- Research Products
- Project Schedule

If there is an experimental intervention, that intervention should be described in full. Protocols for the implementation of the intervention also need to be discussed. If there is to be a control group, clearly identify how the control group will be selected. If the design involves a comparison group rather than a randomly assigned control group, then you will need to discuss your rationale for the selection of the specified group, any shortcomings in using this group, and why this group is preferable to some alternative. For example, if you were to study the psychological consequences of an abortion in an effort to determine the need for follow-up interventions, there are at least four alternative comparison groups: 1) same-aged, never-pregnant women; 2) same-aged women who had a miscarriage; 3) same-aged women who were still pregnant and had not decided how to resolve the pregnancy; or 4) same-aged women who had delivered a baby. Each group might be expected to introduce different types of selection biases, so your rationale for selecting one over the other would be a critical reflection of your conceptualization of the problem and your methodological sophistication.

In quantitative studies, the design section should also indicate how the research situation will be structured to control for extraneous variables. The proposal should specify what variables might represent contaminating sources of influence; which variables will be controlled (and how); why other variables will not be controlled; and what the probable impact of the uncontrolled variables on the study outcome will be. Krathwohl (1988) observed that "probably nobody knows better than the researcher the multiple sources of contamination which might affect the study. Convincingly indicate the nature and basis of the particular compromise which is being proposed and the reasons for accepting it" (p. 31).

A number of things should be included in a section on sampling. The reviewer normally expects to find a description of the population, the proposed sampling design, and the number of subjects to be included in the study. The section should include both a description of the sampling plan and a justification for its use. If you cannot use random sampling, explain the constraints (e.g., the costs of implementing such a design) and discuss steps you would take to make the sample as representative as possible and to document any biases. Increasingly, review panels expect to see a power analysis that justifies the adequacy of the specified sample size in quantitative projects. It is also advisable to document your access to the specified subject pool. For instance, if the proposal indicates that patients and personnel from Park Memorial Hospital will participate in the study, then you should include a letter of cooperation from an administrator of the hospital with the application. The reviewer needs to have confidence that the proposed study, if funded, would actually be done as planned.

Normally, a subsection is devoted to data collection and instrumentation. The use of particular measuring instruments should be justified as appropriate for the purposes of the study. It is inadequate to select a well-known measure without explicitly demonstrating its relevance and valued qualities. For established measures, the proposal should describe reported evidence of the measure's reliability and validity. If a new instrument is to be developed, then the anticipated procedures for its development *and* evaluation should be described. If possible, sample items or the entire instrument should be included in an appendix. In qualitative studies, the data collection section should describe the procedures that will be implemented to enhance and assess the trustworthiness of the data.

A subsection should be devoted to the specific procedures that will be used to collect the research data. This subsection should include such information as where and when the data will be collected, how subjects will be recruited, how research personnel such as interviewers or observers will be trained, whether subjects will be paid a stipend for their time, what quality-control procedures will be implemented to ensure the integrity of the data, and how the security of the data will be maintained. If the study is longitudinal, then it is also important to describe the schedule for waves of data collection (and a rationale for the schedule), as well as information on how the problem of attrition will be managed.

The grant application should include, in as much detail as possible, the plan for the analysis of data. This is typically one of the weakest sections of proposals. Some applications say little more than, "Trust me—I'll figure out what to do with the data once I have collected them." You may not be able to tell in advance every analytic strategy you will try, but you should be able to work through the general procedures you will use in testing the hypotheses or answering the research questions. Earlier in this section, we presented an outline of a grant application relating to parenting among low-income teenaged mothers. The Data Analysis subsection of this grant application described the proposed plan with respect to the following analytic tasks:

a. Data Cleaning and Descriptive Analyses
b. Exploratory Analyses
c. Analysis of Bias
d. Testing Individual Hypotheses
e. Path Analysis

Although the grant application kit does not specifically request a project schedule or work plan, it is often useful to include one (unless the page limitation makes it impossible to do so). A work plan helps reviewers assess how realistic you have been in planning the project, and it should help you to develop an estimate of needed resources (i.e., your budget). Flow charts and other diagrams are often useful for highlighting the sequencing and interrelationships of project activities. One of the simplest and most effective types of charts is called a *Gantt chart,* named after its inventor Henry Gantt. Figure 27-4 presents a Gantt chart for the 30-month study on teenaged parents. Other more sophisticated charting techniques, such as the *Program Evaluation Review Technique* (PERT) and the *Critical Path Method,* are sometimes used for complex projects. These are briefly described by Krathwohl (1988).

5. *Human subjects.* If the research involves data collected from human subjects, then this section must describe the procedures that will be used to protect their rights and to minimize the risks that they will take. The application kit specifies six questions that need to be addressed (an example is presented in Appendix A). This section of the proposal often serves as the cornerstone of the document submitted to the Institutional Review Board of your institution before funding (you should check with your office of research administration for Institutional Review Board requirements).

6. *Vertebrate animals.* If your proposed research involves the use of vertebrate animals, then this section must contain a justification of their use and a description of the procedures used to safeguard their welfare.

7. *Consultants and collaborators.* If you plan to include consultants to help with specific tasks on the proposed project, you must include a letter from each consultant, confirming his or her willingness to serve on the project. Letters are also needed from collaborators on the project, if they are affiliated with an institution different from your own.

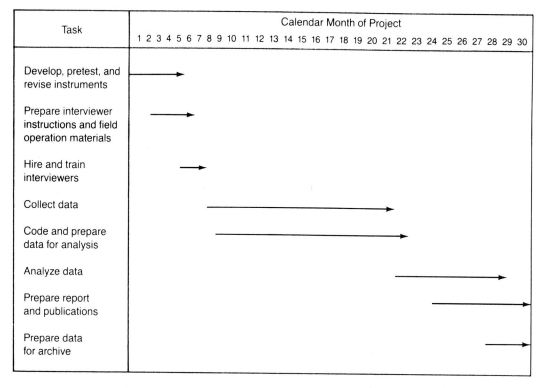

Figure 27-4.   *Example of a Gantt chart*

8. *Consortium or contractual arrangements.* If the proposed project will involve the collaboration of two or more different institutions (e.g., if a separate organization will be used to perform laboratory analyses, under a subcontract agreement), then details about the nature of the arrangements must be described in this section.

9. *Literature cited.* The final subsection of the Research Plan consists of a list of references used in the text of the grant application. Any reference style is acceptable. This section is restricted to six pages.

APPENDIX

The concluding section of the grant application is reserved for appended materials. These materials may include actual instruments to be used in the project, detailed calculations on sample size estimates, scoring or coding instruc-

tions for instruments, proposed letters of consent, letters of cooperation from institutions that will provide access to subjects, complex statistical models, and other supplementary material in support of the application. The researcher can also submit copies of up to 10 published papers or papers accepted for publication (but *not* papers submitted for publication but not yet accepted). The appended materials are not made available to the entire review panel, so essential information should not be relegated to the appendix.

❖ FUNDING FOR RESEARCH PROPOSALS

Funding for research projects is becoming more and more difficult to obtain. The problem lies not only in research cutbacks and inflation but also in the extremely keen and growing competition among researchers. As increasing numbers of nurses become prepared to carry out significant research, so too will applications for research funds increase. Successful proposal writers need to have good research and proposal-writing skills, and they must also know how and from whom funding is available. The combined set of skills and knowledge is sometimes referred to as *grantsmanship.*

Federal Funding

The federal government is the largest contributor to the support of research activities. The two major types of federal disbursements are grants and contracts. *Grants* are awarded for proposals in which the research idea is developed by the investigator. The researcher who identifies an important research problem can seek federal funds through a grant program of one or more agencies of the government.

There are two basic mechanisms for the funding of federal grants. One mechanism is for agencies and institutes to issue broad objectives and priorities through a *program announcement* and to invite grant applications that address these objectives. Researchers apply for funding from this general grants program through the process described in the preceding section.

There are several ways to find out about such grant programs. *The Catalogue of Federal Domestic Assistance* publishes information about all federal programs that provide any kind of aid. The programs of such agencies as NIH, National Institute of Mental Health (NIMH), National Institute on Drug Abuse (NIDA), and so on are described in terms of objectives, types of assistance, award processes, and so on. There are also commercially available guides to programs, such as the annual *Federal Funding Guide.* (This guide, if purchased through Government Information Services in Arlington, Virginia, includes 12 monthly grant updates.) Programs identified as particularly promising through such sources can then be contacted for further information. Many government agen-

cies, including institutes within NIH, also publish information regarding their general funding programs (e.g., NINR distributes a brochure called *Facts about Funding*).

The second grant-funding mechanism offers federal agencies a means of identifying a specific topic area in which they are especially interested in receiving applications. An agency may announce, for instance, that it is soliciting grant applications for studies relating to infertility. Such an announcement is referred to as a *Request for Applications* (RFA). Unlike the more general grants programs, the RFA usually specifies a deadline for the receipt of proposals. General guidelines and goals for the competition are also specified, but the researcher has considerable liberty to develop the specific research problem. Notices of such grant competitions are published in *The Federal Register* and in other publications specific to the funding agency.

The second type of government funding (and this may occur at both the federal and state level) is in the form of *contracts.* An agency that identifies the need for a specific study issues a *Request for Proposals* (RFP), which details the *exact* work that the government wants done and the specific problem to be addressed. Proposals in response to RFPs describe the methods the researcher would use in addressing the research problem, the project staff and facilities, and the cost of doing the study in the proposed way. Contracts are usually awarded to only one of the competitors. The contract method of securing research support severely constrains the kinds of work in which investigators can engage—the researcher responding to an RFP generally has no latitude in developing the research objectives. For this reason, most nurse researchers probably will want to compete for grants rather than contracts. Nevertheless, many interesting RFPs have been issued by NIH and other agencies. For example, one recent NIH RFP called for proposals for a study of "Ethnic Differences in Life Style, Psychological Factors, and Medical Care During Pregnancy."

A summary of each federal RFP is printed in the *Commerce Business Daily,* which is published every government workday. Also, NIH publishes a weekly bulletin called the *NIH Guide for Grants and Contracts*. This bulletin announces new NIH initiatives, including the announcement of RFAs and RFPs issued by NIH.* An example of a portion of an RFA for NINR, listed in the January 7, 1994 issue of the *NIH Guide*, is presented in Figure 27-5.

Private Funds

Health-care research is supported by a number of philanthropic foundations, professional organizations, and corporations. Many investigators prefer private funding to government support because there is often less red tape. Private organizations typically are less rigid in their proposal regulations, reporting requirements, clearance of instruments, and monitoring of progress. Not surprisingly, private organizations are besieged with proposed research projects.

Information about philanthropic foundations that support research is available in *The Foundation Directory,* published by the Foundation Center. This volume, which is updated periodically, lists more than 2500 foundations whose annual grants are at least $500,000. The directory lists the purposes and activities of the foundations and the addresses for contacting them. Also available through the Foundation Center is a directory entitled *National Guide to Foundation Funding in Health*. Information on foundations (as well as federal programs) is also available through the Sponsored Programs Information Network (SPIN), which is a computerized data base to which most universities and research institutions have access.

Professional associations such as the American Nurses' Foundation, Sigma Theta Tau, the American Association of University Women, and the Social Science Research Council offer funds for conducting research. Health organiza-

tions such as the American Heart Association and the American Cancer Society also support research activities. Finally, funds for research are sometimes donated by private corporations, particularly those dealing with health care products. Additional information concerning the requirements and interests of such groups should be obtained either from the organization directly or from personnel in research administration offices of universities, hospitals, or other agencies with which you are affiliated.

Information regarding funding opportunities is also available in a publication offered by the American Association of Colleges of Nursing entitled *The Complete Grants Sourcebook for Nursing and Health*. Finally, announcements relating to grants competitions and funding sources are published in the "Research Reporter" section of the journal *Nursing Research*.

❖ CONCLUSION

Proposals represent the means for opening communication between researchers and parties interested in the conduct of research. Those parties may be funding agencies, faculty advisers, or institutional officers, depending on the circumstances. An accepted proposal is a two-way contract: those accepting the proposal are effectively saying, "We are willing to offer our [emotional or financial] support, as long as the investigation proceeds as proposed," and those writing the proposal are saying, "If you will offer support, then I will conduct the project as proposed." Therefore, the proposal offers some assurance that neither party will be disappointed.

Beginning proposal writers sometimes forget that, in essence, they are selling a product: themselves and their ideas. It is not inappropriate, therefore, to do a little marketing. If the researcher does not sound convinced that the proposed study is important and will be executed with skill, then the reviewers will not be convinced either. The proposal should be written in a positive, confident tone. Instead of saying, "The study will *try* to . . . ," it is better to indicate

---

* The *NIH Guide* is usually available through institutional research offices, or it may be obtained by writing to the NIH Guide Distribution Center, National Institutes of Health, Room B4BN08, Building 31, Bethesda, MD 20892.

SYMPTOM MANAGEMENT: ACUTE PAIN

RFA AVAILABLE: NR-94-003
National Institute of Nursing Research

Letter of Intent Receipt Date: March 15, 1994
Application Receipt Data: April 21, 1994

THIS IS A NOTICE OF AVAILABILITY OF A REQUEST FOR APPLICATIONS (RFA); IT IS ONLY AN ABSTRACT OF THE RFA. POTENTIAL APPLICANTS MUST REQUEST THE COMPLETE RFA, WHICH CONTAINS ESSEN-TIAL INFORMATION FOR THE PREPARATION OF AN APPLICATION, FROM THE CONTACT LISTED IN "IN-QUIRIES," BELOW. FAILURE TO FOLLOW THE INSTRUCTION IN THE COMPLETE RFA MAY RESULT IN AN INCOMPLETE APPLICATION, WHICH WILL BE RETURNED TO THE APPLICANT WITHOUT REVIEW.

PURPOSE
The focus of this RFA is on interventions to improve the assessment, management, and prevention of acute pain. Studies that address the multidimensional nature of pain, which includes a range of physiological, sensory, affective, behavioral, cognitive, and sociocultural factors, are encouraged in order to provide a scientific basis for clinical prac-tice.

ELIGIBILITY REQUIREMENTS
Applications may be submitted by domestic and foreign for-profit and non-profit organizations, public and private, such as universities, colleges, hospitals, laboratories, units of state and local governments, and eligible agencies of the Federal Government. Applications from minority individuals and women are encouraged.

MECHANISM OF SUPPORT
This RFA will use the National Institutes of Health (NIH) individual research project grant (R01)...The total project pe-riod for applications submitted in response to the present RFA may not exceed three years. The anticipated award date is September 30, 1994. Because the nature and scope of the research proposed in response to this RFA may vary, it is anticipated that the size of an award will vary also, but will generally be in the range of $150,000 to $180,000 direct costs. This RFA is a one-time solicitation.

FUNDS AVAILABLE
Approximately $1,200,000 in total costs for the first year will be committed to fund applications submitted in response to this RFA. It is anticipated that four to six applications will be funded.

This is an excerpt from an RFA that appeared in the NIH Guide for Grants and Contracts, Vol. 23, No. 1, January 7, 1994, pp. 36-38.

Figure 27-5.   *Example of a Request for Application*

more positively that the study *will* achieve some goals. Similarly, it is more optimistic to specify what the investigator *will* do, rather than what he or she *would* do, if approved. There is no need to brag or promise what cannot be accomplished. Rather, it is a question of putting the actual project accomplishments and significance in a positive light.

As another aspect of marketing, the proposal should be as physically attractive as possible. A neat and pleasing appearance invites the reviewer to read a proposal and suggests that care has been devoted to its preparation. Flashy and expensive binders, figures, and so forth are unnecessary, but the physical presentation should not leave a bad impression on readers.

Grantsmanship, like research skills, is both a skill and an art. The skill can be acquired through further reading, by attending a course on grantsmanship, or by working with a mentor. We also hope that we have been helpful in communicating some of what goes into the skill part, and we offer all readers our best wishes in cultivating the art of doing and writing about research and acquiring support to pursue it.

❖ SUMMARY

A *research proposal* is a written document specifying what a researcher intends to study and is written with the intent of obtaining approval and support—often financial support. The major components of a research proposal include the following: an abstract, statement of the problem, significance of the problem, background, objectives, methods, work plan, personnel, facilities, and a budget.

A major source of funding for nurse researchers is the National Institutes of Health (NIH), within which is housed the National Institute of Nursing Research (NINR). Nurses can apply for a variety of grants from NIH, the most common being the *Research Project Grant* (R01 grant), *Small Grant, FIRST Grant,* or *AREA Grant.* Grant applications to NIH, which are submitted on special forms and which must fol-

low strict formatting guidelines, are reviewed three times a year in a dual review process. The first phase involves a review by a peer *Study Section* that evaluates each proposal's scientific merit, and the second phase is a review by a National Advisory Council. The Study Section assigns *priority scores* to all approved proposals; a score of 100 represents the most meritorious ranking, and a score of 500 is the lowest possible score. A detailed critique of the proposal, together with information on the priority score and percentile ranking, are sent back to the researcher in the form of a *pink sheet.*

The federal government is the largest source of research funds for health researchers. In addition to regular grants programs, agencies of the federal government announce special funding programs in the form of *Requests for Applications (RFAs)* (for *grants*) and *Requests for Proposals (RFPs)* (for *contracts*). Other sources of funding include foundations, professional associations, and private corporations. The set of skills associated with learning about funding opportunities and developing proposals that can be funded is sometimes referred to as *grantsmanship.*

❖ STUDY SUGGESTIONS

Chapter 27 of the accompanying *Study Guide for Nursing Research: Principles and Methods, 5th ed.,* offers various exercises and study suggestions for reinforcing the concepts taught in this chapter. Additionally, the following study questions can be addressed:

1. Suppose that you were planning to study the problem of role conflict among nursing administrators.
   a. Outline the methods you would recommend adopting.
   b. Develop a work plan.
   c. Prepare a hypothetical budget.
2. Suppose that you were interested in studying separation anxiety in hospitalized children. Using the references cited in this

chapter, identify potential funding sources for your project.

❖ *SUGGESTED READINGS*

Bauer, D. G., & the American Association of Colleges of Nursing (1988). *The complete grants source book for nursing and health.* New York: Macmillan.

Bloch, D. (1990). Strategies for setting and implementing the National Center for Nursing Research priorities. *Applied Nursing Research, 3,* 2–6.

Brodsky, J. (1976). *The proposal writer's swipe file II.* Washington, DC: Taft Products.

Brooten, D., Munro, B. H., Roncoli, M., Arnold, L., Brown, L., York, R., Hollingsworth, A., Cohen, S., & Rubin, M. (1989). Developing a program grant for use in model testing. *Nursing and Health Care, 10,* 315–318.

Clinton, J. (1985). Couvade: Patterns, predictors and nursing management: A research proposal submitted to the Division of Nursing. *Western Journal of Nursing Research, 7,* 221–248.

Cohen, M. Z., Knafl, K., & Dzurec, L. C. (1993). Grant writing for qualitative research. *Image, 25,* 151–156.

Foundation Center Staff. (1989). *National guide to foundation funding in health.* New York: The Foundation Center.

Foundation Center Staff. (1993a). *The foundation directory* (15th ed.). New York: The Foundation Center.

Foundation Center Staff (1993b). *The national directory of corporate giving* (3rd ed.). New York: The Foundation Center.

Fuller, E. O., Hasselmeyer, E. G., Hunter, J. C., Abdellah, F. G., & Hinshaw, A. S. (1991). Summary statements of the NIH nursing research grant applications. *Nursing Research, 40,* 346–351.

Gortner, S. (1980). Researchmanship: The judges and their judgments. *Western Journal of Nursing Research, 2,* 434–437.

Gortner, S. (1982). Research funding sources. *Western Journal of Nursing Research, 4,* 248–250.

Hinshaw, A. S. (1988a). The National Center for Nursing Research: Challenges and initiatives. *Nursing Outlook, 36,* 54, 56.

Hinshaw, A. S. (1988b). The new National Center for Nursing Research: Patient care research programs. *Applied Nursing Research, 1,* 2–4.

Jackson, N. E. (1982). Choosing and using a statistical consultant. *Nursing Research, 31,* 248–250.

Kim, M. J. (1993). The current generation of research proposals: Reviewers' viewpoints. *Nursing Research, 42,* 118–119.

Krathwohl, D. R. (1988). *How to prepare a research proposal* (3rd ed.). Syracuse, NY: Syracuse University Bookstore.

Naylor, M. D. (1990). An example of a research grant application: Comprehensive discharge planning for the elderly. *Research in Nursing and Health, 13,* 327–347.

Sandelowski, M., Davis, D., & Harris, B. (1989). Artful design: Writing the proposal for research in the naturalist paradigm. *Research in Nursing and Health, 12,* 77–84.

Stewart, R., & Stewart, A. L. (1984). *Proposal preparation.* New York: John Wiley and Sons.

Tornquist, E. M., & Funk, S. G. (1990). How to write a research grant proposal. *Image, 22,* 44–51.

White, V. P. (1975). *Grants: How to find out about them and what to do next.* New York: Plenum Press.

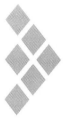

GLOSSARY

abstract A brief description of a completed or proposed research investigation; in research journals, usually located at the beginning of an article.

accessible population The population of subjects available for a particular study; often a nonrandom subset of the target population.

accidental sampling Selection of the most readily available individuals (or units) as subjects in a study; also known as *convenience sampling.*

acquiescence response set A bias in self-report instruments, especially in social psychological scales, created when subjects characteristically agree with statements ("yea-say") independent of their content.

active variable A variable that the researcher creates or manipulates.

adjusted means The mean value of the dependent variable for different groups, after removing the effects of covariates through multiple regression.

after-only design An experimental design in which data are collected from subjects only after the experimental intervention has been introduced; also known as *posttest-only design.*

alpha (α) (1) In tests of statistical significance, the level designating the probability of committing a Type I error, also known as the *p* value; (2) in estimates of internal consistency, a reliability coefficient, as in Cronbach's alpha.

analysis A method of organizing data in such a way that research questions can be answered.

analysis of covariance (ANCOVA) A statistical procedure used to test mean differences among groups on a dependent variable, while controlling for one or more extraneous variables (covariates).

analysis of variance (ANOVA) A statistical procedure for testing mean differences among three or more groups by comparing the variability between groups to the variability within groups.

analytic induction A method of analyzing qualitative data that involves an iterative approach to testing research hypotheses.

anonymity Protection of the participant in a study such that even the researcher cannot link him or her with the information provided.

applications The tasks that computers can be used to perform (e.g., word processing, data base management, statistical analysis).

Polit DF, Hungler BP: NURSING RESEARCH: PRINCIPLES AND METHODS, 5th ed. © 1995 J. B. Lippincott Company.

applied research Research that concentrates on finding a solution to an immediate practical problem.

ASCII format A set of standardized codes used in computers to represent keyboard characters; a file saved in ASCII (an acronym for American Standard Code for Information Interchange) is stripped of proprietary codes specific to the software that created the original file.

assumptions Basic principles that are accepted as being true on the basis of logic or reason, without proof or verification.

asymmetric distribution A distribution of values that is skewed (i.e., has two halves that are not mirror images of each other).

attribute variables Preexisting characteristics of the entity under investigation, which the researcher simply observes and measures.

attrition The loss of participants during the course of a study; can introduce an unknown amount of bias by changing the composition of the sample initially drawn—particularly if more subjects are lost from one group than another; can thereby be a threat to the internal validity of a study.

audit trail The systematic collection and documentation of material that allows an independent auditor (in an inquiry audit of qualitative data) to draw conclusions about the data.

baseline measure The measurement of the dependent variable before the introduction of an experimental intervention.

basic research Research designed to extend the base of knowledge in a discipline for the sake of knowledge production or theory construction rather than for solving an immediate problem.

batch processing mode A method of communicating with a mainframe computer in which a batch of programs is assembled for execution during the same computer run.

before–after design An experimental design in which data are collected from research subjects both before and after the introduction of the experimental intervention; also known as *pretest-posttest design.*

behavioral objective An intended outcome of a program or intervention, stated in terms of the behavior of the individuals at whom the program is aimed.

beneficence A fundamental ethical principle that seeks to prevent harm and exploitation of, and maximize benefits for, human subjects.

beta (β) (1) In multiple regression, the standardized coefficients indicating the relative weights of the independent variables in the regression equation; (2) in statistical testing, the probability of a Type II error.

bias Any influence that produces a distortion in the results of a study.

bimodal distribution A distribution of values with two peaks (high frequencies).

bivariate statistics Statistics derived from the analysis of two variables simultaneously for the purpose of assessing the empirical relationship between them.

blind review The review of a manuscript or proposal such that neither the author nor the reviewer is identified to the other party.

borrowed theory A theory borrowed from another discipline or field to guide nursing practice or research.

bracketing In phenomenological inquiries, the process of identifying and holding in abeyance any preconceived beliefs and opinions one has about the phenomena under study.

byte A single character, such as a number, letter, or specialized symbol, in a computer's memory.

canonical correlation A statistical procedure for examining the relationship between two or more independent variables *and* two or more dependent variables.

case-control study A research design, typically found in retrospective ex post facto research, that involves the comparison of a "case" (i.e., a subject with the condition under scrutiny, such as lung cancer) and a pair-matched control (i.e., a person without the condition).

case study A research method that involves a thorough, in-depth analysis of an individual, group, institution or other social unit.

categorical variable A variable with discrete values rather than incremental placement along a continuum (e.g., a person's marital status).

category system In observational studies,

the prespecified plan for organizing and recording the behaviors and events to be observed.

causal relationship A relationship between two variables such that the presence or absence of one variable (the "cause") determines the presence or absence, or value, of the other (the "effect").

cell (1) The intersection of a row and column in a table with two or more dimensions; (2) in an experimental design, the representation of an experimental condition in a schematic diagram.

census A survey covering an entire population.

central processing unit (CPU) The portion of a computer, comprising the control unit and arithmetic/logic unit, where all decisions and calculations are performed.

central tendency A statistical index of the typicalness of a set of scores that comes from the center of the distribution of scores. The three most common indexes of central tendency are the mode, the median, and the mean.

chi-square test A nonparametric test of statistical significance used to assess whether a relationship exists between two nominal-level variables. Symbolized as χ^2.

clinical research Research designed to generate knowledge to guide nursing practice.

clinical trial An experiment involving a test of the effectiveness of a clinical treatment, generally involving a large and heterogeneous sample of subjects.

closed-ended question A question that offers respondents a set of mutually exclusive and jointly exhaustive alternative replies, from which the one that most closely approximates the "right" answer must be chosen.

cluster analysis A multivariate statistical procedure used to cluster people or things based on patterns of association.

cluster randomization The random assignment of intact groups of subjects to treatment conditions.

cluster sampling A form of multistage sampling in which large groupings ("clusters") are selected first (e.g., nursing schools), with successive subsampling of smaller units (e.g., nursing students).

code of ethics The fundamental ethical principles that are established by a discipline or institution to guide researchers' conduct in research with humans.

codebook The documentation used in data processing that indicates the location and values of all the variables in a data file.

coding The process of transforming raw data into standardized form (usually numerical) for data processing and analysis.

coefficient alpha (Cronbach's alpha) A reliability index that estimates the internal consistency or homogeneity of a measure composed of several items or subparts.

coefficient of determination The proportion of variance in the dependent variable accounted for or explained by a group of independent variables, more commonly referred to as R^2.

coercion In a research context, the explicit or implicit use of threats (or excessive rewards) to get people to agree to participate in a study.

cohort study A kind of trend study that focuses on a specific subpopulation (which is often an age-related subgroup) from which different samples are selected at different points in time (e.g., the cohort of nursing students graduated from 1970 through 1974).

command file In statistical software packages, the file that contains instructions about the data set and the analyses to be performed.

comparison group A group of subjects whose scores on a dependent variable are used as a basis for evaluating the scores of the target group or group of primary interest. The term comparison group is generally used instead of control group when the investigation does not use a true experimental design.

compiler A computer program that translates programming language into machine language.

computer An electronic device that performs simple operations with extreme accuracy and speed.

computer program A set of instructions to a computer.

concealment A tactic involving the unobtrusive collection of research data without the subjects' knowledge or consent, used to obtain an accurate view of naturalistic behavior.

concept An abstraction based on observations of certain behaviors or characteristics (e.g., stress, pain).

conceptual framework (conceptual model) Interrelated concepts or abstractions that are assembled together in some rational scheme by virtue of their relevance to a common theme.

conceptual utilization The use of research findings in a general, conceptual way to broaden one's thinking about an issue, although the knowledge is not put to any specific, documentable use.

concurrent validity The degree to which scores on an instrument are correlated with some external criterion, measured at the same time.

confidence interval The range of values within which a population parameter is estimated to lie.

confidence level The estimated probability that a population parameter lies within a given confidence interval.

confidentiality Protection of participants in a study such that their individual identities will not be linked to the information they provide and will never be publicly divulged

confirmability A criterion for evaluating data quality with qualitative data, referring to the objectivity or neutrality of the data.

consent form A written agreement signed by a subject and a researcher concerning the terms and conditions of a subject's voluntary participation in a study.

consistency check A procedure performed in cleaning a set of data to ensure that the data are internally consistent.

constant comparison A procedure often used in qualitative analysis wherein newly collected data are compared in an ongoing fashion with data obtained earlier, to refine theoretically relevant categories.

construct An abstraction or concept that is deliberately invented (constructed) by researchers for a scientific purpose (e.g., health locus of control).

construct validity The degree to which an instrument measures the construct under investigation.

consumer An individual who reads, reviews, and critiques research findings and who attempts to use and apply the findings in his or her practice.

contact information Information obtained from subjects in longitudinal studies that facilitates their relocation at a future date.

contamination The inadvertent, undesirable influence of one experimental treatment condition on another treatment condition.

content analysis A procedure for analyzing written or verbal communications in a systematic and objective fashion, typically with the goal of quantitatively measuring variables.

content validity The degree to which the items in an instrument adequately represent the universe of content.

contingency table A two-dimensional table that permits a cross-tabulation of the frequencies of two nominal-level or ordinal-level variables.

continuous variable A variable that can take on a large range of values representing a continuum (e.g., height).

control The process of holding constant possible influences on the dependent variable under investigation.

control group Subjects in an experiment who do not receive the experimental treatment and whose performance provides a baseline against which the effects of the treatment can be measured (see also *comparison group*).

convenience sampling Selection of the most readily available individuals (or units) as subjects in a study; also known as *accidental sampling*.

convergent validity An approach to construct validation that involves assessing the degree to which two methods of measuring a construct are similar (i.e., converge).

correlation A tendency for variation in one variable to be related to variation in another variable.

correlational research Investigations that

explore the interrelationships among variables of interest without any active intervention on the part of the researcher.

correlation coefficient An index that summarizes the degree of relationship between two variables. Correlation coefficients typically range from +1.00 (for a perfect direct relationship) through 0.0 (for no relationship) to −1.00 (for a perfect inverse relationship).

correlation matrix A two-dimensional display showing the correlation coefficients between all combinations of variables of interest.

cost/benefit analysis 1) In evaluation research, a comparison of the financial costs of a program or intervention with the financial gains attributable to it; 2) in a utilization project, an assessment of the costs or risks of a new practice or procedure, in relation to its benefits.

counterbalancing The process of systematically varying the order of presentation of stimuli, treatments, or items in a scale to control for ordering effects, as in counterbalancing the order of treatments in a repeated measures design.

covariate A variable that is statistically controlled (held constant) in analysis of covariance. The covariate is typically an extraneous, confounding influence on the dependent variable or a pretest measure of the dependent variable.

covert data collection The collection of information in a study without the subject's knowledge.

Cramer's V An index describing the magnitude of relationship between nominal-level data, used when the contingency table to which it is applied is larger than 2×2.

credibility A criterion for evaluating the data quality of qualitative data, referring to confidence in the truth of the data.

criterion-related validity The degree to which scores on an instrument are correlated with some external criterion.

criterion variable (criterion measure) The quality or attribute used to measure the effect of an independent variable; sometimes used instead of *dependent variable.*

critical incident technique A method of obtaining data from study participants by in-depth exploration of specific incidents and behaviors related to the matter under investigation.

critique An objective, critical, and balanced appraisal of a research report's various dimensions (e.g., conceptual, methodological, ethical).

Cronbach's alpha A widely-used reliability index that estimates the internal consistency or homogeneity of a measure composed of several subparts; also referred to as *coefficient alpha.*

crossover design See *repeated measures design.*

cross-sectional study A study based on observations of different age or developmental groups at a single point in time for the purpose of inferring trends over time.

cross-tabulation A determination of the number of cases occurring when simultaneous consideration is given to the values of two or more variables (e.g., gender—male/female—cross-tabulated with smoking status—smoker/nonsmoker). The results are typically presented in a table with rows and columns divided according to the values of the variables.

data The pieces of information obtained in the course of a study (singular is *datum*).

data analysis The systematic organization and synthesis of research data, and the testing of research hypotheses using those data.

data cleaning The preparation of data for analysis by performing checks to ensure that the data are consistent and correct.

data collection The gathering of information needed to address a research problem.

data entry The process of entering data onto an input medium for computer analysis.

data saturation See *saturation.*

data transformation A step often undertaken before the analysis of research data, to put the data in a form that can be meaningfully analyzed (e.g., recoding of values).

data triangulation See *triangulation.*

debriefing Communication with research subjects, generally after their participation has been completed, regarding various aspects of the study.

deception The deliberate withholding of information, or the provision of false information, to research subjects, usually used to reduce potential biases.

deductive reasoning The process of developing specific predictions from general principles (see also *inductive reasoning*).

degrees of freedom (df) A concept used in tests of statistical significance, referring to the number of sample values that cannot be calculated from knowledge of other values and a calculated statistic (e.g., by knowing a sample mean, all but one value would be free to vary); the number of degrees of freedom is usually $N - 1$, but different formulas are relevant for different tests.

Delphi technique A method of obtaining judgments from a panel of experts. The experts are questioned individually, and a summary of the judgments is circulated to the entire panel. The experts are questioned again, with further iterations introduced as needed until there is some consensus.

demonstration A program or intervention that is being tested, often on a large scale, to determine its effectiveness and the desirability of changing policies or procedures.

dependability A criterion for evaluating data quality in qualitative data, referring to the stability of data over time and over conditions.

dependent variable The outcome variable of interest; the variable that is hypothesized to depend on or be caused by another variable (called the *independent variable*); sometimes referred to as the *criterion variable*.

descriptive research Research studies that have as their main objective the accurate portrayal of the characteristics of individuals, situations, or groups and the frequency with which certain phenomena occur.

descriptive statistics Statistics used to describe and summarize data (e.g., means, standard deviations).

descriptive theory A broad characterization that thoroughly accounts for a single phenomenon.

determinism The belief that phenomena are not haphazard or random but rather have antecedent causes.

deviation score A score computed by subtracting an individual score value from the mean of the distribution of scores.

dichotomous variable A variable having only two values or categories (e.g., gender).

direct costs Specific project-related costs incurred in the course of a study (e.g., for personnel working on the study, supplies, travel, and so on).

directional hypothesis A hypothesis that makes a specific prediction about the direction and nature of the relationship between two variables.

discriminant function analysis A statistical procedure used to predict group membership or status on a categorical (nominal-level) variable on the basis of two or more independent variables.

discriminant validity An approach to construct validation that involves assessing the degree to which a single method of measuring two constructs yields different results (i.e., discriminates the two).

disproportionate sampling design A sampling strategy wherein the researcher samples differing proportions of subjects from different strata in the population to ensure adequate representation of subjects from strata that are comparatively smaller.

double-blind experiment An experiment in which neither the subjects nor those who administer the treatment know who is in the experimental or control group.

dummy variable Dichotomous variables created for use in many multivariate statistical analyses, typically using codes of 0 and 1 (e.g., female = 1, male = 0).

effect size A statistical expression of the magnitude of the relationship between two variables, or the magnitude of the difference between two groups, with regard to some attribute of interest.

eigenvalue In factor analysis, the value equal to the sum of the squared weights for each factor.

element The most basic unit of a population from which a sample will be drawn; in nursing research, the element is typically humans.

eligibility criteria The criteria used by a researcher to designate the specific attributes of the target population, and by which subjects are selected for participation in a study.

emic perspective A term used by ethnographers to refer to the way members of a culture themselves view their world; the "insider's view."

empirical evidence Evidence that is rooted in objective reality and that is gathered through the collection of data using one's senses; used as the basis for generating knowledge through the scientific approach.

endogenous variable In path analysis, a variable whose variation is determined by other variables in the model.

equivalence The degree of similarity between alternate forms of a measuring instrument.

error of measurement The degree of deviation between true scores and obtained scores when measuring a characteristic.

eta squared A statistic calculated, in ANOVA, to indicate the proportion of variance in the dependent variable explained by the independent variables, analogous to R^2 in multiple regression; computed by dividing the sum of squares between groups by the total sum of squares.

ethics A system of moral values that is concerned with the degree to which research procedures adhere to professional, legal, and social obligations to the research subjects.

ethnography A branch of human inquiry, associated with the field of anthropology, that focuses on a culture (or subculture) of a group of people, with an effort to understand the world view of those under study.

ethnomethodology A branch of human inquiry, associated with sociology, that focuses on the way in which people make sense of their everyday activities and come to behave in socially acceptable ways.

ethnonursing research The study of human cultures, with a focus on a group's beliefs and practices relating to nursing care and related health behaviors.

etic perspective A term used by ethnographers to refer to the "outsider's view" of the experiences of a cultural group.

evaluation research Research that investi-

gates how well a program, practice, or policy is working.

event sampling In observational studies, a sampling plan that involves the selection of integral behaviors or events.

exogenous variable In path analysis, a variable whose determinants lie outside the model.

experiment A research study in which the investigator controls (manipulates) the independent variable and randomly assigns subjects to different conditions.

experimental group The subjects who receive the experimental treatment or intervention.

experimental intervention (experimental treatment) See *intervention*; *treatment*.

exploratory research A preliminary study designed to develop or refine hypotheses, or to test and refine the data collection methods.

ex post facto research Research conducted after the variations in the independent variable have occurred in the natural course of events; a form of nonexperimental research in which causal explanations are inferred "after the fact."

external criticism In historical research, the systematic evaluation of the authenticity and genuineness of data.

external storage device A device associated with computers for storage of data and programs (e.g., a floppy disk).

external validity The degree to which the results of a study can be generalized to settings or samples other than the ones studied.

extraneous variable A variable that confounds the relationship between the independent and dependent variables and that needs to be controlled either in the research design or through statistical procedures.

extreme response set A bias in self-report instruments, especially in social psychological scales, created when subjects characteristically express their opinions in terms of extreme response alternatives (e.g., "strongly agree") independent of the question's content.

face validity The extent to which a measuring instrument looks as though it is measuring what it purports to measure.

factor analysis   a statistical procedure for reducing a large set of variables into a smaller set of variables with common characteristics or underlying dimensions.

factorial design   An experimental design in which two or more independent variables are simultaneously manipulated; this design permits an analysis of the main effects of the independent variables separately, plus the interaction effects of these variables.

field notes   The notes taken by researchers regarding the unstructured observations they have made in the field, and their interpretation of those observations.

field study   A study in which the data are collected "in the field" from individuals in their normal roles, with the aim of understanding the practices, behaviors, and beliefs of individuals or groups as they normally function in real life.

file   For computers, a collection of information that can be accessed by the computer by reference to a specific name.

findings   The results of the analysis of the research data; in quantitative studies, the results of the statistical tests.

Fisher's exact test   A statistical procedure used to test the significance of the difference in proportions, used when the sample size is small or cells in the contingency table have no observations.

fixed-alternative question   A question that offers respondents a set of prespecified responses, from which the respondent must choose the alternative that most closely approximates the correct response.

focused interview   A loosely structured interview in which the interviewer guides the respondent through a set of questions using a topic guide.

focus group interview   An interview in which the respondents are a group of individuals assembled to answer questions on a given topic.

follow-up study   A study undertaken to determine the subsequent development of individuals with a specified condition or who have received a specified treatment.

formative evaluation   An ongoing assessment of a product or program as it is being developed, designed to optimize the ultimate quality of that product or program.

F-ratio   The statistic obtained in several statistical tests (e.g., ANOVA) in which variation attributable to different sources (e.g., between groups and within groups) is compared.

frequency distribution   A systematic array of numerical values from the lowest to the highest, together with a count of the number of times each value was obtained.

frequency polygon   Graphic display of a frequency distribution, in which dots connected by a straight line indicate the number of times a score values occur in a set of data.

Friedman test   A nonparametric analogue of ANOVA, used when the researcher is working with paired groups or a repeated measures situation.

full disclosure   The communication of complete information to potential research subjects regarding the nature of the study, the subject's right to refuse participation, and the likely risks and benefits that would be incurred.

functional relationship   A relationship or association between two variables wherein it cannot be assumed that one variable caused the other; however, it can be said that the variable X changes values as a function of changes in variable Y.

Gantt chart   A chart depicting the scheduling of activities (tasks) of a research study and highlighting the sequencing and interrelationships among activities.

generalizability   The degree to which the research procedures justify the inference that the findings represent something beyond the specific observations on which they are based; in particular, the inference that the findings can be generalized from the sample to the entire population.

grand theory   A broad theory aimed at describing large segments of the physical, social, or behavioral world; also referred to as a macrotheory.

grant   An award made to a researcher or team

of researchers, enabling the conduct of a proposed study through the provision of financial support.

grantsmanship The combined set of skills and knowledge needed to secure financial support for one's research ideas.

graphic rating scale A scale in which respondents are asked to rate something (e.g., a concept, issue, institution) along an ordered bipolar continuum (e.g., "excellent" to "very poor").

grounded theory An approach to collecting and analyzing qualitative data with the aim of developing theories and theoretical propositions grounded in real-world observations.

hardware The physical electronic equipment that makes a computer.

Hawthorne effect The effect on the dependent variable caused by subjects' awareness that they are participants under study.

heterogeneity The degree to which objects are dissimilar with respect to some attribute (i.e., characterized by high variability).

histogram A graphic presentation of frequency distribution data.

historical research Systematic studies designed to establish facts and relationships concerning past events.

history threat A threat to the internal validity of a study; refers to the occurrence of events external to the treatment but concurrent with it, which can affect the dependent variable of interest.

homogeneity (1) In terms of the reliability of an instrument, the degree to which the subparts are internally consistent (i.e., are measuring the same critical attribute); (2) more generally, the degree to which objects are similar (i.e., characterized by low variability).

hypothesis A statement of predicted relationships between two or more variables, subjected to testing in empirical studies.

impact analysis An evaluation of the effects of a program or intervention on some outcomes of interest, net of other factors influencing those outcomes.

implementation analysis An evaluation that describes the process by which a program or intervention was implemented in practice.

implementation potential The extent to which an innovation is amenable to implementation in a new setting, an assessment of which is usually made in a research utilization project; includes the criteria of transferability, feasibility, and cost/benefit ratio of the innovation.

independent variable The variable that is believed to cause or influence the dependent variable; in experimental research, the independent variable is the variable that is manipulated.

indirect costs The institutional costs that are included in a research budget, over and above the specific (direct) costs of conducting the study; also referred to as overhead.

inductive reasoning The process of reasoning from specific observations to more general rules (see also *deductive reasoning*).

inferential statistics Statistics that permit inferences on whether relationships observed in a sample are likely to occur in a larger population of concern.

informant A term used to refer to those individuals who provide information to researchers about a phenomenon under study, often used in qualitative studies in lieu of the terms subjects or respondents.

informed consent An ethical principle that requires researchers to obtain the voluntary participation of subjects, after informing them of possible risks and benefits.

input devices Those parts of a computer system that allow data and commands to be entered into the computer.

inquiry audit An independent scrutiny of qualitative data and relevant supporting documents by an external reviewer, a method used to determine the dependability and confirmability of qualitative data.

Institutional Review Board (IRB) A group of individuals who convene to review proposed and ongoing studies with respect to ethical considerations.

instrument The device or technique that a researcher uses to collect data (e.g., questionnaires, tests, observation schedules, etc.).

instrumental utilization   Clearly identifiable attempts to base some specific action or intervention on the results of research findings.

instrumentation system   The entire set of devices and apparatus used to collect in vivo physiologic measurements; includes the subject, stimulus, sensing equipment, signal-conditioning equipment, display equipment, and recording equipment.

instrumentation threat   The threat to the internal validity of the study that can arise if the researcher changes the measuring instrument between two points of data collection.

interaction effect   The effect on a dependent variable of two or more independent variables acting in combination (interactively) rather than as unconnected factors.

interactive mode   A mode of communicating with a computer wherein the user interacts directly with the computer and obtains feedback almost immediately.

intercoder reliability   The degree to which two coders, operating independently, assign the same codes to variables.

internal consistency   A form of reliability, referring to the degree to which the subparts of an instrument are all measuring the same attribute or dimension.

internal criticism   In historical research, an evaluation of the worth of the historical evidence.

internal validity   The degree to which it can be inferred that the experimental treatment (independent variable), rather than uncontrolled, extraneous factors, is responsible for observed effects.

interrater (interobserver) reliability   The degree to which two raters or observers, operating independently, assign the same ratings or values for an attribute being measured; such ratings normally occur in the context of observational research.

interval estimation   A statistical estimation approach in which the researcher establishes a range of values that are likely, within a given level of confidence, to contain the true population parameter.

interval measure   A level of measurement in which an attribute of a variable is rank-ordered on a scale that has equal distances between points on that scale (e.g., Fahrenheit degrees).

intervention   (1) In experimental research, the experimental treatment or manipulation; (2) more generally, the structure the investigator imposes on the research setting before making observations.

interview   A method of data collection in which one person (an interviewer) asks questions of another person (a respondent); interviews are conducted either face to face or by telephone.

interview schedule   The formal instrument, used in structured self-report studies, that specifies the wording of all questions to be asked of respondents.

inverse relationship   A negative correlation between two variables; i.e., a relationship characterized by the tendency of high values on one variable to be associated with low values on a second variable.

isomorphism   In measurement, the correspondence between the measures an instrument yields and reality.

item   A term used to refer to a single question on a test or questionnaire or to a single statement on a social psychological scale (e.g., a final examination might consist of 100 items).

journal club   A group that meets regularly (often in clinical settings) to discuss and critique research reports appearing in research journals, often with the goal of assessing the utilization potential of the findings.

judgmental sampling   A type of nonprobability sampling method in which the researcher selects subjects for the study on the basis of personal judgment about which ones will be most representative or productive; also referred to as *purposive sampling*.

Kendall's tau   A correlation coefficient used to indicate the magnitude of a relationship between ordinal-level data.

key informant   A person well-versed in the phenomenon of research interest and who is willing to share the information and insight with the researcher; key informants are often used in needs assessments.

known-groups technique A technique for estimating the construct validity of an instrument through an analysis of the degree to which the instrument separates groups that are predicted to differ on the basis of some theory or known characteristic.

Kruskal-Wallis test A nonparametric test used to test the difference between three or more independent groups, based on ranked scores.

Kuder-Richardson (KR-20) formula A method of calculating an internal consistency reliability coefficient for a scaled set of items; used when the items are dichotomous.

law A theory that has accrued such persuasive empirical support that it is accepted as truth (e.g., Boyle's law of gases).

least-squares estimation A commonly used method of statistical estimation in which the solution minimizes the sums of squares of error terms; sometimes referred to as OLS (ordinary least squares).

level of measurement A system of classifying measurements according to the nature of the measurement and the type of mathematic operations to which they are amenable; the four levels are nominal, ordinal, interval, and ratio.

level of significance The risk of making a Type I error, established by the researcher before the statistical analysis (e.g., the .05 level).

life history A narrative self-report about a person's life experiences regarding some theme of interest to the researcher.

life table analysis A statistical procedure used when the dependent variable represents a time interval between an initial event (e.g., onset of a disease) and an end event (e.g., death); also referred to as survival analysis.

Likert scale A type of composite measure of attitudes that involves summation of scores on a set of items (statements) to which respondents are asked to indicate their degree of agreement or disagreement.

LISREL The widely used acronym for linear structural relation analysis, typically used for testing causal models using procedures based on maximum likelihood estimation.

listwise deletion A method of dealing with missing values in a data set that involves the elimination of cases with missing data.

literature review A critical summary of research on a topic of interest, generally prepared to put a research problem in context or to identify gaps and weaknesses in prior studies so as to justify a new investigation.

log In participant observation studies, the observer's daily record of events and conversations that took place.

logical positivism The philosophy underlying the traditional scientific approach.

logistic regression A multivariate regression procedure that uses maximum likelihood estimation for analyzing relationships between multiple independent variables and categorical dependent variables; also referred to as logit analysis.

longitudinal study A study designed to collect data at more than one point in time, in contrast to a cross-sectional study.

macrotheory A broad theory aimed at describing large segments of the physical, social, or behavioral world; also referred to as a grand theory.

main effects In a study with multiple independent variables, the effects of a single independent variable on the dependent variable.

mainframe A large, multiuser computer system.

manipulation An intervention or treatment introduced by the researcher in an experimental or quasi-experimental study; the researcher manipulates the independent variable to assess its impact on the dependent variable.

manipulation check In experimental studies, a test to determine whether the manipulation was implemented as intended.

Mann-Whitney U test A nonparametric test used to test the difference between two independent groups, based on ranked scores.

MANOVA See *multivariate analysis of variance.*

matching The pairing of subjects in one group with those in another group based on their similarity in one or more dimension, done to enhance the overall comparability of groups; when matching is performed in the context of an experiment, the procedure results in a randomized block design.

maturation threat   A threat to the internal validity of a study that results when factors influence the outcome measure (dependent variable) as a result of time passing.

maximum likelihood estimation   An estimation approach (sometimes used in lieu of the least squares approach) in which the estimators are ones that estimate the parameters most likely to have generated the observed measurements.

McNemar test   A statistical test for comparing differences in proportions, when the values are derived from paired (nonindependent) groups.

mean   A descriptive statistic that is a measure of central tendency, computed by summing all scores and dividing by the number of subjects.

measurement   The assignment of numbers to objects according to specified rules to characterize quantities of some attribute.

median   A descriptive statistic that is a measure of central tendency, representing the exact middle score or value in a distribution of scores; the median is the value above and below which 50% of the scores lie.

median test   A nonparametric statistical test that involves the comparison of median values of two independent groups to determine if the groups derive from populations with different medians.

mediating variable   A variable that mediates or acts like a "go-between" in a chain linking two other variables (e.g., coping skills may be said to mediate the relationship between stressful events and anxiety).

member check   A method of validating the credibility of qualitative data through debriefings and discussions with informants.

meta-analysis   A technique for quantitatively combining and thus integrating the results of multiple studies on a given topic.

methodological notes   In observational field studies, the notes kept by the researcher regarding the methods used in collecting the data.

methodological research   Research designed to develop or refine procedures for obtaining, organizing, or analyzing data.

methods (research)   The steps, procedures, and strategies for gathering and analyzing the data in a research investigation.

microcomputer   See *personal computer.*

middle-range theory   A theory that focuses on only a piece of reality or human experience, involving a selected number of concepts (e.g., theories of stress).

minimal risk   An anticipated risk that is no greater than one ordinarily encountered in daily life or during the performance of routine tests or procedures.

missing values   Values missing from a data set for some subjects, due, for example, to subject refusals, researcher error, or skip patterns.

modality   A characteristic of a frequency distribution describing the number of peaks; i.e., values with high frequencies.

mode   A descriptive statistic that is a measure of central tendency; the score or value that occurs most frequently in a distribution of scores.

model   A symbolic representation of concepts or variables and interrelationships among them.

molar approach   A way of making observations about behaviors that entails studying large units of behavior and treating them as a whole.

molecular approach   A way of making observations about behavior that uses small and highly specific behaviors as the unit of observation.

mortality threat   A threat to the internal validity of a study, referring to the differential loss of subjects (attrition) from different groups.

multimethod research   Generally, research in which multiple approaches are used to address the research problem; often used to designate research in which both qualitative and quantitative data are collected and analyzed.

multimodal distribution   A distribution of values with more than one peak (high frequency).

multiple classification analysis   A variant of multiple regression and ANCOVA that yields means on the dependent variable adjusted for the effects of covariates.

multiple comparison procedures Statistical tests, normally applied after ANOVA results indicate statistically significant group differences, that compare different pairs of groups.

multiple correlation coefficient An index that summarizes the degree of relationship between two or more independent variables and a dependent variable; symbolized as *R*.

multiple regression A statistical procedure for analyzing the simultaneous effects of two or more independent (or extraneous) variables on a dependent variable; the dependent variable must be measured on an interval or ratio scale.

multi-stage sampling A sampling strategy that proceeds through a set of stages from larger to smaller sampling units (e.g., from states, to nursing schools, to faculty members).

multitrait–multimethod matrix approach A method of establishing the construct validity of an instrument that involves the use of multiple measures for a set of subjects; the target instrument is valid to the extent that there is a strong relationship between it and other measures purporting to measure the same attribute (convergence) and a weak relationship between it and other measures purporting to measure a different attribute (discriminability).

multivariate analysis of variance (MANOVA) A statistical procedure used to test the significance of differences between the means of two or more groups on two or more dependent variables, considered simultanously.

multivariate statistics Statistical procedures designed to analyze the relationships among three or more variables; commonly used multivariate statistics include multiple regression, analysis of covariance, and factor analysis.

N Often used to designate the total number of subjects in a study (e.g., "the total *N* was 500").

n Often used to designate the number of subjects in a subgroup or in a cell of a study (e.g., "each of the four groups had an *n* of 125, for a total *N* of 500").

naturalistic setting A setting for the collection of research data that is natural to those being studied (e.g., homes, places of work, and so on).

needs assessment A study in which a researcher collects data for estimating the needs of a group, community, or organization; usually used as a guide to resource allocation.

negatively skewed distribution An asymmetric distribution of values such that a disproportionately high number of cases have high values—that is, they fall at the upper end of the distribution; when displayed graphically, the tail points to the left.

negative relationship A relationship between two variables in which there is a tendency for higher values on one variable to be associated with lower values on the other (e.g., as temperature increases, people's productivity may decrease); also referred to as an *inverse relationship*.

negative results Research results that fail to support the researcher's hypotheses.

network sampling The sampling of subjects based on referrals from other subjects already in the sample, sometimes referred to as snowballing.

nominal measure The lowest level of measurement that involves the assignment of characteristics into categories (e.g., males, category 1; females, category 2).

nondirectional hypothesis A research hypothesis that does not stipulate in advance the direction and nature of the relationship between variables.

nonequivalent control group A comparison group that was not developed on the basis of random assignment; when randomization is not used, there is no way of ensuring the initial equivalence among different groups.

nonexperimental research Studies in which the researcher collects data without introducing any new treatments or changes.

nonparametric statistics A general class of inferential statistics that does not involve rigorous assumptions about the distribution of the critical variables; most often used when the data are measured on the nominal or ordinal scales.

nonprobability sampling The selection of subjects or sampling units from a population using nonrandom procedures; examples include convenience, judgmental, and quota sampling.

nonsignificant result   The result of a statistical test that indicates that the result could have occurred as a result of chance, given the researcher's level of significance; sometimes abbreviated as *NS* in research journals.

normal distribution   A distribution that is bell-shaped and symmetric; also referred to as a normal curve.

norms   Test-performance standards, based on the collection of test score information from a large, representative sample.

null hypothesis   The hypothesis that states there is no relationship between the variables under study; used primarily in connection with tests of statistical significance as the hypothesis to be rejected.

objectivity   A desired quality of research using the scientific approach; refers to the extent to which two independent researchers would arrive at similar judgments or conclusions (i.e., judgments not biased by personal values or beliefs).

observational notes   In field studies, the observer's descriptions about observed events and conversations.

observational research   Studies in which the data are collected by means of observing and recording behaviors or activities of interest.

obtained (observed) score   The actual score or numerical value assigned to a subject on a measure.

one-tailed test   A test of statistical significance in which only values at one extreme (tail) of a distribution are considered in determining significance; used when the researcher has predicted the direction of a relationship (see *directional hypothesis*).

open-ended question   A question in an interview or questionnaire that does not restrict the respondents' answers to preestablished alternatives.

operating system   The software that controls the overall operation of a computer system; examples for personal computers include MS/DOS and OS/2.

operational definition   The definition of a concept or variable in terms of the operations or procedures by which it is to be measured.

operationalization   The process of translating research concepts into measurable phenomena.

ordinal measure   A level of measurement that yields rank orders of a variable along some dimension.

outcome analysis   An evaluation of what transpires with respect to outcomes of interest after implementing a program or intervention, without use of an experimental design to assess net effects. (See also *impact analysis*)

outcome measure   A term sometimes used to refer to the dependent variable in experimental research, that is, the measure that captures the outcome of the experimental intervention.

outliers   Wild codes or numerical values that are not a part of the coding scheme or numerical values that are extreme.

output devices   Those parts of a computer system that communicate information back to the computer user (e.g., a printer).

p value   In statistical testing, the probability that the obtained results are due to chance alone; the probability of committing a Type I error.

pair matching   See *matching*.

pairwise deletion   A method of dealing with missing values in a data set that involves the deletion of cases with missing data on a selective basis (i.e., deletion of a case only when one variable is paired with another variable that has missing data).

panel study   A type of longitudinal study in which the same subjects are used to provide data at two or more points in time.

paradigm   A way of looking at natural phenomena that encompasses a set of philosophical assumptions and that guides one's approach to inquiry.

parameter   A characteristic of a population (e.g., the mean age of all U.S. citizens).

parametric statistics   A class of inferential statistics that involves (a) assumptions about the distribution of the variables, (b) the estimation of a parameter, and (c) the use of interval or ratio measures.

participant observation A method of collecting data through the observation of a group or organization in which the researcher participates as a member.

path analysis A regression-based procedure for testing causal models, typically using nonexperimental data.

Pearson's r The most widely used correlation coefficient, designating the magnitude of relationship between two variables measured on at least an interval scale; also referred to as the product-moment correlation.

peer reviewer A person who reviews and critiques a research report or research proposal, who also is a researcher (usually working on similar types of research problems as those in the research report under review), and who makes a recommendation about publishing or funding the research.

perfect correlation A correlation between two variables such that the values of one variable permit perfect prediction of the values of the other; designated as 1.00 or −1.00.

personal computer (PC) A small computer used by individual users; also referred to as a microcomputer.

personal notes In field studies, comments about the observer's own feelings during the research process.

personal interview An interview that occurs between an interviewer and a respondent in a face-to-face situation.

phenomenology An approach to human inquiry that emphasizes the complexity of human experience and the need to study that experience holistically as it is actually lived.

phi coefficient An index describing the magnitude of relationship between two dichotomous variables.

pilot study A small-scale version, or trial run, done in preparation for a major study.

pink sheet For grant applications submitted to the National Institutes of Health, the evaluation form containing the comments and priority score of the peer review panel.

point estimation A statistical estimation procedure in which the researcher uses information from a sample to estimate the single value (statistic) that best represents the value of the population parameter.

policy research Research conducted specifically to inform people who create or implement policies, typically policies affecting large groups of people (e.g., federal policies on health care).

population The entire set of individuals (or objects) having some common characteristics (e.g., all RNs in the state of California); sometimes referred to as *universe*.

positively skewed distribution An asymmetric distribution of values such that a disproportionately high number of cases have low values—that is, they fall at the lower end of the distribution; when displayed graphically, the tail points to the right.

positive relationship A relationship between two variables in which there is a tendency for high values on one variable to be associated with high values on the other (e.g., as physical activity increases, pulse rate also increases).

positive results Research results that are consistent with the researcher's hypotheses.

posttest The collection of data after the introduction of an experimental intervention.

posttest-only design An experimental design in which data are collected from subjects only after the experimental intervention has been introduced; also known as *after-only design*.

power In research design, the ability of a design to detect existing relationships among variables.

power analysis A procedure for estimating either the likelihood of committing a Type II error or sample size requirements.

prediction One of the aims of the scientific approach; the use of empirical evidence to make forecasts about how variables of interest will behave in a new setting and with different individuals.

predictive validity The degree to which an instrument can predict some criterion observed at a future time.

pre-experimental design   A research design that does not include controls to compensate for the absence of either randomization or a control group.

pretest   (1) The collection of data before the experimental intervention; sometimes referred to as *baseline data;* (2) the trial administration of a newly developed instrument to identify flaws or assess time requirements.

pretest–posttest design   An experimental design in which data are collected from research subjects both before and after the introduction of the experimental intervention; also known as *before–after design.*

primary source   First-hand reports of facts, findings, or events; in terms of research, the primary source is the original research report as prepared by the investigator who conducted the study.

principal investigator (PI)   In research grants, the person who is the lead researcher and who will have primary responsibility for administering the grant.

probability sampling   The selection of subjects or sampling units from a population using random procedures; examples include simple random sampling, cluster sampling, and systematic sampling.

probing   Eliciting more useful or detailed information from a respondent in an interview than was volunteered in the first reply.

problem statement   The statement of the research problem that identifies the key research variables, specifies the nature of the population, and suggests the possibility of empirical testing.

process analysis   An evaluation focusing on the process by which a program or intervention gets implemented and used in practice.

product–moment correlation coefficient (r)   The most widely used correlation coefficient, designating the magnitude of relationship between two variables measured on at least an interval scale; also referred to as Pearson's *r.*

program   See *computer program.*

projective techniques   Methods for measuring psychological attributes (values, attitudes, personality) by providing respondents with unstructured stimuli to which to respond.

proportional hazards model   A model applied in multivariate analyses in which independent variables are used to predict the risk (hazard) of experiencing an event at a given point in time.

proportionate sampling design   A sampling strategy wherein the researcher samples from different strata of the population in direct proportion to their representation in the population.

proposal   A document specifying what the researcher proposes to study; it communicates the research problem, its significance, planned procedures for solving the problem, and, when funding is sought, how much the research will cost.

prospective study   A study that begins with an examination of presumed causes (e.g., cigarette smoking) and then goes forward in time to observe presumed effects (e.g., lung cancer).

psychometric assessment   An evaluation of the quality of an instrument, based primarily on evidence of its reliability and validity.

psychometrics   The theory underlying principles of measurement and the application of the theory in the development of measuring tools.

purposive sampling   A type of nonprobability sampling method in which the researcher selects subjects for the study on the basis of personal judgment about which ones will be most representative or productive; also referred to as judgmental sampling.

Q-by-Q   The detailed question-by-question instructions that inform interviewers about the intent of questions in an interview schedule and the type of information that should be obtained from respondents.

Q sort   A method of scaling in which the subject sorts statements into a number of piles (usually 9 or 11) according to some bipolar dimension (e.g., most like me/least like me; most useful/least useful).

qualitative analysis   The organization and interpretation of nonnumerical information for the purpose of discovering important underlying dimensions and patterns of relationships.

qualitative data   Information collected in the course of a study that is in narrative (nonnumerical) form, such as the transcript of an unstructured interview.

quantitative analysis The manipulation of numerical data through statistical procedures for the purpose of describing phenomena or assessing the magnitude and reliability of relationships among them.

quantitative data Information collected in the course of a study that is in a quantified (numerical) form.

quasi-experiment A study in which subjects cannot be randomly assigned to treatment conditions, although the researcher manipulates the independent variable and exercises certain controls to enhance the internal validity of the results.

quasi-statistics An "accounting" system used to assess the validity of conclusions derived from qualitative analysis.

questionnaire A method of gathering self-report information from respondents through self-administration of questions in a paper-and-pencil format; sometimes referred to as an SAQ (self-administered questionnaire).

quota sampling The nonrandom selection of subjects in which the researcher prespecifies characteristics of the sample to increase its representativeness.

r The symbol typically used to designate a bivariate correlation coefficient, summarizing the magnitude and direction of a relationship between two variables.

R The symbol used to designate the multiple correlation coefficient, indicating the magnitude (but not direction) of the relationship between the dependent variable and multiple independent variables, taken together.

R^2 The squared multiple correlation coefficient, indicating the proportion of variance in the dependent variable accounted for or explained by a group of independent variables; also referred to as the coefficient of determination.

random assignment The assignment of subjects to treatment conditions in a random manner (i.e., in a manner determined by chance alone); also known as *randomization.*

random number table A table displaying hundreds of digits (from 0 to 9) set up in such a way that each number is equally likely to follow any other; used in randomization or random sampling.

random sampling The selection of a sample such that each member of a population (or subpopulation) has an equal probability of being included.

range A measure of variability, consisting of the difference between the highest and lowest values in a distribution of scores.

ratio measure A level of measurement in which there are equal distances between score units and which has a true meaningful zero point (e.g., weight); the highest level of measurement.

reactivity A measurement distortion arising from the subject's awareness of being observed or, more generally, from the effect of the measurement procedure.

readability The ease with which research materials (e.g., a questionnaire) can be read by people with varying reading skills, often empirically determined through readability formulas.

rectangular matrix A matrix of data (variables by subjects) that contains no missing values for any of the variables.

recursive model A path model in which the causal flow is unidirectional, without any feedback loops; opposite of a nonrecursive model.

refereed journal A journal that makes decisions about the acceptance of manuscripts on the basis of recommendations from peer reviewers.

regression A statistical procedure for predicting values of a dependent variable based on the values of one or more independent variables.

relationship A bond or a connection between two or more variables.

reliability The degree of consistency or dependability with which an instrument measures the attribute it is designed to measure.

reliability coefficient A quantitative index, usually ranging in value from 0.0 to 1.00, that provides an estimate of how reliable an instrument is; computed through such procedures as Cronbach's alpha technique, the split-half technique, test–retest approach, and interrater approaches.

repeated measures design   An experimental design in which one group of subjects is exposed to more than one condition or treatment, in random order; sometimes referred to as a crossover design.

replication   The duplication of research procedures in a second investigation for the purpose of determining if earlier results can be repeated.

representative sample   A sample whose characteristics are highly similar to those of the population from which it is drawn.

research   Systematic inquiry that uses orderly scientific methods to answer questions or solve problems.

research control   See *control*.

research design   The overall plan for collecting and analyzing data, including specifications for enhancing the internal and external validity of the study.

research proposal   See *proposal*.

research report   A document that summarizes the main features of a study, including the research question, the methods used to address it, the findings, and the interpretation and implications of the findings.

research utilization   The use of some aspect of a scientific investigation in an application unrelated to the original research.

residuals   In multiple regression, the error term or unexplained variance.

respondent   In a self-report study, the research subject who responds to questions posed by the researcher.

response rate   The rate of participation in a survey, calculated by dividing the number of people participating by the number of people sampled.

response-set bias   The measurement error introduced by the tendency of some individuals to respond to items in characteristic ways (e.g., always agreeing), independently of the item's content.

results   The answers to research questions, obtained through an analysis of the collected data; in a quantitative study, the information obtained through statistical tests.

retrospective study   A study that begins with the manifestation of the dependent variable in the present (e.g., lung cancer) and then links this effect to some presumed cause occurring in the past (e.g., cigarette smoking).

right justification   A convention used in data entry, when a fixed format mode is used, such that values are placed as far to the right as possible within a designated field (e.g., the value 1 in a two-column field would be entered 01).

risk/benefit ratio   The relative costs and benefits, to an individual subject and to society at large, of participation in a scientific study.

rival hypothesis   An alternative explanation, competing with the researcher's hypothesis, for understanding the results of a study.

sample   A subset of a population selected to participate in a research study.

sampling   The process of selecting a portion of the population to represent the entire population.

sampling bias   Distortions that arise from the selection of a sample that is not representative of the population from which it was drawn.

sampling distribution   A theoretical distribution of a statistic using an infinite number of samples as a basis and the values of the statistic computed from these samples as the data points in the distribution.

sampling error   The fluctuation of the value of a statistic from one sample to another drawn from the same population.

sampling frame   A list of all the elements in the population from which the sample is drawn.

SAQ   See *questionnaire*.

saturation   The process of collecting data in a grounded theory study to the point at which a sense of closure is attained because new data yield only redundant information.

scale   A composite measure of an attribute, consisting of several items that have a logical or empirical relationship to each other; involves the assignment of a score to place subjects on a continuum with respect to the attribute.

scatter plot   A graphic representation of the relationship between two variables.

scientific approach   A set of orderly, systematic, controlled procedures for acquiring dependable, empirical information.

scientific merit The degree to which a study is methodologically and conceptually sound and possesses theoretical relevance and internal and external validity.

screening instrument The instrument used to determine whether potential subjects for a study meet all the eligibility criteria.

secondary analysis A form of research in which the data collected by one researcher are reanalyzed by another investigator, usually to test new research hypotheses.

secondary source Second-hand accounts of events or facts; in a research context, a description of a study or studies prepared by someone other than the original researcher.

selection bias (self-selection) A threat to the internal validity of the study resulting from preexisting differences between the groups under study; the differences affect the dependent variable in ways extraneous to the effect of the independent variable.

self-determination A person's ability to decide voluntarily whether to participate as a subject in a study.

self-report Any procedure for collecting data that involves a direct report of information by the person who is being studied (e.g., by interview or questionnaire).

semantic differential A technique used to measure attitudes that asks respondents to rate a concept of interest on a series of seven-point, bipolar rating scales.

sensitivity In measurement, the ability of the measuring tool to make fine discriminations between objects with differing amounts of the attribute being measured.

setting The physical location and conditions in which data collection takes place in a study.

significance level The probability that an observed relationship could be caused by chance (i.e., because of sampling error); significance at the .05 level indicates the probability that a relationship of the observed magnitude would be found by chance only 5 times out of 100.

sign system In structured observational research, a system for listing the behaviors of interest to the researchers, in situations where the observation focuses on specific behaviors that may or may not be manifested by the subjects.

sign test A nonparametric statistical test for comparing two paired groups, based on the relative ranking of values between the pairs.

simple random sampling The most basic type of probability sampling, wherein a sampling frame is created by enumerating all members of a population of interest and then selecting a sample from the sampling frame through completely random procedures.

skewness A quality of a set of scores relating to their asymmetric distribution around a central point.

snowball sampling The selection of subjects by means of nominations or referrals from earlier subjects; also referred to as *network sampling*.

social desirability response set A bias in self-report instruments created when subjects have a tendency to misrepresent their opinions in the direction of answers consistent with prevailing social norms.

software The instructions for performing operations made to a computer and the documentation for those instructions.

Solomon four-group design An experimental design that uses a before–after design for one pair of experimental and control groups, and an after-only design for a second pair.

Spearman-Brown prophecy formula An equation for making corrections to a reliability estimate that was calculated by the split-half method.

Spearman's rho A correlation coefficient indicating the magnitude of a relationship between variables measured on the ordinal scale.

split-half technique A method for estimating the internal consistency reliability of an instrument by correlating scores on half of the measure with scores on the other half.

standard deviation (SD) The most frequently used statistic for measuring the degree of variability in a set of scores.

standard error   The standard deviation of a theoretical sampling distribution (usually the sampling distribution of means).

standard scores   Scores expressed in terms of standard deviations from the mean; raw scores are transformed to scores with a mean of zero and a standard deviation of one; sometimes referred to as z scores.

statement of purpose   A broad declarative statement of the overall goals of a research project.

statistic   An estimate of a parameter, calculated from sample data.

statistical analysis   The organization and analysis of quantitative data using statistical procedures, including both descriptive and inferential statistics.

statistical inference   The process of inferring attributes about the population based on information from a sample.

statistical significance   A term indicating that the results obtained in an analysis of sample data are unlikely to have been caused by chance, at some specified level of probability.

statistical test   An analytic procedure that allows a researcher to determine the likelihood that obtained results from a sample reflect true population results, according to the laws of probability.

strata   Subdivisions of the population according to some characteristic (e.g., males and females); singular is *stratum.*

stratified random sampling   The random selection of subjects from two or more strata of the population independently.

structured data collection   An approach to collecting information from subjects, either through self-report or observations, wherein the researcher determines in advance the response categories of interest.

Study Section   Within the National Institutes of Health, the Initial Review Group (consisting of peers) that evaluates grant applications.

subgroup effects   The differential effect of the independent variable on the dependent variable for various subsets of the sample.

subject   An individual who participates and provides data in a study; subjects are sometimes designated as ss, as in, "there were 50 ss in the experiment."

subject stipend   A monetary payment to individuals participating in a study to serve as an incentive for participation or to compensate for time and expenses.

summated rating scale   See *Likert scale.*

summative evaluation   Research designed to assess the usefulness or worth of a program or practice after it is already in operation.

survey research   A type of nonexperimental research that focuses on obtaining information regarding the status quo of some situation, often by means of direct questioning of a sample of respondents.

survival analysis   A statistical procedure used when the dependent variable represents a time interval between an initial event (e.g., onset of a disease) and an end event (e.g., death); also referred to as *life table analysis.*

symmetric distribution   A distribution of values that has two halves that are mirror images of the each other; a distribution that is not skewed.

systematic sampling   The selection of subjects such that every kth (e.g., every 10th) person (or element) in a sampling frame or list is chosen.

table of random numbers   See *random number table.*

table shells   A table without any numerical values, prepared in advance of data analysis as a guide to the analyses to be performed.

target population   The entire population in which the researcher is interested and to which he or she would like to generalize the results of a study.

test statistic   A statistic used to test for the statistical significance of relationships between variables; the sampling distributions of test statistics are known for circumstances in which the null hypothesis is true; examples include chi-square, F-ratio, t, and Pearson's r.

testing threat   A threat to the internal validity of a study that occurs when the administration of a pretest or baseline measure of a dependent variable results in changes on the variable, independent of the effect of the independent variable.

test–retest reliability Assessment of the stability of an instrument by correlating the scores obtained on repeated administrations.

theoretical notes In field studies, notes about the observer's interpretations of observed activities.

theoretical sampling In qualitative studies, the selection of sample members based on emerging findings as the study progresses, to ensure adequate representation of important themes.

theory An abstract generalization that presents a systematic explanation about the relationships among phenomena.

time sampling In observational research, the selection of time periods during which observations will take place.

time series design A quasi-experimental design that involves the collection of information over an extended period of time, with multiple data collection points both before and after the introduction of a treatment.

time sharing A method of operating mainframe computers such that several different users have access to the computer in a round-robin fashion, giving the impression of simultaneous use.

topic guide A list of broad question areas to be covered in a semi-structured interview or focus group interview.

transferability (1) A criterion for evaluating the quality of qualitative data, referring to the extent to which the findings from the data can be transferred to other settings or groups—analogous to generalizability; (2) also, a criterion used in assessing implementation potential in the context of a utilization project.

treatment The experimental intervention under study; the condition being manipulated.

treatment group The group receiving the intervention being tested; the experimental group.

trend study A form of longitudinal study in which different samples from a population are studied over time with respect to some phenomenon (e.g., a series of Gallup polls of political preferences).

triangulation The use of multiple methods or perspectives to collect and interpret data about some phenomenon, to converge on an accurate representation of reality.

true score A hypothetical score that would be obtained if a measure were infallible; it is the portion of the observed score not due to random error or measurement bias.

trustworthiness A term used in the evaluation of qualitative data, assessed using the criteria of credibility, transferability, dependability, and confirmability.

t-test A parametric statistical test used for analyzing the difference between two means.

two-tailed test A test of statistical significance in which values at both extremes (tails) of a distribution are considered in determining significance; used when the researcher has not predicted the direction of a relationship (see *nondirectional hypothesis*).

Type I error An error created by rejecting the null hypothesis when it is true (i.e., the researcher concludes that a relationship exists when in fact it does not).

Type II error An error created by accepting the null hypothesis when it is false (i.e., the researcher concludes that *no* relationship exists when in fact it does).

unimodal distribution A distribution of values with one peak (high frequency).

unit of analysis The basic unit or focus of a researcher's analysis; in nursing research, the unit of analysis is typically the individual subject.

univariate descriptive study A study that gathers information on the occurrence, frequency of occurrence, or average value of the variables of interest, one variable at a time, without focusing on interrelationships among variables.

univariate statistics Statistical procedures for analyzing a single variable for purposes of description.

unstructured interview An oral self-report in which the researcher asks respondents questions without preconceived views regarding the specific content or flow of information to be gathered.

unstructured observation   The collection of descriptive information through direct observation, whereby the observer is guided by some general research questions but does not follow a prespecified plan for observing, enumerating, or recording the information.

utilization   See *research utilization*.

utilization criteria   The criteria that are brought to bear in considering whether an innovation is amenable to utilization in a practice setting; includes the criteria of clinical relevance, scientific merit, and implementation potential.

validity   The degree to which an instrument measures what it is intended to measure.

validity coefficient   A quantitative index, usually ranging in value from 0.0 to 1.00, that provides an estimate of how valid an instrument is; usually computed in conjunction with the criterion-related approach to validating an instrument.

variability   The degree to which values on a set of scores are widely different or dispersed.

variable   A characteristic or attribute of a person or object that varies (i.e., takes on different values) within the population under study (e.g., body temperature, age, heart rate).

variance   A measure of variability or dispersion, equal to the square of the standard deviation.

vignette   A brief description of an event, person, or situation to which respondents are asked to react.

visual analogue scale   A scaling procedure used to measure a variety of clinical symptoms (e.g., pain, fatigue) by having subjects indicate on a straight line the intensity of the attribute being measured.

vulnerable subjects   Special groups of people whose rights in research studies need to be protected through additional safeguards because of their inability to provide meaningful informed consent or because their circumstances place them at higher-than-average-risk of adverse effects; examples include young children, the mentally retarded, and unconscious patients.

weighting   A correction procedure used to arrive at population values when a disproportionate sampling design has been used.

Wilcoxon signed ranks test   A nonparametric statistical test for comparing two paired groups, based on the relative ranking of values between the pairs.

Wilk's lambda   An index used in discriminant function analysis to indicate the proportion of variance in the dependent variable *un*accounted for by predictors; $(\lambda) = 1 - R^2$.

windows   A mechanism for dividing a computer's display screen into rectangles for viewing two or more applications or parts of a single application at the same time.

z score   A standard score, expressed in terms of standard deviations from the mean.

Appendix A

HUMAN SUBJECT PROTOCOL*

(1) *Describe the characteristics of the subject population, such as their anticipated number, age ranges, sex, ethnic background, and health status. Identify the criteria for inclusion or exclusion. Explain the rationale for the use of special classes of subjects, such as fetuses, pregnant women, children, institutionalized mentally disabled, prisoners, or others who are likely to be vulnerable.*

1. Characteristics of the population. The sample for the proposed research will consist of approximately 300 women aged 18-22 who first became pregnant before their eighteenth birthday and who subsequently delivered a child. The women were interviewed initially in 1980-1981 as part of an evaluation of the special program for teenage mothers—Project Redirection. At the time of the initial interview, the women were residing in 6 communities: Phoenix, San Antonio, Fresno, Riverside (CA), Harlem and Bedford-Stuyvesant (NY).

The initial eligibility criteria for the Project Redirection study are indicated below:
- either pregnant or a parent;
- living in a household that met certain poverty guidelines;
- 17 years old or younger; and
- without a high school diploma or GED certificate.

The sample size for the proposed study is based on the teens in the six sites who completed three rounds of interviews thus far:

- Phoenix, AZ   81
- San Antonio, TX   86
- Harlem, NY   38
- Bedford-Stuyvesant, NY   54
- Riverside, CA   32
- Fresno, CA   38
- TOTAL   329

(2) *Identify the sources of research material obtained from individually identifiable living human subjects in the form of specimens, records, or data. Indicate whether the material or data will be obtained specif-*

*Grant applications under the Public Health Service (see Chapter 27) must include a section on the protection of human subjects, which must address six specific questions. This appendix contains the actual responses to those six questions for a funded study of parenting among low-income teenage mothers. Such a protocol often serves as the focal point of an evaluation by an Institutional Review Board.

ically for research purposes or whether use will be made of existing specimens, records, or data.

2. Sources of Data. Three rounds of interviews have already been completed with the research sample, and information from these earlier interviews will be used in the present study. Additionally, data will be gathered in a fourth round of in-home interviews, to be collected in 1986–1987 if the proposed research is funded. Data will be gathered by a combined interview/observation approach, using a specially constructed interview schedule and serveral standardized instruments.

(3) Describe plans for the recruitment of subjects and the consent procedures to be followed, including the circumstances under which consent will be sought and obtained, who will seek it, the nature of the information to be provided to prospetive subjects and the method of documenting consent.

3. Recruitment and Consent. Subjects have already been recruited for this study—i.e., they were participants in three earlier rounds of interviewing as part of another research project. For the present study, letters will be mailed to respondents at their most recently known address and they will be asked to verify their current address and telephone number (if available). For respondents for whom there is no return postcard, tracking procedures to ascertain the respondents' present address will be undertaken.

    For those respondents who are located through these procedures, an interviewer will contact them and explain the general nature and purpose of the research, the confidential nature of the interviews, the time commitments, and the stipend ($25) that would be paid to them in compensation for their time. The respondents will also be told that their children should be present at the time of the interview, so that appropriate observations can be made.

Upon consent to be included in this wave of the research, an interview will be scheduled. At the time of the interview, the interviewers, who will receive extensive training for this project, will repeat the description of the research prior to commencing. The respondent will be told that her participation is voluntary; that no information she gives will be divulged to anyone other than research staff; that her participation will have no effect on any services that she might be receiving; that she can stop the interview at any time; and that she can decline to answer individual questions if she so chooses. This information will be included in a Consent Form, which each respondent will be requested to sign prior to the interview.

(4) Describe any potential risks—physical, psychological, social, legal, or other—and assess their likelihood and seriousness. Where appropriate, describe alternative treatments and procedures that might be advantageous to the subjects.

4. Risks. There is relatively minor risk, in interviewing these young women about their family life, that the interview will be stressful to them. Furthermore, our procedures are designed to minimize any discomfort on the respondents' parts. We will use female interviewers who will be trained not only with respect to the research instruments but also with regard to the stresses of parenthood in disadvantaged populations. In the event of any signs of distress during the interview, interviewers will be instructed to refrain from further questioning, proceeding only if the respondent desires. Our experience in dealing with this sample leads us to believe, however, that the women are more likely to find a conversation with an objective but sympathetic listener therapeutic rather than stressful.

(5) Describe the procedures for protecting against or minimizing any potential risks,

including risks to confidentiality, and assess their likely effectiveness. Where appropriate, discuss provisions for inusring necessary medical or professional intervention in the event of adverse effects to the subjects. Also, where appropriate, describe the provisions for monitoring the data collected to insure the safety of subjects.

5. Confidentiality. Measures to protect the confidentiality of the respondents will be instituted throughout the course of this project. Data security procedures to protect the identity of individuals will be implemented during interviewer training, data collection, data analysis, and after completion of the project. Respondents will be fully informed as to these confidentiality procedures at the outset of the interview.

   The issue of confidentiality and data security will be stressed during the training of data collectors. The need for confidentiality and the specific policies and procedures related to this issue will be explained to all interviewers. Thereafter, the interviewers will be required to sign a confidentiality statement prior to conducting interviews.

   All identifying information will be removed from the interview schedule upon receipt from the field staff. Names, addresses, telephone numbers and any other identifying information will be recorded *only* on a cover sheet of the interview. The interview form itself, which will be kept in a locked file, will bear only a numeric identification code. The cover sheet will be removed from completed interviews and kept in a separate locked file. Access to this file will be restricted to key project personnel.

(6) *Discuss why the risks to subjects are reasonable in relation to the anticipated benefits to subjects and in relation to the importance of the knowledge that may reasonably be expected to result.*

6. Anticipated Benefits. In theory, no direct benefits to the respondents are anticipated. However, as mentioned above, we have found that respondents often enjoy the interview experience. Nevertheless, the primary benefit expected from the project is indirect. The study is expected to generate knowledge that will be useful in the formulation of social policy and in the design and delivery of appropriate services for young disadvantaged mothers and their childrenw. Since we believe that the risks to subjects are negligible, we believe that the benefits provide justification for the conduct of this research.

Appendix B

STATISTICAL TABLES

Table B-1.   *Distribution of t Probability*

DF	LEVEL OF SIGNIFICANCE FOR ONE-TAILED TEST					
	.10	.05	.025	.01	.005	.0005
	Level of Significance for Two-Tailed Test					
DF	.20	.10	.05	.02	.01	.001
1	3.078	6.314	12.706	31.821	63.657	636.619
2	1.886	2.920	4.303	6.965	9.925	31.598
3	1.638	2.353	3.182	4.541	5.841	12.941
4	1.533	2.132	2.776	3.747	4.604	8.610
5	1.476	2.015	2.571	3.376	4.032	6.859
6	1.440	1.953	2.447	3.143	3.707	5.959
7	1.415	1.895	2.365	2.998	3.449	5.405
8	1.397	1.860	2.306	2.896	3.355	5.041
9	1.383	1.833	2.262	2.821	3.250	4.781
10	1.372	1.812	2.228	2.765	3.169	4.587
11	1.363	1.796	2.201	2.718	3.106	4.437
12	1.356	1.782	2.179	2.681	3.055	4.318
13	1.350	1.771	2.160	2.650	3.012	4.221
14	1.345	1.761	2.145	2.624	2.977	4.140
15	1.341	1.753	2.131	2.602	2.947	4.073
16	1.337	1.746	2.120	2.583	2.921	4.015
17	1.333	1.740	2.110	2.567	2.898	3.965
18	1.330	1.734	2.101	2.552	2.878	3.922
19	1.328	1.729	2.093	2.539	2.861	3.883
20	1.325	1.725	2.086	2.528	2.845	3.850
21	1.323	1.721	2.080	2.518	2.831	3.819
22	1.321	1.717	2.074	2.508	2.819	3.792
23	1.319	1.714	2.069	2.500	2.807	3.767
24	1.318	1.711	2.064	2.492	2.797	3.745
25	1.316	1.708	2.060	2.485	2.787	3.725
26	1.315	1.706	2.056	2.479	2.779	3.707
27	1.314	1.703	2.052	2.473	2.771	3.690
28	1.313	1.701	2.048	2.467	2.763	3.674
29	1.311	1.699	2.045	2.462	2.756	3.659
30	1.310	1.697	2.042	2.457	2.750	3.646
40	1.303	1.684	2.021	2.423	2.704	3.551
60	1.296	1.671	2.000	2.390	2.660	3.460
120	1.289	1.658	1.980	2.358	2.617	3.373
∞	1.282	1.645	1.960	2.326	2.576	3.291

Table B-2. *Significant Values of F*
α = ·05 (Two-Tailed)   α = ·025 (one-tailed)

df_B / df_w	1	2	3	4	5	6	8	12	24	∞
1	161.4	199.5	215.7	224.6	230.2	234.0	238.9	243.9	249.0	254.3
2	18.51	19.00	19.16	19.25	19.30	19.33	19.37	19.41	19.45	19.50
3	10.13	9.55	9.28	9.12	9.01	8.94	8.84	8.74	8.64	8.53
4	7.71	6.94	6.59	6.39	6.26	6.16	6.04	5.91	5.77	5.63
5	6.61	5.79	5.41	5.19	5.05	4.95	4.82	4.68	4.53	4.36
6	5.99	5.14	4.76	4.53	4.39	4.28	4.15	4.00	3.84	3.67
7	5.59	4.74	4.35	4.12	3.97	3.87	3.73	3.57	3.41	3.23
8	5.32	4.46	4.07	3.84	3.69	3.58	3.44	3.28	3.12	2.93
9	5.12	4.26	3.86	3.63	3.48	3.37	3.23	3.07	2.90	2.71
10	4.96	4.10	3.71	3.48	3.33	3.22	3.07	2.91	2.74	2.54
11	4.84	3.98	3.59	3.36	3.20	3.09	2.95	2.79	2.61	2.40
12	4.75	3.88	3.49	3.26	3.11	3.00	2.85	2.69	2.50	2.30
13	4.67	3.80	3.41	3.18	3.02	2.92	2.77	2.60	2.42	2.21
14	4.60	3.74	3.34	3.11	2.96	2.85	2.70	2.53	2.35	2.13
15	4.54	3.68	3.29	3.06	2.90	2.79	2.64	2.48	2.29	2.07
16	4.49	3.63	3.24	3.01	2.85	2.74	2.59	2.42	2.24	2.01
17	4.45	3.59	3.20	2.96	2.81	2.70	2.55	2.38	2.19	1.96
18	4.41	3.55	3.16	2.93	2.77	2.66	2.51	2.34	2.15	1.92
19	4.38	3.52	3.13	2.90	2.74	2.63	2.48	2.31	2.11	1.88
20	4.35	3.49	3.10	2.87	2.71	2.60	2.45	2.28	2.08	1.84
21	4.32	3.47	3.07	2.84	2.68	2.57	2.42	2.25	2.05	1.81
22	4.30	3.44	3.05	2.82	2.66	2.55	2.40	2.23	2.03	1.78
23	4.28	3.42	3.03	2.80	2.64	2.53	2.38	2.20	2.00	1.76
24	4.26	3.40	3.01	2.78	2.62	2.51	2.36	2.18	1.98	1.73
25	4.24	3.38	2.99	2.76	2.60	2.49	2.34	2.16	1.96	1.71
26	4.22	3.37	2.98	2.74	2.59	2.47	2.32	2.15	1.95	1.69
27	4.21	3.35	2.96	2.73	2.57	2.46	2.30	2.13	1.93	1.67
28	4.20	3.34	2.95	2.71	2.56	2.44	2.29	2.12	1.91	1.65
29	4.18	3.33	2.93	2.70	2.54	2.43	2.28	2.10	1.90	1.64
30	4.17	3.32	2.92	2.69	2.53	2.42	2.27	2.09	1.89	1.62
40	4.08	3.23	2.84	2.61	2.45	2.34	2.18	2.00	1.79	1.51
60	4.00	3.15	2.76	2.52	2.37	2.25	2.10	1.92	1.70	1.39
120	3.92	3.07	2.68	2.45	2.29	2.17	2.02	1.83	1.61	1.25
∞	3.84	2.99	2.60	2.37	2.21	2.09	1.94	1.75	1.52	1.00

(continued)

Table B-2.   *Significant Values of F*
α = ·01 *(Two-Tailed)* *(continued)*   α = ·005 *(one-tailed)*

df_B										
df_w	1	2	3	4	5	6	8	12	24	∞
1	4052	4999	5403	5625	5764	5859	5981	6106	6234	6366
2	98.49	99.00	99.17	99.25	99.30	99.33	99.36	99.42	99.46	99.50
3	34.12	30.81	29.46	28.71	28.24	27.91	27.49	27.05	26.60	26.12
4	21.20	18.00	16.69	15.98	15.52	15.21	14.80	14.37	13.93	13.46
5	16.26	13.27	12.06	11.39	10.97	10.67	10.29	9.89	9.47	9.02
6	13.74	10.92	9.78	9.15	8.75	8.47	8.10	7.72	7.31	6.88
7	12.25	9.55	8.45	7.85	7.46	7.19	6.84	6.47	6.07	5.65
8	11.26	8.65	7.59	7.01	6.63	6.37	6.03	5.67	5.28	4.86
9	10.56	8.02	6.99	6.42	6.06	5.80	5.47	5.11	4.73	4.31
10	10.04	7.56	6.55	5.99	5.64	5.39	5.06	4.71	4.33	3.91
11	9.65	7.20	6.22	5.67	5.32	5.07	4.74	4.40	4.02	3.60
12	9.33	6.93	5.95	5.41	5.06	4.82	4.50	4.16	3.78	3.36
13	9.07	6.70	5.74	5.20	4.86	4.62	4.30	3.96	3.59	3.16
14	8.86	6.51	5.56	5.03	4.69	4.46	4.14	3.80	3.43	3.00
15	8.68	6.36	5.42	4.89	4.56	4.32	4.00	3.67	3.29	2.87
16	8.53	6.23	5.29	4.77	4.44	4.20	3.89	3.55	3.18	2.75
17	8.40	6.11	5.18	4.67	4.34	4.10	3.78	3.45	3.08	2.65
18	8.28	6.01	5.09	4.58	4.29	4.01	3.71	3.37	3.00	2.57
19	8.18	5.93	5.01	4.50	4.17	3.94	3.63	3.30	2.92	2.49
20	8.10	5.85	4.94	4.43	4.10	3.87	3.56	3.23	2.86	2.42
21	8.02	5.78	4.87	4.37	4.04	3.81	3.51	3.17	2.80	2.36
22	7.94	5.72	4.82	4.31	3.99	3.76	3.45	3.12	2.75	2.31
23	7.88	5.66	4.76	4.26	3.94	3.71	3.41	3.07	2.70	2.26
24	7.82	5.61	4.72	4.22	3.90	3.67	3.36	3.03	2.66	2.21
25	7.77	5.57	4.68	4.18	3.86	3.63	3.32	2.99	2.62	2.17
26	7.72	5.53	4.64	4.14	3.82	3.59	3.29	2.96	2.58	2.13
27	7.68	5.49	4.60	4.11	3.78	3.56	3.26	2.93	2.55	2.10
28	7.64	5.45	4.57	4.07	3.75	3.53	3.23	2.90	2.52	2.06
29	7.60	5.42	4.54	4.04	3.73	3.50	3.20	2.87	2.49	2.03
30	7.56	5.39	4.51	4.02	3.70	3.47	3.17	2.84	2.47	2.01
40	7.31	5.18	4.31	3.83	3.51	3.29	2.998	2.66	2.29	1.80
60	7.08	4.98	4.13	3.65	3.34	3.12	2.82	2.50	2.12	1.60
120	6.85	4.79	3.95	3.48	3.17	2.96	2.66	2.34	1.95	1.38
∞	6.64	4.60	3.78	3.32	3.02	2.80	2.51	2.18	1.79	1.00

(continued)

Table B-2.   *Significant Values of F*
α = ·001 *(Two-Tailed)* *(continued)*   α = ·0005 *(one-tailed)*

df_B df_w	1	2	3	4	5	6	8	12	24	∞
1	405284	500000	540379	562500	576405	585937	598144	610667	623497	636619
2	998.5	999.0	999.2	999.2	999.3	999.3	999.4	999.4	999.5	999.5
3	167.5	148.5	141.1	137.1	134.6	132.8	130.6	128.3	125.9	123.5
4	74.14	61.25	56.18	53.44	51.71	50.53	49.00	47.41	45.77	44.05
5	47.04	36.61	33.20	31.09	29.75	28.84	27.64	26.42	25.14	23.78
6	35.51	27.00	23.70	21.90	20.81	20.03	19.03	17.99	16.89	15.75
7	29.22	21.69	18.77	17.19	16.21	15.52	14.63	13.71	12.73	11.69
8	25.42	18.49	15.83	14.39	13.49	12.86	17.04	11.19	10.30	9.34
9	22.86	16.39	13.90	12.56	11.71	11.13	10.37	9.57	8.72	7.81
10	21.04	14.91	12.55	11.28	10.48	9.92	9.20	8.45	7.64	6.76
11	19.69	13.81	11.56	10.35	9.58	9.05	8.35	7.63	6.85	6.00
12	18.64	12.97	10.80	9.63	8.89	8.38	7.71	7.00	6.25	5.42
13	17.81	12.31	10.21	9.07	8.35	7.86	7.21	6.52	5.78	4.97
14	17.14	11.78	9.73	8.62	7.92	7.43	6.80	6.13	5.41	4.60
15	16.59	11.34	9.34	8.25	7.57	7.09	6.47	5.81	5.10	4.31
16	16.12	10.97	9.00	7.94	7.27	6.81	6.19	5.55	4.85	4.06
17	15.72	10.66	8.73	7.68	7.02	6.56	5.96	5.32	4.63	3.85
18	15.38	10.39	8.49	7.46	6.81	6.35	5.76	5.13	4.45	3.67
19	15.08	10.16	8.28	7.26	6.61	6.18	5.59	4.97	4.29	3.52
20	14.82	9.95	8.10	7.10	6.46	6.02	5.44	4.82	4.15	3.38
21	14.59	9.77	7.94	6.95	6.32	5.88	5.31	4.70	4.03	3.26
22	14.38	9.61	7.80	6.81	6.19	5.76	5.19	4.58	3.92	3.15
23	14.19	9.47	7.67	6.69	6.08	5.65	5.09	4.48	3.82	3.05
24	14.03	9.34	7.55	6.59	5.98	5.55	4.99	4.39	3.74	2.97
25	13.88	9.22	7.45	6.49	5.88	5.46	4.91	4.31	3.66	2.89
26	13.74	9.12	7.36	6.41	5.80	5.38	4.83	4.24	3.59	2.82
27	13.61	9.02	7.27	6.33	5.73	5.31	4.76	4.17	3.52	2.75
28	13.50	8.93	7.19	6.25	5.66	5.24	4.69	4.11	3.46	2.70
29	13.39	8.85	7.12	6.19	5.59	5.18	4.64	4.05	3.41	2.64
30	13.29	8.77	7.05	6.12	5.53	5.12	4.58	4.00	3.36	2.59
40	12.61	8.25	6.60	5.70	5.13	4.73	4.21	3.64	3.01	2.23
60	11.97	7.76	6.17	5.31	4.76	4.37	3.87	3.31	2.69	1.90
120	11.38	7.31	5.79	4.95	4.42	4.04	3.55	3.02	2.40	1.56
∞	10.83	6.91	5.42	4.62	4.10	3.74	3.27	2.74	2.13	1.00

Table B-3.   Distribution of χ^2 Probability

	LEVEL OF SIGNIFICANCE				
DF	.10	.05	.02	.01	.001
1	2.71	3.84	5.41	6.63	10.83
2	4.61	5.99	7.82	9.21	13.82
3	6.25	7.82	9.84	11.34	16.27
4	7.78	9.49	11.67	13.28	18.46
5	9.24	11.07	13.39	15.09	20.52
6	10.64	12.59	15.03	16.81	22.46
7	12.02	14.07	16.62	18.48	24.32
8	13.36	15.51	18.17	20.09	26.12
9	14.68	16.92	19.68	21.67	27.88
10	15.99	18.31	21.16	23.21	29.59
11	17.28	19.68	22.62	24.72	31.26
12	18.55	21.03	24.05	26.22	32.91
13	19.81	22.36	25.47	27.69	34.53
14	21.06	23.68	26.87	29.14	36.12
15	22.31	25.00	28.26	30.58	37.70
16	23.54	26.30	29.63	32.00	39.25
17	24.77	27.59	31.00	33.41	40.79
18	25.99	28.87	32.35	34.81	42.31
19	27.20	30.14	33.69	36.19	43.82
20	28.41	31.41	35.02	37.57	45.32
21	29.62	32.67	36.34	38.93	46.80
22	30.81	33.92	37.66	40.29	48.27
23	32.01	35.17	38.97	41.64	49.73
24	33.20	36.42	40.27	42.98	51.18
25	34.38	37.65	41.57	44.31	52.62
26	35.56	38.89	42.86	45.64	54.05
27	36.74	40.11	44.14	46.96	55.48
28	37.92	41.34	45.42	48.28	56.89
29	39.09	42.56	46.69	49.59	58.30
30	40.26	43.77	47.96	50.89	59.70

Table B-4. *Significant Values of the Correlation Coefficient*

| df | **LEVEL OF SIGNIFICANCE FOR ONE-TAILED TEST** | | | | |
	.05	.025	.01	.005	.0005
	Level of Significance for Two-Tailed Test				
	.1	.05	.02	.01	.001
1	.98769	.99692	.999507	.999877	.9999988
2	.90000	.95000	.98000	.990000	.99900
3	.8054	.8783	.93433	.95873	.99116
4	.7293	.8114	.8822	.91720	.97406
5	.6694	.7545	.8329	.8745	.95074
6	.6215	.7067	.7887	.8343	.92493
7	.5822	.6664	.7498	.7977	.8982
8	.5494	.6319	.7155	.7646	.8721
9	.5214	.6021	.6851	.7348	.8471
10	.4973	.5760	.6581	.7079	.8233
11	.4762	.5529	.6339	.6835	.8010
12	.4575	.5324	.6120	.6614	.7800
13	.4409	.5139	.5923	.5411	.7603
14	.4259	.4973	.5742	.6226	.7420
15	.4124	.4821	.5577	.6055	.7246
16	.4000	.4683	.5425	.5897	.7084
17	.3887	.4555	.5285	.5751	.6932
18	.3783	.4438	.5155	.5614	.5687
19	.3687	.4329	.5034	.5487	.6652
20	.3598	.4227	.4921	.5368	.6524
25	.3233	.3809	.4451	.5869	.5974
30	.2960	.3494	.4093	.4487	.5541
35	.2746	.3246	.3810	.4182	.5189
40	.2573	.3044	.3578	.3932	.4896
45	.2428	.2875	.3384	.3721	.4648
50	.2306	.2732	.3218	.3541	.4433
60	.2108	.2500	.2948	.3248	.4078
70	.1954	.2319	.2737	.3017	.3799
80	.1829	.2172	.2565	.2830	.3568
90	.1726	.2050	.2422	.2673	.3375
100	.1638	.1946	.2301	.2540	.3211

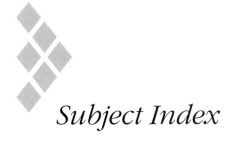

Subject Index

Note: Page numbers followed by n indicate footnotes; page numbers followed by t indicate tables; page numbers in *italic* type indicate figures; page numbers in **boldface** type indicate definitions of terms. Style of alphabetization is letter-by-letter, excluding articles and prepositions.

NAME INDEX

A

Adame, D., 466
Adams, B.N., 285
Addison, R.B., 532
Ager, J., 148
Ahijevych, K., 111, 148, 328
Aldag, J.C., 181
Aldrich, M.S., 143, 324
Alex, C.G., 561
Alexander, D., 328
Algase, D.L., 268
Allen, M., 202, 550
Alligood, M.R., 104
Allison, P.D., 460
American Medical Association, 567
American Nurses' Association, 119
American Nurses' Association Congress for Practice, 593
American Psychological Association, 119, 124, 566
Anderson, G.C., 427
Anderson, M.A., 312
Angel, R., 461
Armstrong, S., 191
Arnaud, S.S., 316
Arnold, L., 51
Aroian, K.J., 316

B

Bach, C.A., 570
Badger, T.A., 174
Bailey, B.J., 51, 562
Baker, C.F., 561
Baldwin, B., 518
Banonis, B.C., 103
Bargagliotti, L.A., 518, 541
Barkman, A., 513
Barnard, K.E., 597
Barton, J.A., 529
Bassford, T.L., 565
Beaver, M., 174
Becker, H.A., 12, 105
Becker, H.S., 529
Becker, M., 104
Becker, M.A., 454, 456, 457
Becker, P.T., 191, 316
Beecroft, P.C., 52
Beel-Bates, C.A., 268
Behm, L.K., 285
Belyea, M.J., 564
Belza, B.L., 466
Benner, P., 108
Bennett, C., 168, 268
Bennett, S.J., 105, 295
Benoliel, J.Q., 517, 518

Bensley, L., 543
Berelson, B., 195
Bernhard, L.A., 395, 396, 397
Betts, D., 327
Betz, M.L., 191
Bingle, J.D., 595, 597
Biocca, L.J., 174
Bishop, B.A., 225
Blalock, H.M., Jr., 453
Bliss-Hotz, J., 327
Bodensteiner, A., 568
Boehm, J., 610
Boehm, S., 328
Boik, R.J., 90, 147
Bond, E.F., 90, 328
Bookbinder, M., 174
Booker, J., 168
Borenstein, M., 454
Borucki, L., 51
Bos, H., 547
Bostrom-Ezrati, J., 465
Bottorff, J.L., 110, 466
Boumans, N.P.G., 247
Bourbonnais, F.F., 103
Bourguignon, C., 174
Boynton, M., 375
Bradle, J.B., 562
Brahim, J.S., 375
Brakey, M.R., 174
Brett, J.L.L., 594, 596, 602, 603
Brewer, J., 541, 544
Bridge, R.G., 337, 338
Bright, M.A., 533
Brittin, M., 168
Brooks, J.A., 62, 285
Brooten, D., 51, 285
Brooten, D.A., 564
Brown, J.S., 188, 241, 255
Brown, L., 532
Brown, L.P., 324
Brown, M.A., 12, 181, 561
Brown, S.J., 203
Bruce, S.L., 141
Buchanan, L.M., 147, 285
Buchko, B.L., 225
Buckwalter, K.C., 174
Buhler-Wilkerson, K., 203
Burgener, S.C., 268, 312
Burke, J., 26
Burr, R., 147, 285

C

Campbell, D.T., 169, 357
Campbell, J.C., 107, 148
Campbell, R.A., 513

Caplan, N., 592
Cardea, J.M., 174
Carlone, J., 466
Carlson, S., 147, 324
Carter, W.B., 544, 545
Caruso, C.C., 133
Cavalieri, T., 331
Cave, G., 547
Chambers, S.B., 569
Champagne, M.T., 599
Champion, V.L., 105, 353, 598
Chan, W., 466
Chance, B., 327
Chang, A., 285, 331
Cheng, G., 328
Chenitz, W.C., 565
Chesla, C.A., 534
Chinn, P.L., 110
Choo, J.T.E., 328
Christian, A., 104
Christian, M., 513
Christman, N.J., 285
Clark, D.C., 285
Clark, J., 561
Clark, V., 460
Cleary, P.D., 461
Clinton, J., 616
Clinton, W., 181
Cloonan, P.A., 564
Cochran, J.F., 225
Coenen, A., 550
Cohen, A.W., 327
Cohen, J., 454, 455, 457, 499
Cohen, M.Z., 108
Cohen, P., 499
Cole, F.L., 324
Coleman, M., 247
Collins, C., 534
Cook, M.A., 168
Cossette, S., 285
Covey, M.K., 561
Cowan, M., 147, 285
Cox, C.L., 111
Coyle, L.A., 594, 595, 596
Crabtree, M., 597
Crane, J., 595, 597
Crase, S.J., 111
Crumley, J., 141
Crumlish, C.M., 285
Curley, M.A., 174
Curry, M.A., 513
Cusack, D., 174

D

Damrosch, S.P., 202, 548
Daun, J.M., 328